Motor Control

Theory and Practical Applications

SECOND EDITION

SECOND EDITION

Motor Control

Theory and Practical Applications

ANNE SHUMWAY-COOK, PT, PhD

Associate Professor
Department of Rehabilitation Medicine
University of Washington
Seattle, Washington

MARJORIE H. WOOLLACOTT, PhD

Professor
Department of Exercise and Movement Science
Institute of Neuroscience
University of Oregon
Eugene, Oregon

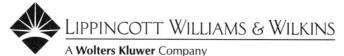

LIPPINCOTT WILLIAMS & WILKINS
A **Wolters Kluwer** Company

Philadelphia · Baltimore · New York · London
Buenos Aires · Hong Kong · Sydney · Tokyo

Editor: Margaret Biblis
Managing Editor: Linda Napora
Marketing Manager: Debby Hartman
Production Editor: Paula C. Williams

351 West Camden Street
Baltimore, Maryland 20201-2436 USA

530 Walnut Street
Philadelphia, Pennsylvania 19106-3621 USA

Printed in the United States of America

First Edition, 1995

Library of Congress Cataloging-in-Publication Data
Shumway-Cook, Anne, 1947-
    Motor control : theory and practical applications / Anne Shumway-Cook, Marjorie H. Woollacott.—2nd ed.
      p. cm.
    Includes index.
    ISBN 0-683-30643-X
    1. Motor ability. 2. Motor learning. 3. Medical rehabilitation. 4. Brain damage—Patients—Rehabilitation. I. Woollacott, Marjorie H., 1946- II. Title.

QP301 .S535 2000
612.7—dc21

                                                                00-064290

To purchase additional copies of this book call our customer service department at **(800) 638-3030** or fax orders to **(301) 824-7390**. International customers should call **(301) 714-2324**.

Visit Lippincott Williams & Wilkins on the Internet: **http://www.lww.com.** Lippincott Williams & Wilkins customer service representatives are available from 8:30 am to 6:00 pm, EST, Monday through Friday, for telephone access.

01 02
2 3 4 5 6 7 8 9 10

It is with great love and gratitude that we dedicate this book
to the many people, including professional colleagues, reviewers, and patients,
who have contributed to the development of the ideas presented here.
We gratefully acknowledge the divine source of our enthusiasm, wisdom, and joy.
We dedicate this book, as we do all our actions,
to the One who set it before us to do
and provided us steadfast wisdom and
support throughout its creation.

In recent years there has been a tremendous interest among clinicians regarding new theories of motor control and the role of these theories in guiding clinical practice. The explosion of new research in the field of neuroscience and motor control has created a gap between research/theory and clinical practices related to helping patients regain motor control. This book is an attempt to bridge the gap between theory and practice. The book stresses the scientific and experimental basis of new motor control theories and explains how principles from this science can be applied to clinical practice. While many theories of motor control are discussed, the major thrust of the book is to present a systems theory of motor control and a clinical approach to examination and intervention based on this model. We refer to this clinical approach as a task-oriented approach.

The book is divided into four sections. Section I, entitled Theoretical Framework, reviews current theories of motor control, motor learning, and recovery of function following neurological insult. The clinical implications of various theories of motor control are discussed. In addition, this section reviews the physiological basis of motor control and motor learning. This section also includes a suggested conceptual framework for clinical practice and a framework for understanding and examining impairments in the neurological patient. The first section is the foundation for the major thrust of the book, which addresses motor control issues as they relate to the control of posture and balance (Section II), mobility (Section III), and upper extremity manipulatory functions (Section IV). The chapters in each of these sections follow a standard format. The first chapter discusses issues related to normal control processes. The second (and in some cases third) chapter describes age-related issues. The third chapter presents research on abnormal function, and the final chapter discusses the clinical applications of current research. This chapter describes the examination and treatment of patients with motor dyscontrol in each of the three functional areas and reviews available outcomes research.

We envision that this text will be of use in both undergraduate and graduate courses on normal motor control, motor development across the life span, and rehabilitation in the areas of physical and occupational therapy as well as kinesiology and exercise science.

This second edition includes major revisions and additions based upon our own use of the textbook in our classes and recent research and clinical findings. These include (a) laboratory activities that are used to demonstrate concepts covered in the chapters, (b) a new chapter reviewing impairments that constrain functional movement in the patient with neurological pathology, (c) major revisions in the section on manipulatory function especially designed for occupational therapy programs, and (d) the use of case studies to help the reader apply concepts to patients with different diagnoses.

Motor Control: Theory and Practical Applications, Second Edition, seeks to provide a framework that will enable the clinician to incorporate current theory and research on motor control into clinical practice. More important, it is our hope that this book will serve as a springboard for developing new, more effective approaches to examining and treating patients with motor dyscontrol.

CONTENTS

SECTION **IV.**

Reach, Grasp, and Manipulation

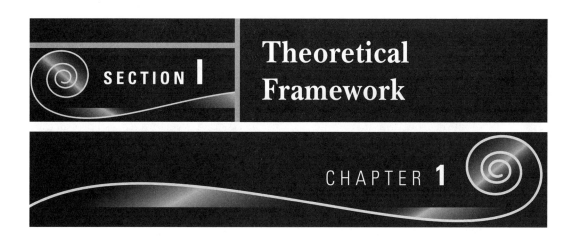

SECTION I

Theoretical Framework

CHAPTER 1

Motor Control: Issues and Theories

@ INTRODUCTION

What Is Motor Control?

Movement is a critical aspect of life. Movement is essential to our ability to walk, run, and play; to seek out and eat the food that nourishes us; to communicate with friends and family; to earn our living; in essence, to survive. The field of motor control is directed at studying the nature of movement and how that movement is controlled. **Motor control** is the ability to regulate or direct the mechanisms essential to movement. It addresses questions such as these: How does the central nervous system (CNS) organize the many individual muscles and joints into coordinated functional movements? How is sensory information from the environment and the body used to select and control movement? What is the best way to study movement? How can movement problems be quantified in patients with motor control problems?

Why Should Therapists Study Motor Control?

Physical and occupational therapists have been referred to as "applied motor control physiologists" (Brooks, 1986). This is because therapists spend a considerable amount of time retraining patients who have motor control problems producing functional movement disorders. Therapeutic intervention is often directed at changing movement or the capacity to move. Therapeutic strategies are designed to improve the quality and quantity of postures and movements essential to function. Thus, understanding motor control and specifically the nature and control of movement is critical to clinical practice.

We begin our study of motor control by discussing important issues related to the nature and control of movement. Following this we explore various theories of motor control, examining their underlying assumptions and clinical implications. Finally we review how theories of motor control relate to past and present clinical practices.

⊘ UNDERSTANDING THE NATURE OF MOVEMENT

Movement emerges from the interaction of three factors: the individual, the task, and the environment. Movement is both task specific and constrained by the environment. The individual generates movement to meet the demands of the task being performed within a specific environment. The individual's capacity to meet interacting task and environmental demands determines that

person's functional capability. Motor control research that focuses only on processes within the individual without taking into account the environment in which one moves or the task one is performing will produce an incomplete picture. Thus, in this book our discussion of motor control focuses on the interaction of the individual, the task, and the environment. Figure 1-1 illustrates this concept.

Factors Within the Individual That Constrain Movement

Within the individual, movement emerges through the cooperative effort of many brain structures and processes. The term motor control in itself is somewhat misleading, since movement arises from the interaction of multiple processes, including those that are related to *perception, cognition,* and *action.*

Movement and Action

Movement is often described within the context of accomplishing a particular action. As a result, motor control is usually studied in relation to specific actions or activities. For example, motor control physiologists might ask how people walk, run, talk, smile, reach, or stand still. Researchers typically study

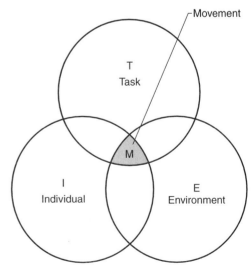

FIGURE 1-1. Movement emerges from an interaction between the individual, the task, and the environment.

movement control within the context of a specific activity, like walking, with the understanding that control processes related to this activity will provide insight into principles for the ways all movement is controlled.

Understanding the control of action implies understanding the motor output from the nervous system to the body's effector systems, or muscles. The body is characterized by a high number of muscles and joints, all of which must be controlled during the execution of coordinated, functional movement. This problem of coordinating many muscles and joints has been called the degrees-of-freedom problem (Bernstein, 1967). It is considered a major issue being studied by motor control researchers and will be discussed in later chapters. So the study of motor control includes the study of the systems that control *action*.

Movement and Perception

Perception is essential to action, just as action is essential to perception. **Perception** is the integration of sensory impressions into psychologically meaningful information. Sensory/perceptual systems provide information about the state of the body (for example, the position of the body in space) and features within the environment critical to the regulation of movement. Therefore, sensory/perceptual information is clearly integral to the ability to act effectively within an environment (Rosenbaum, 1991). Thus, understanding movement requires the study of systems controlling *perception* and the role of perception in determining our actions.

Movement and Cognition

In addition, since movement is not usually performed in the absence of intent, cognitive processes are essential to motor control. In this book we define cognitive processes broadly to include attention, motivation, and emotional aspects of motor control that underlie the establishment of intent or goals. Motor control includes perception and action systems that are organized to achieve specific goals or intents. Thus, the study of motor control must include the

study of *cognitive* processes as they relate to perception and action.

So within the individual, many systems interact in the production of functional movement. While each of these components of motor control—perception, action, and cognition—can be studied in isolation, we believe a true picture of the nature of motor control cannot be achieved without synthesis of information from all three. Figure 1-2 illustrates this concept. In addition to constraints related to the individual, tasks can also impose constraints on motor function.

Task Constraints on Movement

In everyday life we perform a tremendous variety of functional tasks requiring movement. The nature of the task being performed in part determines the type of movement needed. Thus, understanding the control of movement requires an awareness of how tasks regulate, or constrain, movement.

Recovery of function following CNS damage requires that a patient develop movement patterns that meet the demands of functional tasks in the face of sensory/perceptual, motor, and cognitive impairments. Thus, therapeutic strategies that help the patient learn or relearn to perform functional tasks are essential to maximizing recovery of functional independence. But what tasks should be taught, in what order, and at what time? Establishing a therapeutic environment in which functional movement can be mastered requires the therapist to understand the nature of tasks to be taught.

The concept of grouping tasks is not new to clinicians. Within the clinical environment, tasks are routinely grouped into functional categories. Examples of functional task groupings include bed mobility tasks (e.g., moving from supine to sit, moving to the edge of the bed and back, and changing positions within the bed); transfer tasks (e.g., moving from sitting to standing and back, moving from chair to bed and back, moving onto and off a toilet), and activities of daily living (e.g., dressing, toileting, grooming, and feeding). However, classification of movement tasks within a clinical con-

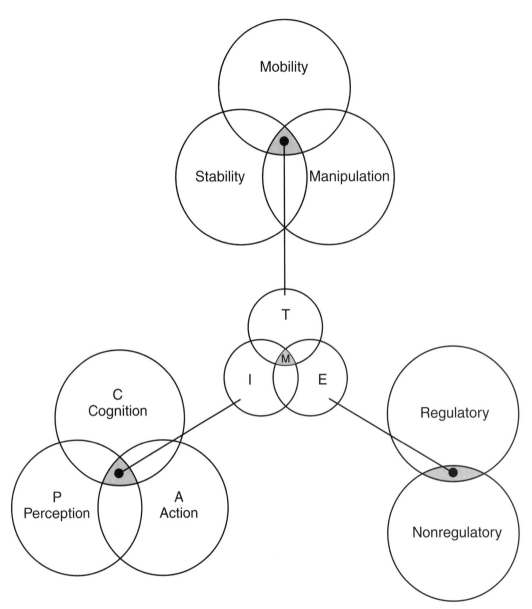

FIGURE 1-2. Factors within the individual, the task, and the environment affect the organization of movement. Factors within the individual include the interaction of *perception, cognition, and action (motor) systems.* Environmental constraints on movement are divided into both regulatory and nonregulatory factors. Finally, attributes of the task contribute to the organization of functional movement.

text is often based on a functional category of tasks rather than on inherent characteristics or attributes of the task itself.

Classification Based on Task Attributes

Tasks can be analyzed and classified using specific attributes that are inherent in the task. This approach to classifying tasks is based on an understanding of the essential attributes of a task that specifically govern or regulate the control of movement. For example, a nonmoving base of support is an attribute of the task of standing; in contrast a moving base of support is an attribute of walking and running. Many task features or attributes can be considered along a continuous scale because they represent continuous variables, such as speed, or accuracy. Other attributes are more discrete.

Discrete Versus Continuous Tasks

Movement tasks can be classified as discrete or continuous. A critical attribute of discrete movement tasks is a recognizable beginning and end. Kicking or throwing a ball, moving from sitting to standing, and lying down in bed are examples of discrete movement tasks. The end point in a discrete task is an inherent attribute of the task itself and cannot be arbitrarily defined by the performer. In contrast to discrete movements, continuous movements have no recognizable beginning or end. Thus the end point of the task is not an inherent characteristic of the task but is decided arbitrarily by the performer (Schmidt, 1988b). Examples of continuous tasks include walking, running, swimming, and biking.

A series of discrete movements that are performed together are referred to as serial movements. Serial movements, while at first appearing continuous, are actually composed of an ordered series of discrete movements (Schmidt, 1988b). Most of the movements involved in basic and instrumental activities of daily life such as dressing, cooking, grooming, and toileting are serial movements.

Stability Versus Mobility Tasks

Movement tasks have also been classified according to whether the base of support is still or in motion (Gentile, 1987). Stability tasks, such as sitting or standing, are performed with a nonmoving base of support. In contrast, a feature or attribute of mobility tasks, such as walking and running, is a moving base of support. Between these two ends are tasks that entail more complex movements over a modified base of support, such as moving from sitting to standing.

Manipulation Continuum

Movement tasks have also been classified using a manipulation component (Gentile, 1987). The amount of upper extremity manipulation involved in the task can range from none to relatively simple manipulation tasks that do not have a large accuracy component to more complex tasks that may require both speed and accuracy. Manipulation tasks that require both speed and accuracy increase the demands on the postural system, since stabilization of the body is critical to the performance of these tasks.

Attention Continuum

Using the attribute of attentional demand to classify movement tasks is relatively new to the field of motor control. Most of the research in this area has examined the attentional demands of postural control tasks. Tasks that have the lowest attentional demand are primarily static postural tasks, such as sitting and standing; attentional demands increase in mobility tasks, such as walking and obstacle clearance (LaJoie et al., 1993; Chen et al., 1996).

Open Versus Closed Tasks

Several researchers have used the term open and closed tasks to describe a classification based on the task–environment interaction (Schmidt, 1988b; Gentile, 1987). In this context, an essential attribute of open movement tasks is variability and flexibility, since they are performed in unpredictable environments. Open movement tasks are performed in a constantly changing environment, making the ability to plan a movement difficult. Playing soccer or tennis requires open movement skills. Open movement skills require performers to adapt their behavior to a constantly changing environment. To be successful performing open movement tasks, performers must develop a broad repertoire of movements allowing quick and responsive adaptation to changing environmental conditions.

Closed movement tasks are characterized by fixed, habitual patterns of movement with minimal variation that are performed in relatively fixed environments. While open movement tasks vary greatly from trial to trial in response to changing environmental features, closed movement tasks are relatively stereotyped, showing little trial to trial variation. Because of their stereotyped nature, closed movement tasks may have lower information processing and attentional demands than open movement tasks, which place larger demands on information processing systems. Between these two extremes are movements carried out in semipredictable environments, for example, walking and carrying a bag of groceries or walking a dog that is fairly well behaved (and thus somewhat predictable) on a leash.

The use of the terms *open task* and *closed task* can be confusing, since these terms are also used in several other contexts related to movement. For example, the terms *open loop* and *closed loop* are used to describe two modes of movement control (Schmidt, 1988b). In open-loop control a movement is not sensitive to environmental feedback; in contrast, closed-loop movements are sensitive to the environment; that is, the loop of control from the environment to centers controlling movement and back to the environment is complete, or "closed" (Schmidt, 1988b).

Finally, the terms *open chain* and *closed chain* have been used to characterize movements. In his 1955 book on kinesiology, Arthur Steindler used the term *open kinetic chain* to describe movements in which the terminal, or distal, joint is free to move. In contrast, a closed kinetic chain movement is one in which the distal segment of the body encounters external resistance within the environment that restrains movement of the distal segment (Steindler, 1955). In all three examples, the role of the environment is central to defining the movement as open or closed.

Creating a Taxonomy of Movement Tasks

Understanding the critical attributes of tasks that govern movement allows the development of a taxonomy of tasks. A taxonomy of tasks can provide a framework for functional examination, since it allows a therapist to identify the specific kinds of tasks that are difficult for the patient. In addition, the set of tasks can serve as a progression for retraining functional movement in the patient with a neurological disorder. The application of this concept can be found in Lab Activity 1-1.

 LAB ACTIVITY 1-1

OBJECTIVE: To develop your own taxonomy of movement tasks.

PROCEDURE: Make a graph like the one illustrated in Table 1-1. Identify two continua you would like to combine. You can begin by using one or more of the continua described above, or alternatively you can create your own continuum based on attributes of movement tasks we have not discussed. In our example we combined the stability–mobility continuum with the open-closed continuum.

ASSIGNMENT: Fill in the boxes with examples of tasks that reflect the demands of each of the continua. Once your taxonomy is filled in, think about ways you could progress a patient through your taxonomy. What assumptions do you have about which tasks are easiest, which the hardest? Is there a "right" way to move through your taxonomy? How will you decide what tasks to use and in what order?

Gentile's Taxonomy of Movement Tasks

Ann Gentile, a motor control scientist from Columbia University in New York, has proposed an approach to categorizing functional movement tasks based on the goals of the task and the environmental context in which the action takes place (Gentile, 1987, 1992). Gentile's taxonomy incorporates three continua: open-closed, stability–mobility, and manipulation continua. Gentile's classification of movement tasks is shown in Table 1-2. One of the limitations of Gentile's classification scheme of movement tasks is that although it represents an interesting theoretical framework for retraining motor control, no formal application of this framework to retraining the patient with movement disorders has yet been proposed.

Environmental Constraints on Movement

Tasks are performed in a wide range of environments. Thus, in addition to attributes of the task, movement is also constrained by features within the environment. To be func-

TABLE 1-1.   A Taxonomy of Tasks Combining the Stability-Mobility and Closed-Open Task Continua

	Stability	Quasi-Mobile	Mobility
Closed predictable environment	Sit/stand/ nonmoving surface	Sit to stand/ Kitchen chair w/arms	Walk/ Nonmoving surface
Open unpredictable environment	Stand/ rocker board	Sit to stand/ Rocking chair	Walk on uneven or moving surface

tional, the CNS must consider attributes of the environment when planning task-specific movement. As shown in Figure 1-2, attributes of the environment that affect movement have been divided into regulatory and nonregulatory features (Gordon, 1987). Regulatory features specify aspects of the environment that shape the movement itself. Task-specific movements must conform to regulatory features of the environment to achieve the goal of the task. Examples of regulatory features of the environment include the size, shape, and weight of a cup to be picked up and the type of surface on which we walk (Gordon, 1987). Nonregulatory features of the environment may affect performance, but movement does not have to conform to these features. Examples of nonregulatory features of the environment include background noise and distractions.

Features of the environment in some instances enable or support performance or alternatively disable or hinder performance. For example, walking in a well-lit environment is much easier than walking in low light or in the dark, since the ability to detect edges, size of small obstacles, and other surface properties is compromised when the light level is low (Patla and Shumway-Cook, 1999).

TABLE 1-2.   Gentile's Taxonomy of Movement Tasks Combining Three Continua to Describe Movement

Environmental Context	Body Stability		Body Transport	
	No Manipulation	Manipulation	No Manipulation	Manipulation
Stationary No intertrial variability	Closed Body stability	Closed Body stability plus manipulation	Closed Body transport	Closed Body transport plus manipulation
Stationary Intertrial variability	Variable Motionless Body stability	Variable Motionless Body stability plus manipulation	Variable Motionless Body stability	Variable Motionless Body stability plus manipulation
Motion No intertrial variability	Consistent Motion Body stability	Consistent Motion Body stability plus manipulation	Consistent Motion Body transport	Consistent Motion Body transport plus manipulation
Motion Intertrial variability	Open Body stability	Open Body stability plus manipulation	Open Body transport	Open Body transport plus manipulation

From Gentile A. Skill acquisition: action, movement, and neuromotor processes. In: Carr J, Shepherd R, Gordon J, et al., eds. Movement science: foundations for physical therapy in rehabilitation. Rockville, MD: Aspen Systems, 1987:115.

Thus, understanding features within the environment that both regulate and affect the performance of movement tasks is essential to planning effective intervention. Preparing patients to perform in a wide variety of environments requires that we understand the features of the environment that will affect movement performance and adequately prepare our patients to meet the demands in various types of environments.

Three Levels for Analyzing Movement

A part of clinical practice is analyzing how and why patients move the way they do. What is the best way to analyze movement behavior? Gentile (1992) suggested that goal-directed functional behavior can be analyzed at three levels: (*a*) action, (*b*) movements, and (*c*) neuromotor processes.

Analysis at the Action Level

According to Gentile, an analysis at the action level examines the behavioral outcome that results from the interaction of the individual, the task, and the environment. For example, analysis of the functional behavior getting out of bed at the action level examines the outcome of the patient performing this task in a particular environment. That is, was the patient able to get out of bed?

Analysis at the Movement Level

Gentile suggests that the second level of analysis focuses on analyzing the movements used to perform the functional tasks. In our example, the movement strategy used to move from lying supine in bed to standing next to the bed can be described. For example, does the patient roll over onto his or her side, use his or her hands to push up to the sitting position, and then stand up from the bed?

Analysis at the Neuromotor Level

Last, Gentile suggests that goal-directed behavior can be analyzed from the perspective of the underlying processes that contribute

to the movement being performed. As we mentioned earlier in this chapter, functional movement emerges through the interaction of many systems. Thus, one can approach the analysis of functional movement by examining the subsystems of movement, both individually and collectively. In our example, we could examine the integrity of individual systems important to movement such as sensation, perception, motor coordination, and strength. We could also examine the interaction of these systems in controlling equilibrium essential to arising from bed. Thus, each of the systems contributing to the behavior getting out of bed could be examined. What is the relationship between these levels? Let's do an experiment and find out. The application of this concept can be found in Lab Activity 1-2.

As you can see from the lab activity, the relationship between these levels is not one to

 LAB ACTIVITY 1-2

OBJECTIVE: To analyze a functional movement task using the three levels of movement analysis described by Gentile.

PROCEDURE: Form a group with three or four people. Pick a functional task, such as moving from supine to standing. Each person in the group should perform the task in his or her own way, with no specific instructions as to how to do this task. Use a stopwatch to time task performance.

ASSIGNMENT: Use Gentile's approach to analyze the functional task. First analyze the behavior from an action perspective. Was everyone in the group able to stand up successfully without assistance and in about the same amount of time? Now analyze the behavior from a movement perspective. Did everyone in the group perform the task in the same way? That is, what kinds of movement strategies were used to accomplish this behavior? Was there variation (movement equivalence) in how people moved from supine to standing? Finally, analyze the underlying components such as strength and coordination that are essential to the movement. Was there variation in strength and coordination in each individual?

one (Gentile, 1992). Many movement strategies can be used to move from supine to standing. This is called movement equivalence (Bernstein, 1967; Gentile, 1992; van Sant, 1988). In addition, there are many ways, called motor equivalence, to organize underlying systems to achieve a specific movement pattern (Bernstein, 1967;Gentile, 1992). Thus, skill in achieving a functional task is not defined by a single movement pattern or a single way to organize underlying elements. Instead, skilled movement behavior is defined by the ability to adapt how we move to achieve the goal of the task consistently and efficiently in a wide variety of environments.

We have explored how the nature of movement is determined by the interaction of three factors, the individual, the task, and the environment. Thus, the movement we observe in patients is shaped not just by factors within the individual such as sensory, motor, and cognitive impairments but also by attributes of the task being performed and the environment in which the individual is moving. We now turn our attention to examining the control of movement from a number of theoretical views.

ℰ THE CONTROL OF MOVEMENT: THEORIES OF MOTOR CONTROL

The field of motor control is directed at studying the nature of movement and how movement is controlled. We have discussed the nature of movement and how it is shaped by attributes of the task, the individual, and the environment. We now turn to issues related to the control of movement. This has been a field of interest in both the research and clinical settings for many years, yet there is no universal agreement among scientists or clinicians about how movement is controlled. Theories of motor control describe viewpoints regarding how movement is controlled. A **theory of motor control** is a group of abstract ideas about the control of movement. A theory is a set of interconnected

statements that describe unobservable structures or processes and relate them to each other and to observable events. Jules Henri Poincare said, "Science is built up of facts, as a house is built of stone; but an accumulation of facts is no more a science than a heap of stones is a house." A theory gives meaning to facts, just as a blueprint provides the structure that transforms stones to a house (Miller, 1983).

However, just as the same stones can be used to make different houses, the same facts are given different meaning and interpretation by different theories of motor control. Different theories of motor control reflect philosophically different views about how the brain controls movement. These theories often reflect differences in opinion about the relative importance of various neural components of movement. For example, some theories stress peripheral influences; others, central influences; still others, the role of information from the environment in controlling behavior. Thus, motor control theories are more than just an approach to explaining action. Often they stress different aspects of the organization of the underlying neurophysiology and neuroanatomy of that action. Some theories of motor control look at the brain as a *black box* and simply study the rules by which this black box interacts with changing environments as a variety of tasks are performed. As you will see, there is no one theory of motor control that everyone accepts.

Value of Theory to Practice

Do theories really influence what therapists do with their patients? YES! Rehabilitation practices reflect theories, or basic ideas, about the cause and nature of function and dysfunction (Shepard, 1991). In general, then, the actions of therapists are based on assumptions that are derived from theories. The specific practices related to examination and intervention used with the patient who has motor dyscontrol are determined by underlying assumptions about the nature and cause of movement. Thus, motor control theory is part of the theoretical basis for clinical practice. This is discussed in more detail in the last section of this chapter.

What are the advantages and disadvantages of using theories in clinical practice? Theories provide the following:

- A framework for interpreting behavior
- A guide for clinical action
- New ideas
- Working hypotheses for examination and intervention

Framework for Interpreting Behavior

Theory can help therapists to interpret the behavior or actions of patients they work with. Theory allows the therapist to go beyond the behavior of one patient and broaden the application to a much larger number of cases (Shepard, 1991).

Theories can be more or less helpful depending on their ability to predict or explain the behavior of an individual patient. When a theory and its associated assumptions does not provide an accurate interpretation of a patient's behavior, it loses its usefulness to the therapist. Thus, theories have the potential to limit a therapist's ability to observe and interpret movement problems in patients.

For example, look at the patient pictured in Figure 1-3. Phoebe J. is a 67-year-old woman referred for rehabilitation following a cerebral vascular accident that produced motor dyscontrol in her left side. The patient habitually sits with her left arm flexed and drawn close to her body. When asked to extend her left arm, she cannot actively extend at the elbow. If you try to extend her arm, there is resistance. In addition, when she walks, her knee is stiff and hyperextended, and she uses a toe–heel pattern.

Prior to deciding how to retrain arm function and gait, as her therapist you must decide what the underlying problems are. What is preventing her from actively extending her arm? Why is she unable to walk with a heel–toe gait? You may assume the patient's inability to extend her arm is the result of spasticity in the elbow flexors. In addition, her inability to walk heel–toe is the result of spasticity (hyperactive stretch re-

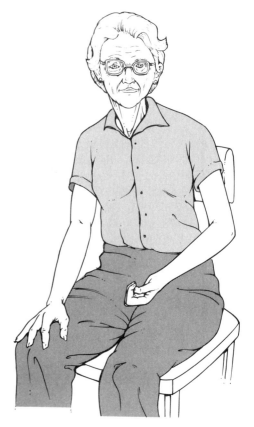

FIGURE 1-3.   Phoebe J. is a 67-year-old woman referred for therapy because of a right cerebral vascular accident resulting in left hemiparesis. Pictured is the habitual upper extremity posture in sitting, which she also typically exhibits in standing.

flexes) in the gastrocnemius muscle. This assumption may be based on a theory of motor control suggesting that reflexes are an important part of movement control and that abnormal reflexes are a major reason patients cannot move normally. In accordance with this theory, you may attribute the loss of arm function, specifically the inability to extend the elbow actively, primarily to spasticity, defined as a release of the stretch reflex, in the elbow flexors.

Has your theoretical framework helped you correctly interpret this patient's behavior? Only if this patient's problems are in fact solely the result of spasticity. The theory has not helped you as a clinician if it has limited your ability to explore other possible explanations for your patient's behavior. What are some of the other factors that may impair arm function in your stroke patient? Later in this chapter we discuss other theories of motor control that provide alternative explanations for loss of function.

Guide for Clinical Action

Theories provide therapists with a possible guide for action (Miller, 1983; Shepard, 1991). Clinical interventions designed to improve motor control in the patient with neurological dysfunction are based on an understanding of the nature and cause of normal movement and an understanding of the basis for abnormal movement. Therapeutic strategies aimed at retraining motor control reflect this basic understanding. In the earlier example, spasticity is assumed to be a major determinant of abnormal function. As a result, numerous interventions have been developed to modify spasticity in the course of retraining function. However, because there are many theories about the nature and control of movement, there are many other therapeutic approaches for retraining motor dyscontrol.

New Ideas: Dynamic and Evolving

Theories are dynamic, and they change to reflect greater knowledge relating to the theory. How does this affect clinical practices related to retraining the patient with motor dyscontrol? Changing and expanding theories of motor control need not be a source of frustration to clinicians. Expanding theories can broaden and enrich the possibilities for clinical practice. New ideas related to examination and intervention will evolve to reflect new ideas about the nature and cause of movement.

Working Hypothesis for Examination and Intervention

A theory is not directly testable, since it is abstract. Rather, theories generate hypotheses, which are testable. Information gained through hypothesis testing is used to validate or invalidate a theory. This same approach is useful in clinical practice. So-called hypothe-

sis-driven clinical practice transforms the therapist into an active problem solver (Rothstein and Echternach, 1986). Using this approach to retrain the patient with motor dyscontrol calls for the therapist to generate multiple hypotheses (explanations) for why patients move or don't move in ways to achieve functional independence. During the course of therapy the therapist tests various hypotheses, discarding some and generating new explanations that are more consistent with their results.

Among the many theories discussed in this chapter, each has made specific contributions to the field of motor control and each has implications for the clinician retraining patients with motor dyscontrol. All models are unified by the desire to understand the nature and control of movement. The differences are in the approach. It is not unlike the story of the group of men trying to understand the nature and function of an elephant. One carefully and systematically studies the trunk and learns everything there is to know about the nature and function of the trunk. Another studies the nature and function of the feet; another, the tail. Each in his own way has provided essential information about the elephant. However, a true understanding about the nature and function of an elephant is made possible only by combining information from all sources. In this spirit, we approach the following section on theories of motor control, their limitations, and possible clinical applications.

Reflex Theory

Sir Charles Sherrington, a neurophysiologist in the late 1800s and early 1900s, wrote the book *The Integrative Action of the Nervous System* in 1906. His research formed the experimental foundation for a classic reflex theory of motor control. For Sherrington, reflexes were the building blocks of complex behavior. He believed that reflexes worked together or in sequence to achieve a common purpose (Sherrington, 1947).

Sherrington performed elegant experiments with cats, dogs, and monkeys to show the existence of the reflex and carefully describe and define reflexes. The conception of a reflex requires three structures, as shown in Figure 1-4: a receptor, a conducting nervous pathway, and an effector. The conductor consists of at least two nerve cells, one connected to the effector and the other connected to the receptor. The reflex arc consists of the receptor, the conductor, and the effector (Gallistel, 1980).

Sherrington went on to describe complex behavior in terms of compound reflexes and their successive combination or chaining together. Sherrington gave the following example of a frog capturing and eating a fly. Picture Mr. Frog sitting in the sun on his lily pad. Along comes the fly; seeing the fly (stimulus) produces the reflex activation of the tongue darting out to capture the fly (response). If he is successful, the contact of the fly on the tongue causes reflex closure of the mouth, and closure of the mouth results in reflex swallowing.

Sherrington concluded that with the whole nervous system intact, the reaction of the various parts of that system, the simple reflexes, are combined into greater actions that constitute the behavior of the individual as a whole. Figure 1-5 represents this concept of reflex chaining. Sherrington's view of a reflexive basis for movement persisted unchallenged by many clinicians for 50 years and continues to influence thinking about motor control today.

Limitations

Because Sherrington looked primarily at reflexes and his questions about the central CNS related to reflexes, he drew a picture of

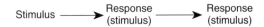

FIGURE 1-5. Reflex chaining as a basis for action. A stimulus leads to a response, which becomes the stimulus for the next response, which becomes the stimulus for the next response.

the CNS and motor control that was skewed toward reflex control. There are a number of limitations to reflex theory of motor control (Rosenbaum, 1991).

First, the reflex cannot be considered the basic unit of behavior if both spontaneous and voluntary movements are recognized as acceptable classes of behavior, since the reflex must be activated by an outside agent. Second, the reflex theory of motor control does not adequately explain and predict movement that occurs in the absence of a sensory stimulus. More recently, it has been shown that animals can move in a relatively coordinated fashion in the absence of sensory input (Taub and Berman, 1968).

Third, Sherrington's theory does not explain fast movements, that is, sequences of movements that occur too rapidly to allow for sensory feedback from the preceding movement to trigger the next. For example, an experienced and proficient typist moves from one key to the next so rapidly that there isn't time for sensory information from one keystroke to activate the next.

Fourth, the reflex chaining model fails to explain the fact that a single stimulus can result in varying responses depending on context and descending commands. For example, there are times when we need to override reflexes to achieve a goal. Thus, normally touching something hot results in the reflexive withdrawal of the hand. However, if a child is in a fire, we may override the reflexive withdrawal to pull the child from the fire.

Finally, reflex chaining does not explain the ability to produce novel movements. Novel movements put together unique combinations of stimuli and responses according to rules previously learned. A violinist who has learned a piece on the violin and also knows the technique of playing the cello can

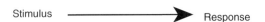

FIGURE 1-4. The basic structure of a reflex consists of a receptor, a conductor, and an effector.

play that piece perfectly on the cello without necessarily having practiced the piece on the cello. The violinist has learned the rules for playing the piece and has applied them to a novel or new situation.

Clinical Implications

How might a reflex theory of motor control be used to interpret a patient's behavior and serve as a guide for the therapist's actions? If chained or compounded reflexes are the basis for functional movement, clinical strategies designed to test reflexes should allow therapists to predict function. In addition, a patient's movement behaviors would be interpreted in terms of the presence or absence of controlling reflexes. Finally, retraining motor control for functional skills would focus on enhancing or reducing the effect of various reflexes during motor tasks.

Applying a reflex theory to interpreting motor dyscontrol was shown in the example of Phoebe J. Clinical strategies for improving motor control using a reflex model focus on methods to reduce flexor spasticity, which should enhance normal movement capacity. Despite the limitations in Sherrington's conclusions, many of his assumptions about how the CNS controls movement have been reinforced and have influenced current clinical practices.

Hierarchical Theory

Many researchers contributed to the view that the nervous system is organized as a hierarchy. Among them, Hughlings Jackson, an English physician, argued that the brain has higher, middle, and lower levels of control, equated with higher association areas, the motor cortex, and spinal levels of motor function (Foerster, 1977).

Hierarchical control in general has been defined as organizational control that is top down. That is, each successively higher level exerts control over the level below it, as shown in Figure 1-6. In a strict vertical hierarchy, lines of control do not cross and there is never bottom-up control.

In the 1920s, Rudolf Magnus began to explore the function of different reflexes

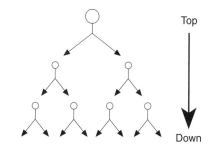

FIGURE 1-6. The hierarchical control model is characterized by a top-down structure, in which higher centers are always in charge of lower centers.

within different parts of the nervous system. He found that reflexes controlled by lower levels of the neural hierarchy are present only when cortical centers are damaged. These results were later interpreted to imply that reflexes are part of a hierarchy of motor control in which higher centers normally inhibit these lower reflex centers (Magnus, 1925, 1926)

Later, Georg Schaltenbrand (1928) used Magnus's concepts to explain the development of mobility in children and adults. He described the development of human mobility in terms of the appearance and disappearance of a progression of reflexes. He went on further to say that pathology of the brain may result in the persistence of primitive reflexes. He suggested that a complete understanding of all the reflexes would allow the determination of the neural age of a child or a patient.

Stephan Weisz (1938) reported on reflex reactions that he thought were the basis for equilibrium in humans. He described the ontogeny of equilibrium reflexes in the normally developing child and proposed a relationship between the maturation of these reflexes and the child's capacity to sit, stand, and walk.

The results of these experiments and observations were drawn together and are often referred to in the clinical literature as a reflex/hierarchical theory of motor control. This theory combines reflex and hierarchical theories into one. This theory suggests that motor control emerges from reflexes that are nested within hierarchically organized levels of the CNS.

In the 1940s, Arnold Gesell (Gesell and Armatruda, 1947; Gesell, 1954) and Myrtle McGraw (1945), two well-known developmental researchers, offered detailed descriptions of the maturation of infants. These researchers applied contemporary scientific thinking about reflex hierarchies of motor control to explain the behaviors they saw in infants. Normal motor development was attributed to increasing corticalization of the CNS resulting in the emergence of higher levels of control over lower-level reflexes. This has been called a neuromaturational theory of development. An example of this model is illustrated in Figure 1-7. This theory assumes that CNS maturation is the primary agent for change in development. It minimizes the importance of other factors, such as musculoskeletal changes during development.

Current Concepts Related to Hierarchical Control

Since Hughlings Jackson's original work, a new concept of hierarchical control has evolved. Modern neuroscientists have confirmed the importance of elements of hierarchical organization in motor control. The concept of a strict hierarchy, in which higher centers are always in control, has been modified. Current concepts describing hierarchical control within the nervous system recognize the fact that each level of the nervous system can act upon other levels (higher and lower) depending on the task. In addition, the role of reflexes in movement has been modified. Reflexes are not considered the sole determinant of motor control but only one of many processes important to the generation and control of movement.

Limitations

One of the limitations of a reflex/hierarchical theory of motor control is that it cannot explain the dominance of reflex behavior in certain situations in normal adults. For example, stepping on a pin results in an immediate withdrawal of the leg. This is an example of a reflex within the lowest level of the hierarchy dominating motor function. It is an example of bottom-up control. Thus, one must be cautious about assumptions that all low-level behaviors are primitive, immature, and nonadaptive, while all higher-level (cortical) behaviors are mature, adaptive, and appropriate.

Clinical Implications

Many clinicians have used abnormalities of reflex organization to explain disordered motor control in the patient with neurologi-

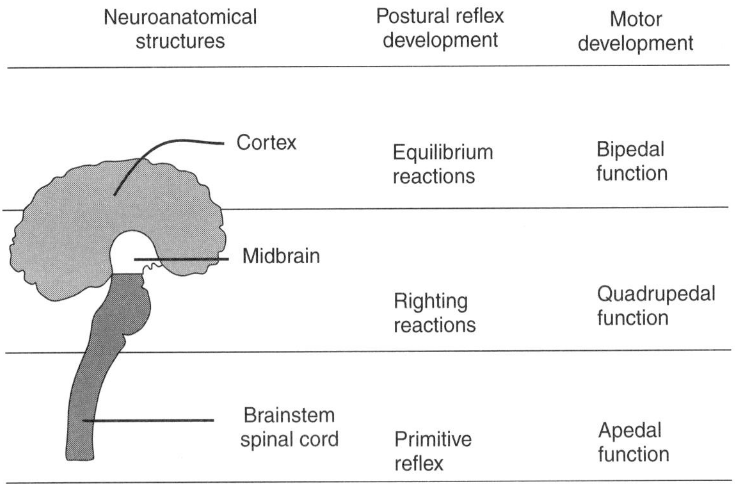

Neuroanatomical structures	Postural reflex development	Motor development
Cortex	Equilibrium reactions	Bipedal function
Midbrain	Righting reactions	Quadrupedal function
Brainstem spinal cord	Primitive reflex	Apedal function

FIGURE 1-7. Neuromaturational theory of motor control attributes motor development to the maturation of neural processes, including the progressive appearance and disappearance of reflexes.

cal disease. Signe Brunnstrom, a physical therapist who pioneered early stroke rehabilitation, used a reflex/hierarchical theory to describe disordered movement following a motor cortex lesion. She stated, "When the influence of higher centers is temporarily or permanently interfered with, normal reflexes become exaggerated and so called pathological reflexes appear" (Brunnstrom, 1970, p. 3).

Berta Bobath, an English physical therapist, in her discussions of abnormal postural reflex activity in children with cerebral palsy, states, "The release of motor responses integrated at lower levels from restraining influences of higher centers, especially that of the cortex, leads to abnormal postural reflex activity" (Bobath, 1965; Mayston, 1992). The clinical applications of the reflex/hierarchical theory are discussed in more detail in the last section of this chapter.

Motor Programming Theories

More recent theories of motor control have expanded our understanding of the CNS. They have moved away from views of the CNS as a mostly reactive system and have begun to explore the physiology of actions rather than the physiology of reactions. Reflex theories have been useful in explaining certain stereotyped patterns of movement. However, an interesting way of viewing reflexes is to consider that one can remove the stimulus, or the afferent input, and still have a patterned motor response (van Sant, 1987). If we remove the motor response from its stimulus, we are left with the concept of a central motor pattern. This concept of a central motor pattern, or motor program, is more flexible than the concept of a reflex because it can be activated either by sensory stimuli or by central processes. Scientists who contributed to the development of this theory include individuals from clinical, psychological, and biological backgrounds (Bernstein, 1967; Keele, 1968; Wilson, 1961).

A motor program theory of motor control has considerable experimental support. For example, experiments in the early 1960s studied motor control in the grasshopper or locust and showed that the timing of the animal's wing beat in flight depended on a rhythmic pattern generator. Even when the sensory nerves were cut, the nervous system by itself could generate the output with no sensory input; however, the wing beat was slowed (Wilson, 1961). This suggested that movement is possible in the absence of reflexive action. Sensory input, while not essential in driving movement, has an important function in modulating action.

These conclusions were further supported by work examining locomotion in cats (Grillner, 1981). The results of these experiments showed that in the cat, spinal neural networks could produce a locomotor rhythm without either sensory inputs or descending patterns from the brain. By changing the intensity of stimulation to the spinal cord, the animal could be made to walk, trot, or gallop. Thus, it was again shown that reflexes do not drive action but that central pattern generators (spinally mediated motor programs) by themselves can generate such complex movements as the walk, trot, and gallop. Further experiments showed the important modulatory effects of incoming sensory inputs on the central pattern generator (Forssberg et al., 1975).

These experiments led to the motor program theory of motor control. This term has been used in a number of ways by different researchers, so take care in determining how the term is being used. The term motor program may be used to identify a central pattern generator (CPG), that is, a specific neural circuit like that for generating walking in the cat. In this case the term represents neural connections that are stereotyped and hardwired.

But the term *motor program* is also used to describe the higher-level motor programs that represent actions in more abstract terms. A significant amount of research in the field of psychology has supported the existence of hierarchically organized motor programs that store the rules for generating movements so that we can perform the tasks with a variety of effector systems (Keele,

1968). The application of this concept can be found in Lab Activity 1-3.

As shown in Figure 1-8, it has been hypothesized that the rules for writing a given word are stored as an abstract motor program at higher levels within the CNS. As a result, neural commands from these higher centers used to write your name may be sent to various parts of the body. Yet, elements of the written signature remain constant regardless of the part of the body used to carry out the task (Bernstein, 1967).

Limitations

The concept of central pattern generators expanded our understanding of the role of the nervous system in the control of movement. However, the central pattern generator concept has never been intended to replace the concept of the importance of sensory input in controlling movement. It simply expanded our understanding of the flexibility of the nervous system in creating movements to include its ability to create movements in isolation from feedback.

An important limitation of the motor program concept is that a central motor program cannot be considered to be the sole determinant of action (Bernstein, 1967). Two identical commands to the elbow flexors, for example, produce very different movements, depending on whether you are resting your arm at your side or holding it out in front of you. The forces of gravity act differently on the limb in the two conditions and thus modify the movement. In addition, if your muscles are fatigued, similar nervous system commands give very different results. Thus, the motor program concept does not take into account the fact that the nervous system must deal with both musculoskeletal and environmental variables in achieving movement control.

Clinical Implications

Motor program theories have allowed clinicians to move beyond a reflex explanation for disordered motor control. Explanations of abnormal movement have been expanded to include problems resulting from abnormalities in central pattern generators and in higher level motor programs.

Phoebe J., our stroke patient, may indeed have flexor spasticity in her arm that affects her ability to move. However, it will be important to determine what levels of motor programming are involved. If her higher levels of motor programming are not affected, she will be able to continue to use such programs as handwriting but will find alternate effectors, for example her unaffected hand, to carry out the tasks. Of course, these less-used lower-level synergy and muscular systems have to be trained to carry out higher-level programs.

In patients whose higher levels of motor programming are affected, motor program theory suggests the importance of helping patients relearn the correct rules for action. In addition, intervention should focus on retraining movements important to a functional task, not just on reeducating specific muscles in isolation.

LAB ACTIVITY 1-3

OBJECTIVE: To apply the concept of motor program to functional movement.

PROCEDURE: Write your signature as you normally would on a small piece of paper. Now write it larger on a blackboard. Now try it with your other hand.

ASSIGNMENT: Examine the three signatures carefully, looking for elements found in all of them. Write down the common elements you found. What do you think are the causes for both the common elements and the differences? How do your results support or contradict the theory of motor programs?

Systems Theory

In the early and mid 1900s Nicolai Bernstein (1896–1966), a Russian scientist, was looking at the nervous system and body in a whole new way. Previous neurophysiologists focused primarily on neural control aspects of movement. Bernstein, who also participated

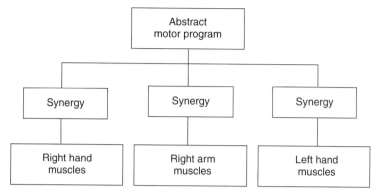

FIGURE 1-8.   Levels of control for motor programs and their output systems. Rules for action are represented at the highest level, in abstract motor programs. Lower levels of the hierarchy contain specific information, including muscle response synergies, essential for effecting action.

in the development of motor program theories, recognized that it is impossible to understand the neural control of movement without understanding the characteristics of the system that is moving and the external and internal forces acting on the body (Bernstein, 1967).

In describing the characteristics of the system being moved, he looked at the whole body as a mechanical system with mass, subject to both external forces, such as gravity, and internal forces, including both inertial and movement-dependent forces. During the course of any movement the amounts of force acting on the body change as potential and kinetic energy change. He thus showed that the same central command could result in quite different movements because of the interplay between external forces and variations in the initial conditions. For the same reasons, different commands could result in the same movement (Bernstein, 1967).

Bernstein also suggested that control of integrated movement was probably distributed throughout many interacting systems working cooperatively to achieve movement. This gave rise to the concept of a distributed model of motor control.

How does Bernstein's approach to motor control differ from the approaches presented previously? Bernstein asked questions about the organism in a continuously changing situation. He found answers about the nature and control of movement that were

different from those of previous researchers, since he asked different questions, such as these: How does the body as a mechanical system influence the control process? How do the initial conditions affect the properties of the movement?

In describing the body as a mechanical system, Bernstein noted that we have many degrees of freedom that must be controlled. For example, we have many joints, all of which flex or extend and many of which can be rotated as well. This complicates movement control incredibly. He said, "Coordination of movement is the process of mastering the redundant degrees of freedom of the moving organism" (Bernstein, 1967). In other words, it involves converting the body into a controllable system.

As a solution to the degrees-of-freedom problem, Bernstein hypothesized that hierarchical control exists to simplify the control of the body's multiple degrees of freedom. In this way, the higher levels of the nervous system activate lower levels. The lower levels activate synergies, or groups of muscles that are constrained to act together as a unit. We can think of our movement repertoire as sentences made up of many words. The letters within the words are the muscles, the words themselves are the synergies, and the sentences are the actions themselves.

Thus, Bernstein believed that synergies play an important role in solving the degrees-of-freedom problem. This is achieved by constraining certain muscles to work together as a unit. He hypothesized that though there are few synergies, they make possible almost the whole variety of movements we know. For example, he considered some simple synergies to be the locomotor, postural, and respiratory synergies.

Limitations

What are the limitations of Bernstein's systems approach? As you can see, it is the broadest of the approaches we have discussed thus far. Since it takes into account not only the contributions of the nervous system to action but also the contributions of the muscle and skeletal systems and the forces of gravity and inertia, it predicts actual behavior much better than previous theories. However, as it is presented today, it does not focus as heavily on the interaction of the organism with the environment, as do some other theories.

Clinical Implications

The systems theory has a number of implications for therapists. First, it stresses the importance of understanding the body as a mechanical system. Movement is not determined solely by the output of the nervous system but is the output of the nervous system as filtered through a mechanical system, the body. When working with the patient who has a CNS deficit, the therapist must be careful to examine the contribution of impairments in the musculoskeletal system to overall loss of motor control.

In the case of Phoebe J., the long-term loss of mobility in her arm and leg may affect the musculoskeletal system. She may show shortening of the elbow flexors and loss of range of motion at the ankle joint. These musculoskeletal limitations will have a significant effect on her ability to recover motor control.

The systems theory suggests that examination and intervention must focus not only on the impairments within individual systems contributing to motor control but also the effect of interacting impairments among multiple systems. A good example of this in

Phoebe J. is the interacting impairments in the musculoskeletal and neuromuscular systems that constrain her ability to move her arm.

Dynamical Action Theory

The dynamical action theory of motor control has begun to look at the moving person from a new perspective (Thelen et al., 1987; Kamm et al., 1991; Kelso and Tuller, 1984; Kugler and Turvey, 1987; Perry, 1998). The perspective, which comes from the broader study of dynamics or synergetics within the physical world, asks these questions: How do the patterns and organization we see in the world come into being from their orderless constituent parts? How do these systems change over time? For example, thousands of muscle cells in the heart work together to make the heart beat. How is this system of thousands of degrees of freedom (each added cell contributes a new degree of freedom to the system) reduced to a system of few degrees of freedom, so that all the cells function as a unit?

This phenomenon, which we see not only in heart muscle but in the patterns of cloud formations and the patterns of movement of water as it goes from ice to liquid to boiling to a gaseous state, are examples of the principle of self-organization, a fundamental dynamical systems principle. It says that when a system of individual parts comes together, its elements behave collectively in an ordered way. There is no need for a "higher" center issuing instructions or commands to achieve coordinated action. This principle applied to motor control predicts that movement can emerge as a result of interacting elements without the need for specific commands or motor programs within the nervous system.

The dynamical action or synergetics perspective also tries to find mathematical descriptions of these self-organizing systems. Critical features that are examined are the nonlinear properties of the system (Kugler and Turvey, 1987). What is nonlinear behavior? A nonlinear behavior is one that transforms into a new configuration when a single

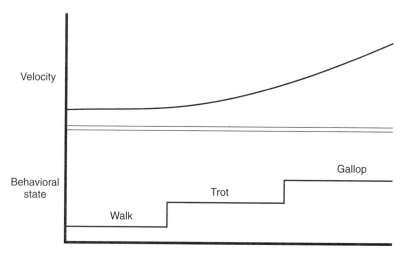

FIGURE 1-9. A dynamical action model predicts discrete changes in behavior resulting from changes in the linear dynamics of a moving system. For example, as velocity increases linearly, the moving animal reaches a threshold that results in a nonlinear change in behavioral state from a walk to a trot to a gallop.

parameter of that behavior is gradually altered and reaches a critical value. For example, as an animal walks faster and faster, there is a point at which suddenly it shifts into a trot. As the animal continues to move faster, it reaches a second point at which it shifts into a gallop. This is shown in Figure 1-9.

What causes this change from one behavioral pattern, for example a walk, to a new behavioral pattern, for example a trot? Dynamical theory suggests that the new movement emerges because of a critical change in one of the systems, called a control parameter. A control parameter is a variable that regulates change in the behavior of the entire system. In our example the control parameter is velocity. When the animal's walking velocity, a control parameter, reaches a critical point, there is a shift in the animal's behavior from a walk to a trot. Thus the dynamical action perspective has deemphasized the notion of commands from the central nervous system in controlling movement and has sought physical explanations that may contribute to movement characteristics as well (Perry, 1998).

An important concept in describing movement from the perspective of dynamical action theory is that of attractor states. Attractor states may be considered preferred patterns of movement used to accomplish common activities of daily life. Animals all habitually walk at a preferred pace that represents an attractor state for walking speed specific to the individual. Walking at other speeds is possible, but barring outside influences, individuals tend to walk at a preferred pace, which is energetically most efficient. The degree to which there is the flexibility to change a preferred pattern of movement is characterized as an attractor well. This concept is shown in Figure 1-10. The deeper the well, the harder it is to change the preferred pattern, suggesting a stable movement pattern. A shallow well suggests an unstable pattern.

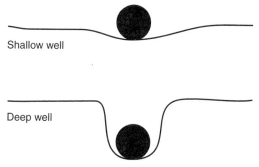

FIGURE 1-10. Attractor wells that describe the variability in preferred pattern of movement.

Attractor wells may be viewed as riverbeds. When a riverbed is quite deep, the likelihood that the river will flow outside the established riverbed is slight. The river flows in the preferred direction established by the riverbed, which is a deep attractor well. Alternatively, if the riverbed is quite shallow, the river is more likely to flow in areas not established by the riverbed. In this case the shallow riverbed is a shallow attractor well. So too, movement patterns in patients can be characterized as stable or unstable based on the difficulty associated with changing them. It is much easier to change an unstable movement pattern that has a shallow attractor well than to change a stable movement pattern that has a deep attractor well.

Kelso and colleagues have shown that stable movement patterns become more variable, or unstable, just prior to a transition to a new movement pattern (Kelso and Tuller, 1984). Researchers have documented an increase in variability prior to the emergence of new, more stable patterns of behavior during the acquisition of new movement skills in both children and adults (Woollacott and Shumway-Cook, 1990; Gordon, 1987). Thus it may be possible for therapists to view variability in movement behavior as an antecedent to change in some patients.

The dynamical action theory has recently been modified to incorporate many of Bernstein's concepts. This has resulted in the blending of these two theories of motor control into a dynamical systems model. This model suggests that movement underlying action results from the interaction of both physical and neural components (Perry, 1998).

Limitations

This approach has added to our understanding of the elements contributing to movement itself and serves as a reminder that understanding the nervous system in isolation will not allow the prediction of movement. However, a limitation of this model can be the presumption that the nervous system has a fairly unimportant role and that the relationship between the physical system of the animal and the environment in which it operates primarily determines the animal's behavior. The focus of the dynamical action theory in the past usually has been at the level of this interface, not at understanding the neural contributions to the system.

Clinical Implications

One of the major implications of the dynamical action theory is the view that movement is an emergent property. That is, it emerges from the interaction of multiple elements that self-organize according to certain dynamic properties of the elements themselves. This means that shifts or alterations in movement behavior can often be explained in terms of physical principles rather than necessarily in terms of neural structures.

What are the implications of this for treating motor dyscontrol in patients? If we clinicians understood more about the physical or dynamic properties of the human body, we could make use of these properties in helping patients to regain motor control. For example, velocity can be an important contributor to the dynamics of movement. Often patients are asked to move slowly in an effort to move safely. Yet this approach to retraining fails to take into account the interaction between physical properties of the body and speed, which produces momentum and therefore can help a weak patient move with greater ease.

For Phoebe J., moving slowly may not be the best strategy for getting up from her chair if weakness is a primary impairment. Instead, teaching her to increase the speed of trunk motion may allow her to generate sufficient momentum to succeed in standing.

Ecological Theory

In the 1960s, independent of the research in physiology, the psychologist James Gibson was beginning to explore the way in which our motor systems allow us to interact most effectively with the environment to perform goal-oriented behavior (Gibson, 1966). His research focused on how we detect environmental information that is relevant to our actions and how we use this information to control our movements (Fig. 1-11). The ability to use to perceptions to guide action emerges early in life. For example, by 15 weeks infants do not automatically reach for every object that passes by but instead use perceptions related to velocity to determine in advance whether they can catch a ball or not (von Hofsten and Lindhagen, 1979).

This view was expanded by the students of Gibson (Lee, 1978; Reed, 1982) and became known as the ecological approach to motor control. It suggests that motor control evolved so that animals could cope with the environment around them, moving in it effectively to find food, run away from predators, build shelter, and even play (Reed, 1982). What is new about this approach? It was the first time researchers began focusing on how actions are geared to the environment. Actions require perceptual information that is specific to a desired goal-directed action performed within a specific environment. The organization of action is specific to the task and the environment in which the task is being performed.

Whereas many previous researchers saw the organism as a sensory–motor system, Gibson stressed that it was not sensation per se but perception that was important to the animal. Specifically, what is needed is the perception of environmental factors important to the task. He stated that perception focuses on detecting information in the environment that will support the actions necessary to achieve the goal. From an ecological perspective, it is important to determine how an organism detects information in the environment that is relevant to action, what form this information takes, and how this information is used to modify and control movement (Lee, 1978).

In summary, the ecological perspective has broadened our understanding of nervous system function from that of a sensory–motor system reacting to environmental variables to that of a perception–action system that actively explores the environment to satisfy its own goals.

Limitations

Although the ecological approach has significantly expanded our knowledge of the interaction of the organism and the environment, it has tended to give less emphasis to the organization and function of the nervous system, which led to this interaction. Thus, the research emphasis has shifted from the nervous system to the organism–environment interface.

Clinical Implications

A major contribution of this view is in describing the individual as an active explorer of the environment. The active exploration of the task and the environment in which the task is performed allow the individual to develop multiple ways to accomplish a task. Adaptability is important not only in the way we organize movements to accomplish a task but also in the way we use perception.

An important part of intervention is helping Phoebe J. explore the possibilities for achieving a functional task in multiple ways. The ability to develop multiple adaptive solutions requires that the patient explore a range of possible ways to accomplish a task and discover the best solution for them, given the patient's set of limitations. In Phoebe J.'s case, this ability to discover a range of solutions is hampered by a reduced

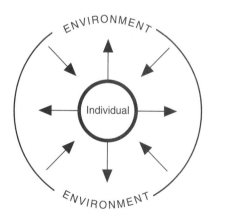

FIGURE 1-11. The ecological approach stresses the interaction between the individual and the environment. The individual actively explores the environment, which in turn supports the individual's actions.

ability to move, inaccurate perceptions, and possibly cognitive limitations.

Which Theory of Motor Control Is Best?

So which motor control theory best suits the theoretical and practical needs of therapists? Which is the most nearly complete theory of motor control, the one that really predicts the nature and cause of movement and is consistent with our knowledge of brain anatomy and physiology?

As you no doubt can already see, no one theory has it all. We believe the best theory of motor control is one that combines elements from all of the presented theories. A comprehensive, or integrated, theory recognizes the elements of motor control we do know about and leaves room for the things we don't. Any current theory of motor control is in a sense unfinished, since there must always be room to revise and incorporate new information.

Many people have been working to develop an integrated theory of motor control (Woollacott and Shumway-Cook, 1990; Horak and Shumway-Cook, 1990; Gordon, 1987). In some cases, as theories are modified, new names are applied. As a result, it becomes difficult to distinguish among evolving theories. For example, systems, dynamical, dynamical action, and dynamical action systems are all terms that are often used interchangeably.

In previous articles we (Woollacott and Shumway-Cook 1990, 1997) have called the theory of motor control on which we base our research and clinical practice a systems approach. We have continued to use this name, though our concept of systems theory differs from Bernstein's systems theory and has evolved to incorporate many of the concepts proposed by other theories of motor control. In this book we continue to refer to our theory of motor control as a systems approach. This approach argues that it is critical to recognize that movement emerges from an interaction between the individual, the task, and the environment in which the task is being carried out. Thus, movement is not solely the result of muscle-specific motor programs, or stereotyped reflexes, but results from a dynamic interplay between perception, cognition, and action systems. This theoretical framework is used throughout this text and is the basis for clinical methods related to the examination and intervention in the patient with neurological problems. We have found it useful in helping us to generate research questions and hypotheses about the nature and cause of movement.

✑ PARALLEL DEVELOPMENT OF CLINICAL PRACTICE AND SCIENTIFIC THEORY

Recently much has been written about the influence of changing scientific theories on the management of patients with movement disorders. Several excellent articles discuss in detail the parallel development between scientific theory and clinical practice (Gordon, 1987; Horak, 1992).

While neuroscience researchers identify the scientific basis for movement and movement disorders, it is up to the clinician to develop the applications of this research. Thus, scientific theory provides a framework that allows the integration of practical ideas into a coherent philosophy for intervention. A theory is not right or wrong in an absolute sense but judged to be more or less useful in solving the problems presented by patients with movement dysfunction (Gordon, 1987; Horak, 1992).

Just as scientific assumptions about the important elements that control movement are changing, clinical practice related to management of the patient with a neurological deficit is changing. New assumptions regarding the nature and cause of movement are replacing old assumptions. Clinical practice evolves in parallel with scientific theory, as clinicians assimilate changes in scientific theory and apply them to practice. This concept is shown in Figure 1-12. Let's explore the evolution of clinical practice in light of changing theories of motor control in more detail.

Motor Control Models

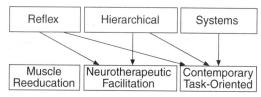

FIGURE 1-12.   The parallel development of theories of motor control and clinical practices designed to examine and treat patients with motor dyscontrol (Reprinted with permission from Horak F. Assumptions underlying motor control for neurologic rehabilitation. In: Contemporary management of motor control problems. Proceedings of the II Step Conference. Alexandria, Va: APTA, 1992:11)

Neurological Rehabilitation: Reflex-Based Neurofacilitation Approaches

In the late 1950s and early 1960s, the so-called neurofacilitation approaches were developed, and they resulted in a dramatic change in clinical interventions directed at the patient with neurological impairments (Gordon, 1987; Horak, 1992). For the most part, these approaches still dominate the way clinicians manage the patient with a neurological deficit.

Neurofacilitation approaches include the Bobath approach, developed by Karl and Berta Bobath (1965), the Rood approach, developed by Margaret Rood (Stockmeyer, 1967), Brunnstrom's approach, developed by Signe Brunnstrom (1966), proprioceptive neuromuscular facilitation (PNF), developed by Kabat and Knott and expanded by Voss (Voss et al., 1985), and sensory integration therapy, developed by Ayres (1972). These approaches were based largely on assumptions drawn from both the reflex and hierarchical theories of motor control.

Prior to the development of the neurofacilitation approaches, therapy for the patient with neurological dysfunction was largely directed at changing function at the level of the muscle itself. This has been referred to as the muscle reeducation approach to intervention (Gordon, 1987; Horak, 1992). While the muscle reeducation approach was effective in managing movement disorders resulting from polio, it was less useful for altering movement patterns in patients with upper motor neuron (UMN) lesions. Thus, the neurofacilitation techniques were developed in response to clinicians' dissatisfaction with previous modes of intervention and a desire to develop approaches that were more effective in solving the movement problems of the patient with neurological dysfunction (Gordon, 1987).

Clinicians working with patients with UMN lesions began to direct clinical efforts toward modifying the CNS itself. Neurofacilitation approaches focused on retraining motor control through techniques designed to facilitate and/or inhibit various movement patterns. Facilitation refers to intervention techniques that increase the patient's ability to move in ways that the clinician judges to be appropriate. Inhibitory techniques decrease the patient's use of movement patterns considered abnormal (Gordon, 1987).

Underlying Assumptions

Neurofacilitation approaches are largely associated with both the reflex and hierarchical theories of motor control. Thus, clinical practices are based on assumptions regarding the nature and cause of normal motor control, abnormal motor control, and the recovery of function.

This approach suggests that *normal movement* results from a chain of reflexes organized hierarchically within the CNS. Thus, control of movement is top down. Normal movement requires that the highest level of the CNS, the cortex, be in control of both intermediate (brainstem) and lower (spinal cord) levels of the CNS. This means that the process of normal development, sometimes called corticalization, is characterized by the emergence of behaviors organized at sequentially higher and higher levels in the CNS. A great emphasis is placed on the understanding that incoming sensory information stimulates and thus drives a normal movement pattern.

Explanations regarding the physiological basis for *abnormal motor control* from a reflex and hierarchical perspective largely suggest that a disruption of normal reflex mechanisms underlies abnormal movement control. It is assumed that lesions at the highest cortical levels of the CNS cause release of abnormal reflexes organized at lower levels within the CNS. The release of these lower level reflexes constrains the patient's ability to move normally.

Another prevalent assumption is that abnormal or atypical patterns of movement seen in the patient with motor cortex lesions are the direct result of the lesion itself, as opposed to considering some behaviors as developing either secondary to or in response to the lesion (i.e., compensatory). Thus, it is predicted that in the child with motor cortex lesions the process of increasing corticalization is disrupted, and as a result, motor control is dominated by primitive patterns of movement organized at lower levels of the CNS. In addition, in the adult with acquired motor cortex lesions, damage to higher levels of the CNS probably results in a release of lower centers from higher-center control. Likewise, primitive and pathological behaviors organized at these levels reemerge to dominate, preventing normal patterns of movement.

A central assumption concerning the *recovery of function* in the patient with a motor cortex lesion is that recovery of normal motor control cannot occur unless higher centers of the CNS once again regain control over lower centers. According to this approach, recovery of function in a sense recapitulates development, with higher centers gradually regaining their dominance over lower centers of the CNS.

Two key assumptions are that (*a*) functional skills will automatically return once abnormal movement patterns are inhibited and normal movement patterns facilitated; and (*b*) repetition of these normal movement patterns will automatically transfer to functional tasks.

Clinical Applications

What are some of the clinical applications of these assumptions? First, examination of motor control should focus on identifying the presence or absence of normal and abnormal reflexes controlling movement. Also, intervention should be directed at modifying the reflexes that control movement. The importance of sensory input for stimulating normal motor output suggests an intervention focus of modifying the CNS through sensory stimulation (Gordon, 1987; Horak, 1992).

A hierarchical theory suggests that one goal of therapy is to regain independent control of movement by higher centers of the CNS. Thus, intervention is geared toward helping the patient regain normal patterns of movement as a way of facilitating functional recovery.

The neurofacilitation approaches still dominate the way clinicians examine and intervene with patients who have central nervous system pathology. However, just as scientific theory about the nature and cause of movement has changed in the past 30 years, so too, many of the neurofacilitation approaches have changed their approach to practice. Currently, within the neurofacilitation approaches, there is a greater emphasis on explicitly training function and less emphasis on inhibiting reflexes and retraining normal patterns of movement. In addition, there is more consideration of motor learning principles when developing intervention plans. The boundaries between approaches are less distinct as each approach integrates into its theoretical base new concepts related to motor control.

Task-Oriented Approach

One of the newer approaches to retraining is the task-oriented approach to clinical intervention, based on newer theories of motor control. In previous publications we have referred to this approach as a systems approach (Woollacott and Shumway-Cook, 1990). Others have called these new clinical methods a motor control, or motor learning, approach (Carr and Shepherd, 1985).

Underlying Assumptions

Assumptions underlying a task-oriented approach are quite different from those underlying the neurofacilitation techniques. In the task-oriented approach it is assumed that *normal movement* emerges as an interaction among many systems, each contributing its own aspects of control. In addition, movement is organized around a behavioral goal and is constrained by the environment. Thus, the role of sensation in normal movement is not limited to a stimulus–response reflex mode but is essential to predictive and adaptive control of movement as well.

Assumptions regarding *abnormal motor control* suggest that movement problems result from impairments within one or more of the systems controlling movement. Movements observed in the patient with a motor cortex lesion constitute behavior that emerges from the best mix of the systems remaining to participate. This means that what is observed is not the result of just the lesion itself but of the efforts of the remaining systems to compensate for the loss and still be functional. However, the compensatory strategies developed by patients are not always optimal. Thus, a goal in intervention may be to improve the efficiency of compensatory strategies used to perform functional tasks.

Clinical Applications

These assumptions suggest that for retraining movement control, it is essential to work on identifiable functional tasks rather than on movement patterns for movement's sake alone. A task-oriented approach to intervention assumes that patients learn by actively attempting to solve the problems inherent in a functional task rather than repetitively practicing normal patterns of movement. Adaptation to changes in the environmental context is a critical part of recovery of function. In this context, patients are helped to learn a variety of ways to solve the task goal rather than a single muscle activation pattern.

℮ SUMMARY

1. Motor control is the ability to regulate the mechanisms essential to movement. Thus, the field of motor control is directed at studying the nature of movement and how that movement is controlled.

2. The specific practices used to examine and treat the patient with motor dyscontrol are determined by underlying assumptions about how movement is controlled, which come from specific theories of motor control.

3. A theory of motor control is a group of abstract ideas about the control of movement. Theories provide the following: (a) a framework for interpreting behavior, (b) a guide for clinical action, (c) new ideas, and (d) working hypotheses for examination and intervention.

4. Rehabilitation practices reflect theories, or basic ideas, about the nature of function and dysfunction.

5. This chapter reviews many motor control theories that influence our perspective regarding examination and intervention, including the reflex theory, hierarchical theory, motor programming theories, systems theory, dynamical action theory, and ecological theory.

6. In this text we use a *systems* theory as the foundation for many clinical applications. According to systems theory, movement arises from the interaction of multiple processes, including (a) *perceptual*, *cognitive*, and *motor* processes within the individual and (b) interactions between the individual, the task, and the environment.

7. Clinical practices evolve in parallel with scientific theory as clinicians assimilate changes in scientific theory and apply them to practice. Neurofacilitation approaches to intervention were developed in parallel with the reflex and hierarchical theories of motor control. New approaches to intervention are being developed in response to changing theories of motor control.

CHAPTER 2

Motor Learning and Recovery of Function

⊚ INTRODUCTION TO MOTOR LEARNING

Phoebe J. has been receiving therapy for 5 weeks now since her stroke. She has gradually regained the ability to stand, walk, and feed herself. What is the cause of her recovery of motor function? How much is due to spontaneous recovery? How much of her recovery may be attributed to therapeutic interventions? How many of her reacquired motor skills will she be able to retain and use when she goes home from the rehabilitation facility? These questions and issues reflect the importance of motor learning to clinicians who retrain the patient with motor control problems.

What Is Motor Learning?

In Chapter 1, we defined the field of motor control as the study of the nature and cause of movement. We define the field of **motor learning** as the study of the acquisition and/or modification of movement. While motor control focuses on understanding the control of movement already acquired, motor learning focuses on understanding the acquisition and/or modification of movement.

The field of motor learning has traditionally referred to the study of the acquisition or modification of movement in normal subjects. In contrast, **recovery of function** has referred to the reacquisition of movement skills lost through injury.

While there is nothing inherent in the term motor learning to distinguish it from processes involved in the recovery of movement function, the two are often thought of as separate. This separation between recovery of function and motor learning may be misleading. Issues facing clinicians concerned with helping patients reacquire skills lost as the result of injury are similar to those faced by people in the field of motor learning. Questions common to both: How can I best structure practice (therapy) to ensure learning? How can I ensure that skills learned in one context transfer to others? Will simplifying a task, that is, making it easier to perform, result in more efficient learning?

In this chapter we use the term motor learning to encompass both the acquisition and reacquisition of movement. We begin our study of motor learning by discussing important issues related to the nature of motor learning. Next we explore various theories of motor learning, examining their underlying assumptions and clinical implications. We discuss the practical applications of motor learning research. Finally we discuss issues related to recovery of function, including the many factors that affect a patient's ability to recover from brain injury.

⊘ NATURE OF MOTOR LEARNING

Early Definitions of Motor Learning

Learning has been described as the process of acquiring knowledge about the world; motor learning has been described as a set of processes associated with practice or experience leading to relatively permanent changes in the capability for producing skilled action. This definition of motor learning reflects four concepts: (*a*) Learning is a process of acquiring the capability for skilled action. (*b*) Learning results from experience or practice. (*c*) Learning cannot be measured directly; instead it is inferred from behavior. (*d*) Learning produces relatively permanent changes in behavior; thus short-

term alterations are not thought of as learning (Schmidt, 1988b).

Broadening the Definition of Motor Learning

In this chapter the definition of motor learning has been expanded to encompass many aspects not traditionally considered part of motor learning.

Motor learning involves more than motor processes. Rather, it involves learning new strategies for sensing as well as moving. Thus, motor learning, like motor control, emerges from a complex of perception–cognition–action processes.

Previous views of motor learning have focused primarily on changes in the individual. But the process of motor learning can be described as the search for a task solution that emerges from an interaction of the individual with the task and the environment. Task solutions are new strategies for perceiving and acting (Newell, 1991).

Similarly, the recovery of function entails the reorganization of both perception and action systems in relation to specific tasks and environments. Thus, one cannot study motor learning or recovery of function outside of the context of the ways individuals are solving functional tasks in specific environments.

Relating Performance and Learning

Traditionally, the study of motor learning has focused solely on motor outcomes. Earlier views of motor learning did not always distinguish it from performance (Schmidt, 1992). Changes in performance that resulted from practice were usually thought to reflect changes in learning. However, this view failed to consider that certain practice effects improved performance initially but were not necessarily retained, a condition of learning. This led to the notion that learning could not be evaluated during practice but rather must be assessed during specific retention or transfer tests. Thus, **learning**, defined as a relatively permanent change, has been distinguished from **performance**, defined as a temporary change in motor behavior seen during practice sessions. For example, Phoebe J. shows an improved ability to stand symmetrically (with weight evenly distributed to both legs) at the end of her daily therapy session, but when she returns to therapy the following day, she again stands with all her weight on her unaffected leg. This suggests that while performance improves in response to therapy, learning has not yet occurred. When on subsequent days Phoebe J. begins to demonstrate a more symmetrical weight-bearing stance, we may infer that learning (a permanent change in behavior) is occurring.

Performance, however, is a complex matter. Performance, whether observed during practice sessions or during retention and transfer tasks, is the result of a complex interaction among many variables, only one of which is the level of learning. Some other variables that may affect performance include fatigue, anxiety, and motivation. Thus, performance is not solely a measure of absolute learning. This is because changes in performance can reflect not only changes in learning but changes in other variables as well.

Forms of Learning

The recovery of function following injury entails the reacquisition of complex tasks. However, it is difficult to understand the processes involved in learning using the study of complex tasks. Therefore, many researchers have begun by exploring simple forms of learning, with the understanding that these simple forms of learning are the basis for the acquisition of skilled behavior. However, there is very little information about how these simple forms of learning contribute to the acquisition of more complex skills.

We begin by reviewing these simple forms of learning and discussing some of their clinical applications. We then consider theories of motor learning that have been developed to describe the acquisition of skilled behavior and suggest how each might be used to explain the acquisition of a skill such as reaching for a glass of water. At the outset, we review simple nonassociative forms of learning, such as habituation and sensitization.

Nonassociative Forms of Learning

Nonassociative learning occurs when animals are given a single stimulus repeatedly. As a result, the nervous system learns about the characteristics of that stimulus. Habituation and sensitization are two very simple forms of nonassociative learning (Kupfermann, 1991b). **Habituation** is a decrease in responsiveness that occurs as a result of repeated exposure to a nonpainful stimulus.

Habituation is used in many ways in the clinical setting. For example, habituation exercises are used to treat dizziness in patients with certain types of vestibular dysfunction. Patients are asked to move repeatedly in ways that provoke their dizziness. This repetition results in habituation to the dizziness response. Habituation also forms the basis of therapy for children who are termed tactile defensive, that is, who show excessive responsiveness to cutaneous stimulation. Children are repeatedly exposed to gradually increasing levels of cutaneous inputs in an effort to decrease their sensitivity to this stimulus.

Sensitization is an increased responsiveness following a threatening or noxious stimulus (Kupfermann, 1991b). For example, if I receive a painful stimulus on the skin and then a light touch, I will react more strongly than normal to the light touch. After a person has habituated to one stimulus, another painful stimulus can dishabituate the first. That is, sensitization counteracts the effects of habituation.

There are times when increasing a patient's sensitivity to a threatening stimulus is important. For example, increasing a patient's awareness of stimuli indicating likelihood of impending falls may be an important aspect of balance retraining.

Not all nonassociative forms of learning are simple. Sensory learning, in which you form a sensory experience, is an example of nonassociative learning. It is learning that relates to understanding about a stimulus, in this case the sensory inputs. Helping patients to explore their perceptual space as it relates to learning a particular skill, such as reaching or transferring, is an example of nonassociative learning.

Associative Forms of Learning

What is *associative learning?* One possible answer is that it involves the association of ideas. For example, if you tell a patient who is having trouble walking to try to associate shifting their center of gravity with lifting their leg, you are helping them combine two aspects of a movement into one integrated whole. It is through associative learning that a person learns to predict relationships, either relationships of one stimulus to another (classical conditioning) or the relationship of one's behavior to a consequence (operant conditioning).

It has been suggested that associative learning has evolved to help animals learn to detect causal relationships in the environment. Establishing lawful and therefore predictive relationships among events is part of the process of making sense and order of our world. Recognizing key relationships between events is an essential part of the ability to adapt behavior to novel situations (Kupfermann, 1991b).

Patients who have an injury that has drastically altered their ability to sense and move in their world must reexplore their body in relation to their world to determine what new relationships exist between the two. Pavlov studied how humans and animals learn the association of two stimuli through the simple form of learning that is now called classical conditioning.

Classical Conditioning

Classical conditioning consists of learning to pair two stimuli. During classical conditioning an initially weak stimulus (the conditioned stimulus, or CS) becomes highly effective in producing a response when it becomes associated with another stronger stimulus (the unconditioned stimulus). The CS is usually something that initially produces no response, such as a bell. In contrast, the unconditioned stimulus (UCS), which may be food, always produces a re-

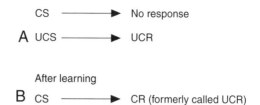

FIGURE 2-1. The process of classical conditioning, showing the relationship between the conditioned stimulus (CS), unconditioned stimulus (UCS), conditioned response (CR), and unconditioned response (UCR) before learning (**A**) and during the course of learning (**B**).

sponse. After repeated pairing of the conditioned and the unconditioned stimulus, one begins to see a conditioned response (CR) to the conditioned stimulus. Remember, it originally produced no response (Kupfermann, 1991b). This relationship is shown in Figure 2-1.

What the subject is doing in this type of learning is predicting an association between two stimuli or events that have occurred and responding accordingly. For example, in a therapy setting, if we repeatedly give patients a verbal cue in conjunction with physical assistance when making a movement, they may eventually begin to make the movement with only the verbal cue.

Thus, as patients gain skills we see them move along the continuum of assistance from hands-on assistance from the therapist to performing the task with verbal cues and eventually to performing the action unassisted.

It has recently been shown that we generally learn relationships that are relevant to our survival; it is more difficult to associate biologically meaningless events. These findings underscore an important learning principle: the brain is most likely to perceive and integrate aspects of the environment that are most pertinent. With regard to therapy, learning in patients is most likely to occur in tasks and environments that are relevant and meaningful to them.

Operant Conditioning

Operant, or instrumental, conditioning is a second type of associational learning (Kupfermann, 1991b). It is basically trial and error learning. During **operant conditioning** we learn to associate a certain response from among many that we have made with a consequence. The classic experiments in this area were done with animals that were given food rewards whenever they randomly pressed a lever inside their cages. They soon learned to associate the lever press with the presentation of food, and lever pressing became very frequent.

The principle of operant conditioning can be stated as follows: behaviors that are rewarded tend to be repeated at the cost of other behaviors. Likewise, behaviors followed by aversive stimuli are not usually repeated. This has been called the *law of effect* (Kupfermann, 1991b).

Operant conditioning plays a major role in determining the behaviors shown by patients referred for therapy. For example, the frail elderly person who leaves her home to go shopping and falls is less likely to repeat that activity. A decrease in activity results in declining physical functions, which in turn increases the likelihood she will fall. This increased likelihood for falls reinforces her desire to be inactive, and on it goes, showing the law of effect in action. Therapists may make use of a variety of interventions to assist this patient in regaining her activity level and reducing her likelihood of falling. One intervention may be the use of desensitization to decrease her anxiety and fear of falling, for example practicing walking outdoors in situations that have engendered fear in the past.

Operant conditioning can be an effective tool during clinical intervention. Verbal praise by a therapist for a job well done serves as a reinforcer for some—though not all—patients. Setting up a therapy session so that a particular movement is rewarded by the successful accomplishment of a task that the patient wants to do is a powerful example of operant conditioning. Using biofeedback to help a patient learn to control the foot during the swing portion of gait is also an example of operant conditioning.

Procedural and Declarative Learning

Some researchers have begun to classify associative learning based on the type of knowledge acquired by the learner. Using this type of classification, researchers have identified two types of learning based on the type and recall of information learned.

Procedural learning refers to learning tasks that can be performed without attention or conscious thought, like a habit. Procedural learning develops slowly through repetition of an act over many trials and is expressed through improved performance of the task. Procedural learning does not depend on awareness, attention, or other higher cognitive processes. During motor skill acquisition, repeating a movement continually under varying circumstances typically leads to procedural learning. That is, one automatically learns the movement itself, or the rules for moving, called a movement schema.

For example, when teaching a patient to transfer from chair to bed, we often have the patient practice an optimal movement strategy to move from one to the other. To prepare to transfer effectively in a wide variety of situations and contexts, patients learn to move from chairs of differing heights and at different positions relative to the bed. They thus begin to form the *rules associated with the task of transfer.* The development of rules for transferring allow them to transfer safely in unfamiliar circumstances. This constant practice and repetition result in efficient procedural learning and effective and safe transfers.

On the other hand, **declarative learning** results in knowledge that can be consciously recalled and thus requires processes such as awareness, attention, and reflection (Kupfermann, 1991b). Declarative learning can be expressed in declarative sentences: first I button the top button, then the next one. Constant repetition can transform declarative into procedural knowledge. For example, when patients are first relearning a skill, they may verbally describe each movement as they do it. However, with repetition, the movement becomes an automatic motor activity, that is, one that does not require conscious attention and monitoring.

The advantage of declarative learning is that it can be practiced in other ways than it was learned. For example, expert ski racers, when preparing to race down a slalom hill at 120 miles an hour, rehearse in their minds the race and how they will run it. Also, figure skaters preparing to perform often mentally practice the sequences to be skated prior to getting on the ice.

In therapy, when clinicians are helping patients reacquire skills lost through injury, the emphasis is often on practices leading to procedural learning rather than on declarative learning. Declarative learning requires the ability to express verbally the process to be performed and is often not possible for patients who have cognitive and language deficits that impair their ability to recall and express knowledge. Teaching movement skills declaratively does, however, allow patients to rehearse their movements mentally, increasing the amount of practice available to them when physical conditions such as fatigue otherwise limit it.

⊘ THEORIES OF MOTOR LEARNING

Just as there are theories of motor control, there are theories of motor learning, that is, a group of abstract ideas about the nature and cause of the acquisition or modification of movement. Theories of motor learning, like theories of motor control, must be based on knowledge regarding the structure and function of the nervous system. The following section reviews current theories of motor learning. Included in this section is a brief discussion of several theories related to recovery of function, the reacquisition of skills lost through injury.

Adams's Closed-Loop Theory

Adams (1971), a researcher in physical education, was the first person to attempt to create a comprehensive theory of motor learning. This theory generated a lot of interest during the 1970s as researchers attempted to determine its applicability to motor skill acquisition.

The most important aspect of Adams's theory was the concept of closed-loop processes in motor control. In a **closed-loop process**, sensory feedback is used for the ongoing production of skilled movement. The idea was that in motor learning, sensory feedback from the ongoing movement was compared within the nervous system with the stored memory of the intended movement (Ivry, 1997). This theory of motor learning stems from some of the principles used by Sherrington, who emphasized the importance of sensory inputs in controlling movement.

The closed-loop theory of motor learning also proposed that two distinct types of memory were important in this process. The first, called the **memory trace**, was used in the selection and initiation of the movement. The second, called the **perceptual trace**, was built up over a period of practice and became the internal reference of correctness. He proposed that after movement is initiated by the memory trace, the perceptual trace takes over to carry out the movement and detect error.

Clinical Implications

What are the clinical implications of the closed-loop theory of motor learning? It suggests that when patients, for example Phoebe J., are learning a new movement skill, such as learning to pick up a glass, with practice they gradually develop a perceptual trace for the movement that serves as a guide for later movements. The more the patient practices the specific movement, the stronger the perceptual trace becomes. In fact, the accuracy of the movement is directly proportional to the strength of the perceptual trace. Thus the closed-loop theory suggests that for retraining motor skills, it is essential to have the patient practice the same exact movement repeatedly to one accurate end point; the more time spent in practicing the movement as accurately as possible, the better the learning.

Limitations

The closed-loop theory of motor learning has been criticized for several reasons. It has been shown that animals and humans can make movements even when they have no sensory feedback (Taub and Berman, 1968; Rothwell et al., 1982; Fentress, 1973). In addition, animals are capable of certain types of learning even after somatosensory deafferentation. As we mentioned in Chapter 1, on theories of motor control, humans can also accurately perform movements that they have never performed before (for example, playing a Bach concerto on the cello, when the person had previously learned and performed it only on the violin). Thus, the closed-loop theory could not explain either the accurate performance of novel movements or of open-loop movements made in the absence of sensory feedback.

It has also been suggested that memory storage processes within the brain would make it impossible to store a separate perceptual trace for every movement ever performed (Schmidt, 1975). Finally, more recent research suggests that variation in movement practice may actually improve motor performance of the task more than practicing moving to a single end point.

Schmidt's Schema Theory

In the 1970s, in response to many of the limitations of the closed-loop theory of motor learning, Richard Schmidt, another researcher from the field of physical education, proposed a new motor learning theory, which he called the schema theory. It emphasized open-loop control processes and the generalized motor program concept (Schmidt, 1975). Though the concept of motor programs was considered essential to understanding motor control, no one had yet addressed how motor programs can be learned. Like other researchers before him, Schmidt proposed that motor programs do not contain the specifics of movements but instead contain general rules for a specific class of movements. He predicted that when learning a new motor program, the individual learns a general set of rules that can be applied to a variety of contexts.

At the heart of this motor learning theory is the concept of **schema**, which has been im-

portant in psychology for many years. The term schema originally referred to an abstract representation stored in memory following multiple presentations of a class of objects. For example, it is proposed that after seeing many types of dogs, we begin to store an abstract set of rules for general *dog* qualities in our brain, so that whenever we see a new dog, no matter what size, color, or shape, we can identify it as a dog. The schema theory of motor learning is equivalent to the motor programming theory of motor control. At the heart of both theories is the **generalized motor program**, which is considered to contain the rules for creating the spatial and temporal patterns of muscle activity needed to carry out a given movement.

Schmidt proposed that after an individual makes a movement, four things are stored in memory: (*a*) the initial movement conditions, such as the position of the body and the weight of the object manipulated; (*b*) the parameters used in the generalized motor program; (*c*) the outcome of the movement in terms of knowledge of results (KR); and (*d*) the sensory consequences of the movement, that is, how it felt, looked, and sounded. This information is abstracted and stored in the form of a recall schema (motor) and a recognition schema (sensory), components of the motor response schema. This is shown in Figure 2-2.

The recall schema is used to select a specific response. When a person makes a given movement, the initial conditions and desired goal of the movement are inputs to the recall schema. Other parts of the schema are the abstract memory of previous response specifications in similar tasks.

The recognition schema is used to evaluate the response. In this case the sensory consequences and outcomes of previous similar movements are coupled with the current initial conditions to create a representation of the expected sensory consequences. This is compared to the sensory information from the ongoing movement to evaluate the efficiency of the response. In Figure 2-2 expected sensory consequences are represented by the boxes EXP PFB (expected

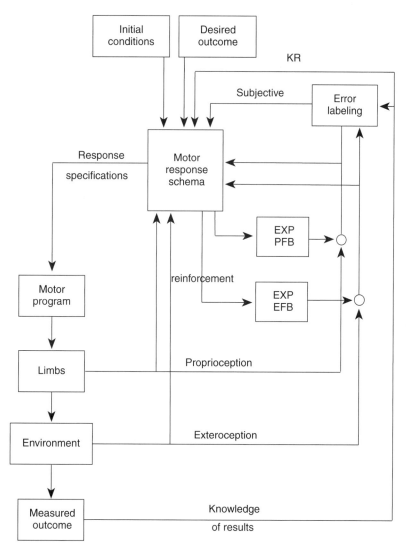

FIGURE 2-2.   Schmidt's schema theory, illustrating the critical elements in the acquisition of movement. EXP PFB, expected proprioceptive feedback; EXP EFB, expected exteroceptive feedback. (Adapted with permission from Schmidt RA. A schema theory of discrete motor skill learning. Psychol Rev 1975;82:225–260.)

proprioceptive feedback) and EXP EFB (expected exteroceptive feedback).

When the movement is over, the error signal is fed back into the schema and the schema is modified as a result of the sensory feedback and KR. Thus, according to this theory, learning consists of the ongoing process of updating the recognition and recall schemas with each movement that is made.

One of the predictions of schema theory is that variability of practice should improve motor learning. Schmidt hypothesized that

learning was not only affected by extent of practice but by the variability of practice. Thus, with increased variability of practice, the generalized motor program rules were made stronger.

Clinical Implications

What are some of the clinical implications of schema theory? According to schema theory, when our patient Phoebe J. is learning a new task such as reaching for a glass of milk with her affected limb, optimal learning occurs if this task is practiced under many conditions. This allows her to develop a set of rules for reaching, which can be applied when reaching for a variety of glasses and cups. As rules for reaching improve, Phoebe J. will become more capable of generating appropriate reaching strategies for picking up an unfamiliar glass, with less likelihood of dropping the glass or spilling the milk.

Limitations

Is schema theory supported by research? Yes and no. As mentioned earlier, one of the predictions of schema theory is that when a person practices a skill, variable forms of practice produce the most effective schema or motor program. Research to test this prediction has used the following paradigms. Two groups of subjects are trained in a new task, one given constant practice conditions and the other given variable practice conditions. Both groups are tested on a new but similar movement. According to schema theory, the second group should show higher level performance than the first, because they have developed a broad set of rules about the task that should allow them to apply the rules to a new situation. On the other hand, the first group should have developed a very narrow schema with limited rules that would not be easily applicable to new situations.

In studies on normal adults, the support is mixed. Many studies show large effects of variable practice, while some studies show very small effects or no effect at all. However, with regard to studies in children, there has been strong support. For example, 7- and 9-year-old children were trained to toss beanbags over a variable distance or a fixed distance. When asked to throw at a new distance, the variable-practice group produced significantly better scores than the fixed-practice group (Kerr and Booth, 1977). Why might there be differences between children and adults in these experiments? It has been suggested that it may be difficult to find experimental tasks at which adults do not already have significant variable practice during normal activities, while

children, with much less experience, are more naive subjects (Shapiro and Schmidt, 1982). Therefore, the experiments may be more valid in children.

Another limitation of the theory is that it lacks specificity. Because of its generality, few recognizable mechanisms can be tested. Thus, it is not clear how schema processing itself interacts with other systems during motor learning and how it aids in the control of that movement.

Another challenge to the schema theory is its inability to account for the immediate acquisition of new types of coordination. For example, researchers have shown that if all of a centipede's limbs except for two pairs are removed, the centipede will immediately produce a quadrupedal gait (Kugler et al., 1980). It has been argued that findings such as these cannot be accounted for by schema theory (Newell, 1991).

Ecological Theory

Karl Newell drew heavily from both systems and ecological motor control theories to create a theory of motor learning based on the concept of search strategies (Newell, 1991). In the learning theories proposed by Adams and Schmidt, practice produced a cumulative continuous change in behavior due to a gradual buildup of the strength of motor programs. It was proposed that with practice a more appropriate representation of action is developed.

In contrast, Newell suggests that motor learning is a process that increases the coordination between perception and action in a way consistent with the task and environmental constraints. What does he mean by this? He proposes that during practice there is a search for optimal strategies to solve the task, given the task constraints. Part of the search for optimal strategies entails not just finding the appropriate motor response for the task but finding the most appropriate perceptual cues as well. Thus, both perception and action systems are incorporated or mapped into an optimal task solution.

Critical to the search for optimal strategies is the exploration of the *perceptual-motor workspace.* Exploring the perceptual workspace requires exploring all possible perceptual cues to identify those that are most relevant to the performance of a specific task. Perceptual cues that are critical to the way in which a task is executed are also called *regulatory* cues (Gentile, 1992). Likewise, exploring the motor workspace involves exploring the range of movements possible to select the optimal or most efficient movements for the task. Optimal solutions incorporate the relevant perceptual cues and optimal movement strategies for a specific task. Newell believes that one useful outcome of his theory will be the impetus to identify critical perceptual variables essential to optimal task-relevant solutions. These critical variables will be useful in designing search strategies that produce efficient mapping of perceptual information and movement parameters.

According to the ecological theory, perceptual information has a number of roles in motor learning. In a prescriptive role, perceptual information relates to understanding the goal of the task and the movements to be learned. This information has typically been given to learners through demonstrations.

Another role of perceptual information is as feedback, both during the movement (concurrent feedback, sometimes called knowledge of performance) and on completion of the movement (knowledge of results). Finally, it is proposed that perceptual information can be used to structure the search for a perceptual-motor solution that is appropriate for the demands of the task. Thus, in this approach, motor learning is characterized by optimal task-relevant mapping of perception and action, not by a rule-based representation of action.

Newell discusses ways to augment skill learning. The first is to help the learner understand the nature of the perceptual motor workspace. The second is to understand the natural search strategies used by performers in exploring space. The third is to provide augmented information to facilitate the search. One central prediction of this theory is that the transfer of motor skills will depend on the similarity between the two tasks of the

optimal perceptual-motor strategies and relatively independent of the muscles used or the objects manipulated in the task.

In summary, this new approach to motor learning emphasizes dynamic exploratory activity of the perceptual-motor workspace to create optimal strategies for performing a task.

Clinical Implications

What are the clinical implications of the ecological theory of motor learning? As in the schema theory, when our patient Phoebe J. is relearning a movement with her affected arm, such as reaching for a glass, repeated practice with reaching for a variety of glasses that contain a variety of substances results in learning to match the appropriate movement dynamics for the task of reaching. But in addition, the ecological theory suggests the patient learns to distinguish the relevant perceptual cues important to organizing action. Relevant perceptual cues for reaching for and lifting a glass of milk include the size of the glass, how slippery the surface is, and how full it is. Thus to relearn to reach, Phoebe J. must not only develop effective motor strategies, she must learn to recognize relevant perceptual cues and match them to optimal motor strategies. If a perceptual cue suggests a heavy glass, she must grasp with more force. If the glass is full, the speed and trajectory of the movement must be modified to avoid spillage. If Phoebe J. is unable to recognize these essential sensory cues, a motor strategy that is less than optimal will be generated. That is, she may spill the fluid, or the glass may slip.

Perceptual cues such as the color of the glass are nonregulatory; that is, they are not essential to the development of optimal movement strategies for grasping. Thus during recovery of motor skills, an important part of motor learning is learning to discriminate relevant from irrelevant perceptual cues. Knowledge of the critical perceptual cues associated with a task is essential in dealing with a new variation of the task. When faced with a novel variation of the task, the patient must actively explore the perceptual cues to find the information necessary to solve the task problem optimally.

Limitations

Though this theory takes into account more of the variables that must be considered in motor learning (dealing with interactions between the individual, the task, and the environment), it is still new. One of its major limitations is that it has yet to be applied to specific examples of motor skill acquisition in any systematic way.

℮ THEORIES RELATED TO STAGES OF LEARNING MOTOR SKILLS

Another set of theories looks at motor learning from a temporal perspective. These theories begin by describing initial stages of skill acquisition and describe how learning occurs over time.

Fitts and Posner Three-Stage Model

Fitts and Posner (1967), two researchers in psychology, described a theory of motor learning related to the stages involved in learning a new skill. They suggest there are three main phases involved in skill learning. In the first stage the learner is concerned with understanding the nature of the task, developing strategies that can be used to carry out the task, and determining how the task should be evaluated. These efforts require a high degree of cognitive activity, such as attention. Accordingly, this stage is called the cognitive stage of learning.

In this stage the person experiments with a variety of strategies, abandoning those that do not work and keeping those that do. Performance tends to be quite variable, perhaps because many strategies for performing the task are being sampled. However, improvements in performance are also quite large in this first stage, perhaps as a result of selecting the most effective strategy for the task.

Fitts and Posner describe the second stage of skill acquisition as the associative stage. By

this time the person has selected the best strategy for the task and now begins to refine the skill. Thus, during this stage there is less variability in performance, and improvement also occurs more slowly. It is proposed that verbal-cognitive aspects of learning are less important at this stage because the person focuses more on refining a particular pattern than on selecting among alternative strategies (Schmidt, 1988b). This stage may last days to weeks or months, depending on the performer and the intensity of practice.

The third stage of skill acquisition has been described as the autonomous stage. Fitts and Posner define this stage by the automaticity of the skill and the low degree of attention required for its performance, as shown in Figure 2-3. Thus, in this stage the person can begin to devote his or her attention to other aspects of the skill in general, like scanning the environment for obstacles that might impede performance, or focusing on a secondary task (like talking to a friend while performing the task), or saving his or her energy so as to avoid fatigue.

Clinical Implications

How can the three-stage model help us to understand the acquisition of motor skills in patients? This theory suggests that Phoebe J. would learn to reach for a glass in the following way. When first learning to reach for the glass, the task would require a great deal of attention and conscious thought. Phoebe J. would initially make a lot of errors and spill a

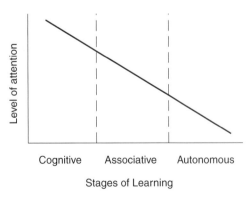

FIGURE 2-3. The changing attentional demands associated with the three stages of motor skill acquisition outlined by Fitts and Posner.

lot of water while she experimented with different movement strategies to accomplish the task. When moving into the second stage, however, her movements toward the glass would become refined as she developed an optimal strategy. At this point the task would not require her full attention. In the third, autonomous, stage, Phoebe J. would be able to reach for the glass while carrying on a conversation or being engaged in other tasks.

Systems Three-Stage Model

Another theory related to stages of motor learning comes from the motor control and development literature (Southard and Higgins, 1987; Newell and van Emmerik, 1989; Fentress, 1973). We have called this theory the systems three-stage theory because, like Bernstein's systems theory of motor control, the emphasis is on controlling degrees of freedom as a central component of learning a new movement skill. This theory suggests that when a novice or an infant is first learning a new skill, the degrees of freedom of the body are constrained as they perform the task to make the task easier to perform. For example, a person learning to use a hammer may contract both agonist and antagonist muscles at the wrist to stiffen it and primarily control hammer movement at the elbow. The learner can reasonably accurately perform the task at this stage, but the movement is not energetically efficient and the performer cannot flexibly deal with environmental changes. As the task is gradually mastered, the learner begins to release the degrees of freedom at the wrist and learns to coordinate the movements at the two joints, which allows for more movement efficiency, freedom, and thus, skill.

This tendency to freeze degrees of freedom during the early stages of learning a task can be seen during the development of balance control. A newly standing infant may freeze the degrees of freedom of the legs and trunk and sway only about the ankle joints in response to threats to balance. Gradually, with experience and practice, infants increase the degrees of freedom used as they learn to control sway at the hip as well (Woollacott et al., 1998).

Vereijken et al. (1992) used this approach to develop a model of the stages of motor learning. They suggest that the first stage of motor learning is the novice stage, in which the learner simplifies the movement to reduce the degrees of freedom. They suggest that this is accomplished by constraining or coupling multiple joints together so they move in unison and by fixing the angles of many of the joints involved in the movement. These constraints are made at the cost of efficiency and flexibility in response to changing task or environmental demands.

The second stage, called the advanced stage, is one in which the performer begins to release additional degrees of freedom by allowing movements at more joints involved in the task. Now the joints can be controlled independently as necessary for the task requirements. Simultaneous contraction of agonist and antagonist muscles at a joint are reduced, and muscle synergies across a number of joints are used to create a well-coordinated movement that is more adaptable to task and environmental demands.

The third stage, called the expert stage, is one in which the individual has released all the degrees of freedom necessary to perform the task in the most efficient and best-coordinated way. In addition, the individual has learned to take advantage of the mechanics of the musculoskeletal system and of the environment and to optimize the efficiency of the movement (Rose, 1997; Vereijken, et al., 1992).

Clinical Implications

The systems three-stage theory has a number of clinical implications. First, it suggests a possible explanation for the coactivation of muscles during the early stages of acquiring a motor skill and as an ongoing strategy for patients who are unable to learn to control a limb dynamically. One explanation is that coactivation stiffens a joint and therefore constrains the degrees of freedom. This strategy may in fact be a reasonable solution to the underlying problem, inability to control the degrees of freedom of a limb segment.

This theory offers a new rationale for using developmental stages in rehabilitation.

Traditionally, recapitulating developmental stages in the adult patient was based on a neuromaturational rationale. Alternatively, motor development could be viewed from a biomechanical perspective as gradual release of degrees of freedom. For example, the progression from all fours to upright kneeling to standing unsupported can be viewed as a gradual increase in the number of degrees of freedom that must be controlled. Thus, according to this theory, having a patient practice kneeling upright before learning to control stance may be justified from a mechanical rather than neural perspective.

Finally, this theory suggests the importance of providing external support during the early phases of learning a motor skill in patients with coordination problems. Providing external support constrains the degrees of freedom that the patient initially has to learn to control. As coordinative abilities improve, support can be systematically withdrawn as the patient learns to control more and more degrees of freedom.

Limitations

Very little research has been focused on the autonomous or expert stage of learning, partly because it would take months or years to bring many subjects to this skill level on a laboratory task. Thus, the principles that govern motor learning processes that lead to this last stage of mastery are largely unknown (Schmidt, 1988b).

Gentile's Two-Stage Model

In contrast to the three-stage theories previously discussed, Gentile (1992, 1987) proposed a two-stage theory of motor skill acquisition that describes the goal of the learner in each stage (Magi, 1998). In the first stage the goal of the learner is to develop an understanding of the task dynamics. At this stage learners are just getting the idea of the requirements of the movement (Gentile, 1992). This includes understanding the goal of the task, developing movement strategies appropriate to achieving the goal, and un-

derstanding the environmental features critical to the organization of the movement. An important feature of this stage of motor learning is learning to distinguish relevant, or regulatory, features of the environment from those that are nonregulatory.

In the second stage, called the fixation/diversification stage, the goal of the learner is to refine the movement. Refining movement includes both developing the capability of *adapting* the movement to changing task and environmental demands and performing the task *consistently* and *efficiently*. The terms fixation and diversification refer to the distinct requirements of open versus closed skills. As discussed in Chapter 1, closed skills have minimal environmental variation and thus require a consistent movement pattern with minimal variation. The concept is illustrated in Figure 2-4, which is a representation of the movement consistency that occurs with repeated practice under unchanging conditions. Movement variability decreases with practice. In contrast, open skills are characterized by changing environmental conditions and therefore require movement diversification. This concept of movement diversification is illustrated in Figure 2-4 (Higgins and Spaeth, 1979).

@ PRACTICAL APPLICATIONS OF MOTOR LEARNING RESEARCH

Therapists often ask themselves questions like these: What is the best way to structure my therapy sessions to optimize learning? How often should my patient practice a particular task? Is the type of feedback that I am giving to my patients concerning the quality of their movements really effective? Could I give a different form of feedback that might be better? Should I give feedback with every trial the patient makes, or would it be better to withhold feedback occasionally and make the patients try to discern by themselves whether their movement is accurate or efficient? What is the best timing for feedback?

In the following section we discuss research in motor learning that has attempted

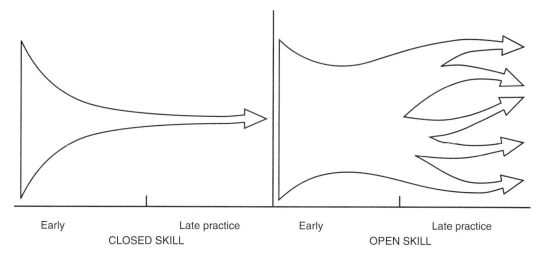

Early   Late practice   Early   Late practice
CLOSED SKILL   OPEN SKILL

FIGURE 2-4.   Movement patterns associated with open versus closed motor skills. Closed skills require refinement of a single or limited number of movement patterns (movement consistency); in contrast, open skills require a diversity of movement patterns (movement diversity). (Reprinted with permission from Higgens JR, Spaeth RA. Relationship between consistency of movement and environmental conditions. Quest 1979;17:65)

to answer these questions. We review the research in relation to specific motor learning factors, including feedback, practice conditions, and variability of practice, that are important to consider in retraining of patients with motor control problems.

Feedback

We have already discussed the importance of feedback in relation to motor learning. Clearly, some form of feedback is essential for learning to take place. In the following section we describe the types of feedback that are available to the performer and the contributions of these different types of feedback to motor learning.

The broadest definition of feedback includes all of the sensory information that is available as the result of a movement. This is typically called **response-produced feedback**. This feedback is usually further divided into two subclasses, intrinsic feedback and extrinsic feedback (Schmidt, 1988b; Shea et al., 1993).

Intrinisic Feedback

Intrinsic feedback is feedback that comes to the individual simply through the various

sensory systems as a result of the normal production of the movement. This includes such things as visual information concerning whether a movement was accurate and somatosensory information concerning the position of the limbs as one was moving (Schmidt, 1988b).

Extrinsic Feedback

Extrinsic feedback is information that supplements intrinsic feedback. For example, when you tell a patient that he or she needs to step higher to clear an object while walking, you are offering extrinsic feedback.

Extrinsic feedback can be given *concurrently* with the task and at the end of the task, in which case it is called *terminal feedback*. An example of concurrent feedback is *verbal* or manual guidance to the hand of a patient learning to reach for objects. An example of terminal feedback is telling a patient who has made a first unsuccessful attempt to rise from a chair that he or she should push harder the next time, using the arms to create more force to stand up.

Knowledge of Results

Knowledge of results (KR) is one important form of extrinsic feedback. It has been defined as terminal feedback about the outcome of the movement in terms of the movement's goal (Schmidt, 1988b; Shea et al., 1993). This is in contrast to knowledge of performance (KP), which is feedback relating to the movement pattern used to achieve the goal.

Research has been performed to determine which types of feedback are best. Almost all of this research addresses the efficacy of different types of knowledge of results. Typically, research has shown that KR is an important learning variable; that is, it is important for learning motor tasks (Bilodeau et al., 1959). However, for certain types of tasks intrinsic feedback, such as visual or kinesthetic feedback, is sufficient to provide most error information, and KR has only minimal effects. For example, in learning tracking tasks KR only minimally improves the performance and learning of a subject.

It has also been shown that KR is a performance variable; that is, it has temporary effects on the ability of the subject to perform a task. This may be due to motivational or alerting effects on the performer and to guidance effects (that is, it tells the subject how to perform the task better in the next trial).

When should KR be given for optimal results? Should it be given right after a movement? What delay is best before the next movement is made, to ensure maximum learning efficiency? Should KR be given after every movement? These are important questions for the therapist who wants to optimize the learning or relearning of motor skills in patients with motor disorders.

Experiments attempting to determine the optimum KR delay interval have found very little effect of KR delay on motor learning efficacy. The same is true of the post-KR delay interval. There may be a slight reduction in learning if the KR delay is very short, but any effects are very small. However, it has been shown that it is good not to fill the KR-delay interval with other movements, since these appear to interfere with the learning of the target movements. Research on the effects of filling the post-KR delay interval with extraneous activities is less clear. Apparently this interval is not as important as the KR-delay

interval for the integration of KR information. It has also been recommended that the *intertrial interval* should not be excessively short, but the literature in this area shows conflicting results (Salmoni et al., 1984) concerning the effects of different lengths of intertrial intervals on learning.

What happens to learning efficacy if KR is not given every trial? For example, if you ask a patient to practice a reaching movement and give the patient feedback on the accuracy of the movement only every 5 or 10 trials, what do you think might happen? One might assume that decreasing the amount of KR given would have a detrimental effect on learning. However, experiments in this area have shown surprising results.

In one study Winstein and Schmidt (1990) manipulated KR to produce what they called a fading schedule, giving more KR early in practice (50% frequency) and gradually reducing it later in practice. They compared the performance of this group to that of a group given 100% frequency feedback (feedback on every trial). No difference in performance was found during acquisition, but the 50% fading frequency condition gave better scores on a delayed retention test. Why would this be the case? They propose that on no-KR trials, the subject must use other cognitive processes, such as those related to error detection. In addition, giving feedback in 100% of trials produces dependency on the KR (Winstein and Schmidt, 1990; Shea et al., 1993).

In another set of studies Lavery (1962) compared the performance of (*a*) subjects who had KR feedback on every trial; (*b*) subjects who had *summary KR*, that is KR for each of the trials only at the end of an entire block of 20 trials; and (*c*) subjects who had both types of feedback. At the end of the acquisition trials, performance was best if KR was given after every trial (groups 1 and 3 were far better than group 2). However, when performance was compared for the groups on transfer tests, in which no KR was given at any time, the group that was originally the least accurate, the summary KR only group (group 2), was the most accurate (Lavery, 1962).

These results suggest that summary KR is the best feedback, but if this were so, group 3 should have been as good as group 2, and this was not the case. It has thus been concluded that immediate KR is detrimental to learning because it provides too much information and allows the subject to rely on the information too strongly (Schmidt, 1988b).

What is the best number of trials to complete before giving KR? This appears to vary with the task. For very simple movement timing tasks, in which KR was given after 1 trial, 5 trials, 10 trials, or 15 trials, the performance on acquisition trials was best for the most frequent feedback, but when a transfer test was given, the performance was best for the 15-trial summary group. In a more complex task, in which a pattern of moving lights had to be intercepted by an arm movement (like intercepting a ball with a bat), the most effective summary length for learning was five trials, and anything more or less was less efficient (Schmidt, 1988b).

How precise must KR be to be most effective? The answer varies between adults and children. For adults, quantitative KR appears to be best, with the more precise KR giving more accurate performance up to a point beyond which there is no further improvement. For adults, units of measure (for example, inches, centimeters, feet, and miles) do not seem to be important, with nonsense units even being effective. However, in children, unfamiliar units or very precise KR can be confusing and degrade learning (Schmidt, 1988b; Newell and Kennedy, 1978).

Practice Conditions

We have discussed the importance of KR to learning. A second important variable is practice. Typically, the more practice you can give a patient, the more the patient learns, other things being equal. Thus, in creating a therapy session, it is desirable to maximize the number of practice attempts. But what about fatigue? How should the therapist schedule practice periods versus rest periods? Research on these questions is summarized in the following sections.

Massed Versus Distributed Practice

To answer these questions researchers have performed experiments comparing two types of practice sessions: massed and distributed. **Massed practice** is defined as a session in which the amount of practice time in a trial is greater than the amount of rest between trials. This may lead to fatigue in some tasks. **Distributed practice** is defined as a session in which the amount of rest between trials equals or is greater than the amount of time for a trial. For continuous tasks, massed practice has been proved to decrease performance markedly while it is present but to affect learning only slightly when learning is measured on a transfer task in distributed conditions. In this case fatigue may mask the original learning effects during massed practice, but they become apparent on the transfer tasks. For discrete tasks, the research results are not as clear; they appear to depend considerably on the task (Schmidt, 1988b).

Keep in mind that in the therapy setting the risk of injury due to fatigue increases during massed practice for tasks that may be somewhat dangerous for the patient, such as tasks that may lead to a fall. In this case, it is best not to overfatigue the patient and risk injury.

Constant Versus Variable Practice

The ability to generalize learning to novel situations is important in motor learning. In general, research has shown that variable practice increases this ability to adapt and generalize learning. For example, in one experiment one group of subjects practiced a timing task (they had to press a button when a moving pattern of lights arrived at a particular point) at variable speeds of 5, 7, 9, and 11 miles per hour, while a second group (constant practice) practiced at only one of those speeds. Then all subjects performed a transfer test, in which they performed at a novel light speed outside their previous range of experience. The absolute errors were smaller for the variable than for the constant practice group (Catalano and Kleiner, 1984). Thus, in this example, variable practice allowed a person to perform significantly better on novel variations of the task. Variable practice may be most important for tasks that are likely to be performed in variable conditions. Tasks that require minimal variation and will be performed in constant conditions may best be practiced in constant conditions (Rose, 1997).

Random Versus Blocked Practice: Contextual Interference

Surprisingly, factors that initially make performing a task more difficult often make learning more effective in the long run. These types of factors have been called *context effects*. For example, suppose you ask a person to practice five tasks in random order, versus blocking the trials—that is, practicing one task for a block of trials then moving on to the next task. You might presume that it would be easier to learn each task in a blocked design. However, this is not the case. While performance is better during the acquisition phase, during testing on a transfer task, performance is actually better in the randomly ordered conditions. Thus contextual interference occurs when multiple skills are practiced within a single session.

Is it always the case that random practice is better than blocked practice? It appears to depend on a number of factors related to both the task and the learner (Magill and Hall, 1990). Random practice appears to be most effective when used with skills that use different patterns of coordination and thus different underlying motor programs (Magill and Hall, 1990). In addition, characteristics of the individual, such as level of experience and intellectual abilities, may also influence the effectiveness of random practice (Rose, 1997). Random practice may be inappropriate until learners understand the dynamics of the task (Del Rey et al., 1983; Goode, 1986). In addition, research by Edward et al. (1986) on motor learning in adolescents with Down's syndrome suggests that random practice was not superior to blocked practice in this group of learners. The application of this concept can be found in Lab Activity 2-1.

What are the clinical implications of research on contextual interference? Tradi-

LAB ACTIVITY 2-1

OBJECTIVE: To understand the clinical applications of contextual interference.

PROCEDURE: Your patient is Zach C, an 18-year-old with a recent closed head injury. He requires moderate assistance of one person to stand and walk because of ataxia, and he is dependent in most of his activities of daily living because he has dysmetria and dyscoordination. Today's therapy session is focusing on transfers (bed to wheelchair and wheelchair to toilet) and bed mobility skills (rolling supine to prone, supine to sitting on edge of bed, and sitting to standing).

ASSIGNMENT: Plan a therapy session showing how your strategies would vary if you were considering context effects on recovery of function. First outline a therapy session to teach these skills on a random practice schedule. How would your therapy session differ if you were using a blocked practice schedule? What will the effects of each approach to practice have on initial acquisition of skills, what effect on long-term retention and transfer to novel conditions? You can repeat this lab to explore how the structure of a therapy session would vary if you were using constant versus variable practice, guided versus discovery learning, knowledge of results versus knowledge of performance.

tional methods for retraining motor skills by having a patient practice one skill repeatedly may initially result in the speedy acquisition of a skill, but long-term learning and the ability to transfer skills to novel conditions is limited. In contrast, encouraging the patient to practice a number of tasks in random order may slow down the initial acquisition of skills but is better for long-term retention (Schmidt, 1988b).

Whole Versus Part Training

One approach to retraining function is to break the task down into interim steps, helping the patient to master each step prior to learning the entire task. This *task analysis* is defined as the process of identifying the components of a skill or movement and then ordering them into a sequence. How are the components of a task defined? They are defined in relation to the goals of the task. So, for example, a task analysis approach to retraining mobility would be to break down the locomotor pattern into naturally occurring components such as step initiation, stability during stance, or push-off to achieve progression. During mobility retraining, the patient would practice each of these components in isolation before combining them into the whole gait pattern. But each of these components must be practiced within the overall context of gait. For example, having a patient practice hip extension while prone will not necessarily increase the patient's ability to achieve stance stability, even though both require hip extension. Part-task training can be an effective way to retrain some tasks if the task itself can be naturally divided into units that reflect the inherent goals of the task (Winstein, 1991; Schmidt, 1991).

Transfer

A critical issue in rehabilitation is how training transfers either to a new task or to a new environment. For example, will learning a task in a clinical environment transfer to the home? Does practice in standing balance transfer to a dynamic balance task such as walking around the house? What determines how well a task learned in one condition will transfer to another? Researchers have determined that the amount of transfer depends on the similarity between the two tasks or the two environments (Schmidt and Young, 1987; Lee, 1988). A critical aspect in both appears to be whether the neural processing demands in the two situations are similar. For example, training a patient to maintain standing balance in a well-controlled environment, such as on a firm, flat surface, in a well-lit clinic, will not necessarily enable the patient to balance in a home that contains thick carpets, uneven surfaces, and visual distractions. The more closely the demands in the practice environment resemble those in the actual environment, the better the transfer (Winstein, 1991; Schmidt, 1991).

Mental Practice

Mentally practicing a skill (the act of performing the skill in one's imagination, without any action involved) can produce large positive effects on the performance of the task. For example, Rawlings et al. (1972) taught subjects a rotary pursuit task. On the first day, all subjects practiced 25 trials. On days 2 to 9, one group of subjects continued with physical practice, while a second group performed only mental practice and a third group was given no practice. On day 10, all subjects were retested, and the mental practice group had improved almost as much as the physical practice group, while the no-practice group showed little improvement.

Why is this the case? One hypothesis is that the neural circuits underlying the motor programs for the movements are actually triggered during mental practice, and the subject either does not activate the final muscle response at all or activates responses at very low levels that do not produce movement. In Chapter 3 we discuss experiments showing that one part of the brain, the supplementary motor cortex, is activated during mental practice.

Guidance Versus Discovery Learning

One technique often used in therapy is guidance; that is, the learner is physically guided through the task to be learned. Research has again explored the efficiency of this form of learning versus other forms of learning that involve trial and error discovery procedures. In one set of experiments (Schmidt, 1988b), various forms of physical guidance were used in teaching a complex elbow movement task. When performance was measured on a no-guidance transfer test, physical guidance was no more effective than simply practicing the task under unguided conditions. In other experiments (Singer, 1980), practice under unguided conditions was found less effective for acquisition of the skill but was more effective for later retention and transfer. This is similar to the results just cited, which showed that those conditions that made the performance acquisition more difficult enhanced performance in transfer tests.

This does not mean that we should never use guidance in teaching skills, but it implies that if guidance is used, it should be used only at the outset of teaching a task, to acquaint the performer with the characteristics of the task to be learned.

☺ RECOVERY OF FUNCTION

Motor learning is the study of the acquisition or modification of movement in normal subjects. In contrast, **recovery of function** has referred to the reacquisition of movement skills lost through injury. Understanding the effect of brain injury on motor control requires a good understanding of issues related to recovery of function.

Concepts Related to Recovery of Function

To understand concepts related to recovery of function it is necessary first to define function and recovery.

Function

Function is defined here as the complex activity of the whole organism that is directed at performing a behavioral task (Craik, 1992). Optimal function is characterized by behaviors that are efficient in accomplishing a task goal in a relevant environment.

Recovery

Recovery has a number of meanings pertaining to regaining function that has been lost following an injury. A stringent definition of recovery requires achieving the functional goal in the same way it was performed before the injury, that is, using the same processes as prior to the injury (Almli and Finger, 1988). Less stringent definitions define recovery as the ability to achieve task goals using effective and efficient means but not necessarily those used before the injury (Slavin et al., 1988).

Recovery Versus Compensation

Is recovery the same as or different from compensation? **Compensation** is defined as behavioral substitution; that is, alternative behavioral strategies are adopted to complete a task. **Recovery** is achieving function through original processes, while compensation is achieving function through alternative processes. Thus function returns but not in its identical premorbid form.

A question of concern to many therapists is whether therapy should be directed at recovery of function or compensation. The response to this question has changed over the years as our knowledge about the plasticity and malleability of the adult central nervous system (CNS) changed (Gordon, 1987). For many years, the adult mammalian CNS was characterized as both rigid and unalterable. Function was believed to be localized to various parts of the CNS upon maturation. Research at the time suggested that regeneration and reorganization were not possible within the adult CNS. This view of the CNS naturally led to therapy directed at compensation, since recovery in the strict sense of the word was not possible. More recent research in the field of neuroscience has begun to show that the adult CNS has great plasticity and capacity for reorganization. Studies on neural mechanisms underlying recovery of function are covered in Chapter 4.

Sparing of Function

When a function is not lost despite a brain injury, it is called a **spared function** (Craik, 1992). For example, when language develops normally in children who had brain damage early in life, retained language function is said to be spared.

Stages of Recovery

Several authors have described stages of recovery from neural injury. Stages of recovery are based on the assumption that the process can be broken down into discrete stages. Classically, it is divided into spontaneous recovery and forced recovery. **Forced recovery** is obtained through specific interventions designed to affect neural mechanisms (Bach-y-Rita and Balliet, 1987).

The presumption is that different neural mechanisms underlie these relatively discrete stages of recovery. Chapter 4 describes how research on neural mechanisms may contribute new methods to improving and speeding the various stages of recovery.

Factors Contributing to Recovery of Function

A number of factors can affect the outcome of damage to the nervous system and the extent of subsequent recovery (Held, 1987; Stein et al., 1995).

Effect of Age

How does age affect recovery? Does outcome vary if brain damage occurs early versus later in life? The age of the individual at the time of the lesion affects recovery of function in a complex manner (Held, 1987; Stein et al., 1995). Early views of age-related effects on recovery of brain function proposed that injury during infancy caused fewer deficits than damage in the adult years. For example, in the 1940s, Kennard (1940, 1942) performed experiments in which she removed the motor cortex of infant and adult monkeys and found that infants were able to feed, climb, walk, and grasp objects, while adults were not. In humans, this effect has been noted in language function: damage to the dominant hemisphere shows little or no effect on speech in infants but causes varying degrees of aphasia in adults.

However, as we understand more about the functions of brain areas, researchers are concluding that not all areas show the same capacity for regeneration. Injury to some areas of the brain shows similar deficits whether it occurs in the infant or adult; damage to other areas show little effect in infancy, but problems develop later in life (Held, 1987; Stein et al., 1995).

Why is this? It has been hypothesized that if an area is mature, injury will cause similar damage in infants and adults. But if another area that is functionally related is not yet mature, it may assume the function of the injured area. In addition, if an immature area is damaged and no other area assumes its function, no problems may be seen in in-

fancy, but in later years, deficits may become apparent.

In addition, when children have brain injuries in the speech areas, there is probably loss of other functions to spare the function of speech. Researchers have found that the IQs of children with spared speech following early brain injury were consistently lower than those of children who had a brain injury when they were older (Woods, 1980). This implies that when a function is spared, a crowding effect may occur at the cost of compromising another behavior (Craik, 1992). In summary, the data on age-related effects on brain injury suggest that "the brain reacts differently to injury at different stages of development" (Stein et al., 1995, p. 77).

Characteristics of the Lesion

In addition to age, characteristics of the lesion affect the extent of recovery (Held, 1987). For example, a small lesion has a greater chance of recovery as long as no functional area has been entirely removed. In addition, slowly developing lesions appear to cause less functional loss than lesions that happen quickly. For example, autopsy has revealed a large lesion in the brain tissue of a person who functioned well until near death.

This phenomenon has been explored experimentally by making serial lesions in animals and allowing the animal to recover between lesions (Craik, 1992). If a single large lesion is made in the motor cortex (Brodmann's areas 4 and 6), animals become immobile; in contrast, function is spared if a similar lesion is produced serially over time. If serial lesions are made, the animal recovers the ability to walk, feed, and right itself with no difficulty (Travis and Woolsey, 1956). Other factors, such as the age of the animal, also influence the effect of serial lesions. In younger animals function is spared even when serial lesions are performed close together. In contrast, older animals may not show any sparing of function regardless of how much time has elapsed between lesions (Stein et al., 1995).

Effect of Experience

Other important factors affecting recovery of function are training and environmental conditions both before and after brain injury (Stein et al., 1995, Held, 1998). Studies in which rats were raised in enriched environments show many resultant changes in the brain morphology and biochemistry, including increased brain weight, dendritic branching, and enzyme activity. As a result of these findings, researchers wondered if this enrichment would improve responses to brain injury. Experiments showed that preinjury environmental enrichment protects animals against certain deficits after brain lesions. For example, two sets of rats, one group with preoperative enrichment and a control group, received lesions of the cortex. After surgery, the enriched animals made fewer mistakes during maze learning and in fact performed better than control animals without brain damage (Held, 1998).

In a second study by Held et al. (1985) the effect of preoperative and postoperative enrichment was compared for a locomotor task following removal of sensorimotor cortex. They found that preoperatively enriched rats were no different from enriched sham-lesioned controls on both behavioral and fine-grained movement analyses. The group that was only postoperatively enriched was mildly impaired in locomotor skills but recovered more quickly than the lesioned controls, though they never regained full locomotor function. Thus, postoperative enrichment is effective but does not allow the same extent of recovery as preoperative enrichment.

Held suggests that enriched subjects may have developed functional neural circuitry that is more varied than that of restricted subjects, and this may provide them with a greater ability to reorganize the nervous system after a lesion or simply to use alternative pathways to perform a task.

It appears that if environmental stimulation is to affect recovery of function, it must incorporate active participation of the patient for full recovery to occur (Stein et al., 1995). When rats with unilateral lesion of the visual cortex were exposed to visual shapes, only rats that were allowed to move freely in the environment and interact with the visual cues showed good recovery of visual function. Rats that were exposed to the visual cues within their environment but restrained from moving were severely impaired (Stein et al., 1995).

Effect of Pharmacology

Another factor that can affect recovery of function following brain injury is the use of pharmacological treatments that reduce the nervous system's reaction to injury and promote recovery of function. Several excellent articles review basic scientific and clinical studies on pharmacological strategies for behavioral restoration following brain damage (Stein et al., 1995; Goldstein, 1993; Feeney and Sutton, 1987). These studies suggest that certain drugs can have profound effects on the recovery process; however, while some drugs are beneficial to the recovery of function, others may be detrimental (Goldstein, 1993).

Scientists are studying the effects of a number of types of drugs on recovery of function following brain injury, including the following:

1. Drugs that affect trophic factors, promoting regeneration and cell survival
2. Drugs that replace neurotransmitters lost because of cell death
3. Drugs that prevent the effects of toxic substances produced or released by dead or dying cells
4. Drugs that restore blood circulation
5. Antioxidants, such as vitamin E, which block the effects of free radicals that destroy cell membranes (Stein et al., 1995)

Amphetamine is a well-studied drug that appears to facilitate recovery from brain injury. Amphetamine works by enhancing the effects of neurotransmitters, such as adrenaline, noradrenaline, serotonin, and dopamine (Stein et al., 1995; Braun et al., 1986; Feeney et al., 1981, 1982; Hovda and Feeney, 1985). Treatment with amphetamine appears to improve cognitive function in young adults with posttraumatic organic brain syndrome (Evans et al., 1987; Kipper and Tuchman, 1976). Several studies have examined the use of amphetamine in conjunction with physical therapy to enhance motor recovery following stroke. Results showed that amphetamine in conjunction with physical therapy produced a significant improvement in motor performance on the Fugl-Meyer test (Crisostomo et al., 1988; Walker-Batson et al., 1992).

In contrast to the positive effects of amphetamine, use of the inhibitory neurotransmitter gamma-aminobutyric acid (GABA) following brain injury has a harmful effect on brain recovery. GABA agonists also impede recovery from brain damage in the rat, while GABA antagonists may be beneficial (Goldstein, 1993). Administration of cholinergic agents appears to facilitate recovery (van Woerkom et al., 1982). However, the administration of various drugs that block specific types of glutamate receptors have had mixed results (Goldstein, 1993).

There is considerable debate about the use of antioxidants such as vitamin E in both traumatic and neurodegenerative diseases such as Parkinson's disease. During early stages of trauma there is considerable destruction of cell tissue that leads to the production of free radicals. Free radicals are molecules of hydrogen, oxygen, and iron that have extra electrons, making them highly destructive to other living cells. Free radicals destroy the lipid membrane of a cell, allowing toxic substances to enter the cell and essential substances inside the cell to leave. Drugs such as vitamin E that block the effects of free radicals are called antioxidants. Stein and colleagues demonstrated that rats given vitamin E directly after frontal lobe damage were able to perform a spatial learning task as well as uninjured rats. A study by Fahn and associates looked at the effect of vitamin E in patients in the early stages of Parkinson's disease and found that it appeared to slow the progression of the disease. Unfortunately, other studies have not been as successful in showing the beneficial effects of vitamin E on slowing the pro-

gression of Parkinson's disease (Stein et al., 1995).

Finally, drugs that are used to treat common comorbidities in older patients can have a deleterious effect on recovery of function following stroke. For example, antihypertensives and sedatives have been shown to slow recovery of motor and language functions following stroke (Goldstein, 1995; Goldstein and Davis, 1988).

Many factors can affect the success of drugs in enhancing recovery of function following brain trauma, including the nature of the drug itself, the patient's history and health status prior to injury, and the environment of the patient after injury.

To be effective a drug has to get across tissue membranes that are biological barriers. Drugs must be absorbed into cell membranes to begin changing cell chemistry. Thus the size of the molecule, its electrical charge, and its solubility in lipid (fatty) membranes determine how well it will be absorbed (Stein et al., 1995). In addition, once in the body, the drug must get through the blood-brain barrier, which protects the brain and spinal cord from toxic substances. Finally, once the drug gets into the brain, it must find a receptor to bind to. The more receptors the drug can bind to, the more potent the effect of the drug. Some drugs are considered agonists. These drugs bind to receptors and enhance a normal biological response. In contrast, an antagonist drug binds to receptors and blocks the effects of naturally occurring neurotransmitters.

In addition to drug-related factors, many factors within the individual influence the effect of drugs on brain recovery. These include age, gender, health status at the time of injury, and type and extent of injury (stroke, trauma, or ischemia). For example, several researchers have shown that hormonal levels have a profound effect on both extent of damage following brain trauma and response to medication. Because of hormonal differences, the effect of a drug varies between males and females. Metabolic status can influence drug reactions as well. This is particularly important in light of the fact that systemic metabolism can change quickly following brain injury (Stein et al., 1995). For example, hypermetabolism can cause the breakdown of a drug too quickly, reducing its effectiveness.

Brain injury is not a single event but a cascade of processes that can continue long after the initial damage. Likewise, the mechanisms underlying recovery of function are multifactorial; they include the growth of new neuronal processes, altered metabolism, and altered neurotransmission. Because of the complexity of the injury and recovery process, the best results may come from combining drugs that influence different mechanisms during the course of injury and recovery. Overall, results from drug studies following brain injury are promising, suggesting that pharmacological treatment can enhance recovery of function following brain injury (Stein et al., 1995; Feeney and Sutton, 1987).

Effect of Training

Training is a different form of exposure to enriched environments in that activities used are specific rather than general (Held, 1998). Ogden and Franz (1917) performed an interesting study in which they produced hemiplegia in monkeys by making lesions in the motor cortex. They then gave four types of postoperative training: (*a*) no treatment, (*b*) general massage of the involved arm, (*c*) restraint of the noninvolved limb, and (*d*) restraint of the noninvolved limb coupled with stimulation of the involved limb to move, along with forced active movement of the animal. The last condition was the only one to show recovery, and in this condition it occurred within 3 weeks.

A study by Black et al. (1975) examined recovery from a motor cortex forelimb area lesion. They initiated training immediately after surgery or at 4 months, with training lasting 6 months. They found that training of the involved hand alone or training of the involved and normal hand together was more effective than training the normal hand alone. When training was delayed, recovery was worse than when it was initiated immediately following the lesion.

These results suggest that recovery is affected by the state of the system at the time of a lesion and that training after the lesion improves recovery best when it occurs immediately after the lesion and is specific to the involved limb (Held, 1987).

Stein et al. (1995) summarize the following critical lessons learned from brain repair and recovery research. First, brain injury must be treated as soon after the damage has occurred to ensure maximal effectiveness. Second, it is not likely that any single approach will be as effective as a combination of interventions. Finally, when developing appropriate treatment strategies, careful attention must be paid to the individual's history, health status, age, and experience.

Clinical Implications

By now it should be clear that the field of rehabilitation has much in common with the field of motor learning, defined as the study of the acquisition of movement. More accurately, therapists involved in management of the adult patient with neurological pathology are concerned with issues related to motor relearning, or the reacquisition of movement. The child who is born with a CNS deficit or is injured early in life faces the task of acquisition of movement in the face of unknown musculoskeletal and neural constraints. In either case, the therapist is concerned with structuring therapy in ways to maximize acquisition and/or recovery of function.

Remember Phoebe J.? She had been receiving therapy for 5 weeks and had recovered much of her ability to function. We wanted to know more about why this happened. What is the cause of her recovery of motor function? How much of her recovery may be attributed to therapeutic interventions? How many of her reacquired motor skills will she be able to retain and use when she leaves the rehabilitation facility and returns home?

Phoebe J.'s reacquisition of function cannot be attributed to any one factor. Some of her functional return is due to recovery, that is, regaining original control of original mechanisms; some is due to compensatory processes. In addition, age, premorbid function, site and size of lesion, and the effect of interventions all interact to determine the degree of function regained.

Phoebe J. has had excellent therapy as well. She has had carefully organized therapy sessions that contributed to her reacquisition of task-relevant behaviors. Both associative and nonassociative forms of learning may have played a role in her recovery. Habituation was used to decrease complaints of dizziness associated with inner ear problems. Trial-and-error learning (operant conditioning) helped her discover optimal solutions to many functional tasks. Her therapist carefully structured her environment so that optimal strategies were reinforced. For example, biofeedback was used to help her develop better foot control during locomotion.

Phoebe J. practiced relevant tasks under wide-ranging conditions. Under optimal conditions this would lead to procedural learning, ensuring that Phoebe J. would be able to transfer many of her newly gained skills to her home. Practicing tasks under varied conditions was aimed at the development of rule-governed action or schemata. Recognizing the importance of developing optimal perceptual and motor strategies, her therapist structured his sessions so that Phoebe J. explored the perceptual environment. This was designed to facilitate the optimal mapping of perceptual and motor strategies for achieving functional goals. Finally, her therapy was directed at helping Phoebe J. repeatedly solve the sensory-motor problems inherent in various functional tasks, rather than teaching her to repeat a single solution.

℮ SUMMARY

1. Motor learning, like motor control, emerges from a complex set of processes, including perception, cognition, and action.
2. Motor learning results from an interaction of the individual with the task and environment.
3. Nonassociative learning occurs when an organism is given a single stimulus repeatedly. As a result, the nervous system learns about the characteristics of that stimulus.
4. Habituation and sensitization are two simple forms of nonassociative learning. Habituation is a decrease in responsiveness that occurs as a result of repeated exposure to a nonpainful stimulus. Sensitization is an increased responsiveness following a threatening or noxious stimulus.
5. In associative learning a person learns to predict relationships, either of one stimulus to another (classical conditioning) or of one's behavior to a consequence (operant conditioning).
6. Classical conditioning consists of learning to pair two stimuli. During operant conditioning we learn to associate with a consequence a certain response from among many that we have made.
7. Procedural learning refers to learning tasks that can be performed without attention or conscious thought, like a habit.
8. Declarative learning results in knowledge that can be consciously recalled and thus requires processes such as awareness, attention, and reflection.
9. Theories of motor control include the closed-loop theory, the schema theory, the ecological theory of learning as exploration, and a number of theories on the stages of motor learning.
10. Classical recovery is divided into spontaneous recovery and forced recovery, that is, recovery obtained through specific interventions designed to affect neural mechanisms.
11. Experiments show that preinjury environmental enrichment protects animals against certain deficits after brain lesions.
12. Training after the lesion improves recovery best when it occurs immediately after the lesion and when it is specific to the involved limb.

CHAPTER 3

Physiology of Motor Control

ⓔ INTRODUCTION AND OVERVIEW

Motor Control Theories and Physiology

As we mentioned in Chapter 1, theories of motor control are not simply a collection of concepts regarding the nature and cause of movement. They must take into consideration research findings about the structure and function of the nervous system. Movement arises from the interaction of both perception and action systems, with cognition affecting both systems at many different levels. Within each of these systems are many levels of processing, which are illustrated in Figure 3-1. For example, perception can be thought of as progressing through various

processing stages. Each stage is controlled by specific brain structures that process sensory information at different levels, from initial stages of sensory processing to increasingly abstract levels of interpretation and integration in higher levels of the brain.

Recent neuroscience research suggests that movement control is achieved through the cooperative effort of many brain structures organized both hierarchically and in parallel. This means that a signal may be processed in two ways. A signal may be processed **hierarchically**, within ascending levels of the central nervous system (CNS). The same signal may be processed simultaneously among many brain structures, showing **parallel distributed processing**. Hierarchical processing, in conjunction with distributed process-

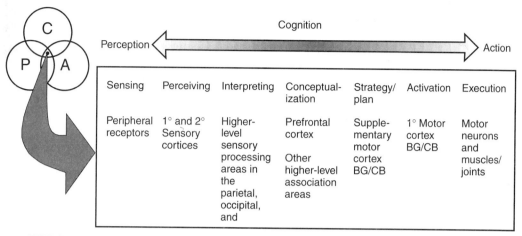

FIGURE 3-1.   Model of the interaction between perceptual, action and cognitive processes involved in motor control. BG, basal ganglia; CB, cerebellum.

ing, occurs in both the perception and action systems of movement control.

When we talk about hierarchical processing in this chapter, we are describing a system in which higher levels of the brain are concerned with issues of abstraction of information. For example, within the perceptual system, hierarchical processing means that higher brain centers integrate inputs from many senses and interpret incoming sensory information. On the action side of movement control, higher levels of brain function form motor plans and strategies for action. Thus, higher levels may select the specific response to accomplish a particular task. Lower levels of processing carry out the detailed monitoring and regulation of the response execution, making it appropriate for the context.

In parallel distributed processing, the same signal is processed simultaneously among many brain structures for different purposes. For example, the cerebellum and the basal ganglia process higher-level motor information simultaneously before sending it back to the motor cortex for action.

This chapter reviews the processes underlying the production of human movement. The first section of this chapter presents an overview of the major components of the CNS and the structure and function of a neuron, the basic unit of the CNS. The remaining sections discuss in more detail the

neural anatomy (the basic circuits) and the physiology (the function) of the systems involved in the production and control of movement. The chapter follows the neural anatomy and physiology of movement control from perception to action, recognizing that it is often difficult to distinguish where one ends and the other begins.

Overview of Brain Function

Brain function underlying motor control is typically divided into multiple processing levels, including the spinal cord, the brainstem, the cerebellum, the diencephalon, and the cerebral hemispheres, comprising the cerebral cortex and basal ganglia (Kandel, 1991a; Patton et al., 1989).

Spinal Cord

At the lowest level of the perception–action hierarchy is the spinal cord. This level also includes the muscles and sensory receptors. The circuitry of the spinal cord is involved in the initial reception and processing of somatosensory information (from the muscles, joints, and skin) contributing to the control of posture and movement. At the level of spinal cord processing, we can expect to see a fairly simple relationship between the sensory input and motor output. At the spinal cord level, we see the organization of reflexes, the most stereotyped responses to sensory stimuli, and the basic flexion and extension patterns of the muscles involved in leg movements, such as kicking and locomotion (Kandel, 1991a).

Sherrington called the motor neurons of the spinal cord the "final common pathway," since they are the last processing level before muscle activation occurs. Figure 3-2A shows the anatomist's view of the nervous system with the spinal cord positioned caudally. Figure 3-2B shows an abstract model of the nervous system with the spinal cord at the bottom of the hierarchy, with its many parallel pathways. In this view, the sensory receptors are represented by input arrows and the muscles by output arrows.

Brainstem

The spinal cord extends rostrally to join the next neural processing level, the brainstem. The brainstem contains important nuclei involved in postural control and locomotion, including the vestibular nuclei, the red nucleus, and the reticular nuclei. The brainstem receives somatosensory input from the skin and muscles of the head and sensory input from the vestibular and visual systems. In addition, nuclei in the brainstem control the output to the neck, face, and eyes and are critical to hearing and taste. In fact, all of the descending motor pathways except the corticospinal tract originate in the brainstem. Finally, the reticular formation, which regulates arousal and awareness, is also found within the brainstem (Kandel, 1991a).

The anatomist's view of the brainstem (Fig. 3-2A) shows divisions from caudal to rostral into the medulla, pons, and midbrain, while the abstract model (Fig. 3-2B) shows its input connections from the spinal cord and higher centers (the cerebellum and motor cortex) and its motor pathways to the spinal cord.

Cerebellum

The cerebellum lies behind the brainstem and is connected to it by tracts called peduncles (Fig. 3-2A). As you can see from Figure 3-2B, the cerebellum receives inputs from

the spinal cord, giving it feedback about movements, and from the cerebral cortex, giving it information on the planning of movements, and it has outputs to the brainstem. The cerebellum has many important functions in motor control. One is to adjust motor responses by comparing the intended output with sensory signals and to update the movement commands if they deviate from the intended path. The cerebellum also modulates the force and range of movements and is involved in motor learning.

Diencephalon

As we move rostrally in the brain, we next find the diencephalon, which contains the thalamus (Fig. 3-2A). The thalamus processes most of the information coming to the cortex from the many parallel input pathways (from the spinal cord, cerebellum, and brainstem) (Fig. 3-2B). These pathways stay segregated during thalamic processing and during the subsequent output to the different parts of the cortex (Kandel, 1991a).

Cerebral Hemispheres: Cerebral Cortex and Basal Ganglia

As we move higher, we find the cerebral hemispheres, which include the cerebral cortex and basal ganglia. Lying at the base of the cerebral cortex, the basal ganglia (Fig. 3-2) receive input from most areas of the cerebral cortex and send their output back to the motor cortex via the thalamus. Some of the functions of the basal ganglia involve higher-order cognitive aspects of motor control, such as the planning of motor strategies (Kandel, 1991a).

The cerebral cortex (Fig. 3-2A) is often considered the highest level of the motor control hierarchy. The parietal and premotor areas, along with other parts of the nervous system, are involved in identifying targets in space, choosing a course of action, and programming movements. The premotor areas send outputs mainly to the motor cortex, which sends its commands on to the brainstem and spinal cord via the corticospinal tract and the corticobulbar system (Fig. 3-2A).

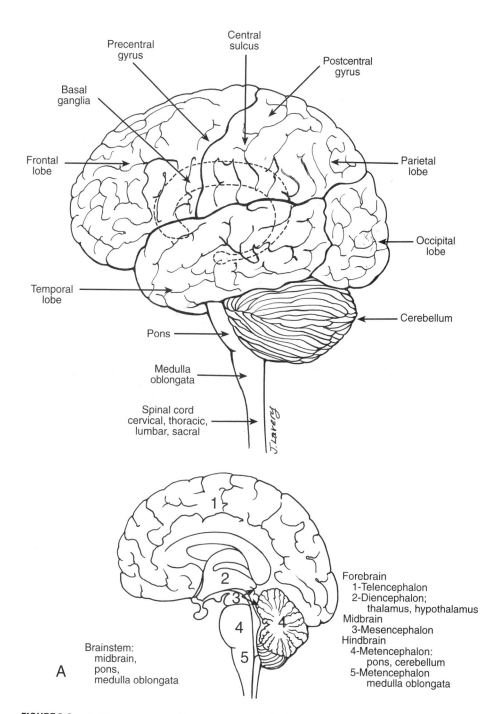

Forebrain
1-Telencephalon
2-Diencephalon;
  thalamus, hypothalamus
Midbrain
3-Mesencephalon
Hindbrain
4-Metencephalon:
  pons, cerebellum
5-Metencephalon
  medulla oblongata

FIGURE 3-2. **A.** Nervous system from an anatomist's view. **B.** An abstract model of the nervous system. (Adapted from Kandel E, Schwartz JH, Jessell TM, eds. Principles of neuroscience. 3rd ed. New York: Elsevier; 1991:8.)

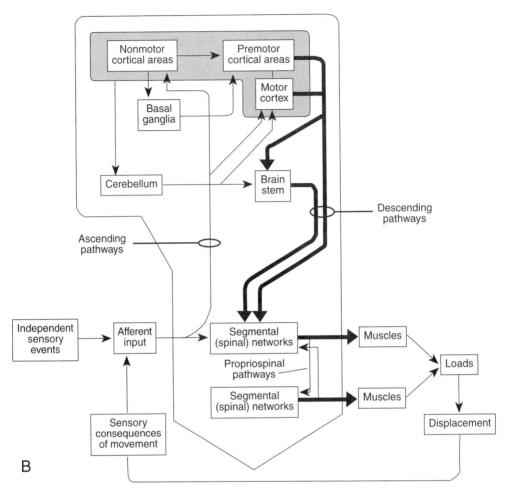

FIGURE 3-2.—*continued*

In light of these various subsystems involved in motor control, clearly the nervous system is organized both hierarchically and in parallel. Thus, the highest levels of control not only affect the next levels down; they also can act independently on the spinal motor neurons. This combination of parallel and hierarchical control allows a certain overlap of functions, so that one system is able to take over from another when environmental or task conditions require it. This also allows a certain amount of recovery from traumatic injury by the use of alternative pathways.

To clarify the function of the different levels of the nervous system, let's examine a specific action and walk through the pathways of the nervous system that contribute to its planning and execution. For example, perhaps you're thirsty and want to pour some milk from the carton in front of you into a glass. Sensory inputs come in from the periphery to tell you what is happening around you, where you are in space, and where your joints are relative to each other: they give you a map of your body in space. In addition, sensory information gives you critical information about the task you are to perform; how big the glass is, what size the milk carton is, and how heavy it is. Higher centers in the cortex make a plan to act on this information in relation to the goal: reaching for the carton of milk.

From your sensory map, you make a movement plan (using possibly the parietal lobes and supplementary and premotor cortex). You're going to reach over the box of corn flakes in front of you. This plan goes to the motor cortex, and muscle groups are specified. The plan is also sent to the cerebellum and basal ganglia, and they modify it to refine the movement. The cerebellum sends an update of the movement output plan to the motor cortex and brainstem. Descending pathways from the motor cortex and brainstem activate spinal cord networks, spinal motor neurons activate the muscles, and you reach for the milk. If the milk carton is full when you thought it was almost empty, spinal reflex pathways will compensate for the extra weight that you did not expect and activate more motor neurons. Then the sensory consequences of your reach will be evaluated, and the cerebellum will update the movement, in this case, to accommodate a heavier milk carton.

Neuron: Basic Unit of the CNS

The lowest level in the hierarchy is the single neuron in the spinal cord. How does it function? What is its structure? To explore more fully the ways that neurons communicate between the levels of the hierarchy of the nervous system, we need to review some of the simple properties of the neuron, including the resting potential, the action potential, and synaptic transmission.

Remember that the neuron, when it is at rest, always has a negative electrical charge or potential on the inside of the cell with respect to the outside. Thus, when physiologists record from a neuron intracellularly with an electrode, they discover that the inside of the cell has a **resting potential** of about −70 mV with respect to the outside (Fig. 3-3). This electrical potential is caused by an unequal concentration of chemical ions on the inside versus the outside of the cell. Thus, K^+ is high on the inside of the cell and Na^+ is high on the outside of the cell, and an electrical pump within the cell membrane keeps the ions in their appropriate concentrations. When the neuron is at rest, K^+ channels are open and keep the neuron at this negative potential (Patton et al., 1989; Koester, 1991; Kandel, 1976).

When a neuron is excited, one sees a series of dramatic jumps in voltage across the cell membrane. These are the **action potentials**, nerve impulses, or spikes. They do not go to zero voltage but to $^+30$ mV (Fig. 3-3). That is, the inside of the neuron becomes positive. Action potentials are also about 1 msec in duration and quickly repolarize. The height of the action potential is always about the same, from −70 to $^+30$ mV, or about 100 mV.

How does the neuron communicate this information to the next cell in line? It does so through the process of **synaptic transmission**. A cleft 200 Å wide separates neurons. Each action potential in a neuron releases a small amount of transmitter substance. It diffuses across the cleft and attaches to receptors on the next cell, which open up channels in the membrane and depolarize the cell. One action potential makes only a small depolarization, called an **excitatory postsynaptic potential**, the EPSP. The EPSP normally dies away after 3 to 4 msec, and as a result, the next cell is not activated (Patton et al., 1989).

However, if the first cell fires enough action potentials, there is a series of EPSPs, and they continue to build up depolarization to the threshold voltage for the action potential in the next neuron. This is called **summation**. There are two kinds of summation, temporal and spatial, and these are illustrated in Figure 3-3. **Temporal summation** results in depolarization because of synaptic potentials that occur close together in time. **Spatial summation** produces depolarization because of the action of multiple cells synapsing on the postsynaptic neuron. Spatial summation is really an example of parallel distributed processing, since multiple pathways are affecting the same neuron (Patton et al., 1989).

The effectiveness of a given synapse changes with experience. For example, if a given neuron is activated over a short period, it may show **synaptic facilitation**, in which it releases more transmitter and therefore more easily depolarizes the next cell. Alternatively, a cell may also show **defacilitation**,

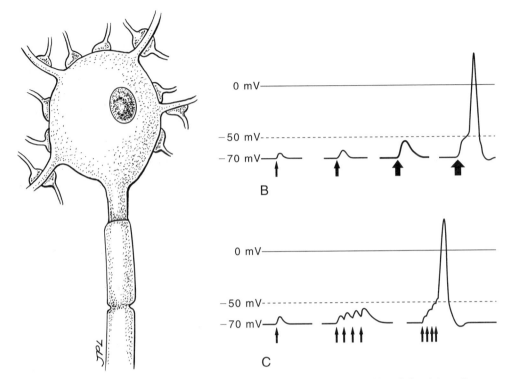

FIGURE 3-3. **A.** Neuron with many synaptic connections on the cell body and dendrites. **B.** Spatial summation, in which progressively larger numbers of presynaptic neurons are activated simultaneously (represented by progressively larger arrows) until sufficient transmitter is released to activate an action potential in the postsynaptic cell. **C.** Temporal summation, in which a single presynaptic neuron is activated once, four times at a low frequency, or four times at a high frequency (arrows indicate timing of presynaptic potentials). With a high-frequency stimulus the postsynaptic potential does not return to resting levels, but each successive potential sums toward threshold to activate an action potential.

or **habituation**. In this case, the cell is depleted of transmitter, hence is less effective in influencing the next cell. Many mechanisms can cause synaptic facilitation or habituation in different parts of the nervous system. Increased use of a given pathway can result in synaptic facilitation. However, in a different pathway, increased use can result in defacilitation or habituation. Variations in the coding within the neuron's internal chemistry and the stimuli activating the neuron determine whether it responds to these signals in one mode or another (Koester et al., 1991).

With this overview of the essential elements of the nervous system, we can now turn our attention to the heart of this chapter, an in-depth discussion of the sensory-motor processes underlying motor control.

❧ SENSORY/PERCEPTUAL SYSTEMS

What is the role of sensation in the production and control of movement? In the chapter on motor control theories, there were divergent views about the importance of sensory input in motor control. Current neuroscience research suggests that sensory information plays many roles in the control of movement.

Sensory inputs serve as the stimuli for reflexive movement organized at the spinal cord level of the nervous system. In addition, sensory information has a vital role in modulating the output of movement that results from the activity of pattern generators in the spinal cord. An example of this type of movement is locomotor output from pattern generators in the spinal cord. Likewise, at the spinal cord level, sensory information can modulate movement that results from commands originating in higher centers of the nervous system. The reason that sensation can modulate all of these types of movement is that sensory receptors converge on the motor neurons, considered the final common pathway. But another role of sensory information in movement control is accomplished via ascending pathways, which contribute to the control of movement in much more complex ways.

Somatosensory System

The somatosensory system, from the lowest to the highest level of the CNS hierarchy, going from the reception of signals in the periphery to the integration and interpretation of those signals relative to other sensory systems, is described in this section. Pay close attention to the way hierarchical and parallel distributed processing contributes to the analysis of somatosensory signals.

Peripheral Receptors

Muscle Spindle

Most muscle spindles are in the belly of skeletal muscles. They consist of specialized muscle fibers, called **intrafusal fibers**, surrounded by a connective tissue capsule (**extrafusal fibers** are the regular muscle fibers). In humans, the muscles with the highest spindle density (spindles per muscle) are the extraocular, hand, and neck muscles. Is it surprising that neck muscles have such a high spindle density? This is because we use these muscles in eye-head coordination as we reach for objects and move about in the environment (Gordon and Ghez, 1991).

Intrafusal muscle fibers are much smaller than extrafusal fibers. There are two types, *nuclear bag* and *nuclear chain* fibers. The bag fiber, which is thicker than the chain fiber, projects beyond the capsule, attaching to the connective tissue surrounding the extrafusal fiber fascicle. The chain fibers attach to the spindle capsule or to the bag fiber (Fig. 3-4A). Each fiber type can be divided into

equatorial, juxtaequatorial, and polar regions. The nuclear bag fiber has many spherical nuclei at the equatorial region and gives a slow twitch contraction, while the nuclear chain fiber has a single row of nuclei and gives a fast twitch contraction. The equatorial region is very elastic, like a balloon full of water.

The muscle spindle sends signals into the nervous system via afferent fibers, and it is controlled by the CNS via efferent fibers. Let's consider the afferent fibers. The muscle spindle sends information to the nervous system via two kinds of afferent fibers, the *group Ia afferents* and the *group II afferents*. The Ia fiber sensory endings wrap around the equatorial region, while the group II endings are on the juxtaequatorial region. The Ia afferents go to both bag and chain fibers, while the group II afferents mainly go to the chain fibers (Fig. 3-4A) (Patton et al., 1989; Gordon and Ghez, 1991).

Both bag and chain muscle fibers are also innervated by efferent fibers, the **γ-motor neurons**. The cell bodies of the γ-motor neurons are inside the ventral horn of the spinal cord, intermingled with the **α-motor neurons**, innervating the extrafusal fibers. The γ-motor neuron endings are at the polar, striated region of the bag and the chain muscle fibers, as shown in Figure 3-4A. There are two types of γ-fibers: (*a*) the γ-dynamic, innervating the bag fiber, and (*b*) the γ-static, innervating the chain fiber.

Passive muscle stretch causes stretch of the equator of intrafusal fibers. The equator of the bag fiber is easily stretched because it is so elastic, while the chain fiber equator stretches less rapidly because it is stiffer, with fewer nuclei. Remember, the Ia fiber endings wrap around the equator of the bag and chain fibers; thus, they have a low threshold to stretch and will follow changes in length easily. This means that the Ia afferents code the rate of stretch (a dynamic response) and the length of the muscle at the end of stretch (static response) (Gordon and Ghez, 1991).

The group II afferents end on the juxtaequatorial region of the chain fiber. This is a stiffer region, and as a result, the group II afferents have a higher threshold than do the

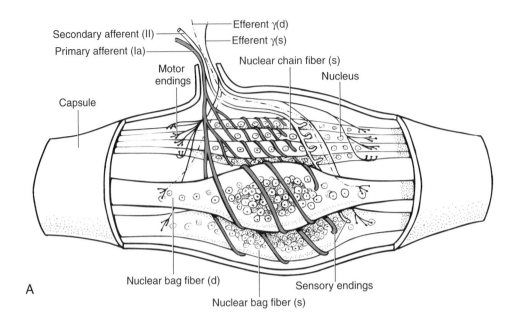

A

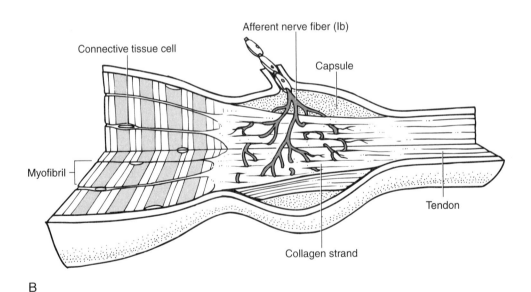

B

FIGURE 3-4. Anatomy of the muscle receptors. **A.** Muscle spindle shows nuclear bag and chain fibers and their group Ia and II afferent and gamma-efferent innervation. **B.** Golgi tendon organ and its Ib afferent innervation. It lies at the muscle-tendon junction and is connected to 15 to 20 muscle fibers.

Ia afferents. The group II afferents code only muscle length and have no dynamic response. Static responses are linearly correlated with the length of the muscle. Thus, the Ia afferents respond well to slight tendon taps, sinusoidal stretches, and even vibration of the muscle tendon, while group II afferents do not respond to these stimuli.

How is information from the muscle spindle used during motor control? Muscle spindle information is employed at many levels of the CNS hierarchy. At the lowest level, it is involved in reflex activation of muscles. However, as the information ascends the CNS hierarchy, it is used in increasingly complex and abstract ways. For example, it may contribute to our perception of effort. In, addition, it is carried over different pathways to different parts of the brain, in this way contributing to the parallel distributed nature of brain processing.

Stretch Reflex Loop. When a muscle is stretched, it stretches the muscle spindle, exciting the Ia afferents. They have excitatory monosynaptic connections to the motor neurons, which activate their own muscle and synergistic muscles. They also excite Ia inhibitory interneurons, which inhibit α-motor neurons to the antagonist muscles. For example, if the gastrocnemius muscle is stretched, the muscle spindle Ia afferents in the muscle are excited, and in turn excite the α-motor neurons of the gastrocnemius, which cause it to contract. The Ia afferent also excites the Ia inhibitory interneuron, which inhibits motor neurons to the antagonist muscle, the tibialis anterior, so that if this muscle was contracting, it now relaxes. The group II afferents also excite their own muscle, but disynaptically (Patton et al., 1989; Gordon and Ghez, 1991).

What is the purpose of γ-fiber activity, and when are these fibers active? Whenever there is a voluntary contraction, there is α–γ coactivation. Without this coactivation, spindle afferents would be silent during muscle contraction. With it, the nuclear bag and chain fibers contract as well as the regular extrafusal fibers of the muscle, and thus the polar region of the muscle spindle cannot go slack. Because of this coactivation, if there is unexpected stretch during the contraction, the group Ia and II afferents will be able to sense it and compensate.

Golgi Tendon Organs

Golgi tendon organs (GTOs), which are spindle-shaped, lie at the muscle–tendon junction (Fig. 3-4*B*). They connect to 15 to 20 muscle fibers. Afferent information from the GTO is carried to the nervous system via the Ib afferent fibers. Unlike the muscle spindles, they have no efferent connections and thus are not subject to CNS modulation.

This is how GTOs function. The GTO is sensitive to tension changes that result from either stretch or contraction of the muscle. The GTO responds to as little as 2 to 25 g of force. The GTO reflex is an inhibitory disynaptic reflex, inhibiting its own muscle and exciting its antagonist.

Researchers used to think that the GTO was active only in response to large amounts of tension, so they hypothesized that the role of the GTO was to protect the muscle from injury. Current research has shown that these receptors constantly monitor muscle tension and are sensitive to even small changes in tension caused by muscle contraction. A newly hypothesized function of the GTO is that it modulates muscle output in response to fatigue. Thus, when muscle tension is reduced by fatigue, the GTO output is reduced, lowering its inhibitory effect on its own muscle (Patton et al., 1989; Gordon and Ghez, 1991).

The GTOs of the extensor muscles of the leg are active during the stance phase of locomotion and act to excite the extensor muscles and inhibit the flexor muscles until the GTO is unloaded (Pearson et al., 1992). This is exactly the opposite of what would be expected from the reflex when it is activated when the animal is passive. Thus, the reflex appears to have different properties under different task conditions.

Researchers have hypothesized that the function of the muscle spindles and GTOs together may be regulation of muscle stiffness. Muscle stiffness may be defined as the force per unit length of a muscle. This is exactly what the GTO and muscle spindle are reciprocally controlling: Force (GTO) per unit length (muscle spindle) (Gordon and Ghez, 1991).

Joint Receptors

How do joint receptors work, and what is their function? There are a number of types of receptors within the joint itself, including Ruffini-type endings or spray endings, paciniform endings, ligament receptors, and free nerve endings, in various portions of the joint capsule. Morphologically, they share the same characteristics as many of the other receptors found in the nervous system. For example, the ligament receptors are almost identical to GTOs, while the paciniform endings are identical to pacinian corpuscles in the skin.

Joint function has a number of intriguing aspects. The joint receptor information is used at several levels of the hierarchy of sensory processing. Some researchers have found that joint receptors appear to be sensitive only to extreme joint angles (Burgess and Clark, 1969). Because of this, the joint receptors may provide a danger signal about extreme joint motion.

Other researchers have reported that many individual joint receptors respond to a limited range of joint motion. This phenomenon has been called *range fractionation,*

with multiple receptors being activated in overlapping ranges. Afferent information from joint receptors ascends to the cerebral cortex and contributes to our perception of our position in space. The CNS determines joint position by monitoring which receptors are activated at the same time, and this allows the determination of exact joint position.

Cutaneous Receptors

There are also several types of cutaneous receptors: (*a*) mechanoreceptors, including pacinian corpuscles, Merkel's discs, Meissner's corpuscles, Ruffini endings, and lanceolate endings around hair follicles, detecting mechanical stimuli; (*b*) thermoreceptors, detecting temperature changes; and (*c*) nociceptors, detecting potential for damage to the skin. Figure 3-5 shows the location of

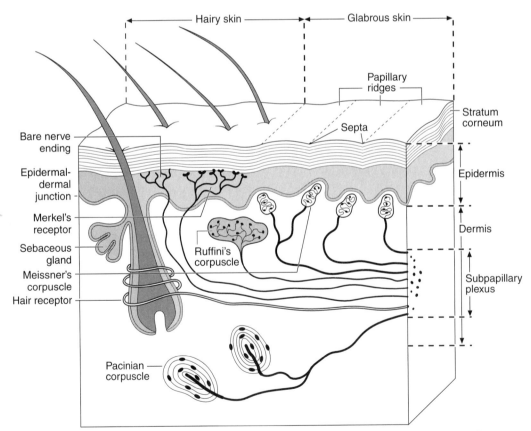

FIGURE 3-5.   Location of cutaneous receptors in the skin. (Reprinted with permission from Kandel E, Schwartz JH, Jessell TM, eds. Principles of neuroscience. 3rd ed. New York: Elsevier, 1991.)

these receptors in the skin. The number of receptors within the sensitive areas of the skin, such as the tips of the fingers, is very high, on the order of 2500 per square centimeter (Kandel and Jessel, 1991).

Information from the cutaneous system is also used in hierarchical processing in several ways. At lower levels of the CNS hierarchy, cutaneous information gives rise to reflex movements. Information from the cutaneous system also ascends and provides information concerning body position essential for orientation within the immediate environment.

The nervous system uses cutaneous information for reflex responses in various ways, depending on the extent and type of cutaneous input. A light diffuse stimulus to the bottom of the foot tends to produce extension in the limb; for example when you touch the pad of a cat's foot lightly, it will extend it. This is called the placing reaction, and it is found in human infants as well. In contrast, a sharp focal stimulus tends to produce withdrawal, or flexion, even when it is applied to exactly the same area of the foot. This flexor withdrawal reflex protects us from injury. The typical pattern of response in the cutaneous reflex is ipsilateral flexion and contralateral extension, which allows you to support your weight on the opposite limb (mediated by group III and IV afferents).

Even though we consider reflexes to be stereotyped, they are modulated by higher centers, depending on the task and the context. Remember the flexor reflex, which typically causes withdrawal of a limb from a noxious stimulus. However, if there is more at stake than not hurting yourself, such as saving the life of your child, the CNS inhibits the activation of this reflex movement in favor of actions more appropriate to the situation.

Role of Somatosensation at the Spinal Cord Level

Information from cutaneous, muscle, and joint receptors modifies the output of circuits at the spinal cord level that control

such basic activities as locomotion. In the late 1960s, Grillner performed experiments in which he cut the dorsal roots to the cat spinal cord to eliminate sensory feedback from the periphery (Grillner and Wallen, 1985). He stimulated the spinal cord and was able to activate the neural pattern generator for locomotor patterns. He found that low rates of repetitive stimulation gave rise to a walk; higher rates, to a trot; and still higher ones, to a gallop. This suggests that complex movements, such as locomotion, can be generated at the spinal cord level without supraspinal influences or inputs from the periphery.

If we do not need sensory information to generate complex movement, does that mean there is no role for sensory information in its execution? No. Forssberg et al. (1977a) have shown that sensory information modulates locomotor output in a very elegant way. When he brushed the paw of a spinalized cat with a stick during the swing phase of walking, it caused the paw to flex more strongly and get out of the way of the stick. But during stance, the same stimulation caused stronger extension, to push off more quickly and avoid the stick in this way. Thus, he found that the same cutaneous input could modulate the step cycle in different functional ways, depending on the context in which it was used.

Ascending Pathways

Information from the trunk and limbs is also carried to the sensory cortex and cerebellum. Two systems ascend to the cerebral cortex: the *dorsal column–medial lemniscal* (DC-ML) *system* and the *anterolateral system.* (Systems that ascend to the cerebellum are discussed later in the chapter.) The DC-ML and anterolateral systems are shown in Figures 3-6 and 3-7. They are examples of parallel ascending systems. Each relays information about somewhat different functions, but there is some redundancy between the two pathways. What is the advantage of parallel systems? They give extra subtlety and richness to perception by using multiple modes of processing information. They also give a

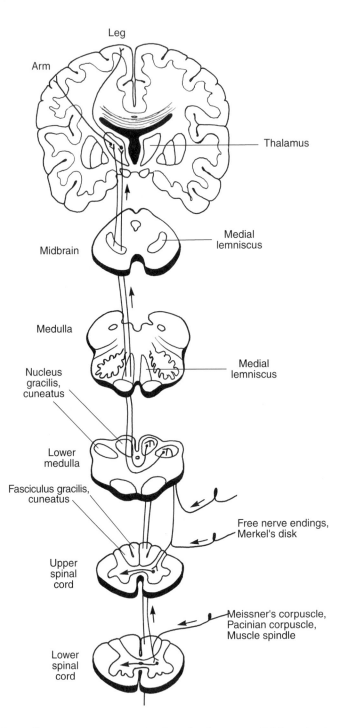

FIGURE 3-6. Ascending sensory systems: the dorsal column–medial lemniscal pathway containing information from touch and pressure receptors.

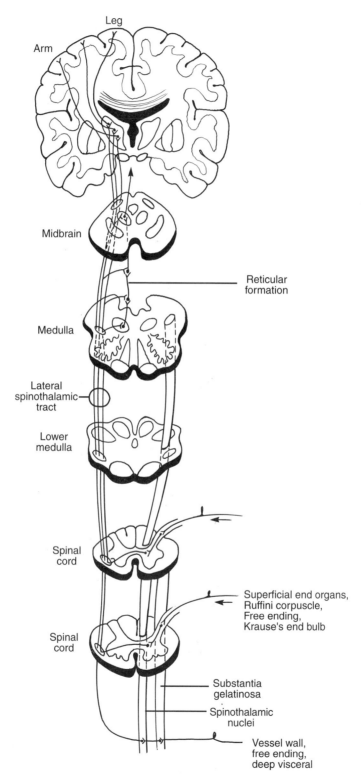

FIGURE 3-7.   Ascending sensory systems: the anterolateral system, containing information on pain and temperature.

measure of insurance of continued function in case of injury (Patton et al., 1989; Martin and Jessel, 1991).

Dorsal Column–Medial Lemniscal System

The *dorsal columns* are formed mainly by dorsal root neurons and thus are first-order neurons. The majority of the fibers branch on entering the spinal cord, synapsing on interneurons and motor neurons to modulate spinal activity, and send branches to ascend in the dorsal column pathway toward the brain. What are the functions of the dorsal column neurons? They send information on muscle, tendon, and joint sensibility up to the somatosensory cortex and other higher brain centers. There is an interesting exception, however. Leg proprioceptors have their own private pathway to the brainstem, the lateral column. They join the dorsal column pathway in the brainstem. The dorsal column pathway also contains information from touch and pressure receptors and codes especially for discriminative fine touch. This pathway is shown in Figure 3-6 (Martin and Jessel, 1991).

Where does this information go, and how is it processed? The pathways synapse at multiple levels in the nervous system, including the medulla, where second-order neurons become the *medial lemniscal* pathway and cross over to the thalamus, synapsing with third-order neurons, which proceed to the somatosensory cortex. Every level of the hierarchy can modulate the information coming into it from below. Through synaptic excitation and inhibition, higher centers can shut off or enhance ascending information. This lets higher centers selectively tune (up or down) the information coming from lower centers.

As the neurons ascend through each level to the brain, the information from the receptors is increasingly processed to allow for interpretation. This is done by selectively enlarging the receptive field of each successive neuron.

Anterolateral System

The second ascending system, shown in Figure 3-7, is the *anterolateral* (AL) system. It consists of the spinothalamic, spinoreticular,

and spinomesencephalic tracts. These fibers cross over upon entering the spinal cord and then ascend to brainstem centers. The anterolateral system has a dual function. First, it transmits information on crude touch and pressure and thus contributes in a minor way to touch and limb proprioception. It also plays a major role in relaying information related to thermal and nociception to higher brain centers. All levels of the sensory processing hierarchy act on the AL system in the same manner as for the DC-ML system (Martin and Jessel, 1991).

There is redundancy of information in both tracts. A lesion in one tract does not cause complete loss of discrimination in any of these senses. However, a lesion in both tracts causes severe loss. Hemisection of the spinal cord (caused by a serious accident, for example) causes loss of tactile sensation and proprioception in the ipsilateral arm (fibers have not crossed yet), while pain and temperature sensation are lost on the contralateral side (fibers crossed upon entering the spinal cord) (Martin and Jessel, 1991).

Thalamus

Information from both the ascending somatosensory tracts, like information from virtually all sensory systems, goes through the *thalamus*. In addition, the thalamus receives information from a number of other areas of the brain, including the basal ganglia and the cerebellum. Thus the thalamus is a major processing center of the brain. In general, a lesion in this area causes severe sensory and motor problems. Recently the thalamus has become a target for treatments aimed at decreasing tremor in patients with Parkinson's disease.

Somatosensory Cortex

The *somatosensory cortex* is a major processing area for all the somatosensory modalities, and marks the beginning of conscious awareness of somatosensation. The somatosensory cortex is divided into two major areas: *primary somatosensory cortex* (SI) (also called Brodmann's area 1, 2, 3a, and 3b); and *secondary somatosensory cortex* (SII) (Fig. 3-8A).

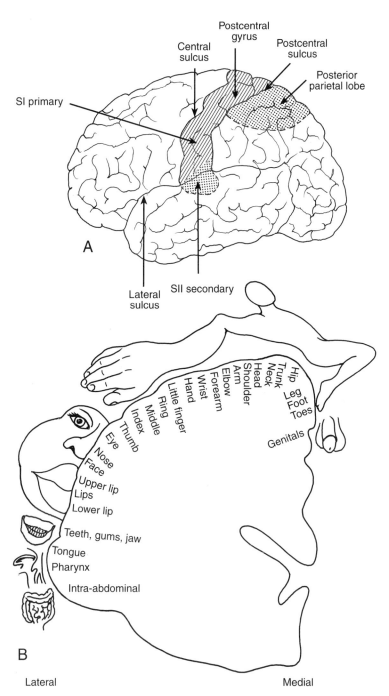

FIGURE 3-8. Somatosensory cortex and association areas. **A.** Located in the parietal lobe, the somatosensory cortex contains three major divisions: the primary (SI), secondary (SII), and posterior parietal cortex. **B.** Sensory homunculus showing the somatic sensory projections from the body surface. (Adapted from Kandel E, Schwartz JH, Jessell TM, eds. Principles of neuroscience. 3rd ed. New York: Elsevier, 1991:368, 372.)

In SI, kinesthetic and touch information from the contralateral side of the body is organized somatotopically and spans four cytoarchitectural areas, Brodmann's areas 1, 2, 3a, and 3b.

It is in this area that we begin to see cross-modality processing. This means that information from joint receptors, muscle spindles, and cutaneous receptors is now integrated to give us information about movement in a given body area. This information is laid on top of a map of the entire body, which is distorted to reflect the relative weight given sensory information from certain areas, as you see in Figure 3-8*B*. For example, the throat, mouth, and hands are heavily represented because we need more detailed information to support the movements executed by these structures. This is the beginning of the spatial processing that is essential to the coordination of movements in space. Coordinated movement requires information about the position of the body relative to the environment and the position of one body segment relative to another (Martin, 1991).

Contrast sensitivity is important to movement control, since it allows the detection of the shape and edges of objects. The somatosensory cortex processes incoming information to increase contrast sensitivity so that we can more easily identify and discriminate between objects through touch. How does it do this? The receptive fields of the somatosensory neurons have an excitatory center and inhibitory surround. This inhibitory surround aids in two-point discrimination through *lateral inhibition.*

How does lateral inhibition work? The cell that is excited inhibits the cells next to it, enhancing contrast between excited and nonexcited regions of the body. The receptors have no lateral inhibition. But it comes in at the level of the dorsal columns and at each subsequent step in the relay. In fact, humans have a sufficiently sensitive somatosensory system to perceive the activation of a single tactile receptor in the hand (Martin, 1991).

Also, special cells within the somatosensory cortex respond best to moving stimuli and are directionally sensitive. One does not find this feature in the dorsal columns or in the thalamus. These higher-level processing cells also have larger receptive fields than the typical cells in the somatosensory cortex, often encompassing a number of fingers. These cells appear to respond preferentially when neighboring fingers are stimulated. This may indicate their participation in such functions as the grasp of objects.

It has recently been found that the receptive fields of neurons in the somatosensory cortex are not fixed in size. Both injury and experience can change their dimensions considerably. The implications of these studies are considered in the motor learning sections of this book.

Somatosensory cortex also has descending connections to the thalamus, dorsal column nucleus, and the spinal cord, and thus has the ability to modulate ascending information coming through these structures.

Association Cortices

It is in the many association cortices that we begin to see the transition from perception to action. It is here too that we see the interplay between cognitive and perceptual processing. The association cortices, found in parietal, temporal, and occipital lobes, include centers for higher-level sensory processing and higher-level abstract cognitive processing. The locations of these various areas are shown in Figure 3-9.

Within the parietal, temporal, and occipital cortices are association areas, which are hypothesized to link information from several senses. Area 5 of the parietal cortex is a thin strip posterior to the postcentral gyrus. After intermodality processing has taken place within area SI, outputs are sent to area 5, which integrates information between body parts. Area 5 connects to area 7 of the parietal lobe. Area 7 also receives processed visual information. Thus, area 7 combines eye–limb processing in most visually triggered or guided activities.

Lesions in area 5 or 7 in either humans or other animals cause problems with the learning of skills that use information regarding

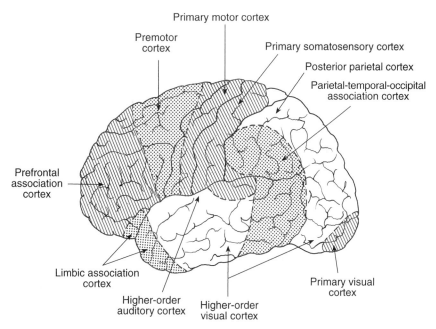

FIGURE 3-9. Locations of primary sensory areas, higher-level sensory association areas, and higher-level cognitive (abstract) association cortices. (Adapted with permission from Kandel E, Schwartz JH, Jessell TM, eds. Principles of neuroscience. 3rd ed. New York: Elsevier, 1991 : 825.)

the position of the body in space. In addition, certain cells in these areas are activated during visually guided movements, with their activity becoming more intense when the animal attends to the movement. These findings support the hypothesis that the parietal lobe participates in processes involving attention to the position of and manipulation of objects in space.

These experimental results are further supported by observations of patients with damage to the parietal lobes. Their deficits include problems with body image and perception of spatial relations, which may be very important in both postural control and voluntary movements. Clearly, lesions to this area do not simply reduce the ability to perceive information coming in from one part of the body; in addition, they can affect the ability to interpret this information.

For example, people with lesions in the right angular gyrus (the nondominant hemisphere), just behind area 7, show complete neglect of the contralateral side, including body, objects, and drawings. This is called **agnosia**, or the lack of recognition. When their own arm or leg is passively moved into their visual field, they may claim that it is not theirs. In certain cases, patients may be totally unaware of the hemiplegia that accompanies the lesion and may thus desire to leave the hospital early, since they are unaware that they have any problem (Kupfermann, 1991a). Many of these same patients show problems when asked to copy drawn figures. They may make a drawing in which half of the object is missing. This is called *constructional apraxia.* Larger lesions may cause the inability to operate and orient in space or the inability to perform complex sequential tasks.

Right-handed patients who have lesions in the left angular gyrus (the dominant hemisphere) show such symptoms as confusion between left and right; difficulty in naming their fingers, though they can sense touch; and difficulty in writing, though their motor and sensory functions are normal for the hands. Alternatively, patients who have lesions to both sides of these areas commonly have problems attending to visual stimuli, using vision to grasp an object, and making voluntary eye movements to a point in space (Kupfermann, 1991a).

We have just taken one sensory system, the somatosensory system, from the lowest to the highest level of the CNS hierarchy, going from the reception of signals in the periphery to the integration and interpretation of those signals relative to other sensory systems. We have also looked at how hierarchical and parallel distributed processing have contributed to the analysis of these signals. We are now going to look at a second sensory system, the visual system, in the same way.

Visual System

Vision serves motor control in a number of ways. Vision allows us to identify objects in space and to determine their movement. When vision plays this role, it is considered an exteroceptive sense. But vision also gives us information about where our body is in space, about the relation of one body part to another, and the motion of our body. When vision plays this role, it is called visual proprioception, which means that it gives us information not only about the environment but also about our own body. Later chapters show how vision plays a key role in the control of posture, locomotion, and manipulatory function. In the following sections, we consider the anatomy and physiology of the visual system to show how it supports these roles in motor control.

Peripheral Visual System

Photoreceptors

Let's first look at an overall view of the eye. The eye is a great instrument, designed to focus the image of the world on the retina with high precision. As illustrated in Figure 3-10*A*, light enters the eye through the cornea and is focused by the cornea and lens on the retina at the back of the eye. An interesting feature of the retina is that light must travel through all of the layers of the eye and the neural layers of the retina before it hits the photoreceptors, which are at the back of the retina, facing away from the light source. Luckily, these layers are nearly transparent.

There are two types of photoreceptor cells: the *rods* and the *cones*. The cones are functional for vision in normal daylight and are responsible for color vision. The rods are responsible for vision at night, when the amount of light is very low and too weak to activate the cones. Right at the fovea, the rest of the layers are pushed aside so the cones can receive the light in its clearest form. The blind spot (where the optic nerve leaves the retina) has no photoreceptors, and therefore we are blind in this one part of the retina. Except for the fovea, there are 20 times as many rods as cones in the retina. However, cones are more important for normal vision, because their loss causes legal blindness, while total loss of rods causes only night blindness (Tessier-Lavigne, 1991).

Remember that sensory differentiation is a key aspect of sensory processing that supports motor control. To accomplish this, the visual system has to identify objects and determine whether they are moving. So how are *object identification* and *motion sense* accomplished in the visual system? Two separate pathways process them. We will follow these pathways from the retina to the visual cortex. We will see that *contrast sensitivity* is used in both pathways to identify objects and sense motion. Contrast sensitivity enhances the edges of objects, giving us greater precision in perception. As in the somatosensory system, all three processes are used extensively in the visual system. This processing begins in the retina. So let's first look at the cells of the retina, so that we can understand how they work together to process information (Tessier-Lavigne, 1991).

Vertical Cells

In addition to the rods and cones, the retina contains *bipolar cells* and *ganglion cells*, which you may consider vertical cells, since they connect in series to one another but have no lateral connections (Fig. 3-10). For example, the rods and cones make direct synaptic contact with bipolar cells. The bipolar cells in turn connect to the ganglion cells, which relay visual information to the CNS by sending axons to the lateral geniculate nucleus (LGN) and superior colliculus as well as to brainstem nuclei (Tessier-Lavigne, 1991; Dowling, 1987).

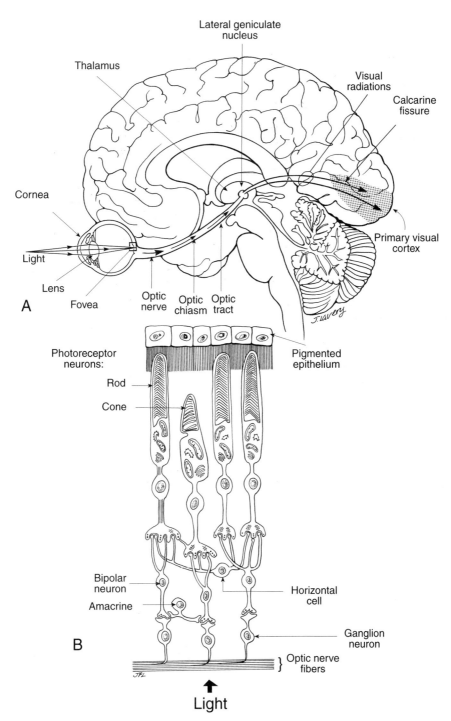

FIGURE 3-10. **A.** The eye, and the visual pathways from the retina to the thalamus and the primary visual cortex (area 17). **B.** Magnification of retina to show specific neurons (Adapted with permission from Kandel E, Schwartz JH, Jessell TM, eds. Principles of neuroscience. 3rd ed. New York: Elsevier, 1991:401, 415, 423.)

Horizontal Cells

There is another class of neurons in the retina, which we call horizontal cells. These neurons modulate the flow of information within the retina by connecting the vertical cells laterally. These are called the *horizontal* and *amacrine cells*. The horizontal cells mediate interactions between the receptors and bipolar cells, while the amacrine cells mediate interactions between bipolar and ganglion cells. The horizontal cells and amacrine cells are critical for achieving contrast sensitivity. Though it may appear that there are complex interconnections between the receptor cells and other neurons before the final output of the ganglion cells is reached, the pathways and functions of the different classes of cells are straightforward.

Let's first look at the bipolar cell pathway. There are two types of pathways that involve bipolar cells, a direct pathway and a lateral pathway. In the direct pathway, a cone, for example, makes a direct connection with a bipolar cell, which makes a direct connection with a ganglion cell. In the lateral pathway, activity of cones is transmitted to the ganglion cells lateral to them through horizontal cells or amacrine cells. Figure 3-10*B* shows these organizational possibilities (Dowling, 1987).

In the direct pathway, cones (or rods) connect directly to bipolar cells with either on-center or off-center receptive fields. The **receptive field** of a cell is the specific area of the retina to which the cell is sensitive when that part of the retina is illuminated. The receptive field can be either excitatory or inhibitory, increasing or decreasing the cell's membrane potential. The receptive fields of bipolar cells and ganglion cells are circular. At the center of the retina the receptive fields are small, while in the periphery receptive fields are large. The term on-center means that the cell has an excitatory central portion of the receptive field with an inhibitory surrounding area. Off-center refers to the opposite case, an inhibitory center and excitatory surround (Dowling, 1987).

How do the cells take on their antagonistic surround characteristics? It appears that horizontal cells in the surround area of the bipolar cell receptive field (RF) make connections to cones in the center of the field. When light shines on the periphery of the receptive field, the horizontal cells inhibit the cones adjacent to them. Each type of bipolar cell then synapses with a corresponding type of ganglion cell, on-center and off-center, and makes excitatory connections with that ganglion cell.

On-center cells give very few action potentials in the dark, and they are activated when their RF is illuminated. When the periphery of their RF is illuminated, it inhibits the effect of stimulating the center. Off-center ganglion cells likewise show inhibition when light is applied to the center of their RF, and they fire at the fastest rate just after the light is turned off. They also are activated if light is applied only to the periphery of their RF.

Ganglion cells are also influenced by the activity of amacrine cells. Many of the amacrine cells function in a similar manner to horizontal cells, transmitting inhibitory inputs from nearby bipolar cells to the ganglion cell, increasing contrast sensitivity.

These two types of pathways, on- and off-center, for processing retinal information are two examples of *parallel distributed processing* of similar information within the nervous system. We talked about a similar *center-surround inhibition* in cutaneous receptor receptive fields. What is the purpose of this type of inhibition? It appears to be important in detecting contrasts between objects, rather than the absolute intensity of light produced or reflected by an object. This inhibition allows us to detect edges of objects easily. It is important in locomotion, when we are walking downstairs and need to see the edge of the step. It is also important in manipulatory function in being able to determine the exact shape of an object for grasping.

The ganglion cells send their axons via the optic nerve to three regions in the brain, the LGN, the pretectum, and the superior colliculus (Mason and Kandel, 1991). Figure 3-10*A* shows connections to the LGN of the thalamus.

Central Visual Pathways

Lateral Geniculate Nucleus

To determine what parts of the retina and visual field are represented in these areas of the brain, let's first discuss the configuration of the visual fields and hemiretina. The left half of the visual field projects on the nasal (medial, next to the nose) half of the retina of the left eye and the temporal (lateral) half of the retina of the right eye. The right visual field projects on the nasal half of the retina of the right eye and the temporal half of the retina of the left eye (Mason and Kandel, 1991).

Thus, the optic nerves from the left and right eyes leave the retina at the optic disc in the back of the eye. They travel to the optic chiasm, where the nerves from each eye come together and axons from the nasal side of the eyes cross, while those from the temporal side do not cross. At this point, the optic nerve becomes the optic tract. Because of this re-sorting of the optic nerves, the left optic tract has a map of the right visual field. This is similar to what we found for the somatosensory system, in which information from the opposite side of the body was represented in the thalamus and cortex.

One of the targets of cells in the optic tract is the LGN of the thalamus (Fig. 3-10*A*). The LGN has six layers of cells, which map the contralateral visual field. The ganglion cells from different areas project onto specific points in the LGN, but just as we find for somatosensory maps of the body, certain areas are represented much more strongly than others. The fovea of the retina, which we use for high-acuity vision, is represented to a far greater degree than the peripheral area. Each layer of the LGN gets input from only one eye. The first two layers (most ventral) are called the *magnocellular* (large cell) layers, and layers three through six are called the *parvocellular* (small cell) layers. The projection cells of each layer send axons to the visual cortex (Mason and Kandel, 1991).

The receptive fields of neurons in the LGN are similar to those found in the ganglion cells of the retina. There are separate on-center and off-center receptive field pathways. The magnocellular layers appear to be involved in the analysis of movement of the visual image and the coarse details of an object, while the parvocellular layers function in color vision and a more detailed structural analysis. Thus, magnocellular layers are more important in motor functions, such as balance control, in which movement of the visual field gives us information about our body sway, and in reaching for moving objects. The parvocellular layers are more important in the final phases of reaching for an object, when we need to grasp it accurately.

Superior Colliculus

Ganglion cell axons in the optic tract also terminate in the *superior colliculus* (in addition to indirect visual inputs coming from the visual cortex). The superior colliculus is in the midbrain posterior to the thalamus. It has been hypothesized that the superior colliculus maps the visual space around us in terms of not only visual but also auditory and somatosensory cues. The three sensory maps in the superior colliculus are different from those in the sensory cortex. Body areas here are not mapped in terms of density of receptor cells in a particular area, but in terms of their relationship to the retina. Areas close to the retina (e.g., the nose) are given more representation than areas far away (e.g., the hand). For any part of the body, the visual, auditory, and somatosensory maps are aligned in the different layers of the colliculus (Mason and Kandel, 1991).

In addition to these three maps in the upper and middle of the seven layers of the colliculus, there is a motor map in the deeper layers of the colliculus. Through these output neurons, the colliculus controls saccadic eye movements, which cause the eye to move toward a specific stimulus. The superior colliculus then sends outputs to (*a*) regions of the brainstem that control eye movements, (*b*) the tectospinal tract, mediating the reflex control of the neck and head, and (*c*) the tectopontine tract, which projects to the cerebellum, for further processing of eye–head control.

Recent research (Cowie and Robinson, 1994; Werner et al., 1997) has also shown that superior colliculus output neurons control head, trunk, and arm movements. One study on primates has shown that during reaching, the temporal patterns of neurons of the superior colliculus and muscles of the arm, shoulder, and trunk were similar, with most neurons active in advance of the arm movement and often before muscle activity onset. The properties of these cells are more like those of the skeletomotor than the oculomotor system. What might be the functional significance of these movement related neurons in the superior colliculus? It has been suggested that they may reflect an upcoming movement via efference copy, used to coordinate eye, head, and arm movements. It is also possible that they are part of the output leading to movement via tectoreticulospinal pathways (Werner et al., 1997).

Pretectal Region

Ganglion cells also terminate in the *pretectal* region, which is just anterior to the superior colliculus. The pretectal region is an important visual reflex center involved in pupillary eye reflexes, in which the pupil constricts in response to light shining on the retina.

Primary Visual Cortex

From the LGN, axons project to the *primary visual cortex* (also called striate cortex) to Brodmann's area 17, in the occipital lobe (Fig. 3-10). The inputs from the two eyes alternate throughout the striate cortex, producing *ocular dominance columns.* Output cells from primary visual cortex (V1) then project to Brodmann's area 18 (V2). From area 18 neurons project to medial temporal (MT) cortex (area 19), to inferotemporal cortex (areas 20 and 21) and posterior parietal cortex (area 7). In addition, outputs go to the superior colliculus and back to the LGN (feedback control). The primary visual cortex contains a topographic map of the retina. In addition, the occipital lobe alone has six other representations of the retina.

The receptive fields of cells in the visual cortex are not circular but linear: the light must be in the shape of a line, a bar, or an edge to excite them. These are classified as *simple cells* or *complex cells.* Simple cells respond to bars, with an excitatory center and an inhibitory surround, or vice versa. They also have a specific axis of orientation for which the bar is most effective in exciting the cell. All axes of orientation for all parts of the retina are represented in the visual cortex. Results of experiments by Hubel and Wiesel (1959, 1962) suggest that this bar-shaped receptive field is created from many geniculate neurons with partially overlapping circular receptive fields in one line, converging onto a simple cortical cell. It has been suggested that complex cells have convergent input from many simple cells. Thus, their receptive fields are larger than simple cells and have a critical axis of orientation. For many complex cells, the most useful stimulus is movement across the field.

The visual cortex is divided into columns, with each column consisting of cells with one axis of orientation and neighboring columns receiving input from the left or right eye. Hubel and Wiesel used the name *hypercolumn* to describe a set of columns from one part of the retina, including all orientation angles for the two eyes (Hubel and Weisel, 1959, 1962).

Higher-Order Visual Cortex

Central visual processing pathways also include cells in the primary visual cortex in the occipital lobe and cells in the higher-order visual cortices in the temporal and parietal cortex. Higher-order cortices are involved in the integration of somatosensory and visual information underlying spatial orientation, an essential part of all actions. This interaction between visual and somatosensory inputs within higher-order association cortices was discussed in the somatosensory section of this chapter.

The cells within the visual pathways contribute to a *hierarchy* within the visual system, with each level of the hierarchy increasing the visual abstraction (Hubel, 1988). In addition, Ungerleider and Brody (1977) have proposed a model of two visual systems, with *parallel pathways* through which visual information is processed. It has been proposed that these two pathways can be traced to two main subdivisions of retinal ganglion cells, one of which synapses on the magnocellular layers (processing movement and coarse detail, or processing "where") and the other on the parvocellular layers (processing fine detail and color, or processing "what") of the LGN (Livingstone and Hubel, 1988).

One of these pathways, called the dorsal stream, terminates finally in the posterior parietal region. The second pathway, the ventral stream, terminates in the inferotemporal cortex. The authors noted that monkeys with lesions in the inferotemporal cortex were severely impaired in visual pattern discrimination and recognition but less impaired in solving tasks involving spatial visual cues. The opposite pattern of results was seen for monkeys with posterior parietal lesions (Ungerleider and Brody, 1977; Milner et al., 1977).

Interesting clinical evidence supports the existence of these parallel processing pathways. A perceptual deficit, movement agnosia, occurs after damage to the MT area or the medial superior temporal (MST) region of the cortex, which are part of the dorsal stream. Patients show a specific loss of motion perception without any other perceptual problems. Other patients with damage to Brodmann's area 18 or 37 (part of the ventral stream) lose only color vision (achromatopsia); they can still identify form. Still other patients lose the ability to identify forms with damage to areas 18, 20, and 21 (Kandel, 1991b).

How do we sense motion? The magnocellular pathway continues to areas MT and MST and the visual motor area of the parietal lobe (the dorsal stream). In MT the activity in the neurons is related to the velocity and movement direction of objects. This information is further processed in MST for visual perception, pursuit eye movements, and guiding the movements of the body through space. Area MST has also been implicated in the processing of optic flow, which plays a role in posture and balance control (Duffy and Wurtz, 1997).

More recent research (Goodale and Milner, 1992; Goodale et al., 1991) suggests

other functions for the dorsal and ventral streams. They suggest that the visual projection to the parietal cortex provides action-relevant information about the structure and orientation of objects and not just about their position. They also propose that projections to the temporal lobe may provide our conscious experience of visual perception.

Observations that support this model draw on the fact that most neurons in the dorsal stream area show both sensory-related and movement-related activity (Andersen, 1987). In addition, patients with optic ataxia due to lesions in the parietal areas have problems not only with reaching in the right direction but also with positioning their fingers or adjusting the orientation of their hand when reaching toward an object. They also have trouble adjusting their grasp to reflect the size of the object they are picking up. Goodale and colleagues note that damage to the parietal lobe can impair the ability of patients to use information about the size, shape, and orientation of an object to control the hand and fingers during a grasping movement, even though this same information can be used to identify and describe objects.

It is also interesting that the two cortical pathways are different with respect to their access to consciousness. One patient with ventral stream lesions had no conscious perception of the orientation or dimension of objects, but she could pick them up with great adeptness. Thus it may be that information in the dorsal system can be processed without reaching conscious perception (Goodale and Milner, 1992). As a result of their analysis of these observations, the authors propose that the ventral stream of projections plays a major role in the perceptual identification of objects, while the dorsal stream mediates the required sensorimotor transformations for visually guided actions directed at those objects (Goodale and Milner, 1992).

How do we take the information processed by these parallel pathways and organize it into a perceptual whole? This process by which the brain recombines information in its different regions is called the binding problem. The recombination of this information appears to require attention, which may be mediated by subcortical structures, such as the superior colliculus, and cortical areas, such as the posterior parietal and prefrontal cortex. It has been hypothesized that the CNS takes information related to color, size, distance, and orientation and organizes it into a master map of the image (Treisman, 1988). Our attentional systems allow us to focus on one small part of the master map as we identify objects or move through space.

Vestibular System

The vestibular system is sensitive to two types of information: the position of the head in space and sudden changes in the direction of movement of the head. Although we are not consciously aware of vestibular sensation as we are of the other senses, vestibular inputs are important for the coordination of many motor responses and help to stabilize the eyes and to maintain postural stability during standing and walking. Abnormalities within the vestibular system result in sensations such as dizziness or unsteadiness, which do reach our awareness, as well as problems with focusing our eyes and keeping our balance.

Like other sensory systems, the vestibular system can be divided into two parts, a peripheral and a central component. The peripheral component consists of the sensory receptors and eighth cranial nerve, while the central part consists of the four vestibular nuclei and the ascending and descending tracts.

Peripheral Receptors

Let's first look at the anatomy of the vestibular system (Fig. 3-11A). The vestibular system is part of the *membranous labyrinth* of the inner ear (right side of Fig. 3-11A). The other part of the labyrinth is the *cochlea*, which is concerned with hearing. The membranous labyrinth consists of a continuous series of tubes and sacs in the temporal bone of the skull. The membranous labyrinth is sur-

rounded by a fluid called the *perilymph* and filled with a fluid called the *endolymph*. The endolymph has a density greater than that of water, giving it inertial characteristics that are important to the way the vestibular system functions. The vestibular portion of the labyrinth includes five receptors: three *semicircular canals*, the *utricle*, and the *saccule*.

Semicircular Canals

The semicircular canals function as angular accelerometers. They lie at right angles to each other on either side of the head and are named the anterior, posterior, and horizontal canals (Fig. 3-11). At least one pair is affected by any given angular acceleration of the head or body. The sensory endings of the semicircular canals are in the enlarged end of each canal, the *ampulla*, near its junction with the utricle. Each ampulla has an *ampullary crest*, which contains the vestibular hair cells. The hair cells project upward into the *cupula* (Latin for small inverted cup), made of gelatinous material and extending to the top of the ampulla, preventing movement of the endolymph past the cupula. The hair cells are the vestibular receptors and are innervated by bipolar sensory neurons, which are part of the eighth nerve. Their cell bodies are in the vestibular ganglion (Kelly, 1991; Baloh, 1984).

How do the semicircular canals signal head motion to the nervous system? When the head starts to rotate, the fluid in the canals does not move initially because of its inertial characteristics. As a result, the cupula, along with its hair cells, bends in the direction opposite to head movement. When head motion stops, the cupula and hair cells are deflected in the opposite direction, that is, the direction in which the head was moving.

When the hair cells bend, they cause a change in the firing frequency of the nerve, depending on which way the hair cells bend. Each hair cell has a *kinocilium* (the tallest tuft) and 40 to 70 *stereocilia*, which increase in length as they get closer to the kinocilium. Bending the hair cell toward the kinocilium causes a depolarization of the hair cell and an increase in firing rate of the bipolar cells

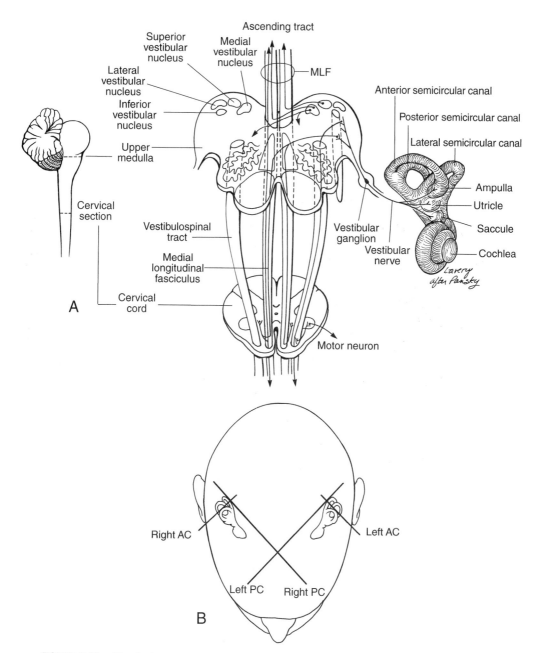

FIGURE 3-11. Vestibular system. **A.** The membranous labyrinth (otoliths and semicircular canals) and the central connections of the vestibular system with the ascending vestibular inputs to the oculomotor complex, important for stabilizing gaze, and the descending vestibulospinal system, important for posture and balance. **B.** The paired semicircular canals within the temporal bone of the skull. Lines show their orientation. AC, anterior canal; PC, posterior canal.

of the eighth nerve, and bending away causes hyperpolarization and a decrease in firing rate of bipolar cells. At rest the hair cells fire at 100 Hz, so they have a wide range of frequencies for modulation. Thus, changes in firing frequency of the neurons either up or down are possible because of this tonic resting discharge, which occurs in the absence of head motion (Kelly, 1991; Baloh, 1984).

Because canals on each side of the head are approximately parallel to one another, they work together in a reciprocal fashion. The two horizontal canals work together, while each anterior canal is paired with a posterior canal on the opposite side of the head, as you see in Figure 3-11*B*. When head motion occurs in a plane specific to a pair of canals, one canal is excited and its paired opposite canal is hyperpolarized.

Thus, angular motion of the head, either horizontal or vertical, results in either an increase or decrease in hair cell activity, which produces a parallel change in the frequency of neuronal activity in paired canals. Receptors in the semicircular canal are very sensitive: they respond to angular accelerations of 0.1 degree per second squared but do not respond to steady-state motion of the head. During prolonged motion of the head, the cupula returns to its resting position and firing frequency in the neurons returns to its steady state.

Utricle and Saccule

The utricle and saccule provide information about body position with reference to the force of gravity and linear acceleration or movement of the head in a straight line. On the wall of these structures is a thickening where the epithelium contains hair cells. The receptor cells are in this area, called the *macula* (Latin for spot). The hair cells project tufts or processes up into a gelatinous membrane, the *otolith organ* (Greek, from *lithos*, stone). The otolith organ has many calcium carbonate crystals called *otoconia*, or otoliths (Kelly, 1991).

The macula of the utricle lies in the horizontal plane when the head is held horizontally (normal position), so the otoliths rest upon it. But if the head is tilted or acceler-

ates, the movement of the gelatinous mass bends the hair cells. The macula of the saccule lies in the vertical plane when the head is positioned normally, so it responds selectively to vertical linear forces. As in the semicircular canals, hair cells in the otoliths respond to bending in a directional manner.

Central Connections

Vestibular Nuclei

Neurons from both the otoliths and the semicircular canals go through the eighth nerve and have their cell bodies in the vestibular ganglion (Scarpa's ganglion). The axons enter the brain in the pons and most go to the floor of the medulla, where the vestibular nuclei are, as you see in Figure 3-11*A*, center. There are four nuclei in the complex: the *lateral vestibular nucleus* (Deiters' nucleus), the *medial vestibular nucleus*, the *superior vestibular nucleus*, and the *inferior*, or *descending, vestibular nucleus*. A certain portion of the vestibular sensory receptors goes directly to the cerebellum, the reticular formation, the thalamus, and the cerebral cortex.

The lateral vestibular nucleus receives input from the utricle, semicircular canals, cerebellum, and spinal cord. The output contributes to vestibulo-ocular tracts and to the lateral vestibulospinal tract, which activates antigravity muscles in the neck, trunk, and limbs.

Inputs to the medial and superior nuclei are from the semicircular canals. The outputs of the medial nucleus are to the medial vestibulospinal tract (MVST), with connections to the cervical spinal cord, controlling the neck muscles. The MVST plays an important role in coordinating interactions between head and eye movements. In addition, neurons from the medial and superior nuclei ascend to motor nuclei of the eye muscles and aid in stabilizing gaze during head motions.

The inputs to the inferior vestibular nucleus include neurons from the semicircular canals, utricle, saccule, and cerebellar vermis, while the outputs are part of the vestibulospinal tract and vestibuloreticular tracts.

Ascending information from the vestibular system to the oculomotor complex is responsible for the *vestibulo-ocular reflex* (VOR), which rotates the eyes opposite to head movement, allowing the gaze to remain steady on an image even when the head is moving.

Vestibular nystagmus is the rapid alternating movement of the eyes in response to continued rotation of the body. One can create vestibular nystagmus in a subject by rotating to the left a person seated on a stool: when the acceleration first begins, the eyes go slowly to the right, to keep the eyes on a single point in space. When the eyes reach the end of the orbit, they reset by moving rapidly to the left; then they move again slowly to the right.

This alternating slow movement of the eyes in the direction opposite to head movement and rapid resetting of the eyes in the direction of head movement is called *nystagmus*. It is a normal consequence of acceleration of the head. However, when nystagmus occurs without head movement, it is usually an indication of dysfunction in the peripheral nervous system or CNS.

Postrotatory nystagmus, a reversal in the direction of nystagmus, occurs when a person who is spinning stops abruptly. Postrotatory nystagmus has been used clinically to evaluate the function of the vestibular system (Ayres, 1972).

The vestibular apparatus has both static and dynamic functions. The dynamic functions are controlled mainly by the semicircular canals, allowing us to sense head rotation and angular accelerations and to control the eyes through the VOR. The static functions are controlled by the utricle and saccule, allowing us to monitor absolute position of the head in space, and they are important in posture. (The utricle and saccule also detect linear acceleration, a dynamic function.)

✆ ACTION SYSTEMS

The action system includes areas of the nervous system such as motor cortex, cerebellum, and basal ganglia, which perform processing essential to the coordination of movement.

Remember the example presented in the beginning of this chapter. You're thirsty and want to pour some milk from the carton in front of you into a glass. We have already seen how sensory structures help you form the map of your body in space and locate the milk carton relative to your arm. Now you need to generate the movements that will allow you to pick up the carton and pour the milk. You need a plan to move, you need to specify specific muscles (both timing and force), and you need a way to modify and refine the movement. So let's look at the structures that allow you to do that.

Motor Cortex

Primary Motor Cortex and Corticospinal Tract

The motor cortex, which is in the frontal lobe, consists of a number of processing areas, including the *primary motor cortex* (MI) the *supplementary motor area*, (occasionally called MII), and the *premotor cortex*, shown in Figure 3-12A. These areas interact with sensory processing areas in the parietal lobe and with basal ganglia and cerebellar areas to identify where we want to move, to plan the movement, and finally to execute our actions (Ghez, 1991c).

All three of these areas have their own somatotopic maps of the body, so that if different regions are stimulated, different muscles and body parts move. The primary motor cortex (Brodmann's area 4) contains a complex map of the body. There is often a one-to-one correspondence between cells stimulated and the activation of individual α-motor neurons in the spinal cord. In contrast to a one-to-one activation pattern typical of neurons in the primary motor cortex, stimulation of neurons in the premotor and supplementary motor areas (Brodmann's area 6) typically activates multiple muscles at multiple joints, giving coordinated actions.

The motor map, or motor homunculus (Fig. 3-12B), is similar to the sensory map in the way it distorts the representations of the body. In both cases, the areas that require the most detailed control (the mouth, throat, and hand), allowing finely graded

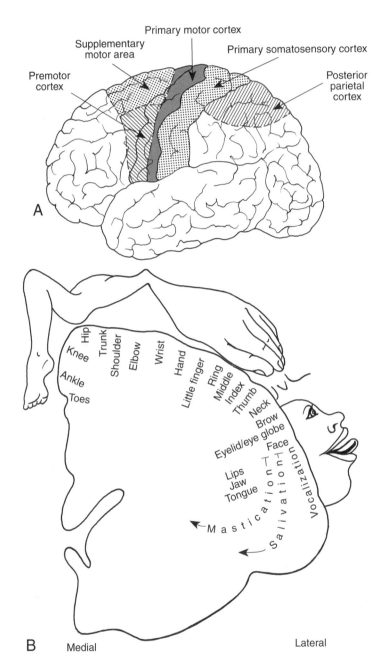

FIGURE 3-12. Motor cortex. **A.** Lateral view of the brain showing the location of the primary motor cortex, supplementary motor area, and premotor cortex. **B.** Motor homunculus. (Adapted from Kandel E, Schwartz JH, Jessell TM, eds. Principles of neuroscience. 3rd ed. New York: Elsevier, 1991:610, 613.)

movements, are most highly represented (Penfield and Rassmussen, 1950).

Inputs to the motor areas come from the basal ganglia, the cerebellum, and sensory areas, including the periphery via the thalamus, SI, and sensory association areas in the parietal lobe. Interestingly, MI neurons receive sensory inputs from their own muscles and from the skin above the muscles. It has been suggested that this transcortical pathway may be used in parallel with the spinal reflex pathway to give additional force output in the muscles when an unexpected load is encountered during a movement. This pathway has also been hypothesized to be an important proprioceptive pathway functioning in postural control.

Outputs from the motor cortex contribute to the *corticospinal tract* (also called the *pyramidal tract*) and often make excitatory monosynaptic connections onto α-motor neurons, in addition to polysynaptic connections to γ-motor neurons, which control muscle spindle length. In addition to their monosynaptic connections, corticospinal neurons make many polysynaptic connections through interneurons within the spinal cord.

The corticospinal tract, shown in Figure 3-13, includes neurons from primary motor cortex (about 50%), supplementary motor cortex, premotor areas, and even somatosensory cortex. The fibers descend ipsilaterally from the cortex through the internal capsule, the midbrain, and the medulla. In the medulla, the fibers concentrate to form pyramids, and near the junction of the medulla and the spinal cord, most (90%) cross to form the lateral corticospinal tract. The remaining 10% continue uncrossed to form the anterior corticospinal tract. Most of the anterior corticospinal neurons cross just before they terminate in the ventral horn of the spinal cord. Most axons enter the ventral horn and terminate in the intermediate and ventral areas on interneurons and motor neurons.

What is the specific function of primary motor cortex and corticospinal tract in movement control? Evarts (1968) recorded the activity of corticospinal neurons in mon-

keys while they made wrist flexion and extension movements. He found that the firing rate of the corticospinal neurons codes (*a*) the force used to move a limb, and (*b*) in some cases, the rate of change of force. Thus, both absolute force and the speed of a movement are controlled by the primary motor cortex.

Now, think about a typical movement that we make—reaching for the carton of milk, for example. How does the motor cortex encode the execution of such a complex movement? Researchers performed experiments in which a monkey made arm movements to many targets around a central starting point (Georgopoulos et al., 1982). They found specific movement directions for which each neuron was activated maximally, yet each responded for a wide range of movement directions. To explain how movements can be finely controlled when neurons are so broadly tuned, these researchers suggested that actions are controlled by a population of neurons. The activity of each of the neurons can be represented as a vector whose length represents the degree of activity in any direction. The sum of the vectors of all of the neurons predicts the direction and amplitude of the movement.

If this is the case, does it mean that whenever we make a movement, for example with our hand, the exact same neurons are activated in the primary motor cortex? No. Specific neurons in the cortex, activated when we pick up an object, may remain silent when we make a similar movement, such as a gesture in anger. This is a very important point because it implies many parallel motor pathways for carrying out an action sequence, just as there are parallel pathways for sensory processing. Thus, simply by training a patient in one situation, we cannot automatically assume that the training will transfer to all other activities requiring the same set of muscles (Ghez, 1991c).

Supplementary and Premotor Areas

What are the functions of the supplementary and premotor areas? Both the premotor area and the supplementary motor areas

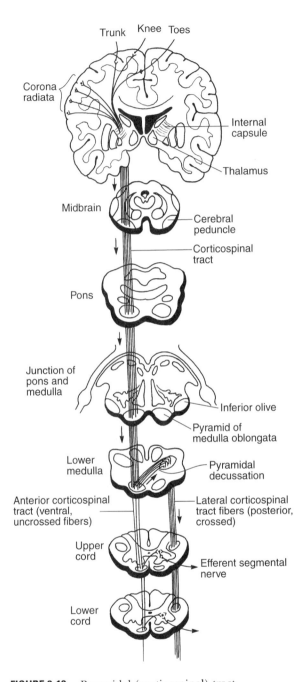

FIGURE 3-13.   Pyramidal (corticospinal) tract.

send projections to primary motor cortex; however, they receive largely distinct inputs from the thalamus and other cortical areas. This suggests that they may have very different functions.

Researchers (Roland et al., 1980; Lang et al., 1990) have examined the role of the supplementary cortex in humans and have begun to clarify its functions. Roland et al. (1980) asked subjects to perform tasks ranging from very simple to complex movements, and while the subjects were making the movements, the investigators assessed the amount of cerebral blood flow in different areas of the brain. (To measure blood flow one injects short-lived radioactive tracer into the blood, then measures the radioactivity in different brain areas with detectors on the scalp).

As shown in Figure 3-14, when subjects were asked to perform a simple task (simple repetitive movements of the index finger or pressing a spring between the thumb and index finger) the blood flow increase was only in primary motor and sensory cortex. In contrast, when they were asked to perform a complex task (a sequence of movements involving all four fingers, touching the thumb in different orders), subjects showed a blood flow increase in the supplementary motor area bilaterally and in the primary motor and sensory areas. Finally, when they were asked to rehearse the task but not perform it, the blood flow increase was only in the supplementary motor area, not the primary sensory or motor cortex. Roland concluded that the supplementary motor area is active when a sequence of simple ballistic movements is planned. Thus he proposed that it participates in the assembly of the central motor program or forms a motor subroutine.

More recent work by Mushiake et al. (1991) has suggested that both premotor and supplementary motor areas may be involved in the performance of a sequential motor task. However, neurons in premotor and supplementary motor areas differed in their activity depending on how the movement was initiated and guided. Premotor neurons were more active when the sequential task was visually guided, while supple-

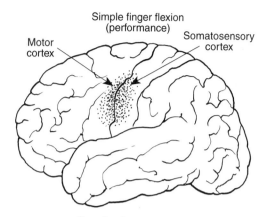
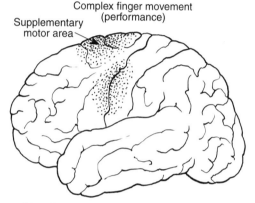
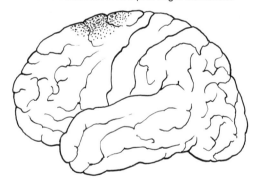

FIGURE 3-14. Changes in blood flow during different motor behaviors indicating the areas of the motor cortex involved in the behavior. (Adapted with permission from Roland PE, Larsen B, Lassen NA, Skinhof E. Supplementary motor area and other cortical areas in organization of voluntary movements in man. J Neurophysiol 1980;43: 118–136.)

mentary motor area neurons were more active when the sequence was remembered and self determined. Previous researchers proposed a hypothesis about the functional specialization of the supplementary motor area and premotor cortex, based on different phylogenetic origins, with the supplementary motor area being specialized for controlling internally referenced motor output and the premotor cortex specialized for control of externally referenced motor acts (Roland et al., 1980; Passingham, 1985). Studies also indicate that premotor lesions cause impairment of retrieval of movements in accordance with visual cues, while supplementary motor area lesions disrupt retrieval of self-initiated movements (Passingham, 1985; Passingham et al., 1989).

Interestingly, the supplementary motor area receives inputs from the putamen of the basal ganglia complex, while the premotor area receives inputs from the cerebellum. In Parkinson's disease there is massive depletion of dopamine in the putamen, and patients with Parkinson's disease have difficulty initiating movements such as walking. Thus Parkinson's disease may cause impaired input to the supplementary cortex, which results in bradykinesia, or slowness in initiating movement (Marsden, 1989).

Work by Rizzolatti et al. (1988) suggests an interesting function of the premotor area F5 in reaching. They recorded from single neurons in F5 in monkeys during reaching. They found that an important property of most (85%) of these neurons was their selectivity for different types of hand grip: precision grip (most common), finger prehension and whole-hand prehension. Interestingly, precision grip neurons were activated only by small visual objects. Recent research on hand movements has also found neurons in the anterior intraparietal cortex (AIP) that are connected closely with area F5. These AIP neurons could be either visually or motor dominant and appeared to encode the three-dimensional (3D) features of objects in a way that was suitable to guide the movements for grasping them (Jeannerod et al., 1995; Taira et al., 1990).

When the properties of parietal and F5 premotor neurons were compared, they were found to be similar, but visual responses to 3D objects were more common in the parietal cortex. The motor-dominant neurons in the parietal lobe appeared to encode precision grip, whole hand prehension, etc., but were activated during the entire action, while F5 premotor area neurons were activated only during a segment of the action. Interestingly, neurons in the primary motor cortex to which F5 projects, code for even smaller fragments of movements. This suggests that the parietal neurons involved in manipulation (in area AIP) play a role in the visuomotor transformation involved in grasping objects (Jeannerod et al., 1995).

Higher-Level Association Areas

Association Areas of the Frontal Region

The association areas of the frontal regions (areas rostral to Brodmann's area 6) are important for motor planning and other cognitive behaviors. For example, these areas have been hypothesized to integrate sensory information and then select the appropriate motor response from the many possible responses (Fuster, 1989).

The prefrontal cortex may be divided into the principal sulcus and the prefrontal convexities. Experiments have indicated that the neurons of the principal sulcus are involved in the strategic planning of higher motor functions. For example, monkeys with lesions in this area had difficulty performing spatial tasks in which information had to be stored in working memory to guide future action. This area is densely interconnected with the posterior parietal areas. These areas are hypothesized to work closely together in spatial tasks that require attention.

Lesions in the prefrontal convexity, by contrast, cause problems in performing any kind of delayed-response task. Animals with these lesions have problems with tasks for which they have to inhibit certain motor responses at specific moments. Lesions in adjacent areas cause problems with a monkey's ability to select from a variety of motor responses when they are given different sensory cues (Kupfermann, 1991a).

Lesions in other prefrontal regions cause patients to have difficulty changing strategies when they are asked to. Even when they are shown their errors, they fail to correct them.

Cerebellum

The cerebellum is considered one of three important brain areas contributing to coordination of movement, in addition to the motor cortex and basal ganglia. Yet despite its important role in the coordination of movement, the cerebellum does not play a primary role in either sensory or motor function. If the cerebellum is destroyed, we do not lose sensation or become paralyzed. However, lesions of the cerebellum do produce devastating changes in our ability to perform movements, from the very simple to the most elegant. The cerebellum receives afferent information from almost every sensory system, consistent with its role as a regulator of motor output (Ghez, 1991c; Ito, 1984).

How does the cerebellum adjust the output of the motor systems? Its function is related to its neuronal circuitry. It appears that through this circuitry and its input and output connections, it acts as a comparator, a system that compensates for errors by comparing intention with performance.

The cerebellum's input and output connections are vital to its role as error detector; they are summarized in Figure 3-15. It receives information from other modules of the brain related to the programming and execution of movements (corticopontine areas). This information is often called *efference copy* or *corollary discharge* when it comes from the primary motor cortex, since it is hypothesized to be a direct copy of the motor cortex output to the spinal cord. The cerebellum also receives sensory feedback information (reafference) from the receptors about the movements as they are being made (spinal and trigeminal somatosensory inputs; visual, auditory, and vestibular inputs). After processing this information, outputs (Fig. 3-

15*B*) from the cerebellum go to the motor cortex and other systems within the brainstem to modulate their motor output. In addition to its role in motor control processes, research has recently suggested that the cerebellum may have important nonmotor functions, including cognition, discussed later in the chapter (Fiez et al., 1992).

Anatomy of the Cerebellum

An understanding of the anatomy of the cerebellum is helpful in explaining its function. The cerebellum consists of an outer layer of gray matter (the cortex), internal white matter (input and output fibers), and three pairs of *deep nuclei*: the *fastigial nucleus*, the *interposed nucleus*, and the *dentate nucleus*. All inputs to the cerebellum go first to one of these three deep cerebellar nuclei and then go on to the cortex. All outputs of the cerebellum go back to the deep nuclei before going on to the cerebral cortex or the brainstem (Ghez, 1991c; Ito, 1984).

The cerebellum can be divided into three phylogenetic zones (Fig. 3-15). The oldest zone corresponds to the *flocculonodular lobe* and is functionally related to the vestibular system. The phylogenetically more recent areas to develop are the (*a*) *vermis* and *intermediate* part of the hemispheres and the (*b*) *lateral hemispheres*. These three parts of the cerebellum have distinct functions and distinct input–output connections, as you see in Figure 3-15.

Flocculonodular Lobe

The flocculonodular lobe receives inputs from both the visual system and the vestibular system, and its outputs return to the vestibular nuclei. It functions in the control of the axial muscles, which are used in equilibrium control. A dysfunction in this system produces an ataxic gait, wide-based stance, and nystagmus.

Vermis and Intermediate Hemispheres

The vermis and intermediate hemispheres receive proprioceptive and cutaneous inputs from the spinal cord via the spinocerebellar tracts in addition to visual, vestibular, and auditory information. Re-

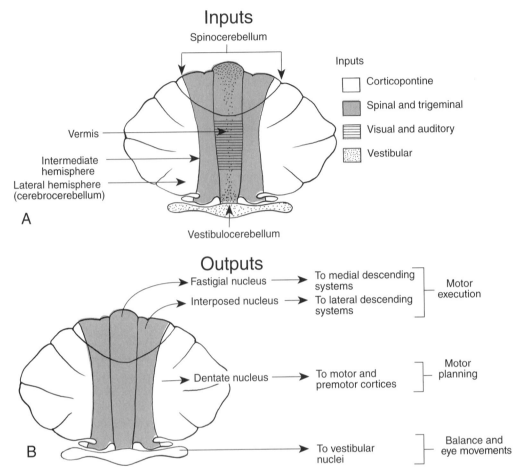

FIGURE 3-15.   The basic anatomy of the cerebellum, including **(A)** its inputs and **(B)** its outputs. The white area represents the lateral cerebellum with inputs from the corticopontine systems. The shaded area represents the spinocerebellum with inputs from the spinal and trigeminal somatosensory systems. The stippled (visual and auditory) and lined (vestibular) areas receive inputs from other sensory systems. (Adapted with permission from Ghez C. The cerebellum. In: Kandel E, Schwartz JH, Jessell TM, eds. Principles of neuroscience. 3rd ed. New York: Elsevier, 1991:633.)

searchers used to think that there were two maps of the complete body in the cerebellum, but now it has been shown that the maps are much more complex and can be divided into many smaller maps. This has been called *fractured somatotopy*. These smaller maps appear to be related to functional activities: thus, in the rat, the mouth and paw receptive fields are close together, possibly to contribute to the control of grooming behavior. Inputs to this part of the cerebellum go through the fastigial nucleus (vermis) and interposed nucleus (intermediate lobes) (Shambes et al., 1978).

Four spinocerebellar tracts relay informa-

tion from the spinal cord to the cerebellum. Two tracts relay information from the arms and the neck and two relay information from the trunk and legs. Inputs also come from the spino-olivocerebellar tract through the inferior olivary nucleus (climbing fibers). These inputs, which are important in learning, are discussed later.

What are the output pathways of this part of the cerebellum? The outputs go to the (*a*) brainstem reticular formation, (*b*) vestibular nuclei, (*c*) thalamus and motor cortex, and (*d*) red nucleus in the midbrain.

What are the functions of the vermis and intermediate lobes? First, they appear to function in the control of the actual execution of movement: they correct for deviations from an intended movement by comparing feedback from the spinal cord with the intended motor command. They also modulate muscle tone. This occurs through the continuous output of excitatory activity from the fastigial and interpositus nucleus, which modulates the activity of the γ-motor neurons to the muscle spindles. When there are lesions in these nuclei, there is a significant drop in muscle tone (hypotonia) (Ghez, 1991c).

Lateral Hemispheres

The last part of the cerebellum and the newest phylogenetically is the lateral zone of the cerebellar hemispheres (Fig. 3-15). It has undergone a marked expansion in the course of human evolution, which has added many nonmotor functions to its repertoire. It receives inputs from the pontine nuclei in the brainstem that relay information from wide areas of the cerebral cortex (sensory, motor, premotor, and posterior parietal). Its outputs are to the thalamus and then to the motor, premotor, and prefrontal cortex (Middleton and Strick, 1994).

What is the function of the lateral hemispheres? This part of the cerebellum appears to have a number of higher-level functions involving both motor and nonmotor skills. First, research suggests that it is involved in the preparation of movement, whereas the intermediate lobes function in movement execution and fine tuning of ongoing movement via feedback information. It appears that the lateral hemispheres of the cerebellum participate in programming the motor cortex for the execution of movement. The cerebellar pathways are a part of many parallel pathways affecting the motor cortex.

The lateral hemispheres also appear to function in the coordination of ongoing movements. Cooling parts of the cerebellum disturbs the timing of agonist and antagonist muscle responses during rapid movements (Brooks and Thatch, 1981). The antagonist activity is delayed, giving a hypermetric, or overshooting, movement. As corrections are attempted in patients with cerebellar lesions,

one sees unintended movements in the opposite direction, giving intention tremor.

Cerebellar Involvement in Nonmotor Tasks

Recent research has suggested that the lateral cerebellum, in addition to its role in motor control processes, may have important nonmotor functions, including cognition (Fiez et al., 1992). Neuroanatomical experiments have shown projections from the lateral dentate nucleus of the cerebellum to frontal association areas known to be involved in higher-level cognitive processing (Middleton and Strick, 1994). These connections suggest that subjects do not have to make a movement to activate the cerebellum; research measuring cerebral blood flow has shown an increase in cerebellar activity when subjects are asked only to imagine making a movement (Decety et al., 1990).

Ivry and Keele (1989) have shown that the cerebellum has important timing functions, with patients with cerebellar lesions showing problems in both timing production and perception. Patients with lateral-hemisphere lesions showed errors in timing related to perceptual abilities, which researchers think may be related to a central clocklike mechanism. In contrast, patients with intermediate-lobe lesions made errors related to movement execution.

Many parts of the cerebellum, including the lateral cerebellum, seem to be important in both motor and nonmotor learning. The unique cellular circuitry of the cerebellum has been shown to be perfect for the long-term modification of motor responses. As animals learn a new task, the climbing fiber, which detects movement error, changes the effectiveness of the synapse between the granule cell parallel fiber and the Purkinje cells (the main output cells of the cerebellum) (Gilbert and Thatch, 1977).

This type of cerebellar learning also appears to occur in the VOR circuitry, which includes cerebellar pathways. The VOR keeps the eyes fixed on an object when the head turns. In experiments in which humans wore prismatic lenses that reversed the image on the eye, the gain of the VOR was altered over time. This modification of the VOR did not occur in patients with cerebellar lesions (Gonshor and Melville-Jones, 1976).

The right lateral cerebellum becomes active when subjects read aloud verbs but not when they read nouns, implying that something about the cognitive processing of verb generation requires the cerebellum, where the same processing of other words does not. Correlated with this, certain patients with cerebellar deficits also showed difficulty in these verb generation tasks and in learning and performing a variety of tasks involving complex nonmotor (cognitive) cortical processing. This is the case even though scores on intelligence, language, frontal function, and memory were normal. For example, patients showed problems in detecting errors they made in nonmotor and motor tasks. This implies that they had problems with both perception and production processes in higher-order analyses, including those involving language (Fiez et al., 1992).

Research on learning problems in patients with cerebellar lesions has shown that while they had normal scores on the Wechsler Memory Scale, they had problems with some types of learned responses. Problems were found particularly in recalling habits, defined as automatic responses learned though repetition. This is opposite to the learning problems seen in patients with severe amnesia resulting from hippocampal and/or midline diencephalic damage, who do not learn tasks that rely upon conscious recall of previous experience but who show normal improvement on a variety of skill learning tasks that involve repetition (Squire, 1986; Fiez et al., 1992).

Certain neurons in the dentate nucleus of the cerebellum are preferentially involved in the generation and/or guidance of movement based on visual cues. As mentioned earlier, these neurons project to the premotor areas of the cerebral cortex (Mushiake and Strick, 1993). Patients with cerebellar deficits showed improved motor performance when their eyes were closed or when visual feedback was reduced. In fact, Sanes et al. (1988) noted that cerebellar tremor was greatest when patients used visual cues to guide movements.

Basal Ganglia

The basal ganglia complex consists of a set of nuclei at the base of the cerebral cortex, including the *putamen, caudate nucleus, globus pallidus, subthalamic nucleus*, and *substantia nigra*. Basal literally means at the base, in other words, just below the cortex. As with patients with cerebellar lesions, patients with basal ganglia damage are not paralyzed, but they have problems with the coordination of movement. Advancement in our understanding of basal ganglia function first came from clinicians, especially James Parkinson, who in 1817 first described Parkinson's disease as "the shaking palsy" (Cote and Crutcher, 1991).

The basal ganglia were once believed to be part of the extrapyramidal motor system, which was believed to act in parallel with the pyramidal system (the corticospinal tract) in movement control. Thus clinicians defined pyramidal problems as relating to spasticity and paralysis, while extrapyramidal problems were defined as involuntary movements and rigidity. As we have seen in this chapter, this distinction is not valid, since many other brain systems also control movement. In addition, the pyramidal and extrapyramidal systems are not independent but work together in controlling movements.

Anatomy of the Basal Ganglia

The major connections of the basal ganglia are summarized in Figure 3-16. They include the major afferent (Fig. 3-16A), internal (Fig. 3-16B), and efferent (Fig. 3-16C) connections. The main input nuclei of the basal ganglia complex are the caudate and the putamen. The caudate and the putamen develop from the same structure and are often discussed as a single unit, the *striatum*. Their primary inputs are from widespread areas of the neocortex, including sensory, motor, and association areas (Alexander and Crutcher, 1990).

The globus pallidus has two segments, internal and external, and it lies next to the

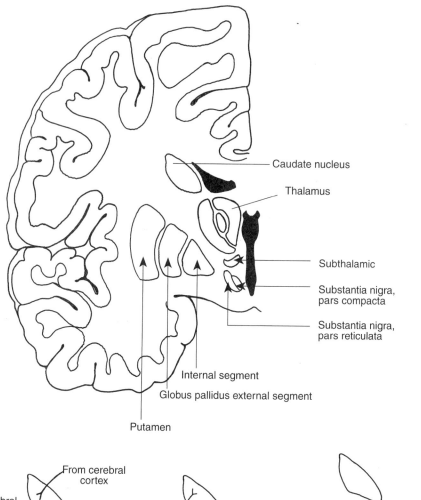

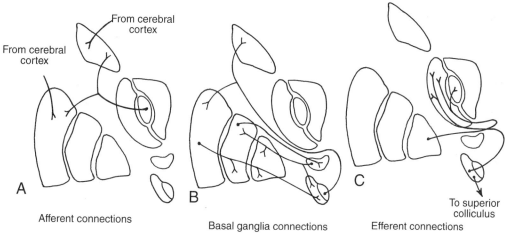

FIGURE 3-16. *Top.* Locations of the nuclei of the basal ganglia complex. *Bottom.* The major afferent (**A**), internal (**B**), and efferent (**C**) connections of the basal ganglia. (Adapted with permission from Cote L, Crutcher MD. The basal ganglia. In: Kandel E, Schwartz JH, Jessell TM, eds. Principles of neuroscience. 3rd ed. New York: Elsevier, 1991:649.)

putamen, while the substantia nigra is a little more caudal, in the midbrain, as shown in the top half of Figure 3-16. The internal segment of the globus pallidus and the substantia nigra are the major output areas of the basal ganglia. Their outputs terminate in the prefrontal, supplementary, and premotor cortex areas by way of the thalamus. The final nucleus, the subthalamic nucleus, is just below the thalamus.

The connections within the basal ganglia complex are as follows: Cells in both the caudate and putamen terminate in the globus pallidus and the substantia nigra in a somatotopic manner, as seen for other pathways in the brain. Cells from the external segment of the globus pallidus terminate in the subthalamic nucleus, while the subthalamic nucleus in turn projects to the globus pallidus and substantia nigra. Other inputs to the subthalamic nucleus include direct inputs from the motor and premotor cortex.

Role of the Basal Ganglia

The basal ganglia and cerebellum have many similarities in the way they interact with the rest of the elements of the motor system. But what are their differences? First, their input connections are different. The cerebellum receives input only from the sensory and motor areas of the cerebral cortex, and it receives visual, auditory, vestibular, and somatosensory information directly from the spinal cord. However, the basal ganglia complex is the termination site for tracts from the entire cerebral cortex but not the spinal cord (Alexander and Crutcher, 1990; Cote and Crutcher, 1991).

Their outputs also influence different parts of the motor system. The basal ganglia complex sends its outputs to the prefrontal, premotor and supplementary motor cortex areas, which are involved in higher-level processing of movement. The cerebellar output goes to prefrontal and premotor areas, the motor cortex, and also to the spinal cord via brainstem pathways. As was noted in the section on premotor versus supplementary motor areas of the cortex, premotor areas are

more involved with visually triggered and guided movements, while supplementary motor areas are more involved in self-initiated movements.

This research suggests that the basal ganglia may be particularly concerned with internally generated movements, while the cerebellum is involved in visually triggered and guided movements. Experiments have shown that in the internal globus pallidus, cells that project to the supplementary motor area are activated during internally generated movements (Mushiake and Strick, 1995). This is consistent with clinical data demonstrating that persons with Parkinson's disease have a great deal of difficulty with internally generated movements (Georgiou et al., 1993; Morris et al., 1996a,b). Patients with Parkinson's disease who have frozen gait syndrome (difficulty initiating or maintaining gait) are able to use visual cues to improve their walking abilities. This research suggests that this may be due to the use of alternative pathways from the cerebellum to trigger and guide the movements.

It has been hypothesized that the basal ganglia may play a role in selectively activating some movements as they suppress others (Alexander and Crutcher, 1990). Diseases of the basal ganglia typically produce involuntary movements (dyskinesia), poverty and slowness of movement, and disorders of muscle tone and postural reflexes. Parkinson's disease symptoms include resting tremor, increased muscle tone or rigidity, and slowness in the initiation of movement (akinesia) and in the execution of movement (bradykinesia). The site of the lesion is in the dopaminergic pathway from the substantia nigra to the striatum. The tremor and rigidity may be due to loss of inhibitory influences within the basal ganglia. Huntington's disease characteristics include chorea and dementia. Symptoms appear to be caused by loss of cholinergic neurons and GABA-ergic neurons in the striatum (Alexander and Crutcher, 1990; Cote and Crutcher, 1991).

This concludes our review of the physiological basis for motor control. In this chapter we showed you the neural substrates for movement. This involved a review of the perception and action systems and of the higher-level cognitive processes that play a part in their elaboration. We showed the importance of both the hierarchical and distributed nature of these systems. The presentation of the perception and action systems separately is somewhat misleading. In real life, as movements arc generated to accomplish tasks in varied environments, the boundaries between perception, action, and cognition are blurred.

☺ SUMMARY

1. Movement control is achieved through the cooperative effort of many brain structures, which are organized both hierarchically and in parallel.

2. Sensory inputs perform many functions in the control of movement. They (*a*) serve as the stimuli for reflexive movement organized in the spinal cord, (*b*) modulate the output of movement that results from the activity of pattern generators in the spinal cord, (*c*) modulate commands that originate in higher centers of the nervous system, and (*d*) contribute to the perception and control of movement through ascending pathways in much more complex ways.

3. In the somatosensory system, muscle spindles, GTOs, joint receptors, and cutaneous receptors contribute to spinal reflex control, modulate spinal pattern generator output, modulate descending commands, and contribute to perception and control of movement through ascending pathways.

4. Vision (*a*) allows us to identify objects in space and to determine their movement (exteroceptive sensation) and (*b*) gives us information about where our body is in space, the relation of one body part to another, and the motion of our body (visual proprioception).

5. The vestibular system is sensitive to two types of information: the position of the head in space and sudden changes in the direction of movement of the head.

6. As sensory information ascends to higher levels of processing, every level of the hierarchy can modulate the information coming into it from below, letting higher centers selectively tune (up or down) the information coming from lower centers.

7. Information from sensory receptors is increasingly processed as it ascends the neural hierarchy, enabling meaningful interpretation of the information. This is done by selectively enlarging the receptive field of each successively higher neuron.

8. The somatosensory and visual systems process incoming information to increase contrast sensitivity so that we can more easily identify and discriminate between different objects. This is done through lateral inhibition, in which the cell that is excited inhibits the cells next to it, enhancing contrast between excited and nonexcited regions of the body or visual field.

9. There are special cells within the somatosensory cortex and visual systems that respond best to moving stimuli and that are directionally sensitive.

10. In the association cortices we begin to see the transition from perception to action. The parietal lobe participates in processes involving attention to the position and manipulation of objects in space.

11. The action system includes areas of the nervous system such as motor cortex, cerebellum and basal ganglia.

12. The motor cortex interacts with sensory processing areas in the parietal lobe and also with basal ganglia and cerebellar areas to identify where we want to move, to plan the movement, and finally, to execute our actions.

13. The cerebellum appears to act as a comparator, a system that compensates for errors by comparing intention with performance. In addition, it modulates muscle tone, participates in the programming of the motor cortex for the execution of movement, and contributes to the timing of movement and

to motor and nonmotor learning. It is involved in the control of visually triggered and guided movements.

14. Basal ganglia function is related to the planning and control of complex motor behavior, controlling self-initiated movements through outputs to supplementary motor areas. In addition, it may play a role in selectively activating some movements and suppressing others.

CHAPTER 4

Physiological Basis of Motor Learning and Recovery of Function

✆ INTRODUCTION

In Chapter 2 we defined *learning* as the process of acquiring knowledge about the world and *motor learning* as the process of the acquisition and/or modification of movement. We also mentioned that just as motor control must be seen in light of the interaction between the individual, the task, and the environment, this also applies to motor learning.

In this chapter we extend our discussion of the physiological basis of motor control to include motor learning. We show that the physiological basis for motor learning, like motor control, is distributed among many brain structures and processing levels, rather than being localized to a particular learning site of the brain. Likewise, the physiological basis for the recovery of function is similar to learning in that recovery involves processes occurring throughout the nervous system and not just at the lesioned site. These processes have many properties in common with those occurring during learning.

This chapter focuses on the physiological basis of motor learning and recovery of function, showing the similarities and differences between these important functions. The material in this chapter builds on material presented in the chapter on the physiological basis of motor control. Since we assume that the reader has a basic familiarity with the concepts presented in Chapter 3, these concepts will not be reviewed again in this chapter.

Integral to a discussion on the physiological basis of motor learning are issues related to neural plasticity. A fundamental question addressed in this chapter is what is the relationship between neural plasticity and motor learning? Specifically we want to know how learning modifies the structure and function of neurons in the brain. Of equal concern is understanding the relationship between neural plasticity and recovery of function. Specifically we want to know what changes in the structure and function of neurons underlie the recovery of function following injury. We will also look at research that explores whether physiological plasticity associated with recovery of function is the same or different from that involved with learning. Previous views have typically held that recovery of function and learning are served by different neural mechanisms. More recent physiological studies suggest that the same mechanisms of neural plasticity underlie both recovery of function and learning. Finally, in this chapter we consider how developmental processes modify the neural mechanisms underlying both learning and recovery of function. During development, synaptic connectivity develops and is fine-tuned during critical periods by interacting environmental and genetic factors. Thus developmental factors play a significant role in how plasticity manifests throughout life.

Defining Neural Plasticity

Plasticity is a general term describing the ability to show modification. Throughout this book we use the term plasticity in reference to mechanisms related to neural modifiability. Plasticity, or neural modifiability, may be seen as a continuum from short-term changes in the efficiency or strength of synaptic connections to long-term structural changes in the organization and numbers of connections among neurons.

Learning also can be seen as a continuum of short-term to long-term changes in the ability to produce skilled actions. The gradual shift from short-term to long-term learning reflects a move along the continuum of neural modifiability, as increased synaptic efficiency gradually gives way to structural changes, which are the underpinning of long-term modification of behavior. This relationship is shown in Figure 4-1.

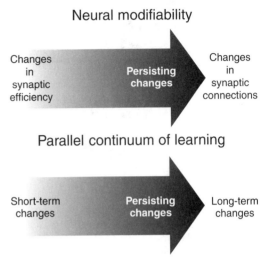

FIGURE 4-1. The gradual shift from short-term to long-term learning reflected in a move along the continuum of neural modifiability. Short-term changes, associated with an increased synaptic efficiency, persist and gradually give way to structural changes, the underpinning of long-term learning.

Like learning, recovery of function can be characterized by a continuum of changes from short-term functional changes that immediately follow injury, like unmasking of existing but weak connections, to long-term structural changes, such as remapping of sensory or motor cortex.

Learning and Memory

Learning is defined as the acquisition of knowledge or ability; memory is the retention and storage of that knowledge or ability (Kupfermann, 1991b). Learning reflects the *process* by which we acquire knowledge; memory is the *product* of that process. Memory storage is often divided into short-term and long-term components. **Short-term memory** refers to *working* memory, which has a limited capacity for information and lasts for only a few moments. Short-term memory reflects momentary attention to something, such as when we remember a phone number only long enough to dial it and then it's gone.

Long-term memory is intimately related to the process of learning. Long-term memory can also be seen as a continuum. Initial stages of long-term memory formation reflect functional changes in the efficiency of synapses. Later stages of memory formation reflect structural changes in synaptic connections. These memories are less subject to disruption.

Localization of Learning and Memory

Are learning and memory localized in a specific brain structure? It appears that they are not. In fact, learning can occur in all parts of the brain. Learning and the storage of that learning, memory, appear to involve both parallel and hierarchical processing within the central nervous system (CNS). Even for relatively simple learning tasks, multiple parallel channels of information are used. In addition, the information can be stored in many areas of the brain.

Apparently, mechanisms underlying learning and memory are the same whether the learning is occurring in fairly simple circuits or in complex circuits incorporating many aspects of the CNS hierarchy. Thus, current neuronal models of memory suggest that a memory consists of a pattern of changes in synaptic connections among networks of neurons distributed throughout the brain. It is interesting to note that Lashley, in 1929, was the first to hypothesize that memory was stored throughout the nervous system (Lashley, 1929, 1950). To try to find the location of memory storage, he performed experiments in which he made lesions to many areas of the cortex of animals. To his surprise he found that loss of memory abilities was not related to the site of the lesion but to the amount of cortex lesioned.

This chapter describes the continuum of plasticity within the nervous system that represents learning and specifically motor learning. It describes the processes underlying learning in the nervous system and those that underlie recovery of function. Once these processes are understood, principles of plasticity related to learning and recovery of function can be derived. Then, in later chapters, we apply these principles to therapy settings.

☺ PLASTICITY AND LEARNING

Many factors potentially modify synaptic connections. We are concerned in this chapter with *activity-dependent* modifications of synaptic connections, that is, both the *transient* and *long-term modulation* of synapses resulting from experience. Learning alters our capability for acting by changing both the effectiveness and anatomic connections of neural pathways. We discuss modifications of synaptic connections at both the cellular level and at the level of whole networks of neurons.

Plasticity and Nonassociative Forms of Learning

Remember that in *nonassociative* forms of learning, the person is learning about the properties of a stimulus that is repeated. The learned suppression of a response to a nonnoxious stimulus is called *habituation*. In contrast, an increased response to one stimulus that is consistently preceded by a noxious stimulus is called *sensitization*. Keep in mind that nonassociative forms of learning can be short term or long lasting. What are the neural mechanisms underlying these simple forms of learning, and do the same neural mechanisms underlie both short-term and long-term changes?

Habituation

Habituation was first studied by Sherrington, who found that the flexion reflex habituated with many stimulus repetitions. More recent research examining habituation in relatively simple networks of neurons in invertebrate animals has shown that habituation is related to a decrease in synaptic activity between sensory neurons and their connections to interneurons and motor neurons (Kandel and Schwarz, 1982; Kandel, 1991c).

During habituation, there is a reduction in the amplitude of synaptic potentials (a decreased excitatory postsynaptic potential, or EPSP) produced by the sensory neuron on the interneuron and motor neuron. This short-term change in EPSP amplitude during habituation is illustrated in Figure 4-2*A*. During initial stages of learning, the decreased size of the EPSP may last for only several minutes. With continued presentation of the stimulus, persisting changes in synaptic efficacy occur, representing longer-term memory for habituation.

During the course of learning, continued presentation of the stimulus results in structural changes in the sensory cells themselves. Structural changes include a decrease in the number of synaptic connections between the sensory neuron and interneurons and motor neurons, shown in Figure 4-2*B*. In addition, the number of active transmitting zones within existing connections decreases. As a result of these structural changes, habituation persists over weeks and months, representing long-term memory for habituation. Thus, the process of habituation does not involve specific memory storage neurons found in specialized parts of the CNS. Rather, memory (retention of habituation) results from a change in the neurons that are normal components of the response pathway.

How might this research apply to intervention strategies used by therapists in the clinic? As we mentioned earlier, habituation exercises are given to patients who have certain types of inner ear disorders resulting in complaints of dizziness when they move their head in certain ways. When patients begin therapy, they may experience an initial decline in the intensity of their dizziness symptoms during the course of one session of exercise. But the next day, dizziness is back at the same level. Gradually, over days and weeks of practicing the exercises, the patient begins to see that decreases in dizziness persist across sessions (Shumway-Cook and Horak, 1990).

Application of Kandel's research to patients with inner ear disorders suggests that initially with exercise there is a temporary decrease in the synaptic effectiveness of certain vestibular neurons and their connections because of a decrease in the size of the EPSPs. With continued exercise, changes in synaptic effectiveness would become more permanent. In addition, structural changes, including a reduction in the number of vestibular neuron synapses connecting to interneurons, would occur. With the advent of structural changes, the decline in dizziness in response to the repeated head movement

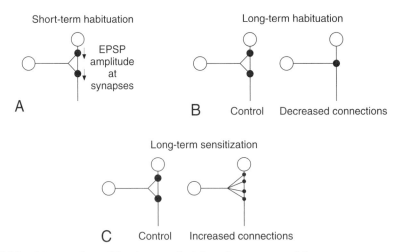

FIGURE 4-2. Neuronal modifications underlying short-term and long-term nonassociative learning. **A.** Short-term habituation results from a decrease in EPSP amplitude at the synapse between the sensory and motor neuron. **B.** Long-term habituation results in a decrease in numbers of connections. **C.** Long-term sensitization results in an increase in numbers of connections. (Adapted with permission from Kandel ER. Cellular mechanisms of learning and the biological basis of individuality. In: Kandel ER, Schwartz JH, Jessell TM, eds. Principles of neuroscience. 3rd ed. New York: Elsevier, 1991:1009–1031.)

would persist, allowing the patient to discontinue the exercise without recurrence of dizziness. It is possible that if exercises were discontinued too soon, before structural changes had occurred in the sensory connections, dizziness symptoms would recur because of the loss of habituation.

Sensitization

As we mentioned in Chapter 2, sensitization is caused by a strengthening of responses to potentially injurious stimuli. Sensitization may also be short-term or long-term, and it may involve the exact set of synapses that show habituation. However, the mechanisms involved in sensitization are a little more complex than those involved in habituation. One way that sensitization may occur is by prolonging the action potential through changes in potassium conductance. This allows more transmitter to be released from the terminals, giving an increased EPSP. It also appears to improve the mobilization of transmitter, making it more available for release (Kandel, 1991c).

Sensitization, like habituation, can be short-term or long-term. Mechanisms for long-term memory of sensitization involve the same cells as short-term memory but now reflect structural changes in these cells (Kandel and Schwarz, 1982; Sweatt and Kandel, 1989). Kandel (1989) has shown that in invertebrates short-term sensitization involves changes in preexisting protein structures, while long-term sensitization involves the synthesis of new protein. This synthesis of new protein at the synapse implies that long-term sensitization involves changes that are genetically influenced.

This genetic influence also encompasses the growth of new synaptic connections, as illustrated in Figure 4-2C. Animals who showed long-term sensitization were found to have twice as many synaptic terminals as untrained animals, increased dendrites in the postsynaptic cells, and an increase in numbers of active zones at synaptic terminals from 40 to 65% (Bailey and Chen, 1983).

In summary, the research on habituation and sensitization suggests that short-term

and long-term memory may not be separate categories but may be part of a single graded memory function. With sensitization, as with habituation, long-term and short-term memory involves change at the same synapses. While short-term changes reflect relatively temporary changes in synaptic effectiveness, structural changes are the hallmark of long-term memory (Kandel, 1991).

Neural Plasticity and Associative Learning

Remember that during *associative learning* a person learns to predict relationships, either relationships of one stimulus to another (*classical conditioning*) or the relationship of one's behavior to a consequence (*operant conditioning*). Through associative learning we learn to form key relationships that help us adapt our actions to the environment.

Researchers examining the physiological basis for associative learning have found that it can take place through simple changes in synaptic efficiency without requiring complex learning networks. Associative learning, whether short-term or long-term, uses common cellular processes. Initially, when two neurons are active at the same time (that is, in association), there is a modification of existing proteins within these two neurons that produces a change in synaptic efficiency. Long-term association results in the synthesis of new proteins and the subsequent formation of new synaptic connections between the neurons.

Classical Conditioning

During classical conditioning, an initially weak stimulus (the conditioned stimulus) becomes highly effective in producing a response when it becomes associated with another stronger stimulus (the unconditioned stimulus). It is similar to though more complex than sensitization. In fact, it may be that classical conditioning is simply an extension of the processes involved in sensitization.

Remember that in classical conditioning, timing is critical. When conditioned and unconditioned stimuli converge on the same neurons, facilitation occurs if the conditioned stimulus causes action potentials in the neurons just before the unconditioned stimulus arrives. This is because action potentials allow Ca^+ to move into the presynaptic neuron and this Ca^+ activates special modulatory transmitters involved in classical conditioning. If the activity occurs after the unconditioned stimulus, Ca^+ is not released at the right time and the stimulus has no effect (Abrams and Kandel, 1988; Kandel, 1991).

Operant Conditioning

Although operant conditioning and classical conditioning may seem to be two different processes, in fact, the laws that govern the two are similar, indicating that the same neural mechanisms may control them. In each type of conditioning, learning involves the development of predictive relationships. In classical conditioning, a specific stimulus predicts a specific response. In operant conditioning, we learn to predict the outcome of specific behaviors. However, the same cellular mechanisms that underlie classical conditioning are also responsible for operant conditioning.

Declarative Learning

Remember that associative learning can also be thought of in terms of the type of knowledge acquired. *Procedural learning* (resulting in implicit knowledge) refers to learning tasks that can be performed automatically, without attention or conscious thought. In contrast, *declarative learning* (resulting in explicit knowledge) requires conscious processes such as awareness and attention, and it results in knowledge that can be expressed consciously. Procedural learning is expressed through improved performance of the task learned, while declarative learning can be expressed in a form other than that in which it was learned.

Consistent with the two types of associative learning described, scientists believe that the circuits involved in the storage of these two types of learning are different. Procedural memory involves primarily cerebellar circuitry, while declarative memory in-

volves temporal lobe circuitry (Kupfermann, 1991b).

Wilder Penfield, a neurosurgeon, was one of the first researchers to understand the important role of the temporal lobes in memory function. While performing temporal lobe surgery in patients with epilepsy, he stimulated the temporal lobes of the conscious patients to determine the location of the diseased versus normal tissue. The patients relived memories from the past as if they were happening again. For example, one patient heard music from an event long ago and saw the situation and felt the emotions that surrounded the singing of that music, with everything happening in real time (Penfield, 1958).

In humans, lesions in the temporal lobe of the cortex and the hippocampus may interfere with the laying down of declarative memory. A few patients have been studied after having the hippocampus and related temporal lobe areas removed because of epilepsy. After surgery, the patients were no longer able to acquire long-term declarative memories, though they retained old memories. Their short-term memory was normal, but if their attention was distracted from an item held in short-term memory, they forgot it completely. However, skill learning was unaffected in these patients. They would often learn a complex task but be unable to remember the procedures that made up the task or the events surrounding learning the task (Milner, 1966). This work suggests that the temporal lobes and hippocampus may be important to the establishment of memory but are not a part of the memory storage area.

The hippocampus, which is a subcortical structure and part of the temporal lobe circuitry, is critical for declarative learning. Research has shown evidence of plastic changes in hippocampal neurons similar to those found in neural circuits of simpler animals when learning takes place.

Researchers have shown that pathways in the hippocampus show a facilitation that has been called **long-term potentiation** (LTP), which is similar to the mechanisms causing sensitization (Bliss and Lomo, 1973). For example, in one region of the hippocampus LTP occurs when a weak and an excitatory input arrive at the same region of a neuron's dendrite. The weak input will be enhanced if it is activated in association with the strong one. This process is shown in Figure 4-3. LTP appears to require the simultaneous firing of both presynaptic and postsynaptic cells. After this occurs, LTP is maintained through an increase in presynaptic transmitter release.

Long-term potentiation has been found in many areas of the brain in addition to the hippocampus, and it has been shown that it is involved in *spatial memory* (Kandel, 1991). For example, Morris et al. (1986) performed an experiment in which rats swam a water maze to find a platform under the water. The water was made opaque to block the use of vision in finding the target. The rats were released in different parts of the maze and were required to use spatial cues related to the position of the walls to find the target. They also performed a nonspatial task with the platform above the water, so that the rat could simply use visual cues to swim to the target. These experimenters showed that blocking special receptors in hippocampal neurons caused the rats to fail to learn the spatial version of the task. This finding suggests that certain hippocampal neurons are involved in spatial learning through LTP.

Procedural Learning

Experiments by a number of scientists support the hypothesis that procedural learning (resulting in implicit knowledge) appears to involve the cerebellum and/or the motor cortex. Gilbert and Thach (1977) examined the involvement of the cerebellum in a very simple form of procedural learning. You will recall that the cerebellum has two types of input fibers, the climbing fibers and the mossy fibers, and one type of output fiber, the Purkinje cells. Climbing fiber inputs to the Purkinje cells typically signal error and are important in the correction of ongoing movements. In contrast, mossy fiber inputs to the Purkinje cells provide kinesthetic information about ongoing movements, im-

portant in the control of those movements. Figure 4-4*B* reviews the relationship of these fibers. It has been shown that the climbing fiber inputs signaling error to the Purkinje cells may increase or decrease the strength of mossy fiber synapses onto the same Purkinje cells. This produces a long-term change in Purkinje cell output, which contributes to motor learning.

Gilbert and Thach (1977) examined the role of the cerebellum in motor learning during experiments in which monkeys were trained to return a handle to a central position whenever it was moved to the left or right. During the sessions, they recorded the activity of Purkinje neurons in the arm area of the anterior lobe of the cerebellum. Once the task was learned and repeatedly performed in the same way, the arm movement was accompanied by predictable changes occurring primarily in mossy fiber inputs reporting the kinesthetics of the movement, with occasional climbing fiber input. Figure 4-4*A1* shows the activity of the mossy fibers (simple spikes) and climbing fibers (complex spikes) during the wrist flexion movements when the monkeys were moving against an expected force or load.

Then the experimenters modified the task, requiring the monkeys to use more force to return the handle to the original position. At first the animal was unable to return the handle in one simple movement, but gradually the animal learned to respond correctly. On the first few trials of the new task, there was a sudden increase in activity in the climbing fibers, signaling the error, as you see in Figure 4-4*A2*.

This increase in climbing fiber activity was associated with a reduction in the efficiency of the mossy fiber connections to the Purkinje cells. The reduction in Purkinje cell output in turn was associated with an increase in force generation, allowing the monkey to complete the task, as you see in Figure 4-4*A3*. Thus, it appears that changes in synaptic efficiency between these neurons in the cerebellum are an important link in the modification of movements through procedural learning.

This type of cerebellar learning may also

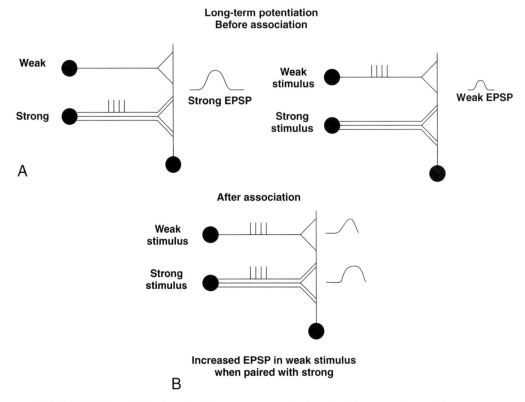

Long-term potentiation
Before association

FIGURE 4-3.   The cellular basis for long-term potentiation. **A.** Prior to pairing with a strong stimulus, the weak stimulus produces only a weak EPSP. **B.** After association, there is an increased EPSP produced by the weak stimulus when paired with the strong. (Adapted with permission from Kandel ER. Cellular mechanisms of learning and the biological basis of individuality. In: Kandel ER, Schwartz JH, Jessell TM, eds. Principles of neuroscience. 3rd ed. New York: Elsevier, 1991:1009–1031.)

occur in the vestibulo-ocular reflex circuitry, which includes cerebellar pathways. This reflex keeps the eyes fixed on an object when the head turns. In experiments in which humans wore prismatic lenses that reversed the image on the eye, the vestibulo-ocular reflex was reversed over time. This modification of the reflex did not occur with cerebellar lesions (Melville-Jones and Mandl, 1983).

Motor Cortex Contributions to Procedural Learning and the Shift From Implicit to Explicit Knowledge

Pascual-Leone et al. (1994) have shown that modulation of motor cortex outputs occurs when explicit knowledge is associated with improved motor performance. In addition, they have now explored the changes in motor cortical outputs when implicit knowledge is transformed into explicit knowledge.

They used a sequential finger movement task in which the subject sat in front of the computer with a response pad with four buttons to be pressed by the four fingers of the hand. When a number was displayed on the screen, the subject was to press the appropriate button as fast as possible. A group of experimental subjects was given a repeating sequence of cues but not told of the repetitive nature. Their performance was compared to that of a control group given a random sequence. Subjects were asked if the sequence was random or repeating at the end of each block of 10 repetitions of the sequence.

Pascual-Leone et al. (1994) found that as the subjects learned the sequence of finger movement, their reaction times became shorter and the cortical maps representing the finger muscles involved in the movement became progressively larger (measured by transcranial magnetic stimulation).

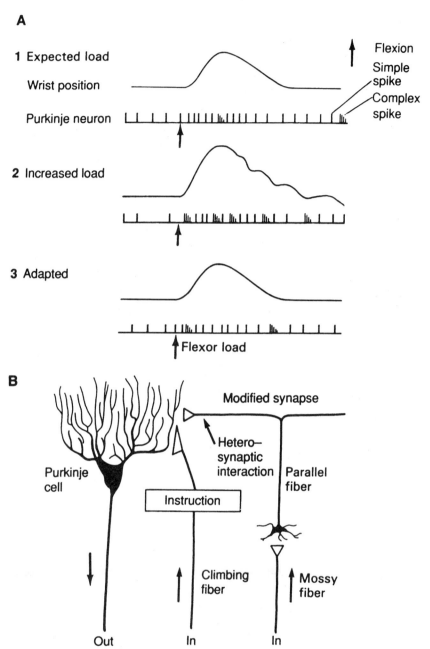

FIGURE 4-4. A.   Activity of mossy fibers (simple spikes) and climbing fibers (complex spikes) during wrist flexion movements when monkeys were moving against (*1*) an expected load; (*2*) an unexpectedly increased load; (*3*) the increased load after practice (adapted). Climbing fiber (complex spike) activity increased with the increase in load, signaling error in returning the handle to its original position and reducing the efficiency of the mossy fiber–Purkinje cell synapse. After adaptation the simple spike activity is reduced and complex spike activity is back to low levels. **B.** The cerebellum, showing the relationship between mossy input via parallel fibers and climbing fiber input important to learning. (Reprinted with permission from Kandel ER, Schwartz JH, Jessell TM. Principles of Neuroscience, 3rd ed. Norwalk, CT: Appleton & Lange, 1991:643.)

After four blocks of trials, reaction time was significantly shorter and peak amplitudes and size of the cortical outputs to the muscles were significantly higher. At this point all subjects knew that the sequences were not random but did not yet know the entire sequence. The maps of cortical output to the muscles continued to enlarge until the subjects attained explicit knowledge of the sequence (6 to 9 blocks). At this point the maps returned to baseline size within three additional blocks of trials, as subjects also began to anticipate the cues for the finger presses. The authors suggest that after explicit learning of a sequence the contribution of the motor cortex is attenuated and other brain structures begin to assume a more active role in task execution (Pascual-Leone et al., 1994).

Complex Forms of Motor Learning

Motor learning includes both simple forms, such as both instrumental and classical conditioning, and more complex forms involving the acquisition of skilled movements. Asanuma and Keller (1991) have begun to examine the neural mechanisms underlying these more complex motor skills. In an initial study they noted that removal of somatosensory cortex in monkeys did not produce overt motor deficits in previously learned motor skills but slowed the learning of new motor skills. They hypothesized that one mechanism underlying motor learning involved LTP of specific cells in the motor cortex by cells in the somatosensory cortex. To test this hypothesis, they stimulated cells in the somatosensory cortex. Whenever they saw short-latency EPSPs in the motor cortex cells, they gave a tetanic stimulus through the somatosensory cortex electrode (50 Hz, 5 seconds). They found that the amplitude of the EPSPs was increased to about twice control levels. This supports the idea that repeated practice of a motor skill results in improved synaptic efficiency between the sensory and motor cortex.

These results seemed to contradict the finding that somatosensory cortex lesions did not seem to affect the performance of previously learned skills. To explain this apparent contradiction, the authors hypothesized that during learning, changes in the sensory-motor cortical pathways also increase the efficiency of the thalamocortical pathways that are coactivated during the learning process. Thus, with training, these alternative pathways could take over activation of the motor cortex. Subsequent experiments found that after repeated practice, the efficiency of the thalamic input to the motor cortex was facilitated and remained so, even when the sensory-motor cortical inputs were no longer activated (Asanuma and Keller, 1991). This could thus explain the lack of sensory input required in making movements after learning, since the somatosensory cortex could be bypassed and other pathways could take over.

When learning a new motor skill, a beginner tends to coactivate many muscles simultaneously, and then with practice, these less efficient contractions are eliminated and only the necessary muscles contract. Can LTP between the sensory and motor cortex explain this change with motor learning?

To answer this question, Asanuma and colleagues carried out the following experiment (Asanuma and Keller, 1991). A cat was placed in a clear plastic box with a small opening in the front, as shown in Figure 4-5. In front of the box was a rotating beaker in which a biscuit was placed. There was a gap between the beaker and the box, so the cat would drop the food unless it learned a new technique of supinating the wrist while picking up the food. Prior to training, the somatosensory cortex in one hemisphere was removed. Acquisition of the skill by the limb contralateral to the lesion was severely affected compared to the control limb. After training, the other somatosensory cortex was removed. Interestingly, the previously learned skill was not affected. This suggests that the somatosensory cortex participates in the learning of motor skills through LTP and that after learning, other areas, such as the thalamus, may take over (Asanuma and Keller, 1991).

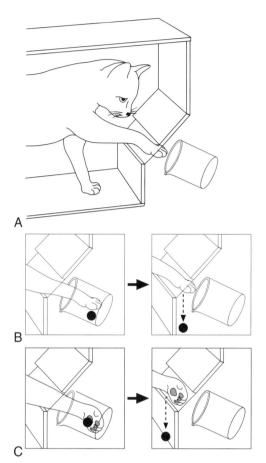

A

B

C

FIGURE 4-5.   Paradigm used to study the role of somatosensory cortex in learning complex motor skills in the cat. **A.** The cat reaches through a slit in a clear plastic training box to retrieve a food pellet in a rotating beaker. **B.** Untrained cats flex the paw, and the pellet drops between the beaker and the box. **C.** Trained cats learn to supinate and flex the paw to retrieve the pellet (Adapted with permission from Asanuma and Keller, 1991: 221.)

Perceptual Learning

Perceptual learning, or the formation of sensory memories, is actually a form of nonassociative learning (Kupfermann, 1991b). It is a more complex form of nonassociative learning than either habituation or sensitization, so it is presented separately. How does perceptual learning actually occur? For example, a person who is first introduced to a new skill and sees someone perform it often can remember the essence of the skill after only one exposure. One hypothesis is that in the process of viewing a new scene, the brain stores a coded representation of it in the visual cortex and we recognize that stimulus when this visual representation is reactivated by the same scene at a later time.

Experiments on monkeys by Mishkin et al. (1984) support this hypothesis and indicate that these coded representations of visual stimuli are stored in higher-order sensory association areas of the visual cortex. How does this representation get stored? When we see a unique scene, this new set of visual stimuli is coded by parallel neural circuits in the visual cortex, coding for size, color, texture, and shape of the stimulus. These circuits are in such places as Brodmann's areas, 18, 20, 21, and 37 of higher visual cortex. These parallel pathways converge on a single set of inferior temporal cortex neurons, and they in turn stimulate a reverberating circuit that includes neurons in a corticolimbothalamocortical pathway (including neurons in the amygdala, hippocampus, thalamus, returning to the visual cortex). This circuit is a spontaneous rehearsal mechanism that serves to strengthen the connections that were part of the first activation of the circuit.

When the neurons are later reactivated, the pathway can be considered the stored representation of that scene. This visual memory also interacts with other memories that were laid down at the same time, such as sensory memories, emotional memories, spatial memories, and motor memories. Thus, the first pathway can arouse the other pathways or be aroused by them through reciprocal connections between these different parts of the cortex.

✆ INJURY-INDUCED PLASTICITY AND RECOVERY OF FUNCTION

In the early part of this century, Ramon y Cajal performed experiments suggesting that growth was not possible in neurons in the adult mammalian CNS. In a 1928 paper he said that when development was complete, the growth and regeneration of axons and dendrites ceased. He asserted that in the adult brain, nervous system pathways were fixed and unmodifiable (Ramon y Cajal, 1928). This led to a view of the CNS as a static structure with rigid and unalterable connections (Gordon, 1987; Stein et al., 1995). This view persisted until the late 1960s and 1970s, when researchers began to discover growth and reorganization of neurons in the adult CNS after injury. The latest research on injury-induced plasticity underlying recovery of function is discussed later in the chapter.

Injury to the CNS can affect neuronal function through direct damage to the neurons themselves. In addition, disruption of neuronal function can occur as the result of indirect effects of injuries that impair cerebral blood flow, control of the cerebrospinal fluid, or cerebral metabolism. As shown in Figure 4-6, whether the trauma occurs through a direct or indirect mechanism, the effect on neuronal function can include interrupting axonal projections from areas injured (Fig. 4-6*A*), denervation of the population of neurons innervated by the injured neurons (Fig. 4-6*B*), and removing some neurons entirely (Fig. 4-6*C*) (Steward, 1989).

Aside from the loss of neurons damaged at the site of injury, the consequences of synaptic loss from these neurons produces a cascading degeneration along neuronal pathways, increasing the extent of neuronal disruption with time (Steward, 1989).

Cellular Responses to Injury

The following sections review some of the events occurring within the nervous system following injury. These injury-induced events may in some cases contribute to recovery of function, while others limit the recovery of function.

Diaschisis

One of the first events following nervous system injury is *diaschisis* (Goldstein, 1990; Held, 1987; Craik, 1992; Stein et al., 1995). Diaschisis is the temporary disruption of function produced by the shock of damage to the brain tissue (Stein et al., 1995). The sudden functional depression of brain regions distant from the primary site of injury can be due to a reduction in blood flow and/or metabolism. Recent research using positron emission tomography (PET) to

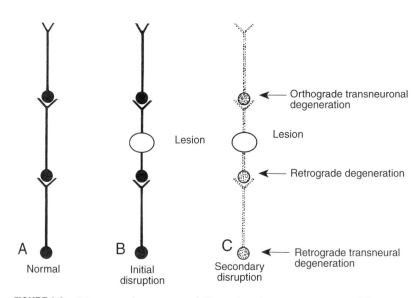

FIGURE 4-6. The secondary neuronal disruption that occurs as part of the cascade of events following neural injury. **A.** Normal neuronal function. **B.** Interruption of axonal projections from injured area. **C.** Secondary neuronal disruption.

measure blood flow to various parts of the brain, and thus neural activity indicates that in many cases, with time the patient recovers to normal activity levels (Stein et al., 1995). It has been proposed that drugs such as amphetamine may promote recovery of function by accelerating the resolution of diaschisis (Feeney et al., 1985).

Edema

Cerebral edema commonly follows brain injury. Cytotoxic cerebral edema is the accumulation of intracellular fluid, whereas vasogenic edema entails leakage of proteins and fluid from damaged blood vessels. Cerebral edema can be local, that is, adjacent to the primary injury site, or remote, producing a functional depression in brain tissue not part of the primary injury (Goldstein, 1993).

Edema at the site of neuronal injury may lead to a compression of axons and physiological blocking of neuronal conduction (Craik, 1992). Reduction of the edema restores a portion of the functional loss. This process is shown in Figure 4-7.

Denervation Supersensitivity

Denervation supersensitivity can occur when neurons show a loss of input from another brain region. In this case, the postsynaptic

membrane of a neuron becomes hyperactive to a released transmitter substance. For example, Parkinson's disease causes a loss of dopamine-producing neurons in the substantia nigra of the basal ganglia. In response to this disease-induced denervation, their postsynaptic target neurons in the striatum become hypersensitive to the dopamine that is released by the remaining substantia nigra neurons. This occurs through the postsynaptic cells forming more receptors to capture more dopamine. It is interesting that this denervation supersensitivity occurs only when at least 90% of the nerve fibers in the substantia nigra are gone. Thus, it occurs only when a critical number of neurons have been destroyed (Stein et al., 1995).

Unmasking of Silent Synapses

Recruitment of previously silent synapses also occurs during recovery of function. This suggests that structural synapses are present in many areas of the brain that may not normally be functional because of competition within neuronal pathways. However, experiential factors or lesions may lead to their being unmasked when they are released from these previous effects. Certain drugs, such as amphetamines, may promote recovery of function by facilitating unmasking (Goldstein, 1990).

Neural Regeneration: Regenerative Synaptogenesis

Neural regeneration, or **regenerative synaptogenesis**, occurs when injured axons begin sprouting. An example of regenerative synaptogenesis is shown in Figure 4-8 (Held, 1987; Craik, 1992). Bjorklund, a neurologist from Sweden, was one of the first scientists to perform research providing evidence that neural growth and regeneration were possible after brain damage. He and his colleagues made lesions in nigrostriatal pathways within the basal ganglia of rats, trying to simulate the degeneration of the pathway that occurs with Parkinson's disease. They then examined the brains with special histological florescence techniques at various times after the lesions. They found that

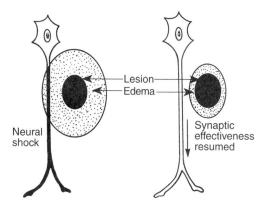

FIGURE 4-7. Recovery of synaptic effectiveness with the resolution of edema, allowing nerve conduction to resume. (Adapted with permission from Craik RL. Recovery processes: maximizing function. In: Contemporary management of motor control problems. Proc. II Step Conference. Alexandria, VA: APTA, 1992:165–173.)

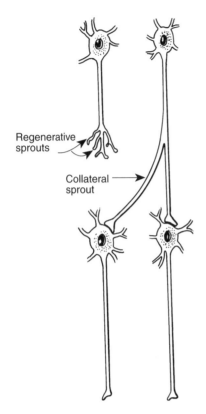

Regenerative
sprouts

Collateral
sprout

FIGURE 4-8. Regenerative and reactive synaptogenesis in related neurons following injury.
(Adapted with permission from Held JM. Recovery of function after brain damage: theoretical
implications for therapeutic intervention. In:
Carr JH, Shepherd RB, Gordon F, et al., eds.
Movement sciences: foundations for physical
therapy in rehabilitation. Rockville, MD: Aspen
Systems, 1987:155–177.)

within 3 to 7 days neurons had begun to
grow across the cut area and eventually
reestablished their connections with their
target neurons in the caudate nucleus of the
basal ganglia (Bjorklund, 1994).

In addition, Albert Aguayo and colleagues
from McGill University tried to determine
why it is difficult for neurons to regenerate
axons over long distances, as in the spinal
cord. They hypothesized that one problem
may be mechanical factors at the site of damage, so they created a bridge of sciatic nerve
to help the regenerating nerve fibers grow
across the site of the lesion. In a series of experiments they showed that when they used
a long sciatic nerve bridge between the
spinal cord and the brainstem (the length of

the bridge lay outside the spinal cord, with
the ends inserted into the spinal cord or the
brainstem) both brainstem and spinal cord
neurons did grow over distances of about 3
cm in the adult rat. However, their penetra-
tion into the nervous system was only about 2
mm. In another set of experiments they
showed that a portion of the retinal neurons
(about 10%) could also grow across a sciatic
nerve bridge into the superior colliculus and
make connections in the appropriate layers.
When they recorded from these neurons
when shining light on the retina, they found
that they did respond, though not completely normally (Aguayo et al., 1996).

Though that work was performed on rats,
other experiments have shown that human
adult retinal nerve cells can also be induced
to regenerate in vitro. Stein et al. (1995)
note that though this work may be promising, it is not yet clear whether regenerative
growth will help patients with lesions, lead to
a return of previous behaviors, and remain
functional throughout the lifetime of the patient. Can postinjury reorganizational processes be manipulated to facilitate CNS reorganization? These and other questions have
critical importance for basic scientists and
clinicians involved in the rehabilitation of
brain-injured patients.

Collateral Sprouting: Reactive Synaptogenesis

Collateral sprouting, or **reactive synaptogenesis**, may occur when neighboring normal
axons sprout to innervate synaptic sites that
were previously activated by the injured axons. Typically the axons that begin to sprout
belong to the same neural system that originally innervated the synaptic sites. Steward,
working with rats, decided to determine
whether collateral sprouting could occur in
the entorhinal-hippocampal circuitry involved in short-term memory. He showed
that when lesions were made in the entorhinal cortex on one side of the brain, fibers
from the intact entorhinal cortex on the opposite side of the brain sprouted branches
that crossed over and innervated the hippocampal sites damaged by the lesion. The

new connections were similar in organization to the original ones. They also noted that the time for the fibers to sprout and make connections was about the same as the time for the return of the behaviors used to indicate the return of short-term memory (Steward, 1989; Stein et al., 1995).

Changes in Cortical Maps After Lesions and During Recovery of Function

With this understanding of some of the responses of neurons to injury, we might ask how this contributes to more global aspects of plasticity within the nervous system. For example, how modifiable are the sensory-motor maps of our brain?

Research on the development of the visual system has shown that the visual cortex is highly modifiable by experience during certain critical periods shortly after birth. Experiments on cats that were visually deprived from birth have shown that they have improved auditory location abilities. For example, when required to localize a sound source at one of eight locations around them to obtain a food reward, they are much better than control cats (Rauschecker and Kniepert, 1994). In addition, the animals show hypertrophy of the facial vibrissae, which helps the animals to locate themselves in space. When neural recordings were made in the anterior ectosylvian cortex, where visual, auditory, and somatosensory representations occur, it was found that there was an expansion of auditory and somatosensory regions into normally visual territory.

It has also been shown that the visual cortex receives input from the somatosensory system in blind subjects (Sadato et al., 1996). Using PET, these authors showed that primary and secondary visual cortex areas are activated in blind subjects during tactile tasks (e.g., Braille reading), whereas subjects with normal vision showed deactivation. A simple tactile task that required no discrimination showed no activation of visual areas in either group.

Is this modifiability also possible in other sensory and motor systems, and is it possible to change these systems in the adult as well as early in the developmental process? The answers to these questions are YES!

In Chapter 3, we talked about the primary somatosensory cortex areas 1, 2, 3a, and 3b, each having a separate sensory map of the body. Research (Merzenich, 1985; Kaas, 1988) has shown that these maps of the somatosensory cortex vary from individual to individual according to experience.

Remapping Following Peripheral Lesions

What have researchers learned about how these maps change during recovery of function? When the monkey's median nerve, which innervates the radial part of the glabrous (nonhairy) regions of the hand, is severed, one might expect that its corresponding parts of the somatosensory cortex would become silent, since there would be no input coming into them. Immediately after the lesion, much of the deprived cortex did not respond to light cutaneous stimulation, but over the next days and weeks, the neurons began to respond again. Now they responded when the hairy dorsal surface was stimulated. When experiments were performed to test the mapping of the cortex after surgery, it was found that neighboring maps had expanded their receptive fields to cover much of the denervated region. These representations increased further in the weeks following denervation (Merzenich et al., 1983a, b). Since the extent of the reorganization of cortex was a few millimeters, it was assumed that it was due to the increased responsiveness of existing but previously weak connections.

However, if nerves to matching parts of the back and front of the hand were cut, some zones of cortex remained unresponsive even months after the lesion (Garraghty et al., 1994; Kaas et al., 1997). These studies supported the proposal that the reactivation of the cortex was due to the increased responsiveness of weak inputs from neighboring areas, and if the denervation exceeded a certain distance, silent areas would remain (Kaas et al., 1997).

Other related work suggests that there can be reactivation of cortex in areas that are too large to be explained by the strengthening of existing connections. For example, Taub (1976) showed that at least 12 years after a dorsal rhizotomy to eliminate sensory input from the arm of the monkey, the somatosensory cortex had been completely reactivated by remaining inputs, mainly from the face. Since this area covered more than 10 mm of area 3b, it was too large to have occurred through the increased effectiveness of previous weak connections. New connections formed somewhere in the nervous system.

To determine where these connections occurred, Florence and Kaas (1995) studied the reorganization of the spinal cord, brainstem, and cortex in monkeys with amputation of the hand or forearm. They found that the central termination of the nerves that had not been injured by the amputation had sprouted into territories of the spinal cord and brainstem that were no longer in use because of the amputation. They believe that the expansion of the arm representation in the cortex after amputation was due to the growth of axons that relay information about the arms into the parts of the spinal cord and brainstem previously occupied by the hand. Thus, the researchers hypothesized that the key to the large-scale reorganization following amputations and dorsal root damage is due to sensory neuron loss and the creation of space in the spinal cord and cuneate nucleus, allowing new growth that leads to reactivation of cortex (Kaas et al., 1997).

Similar results have been observed in humans who had forearm amputations as a result of disease or injury. Researchers used transcranial magnetic stimulation to map motor responses of different muscles activated by cortical areas. They found that muscles proximal to the amputation showed evoked potentials that were larger than those of the equivalent muscles on the opposite side of the body. These muscles were also activated at lower stimulation levels and over a wider area of cortex than those on the opposite side (Cohen et al., 1991, 1993; Lee and van Donkelaar, 1995). This research demonstrates that alterations in cortical mapping follow peripheral nerve lesions or amputation.

Remapping Following Central Lesions

Are there similar changes in response to central lesions? To answer this question Jenkins and Merzenich (1987) performed a study in the monkey in which they made ablations in the sensory cortex area representing one of the fingers. They found that skin surfaces originally represented in the ablated area were now represented in the nearby intact somatosensory areas. Studies of human subjects with infarcts in the internal capsule have shown that recovery of hand function was associated with a ventral extension of the hand area of the cortex into the area normally controlled by the face (Weiller et al., 1993). In a second study Pons et al. (1988) selectively removed the hand area of primary somatosensory cortex (SI), which is the input to the secondary somatosensory area (SII). They found that the hand areas of SII no longer responded to cutaneous stimulation of the hand, but after a number of weeks of recovery the area became responsive to light touch of the foot. These results demonstrate that the nervous system is capable of reorganization following central as well as peripheral lesions.

Does this reorganization occur slowly, as a result of synaptic sprouting and growth of new axons, or does it occur more quickly by other mechanisms? It appears that there are both long-term and short-term responses to these lesions. For example, Donoghue et al. (1990) observed short-term changes. They noted that only 95 minutes after the facial nerve of rats was lesioned, activation of the vibrissa (whisker) area of motor cortex elicited forelimb activity rather than activity in the vibrissae. Since it seems unlikely that collateral sprouting of neurons from the forelimb area could occur this quickly, it has been hypothesized that the synapses already existed but were nonfunctional or weak under normal conditions. Thus, when the proper conditions occurred, the synapses were unmasked or disinhibited. Experiments have shown that neurons in the motor cortex have axon collaterals extending to nearby areas and synapsing on inhibitory interneurons (Gosh and Porter, 1988; Lee and van Donkelaar, 1995).

Reorganization Following Lesions to Large Areas of Cortex

This type of cortex reorganization may not be possible when large areas of the cortex are damaged. In this case it has been suggested that representations may shift to areas that are functionally related but farther from the original site. This could cause a shift in the hierarchical organization of the cortex, with supplementary motor cortex descending pathways taking over for the primary corticomotor pathways (corticospinal tract) (Lee and van Donkelaar, 1995). Support for this idea comes from studies with patients who recover motor function, though tests show that a capsular infarct has completely destroyed the corticospinal tract from the primary motor cortex. In this condition, existing descending pathways from premotor and supplementary motor cortex that have direct projections to brainstem areas involved in motor control take over (Alexander and Crutcher, 1990; Strick, 1988; Fries et al., 1993).

Contributions of Ipsilateral (Uncrossed) Motor Pathways to Recovery of Function

Do uncrossed pathways play an important role in recovery of function? In many patients this appears to be the case. For example, in certain patients a complete cerebral hemisphere was removed to control intractable epilepsy, but no significant hemiplegia was seen. This unusual occurrence may have been due to the fact that the hemisphere had been abnormal since early childhood, and thus there were many years in which the ipsilateral hemisphere could gradually take control of the limbs (Lee and van Donkelaar, 1995).

Weiller et al. (1992) used PET to examine ipsilateral motor activity in patients who had a capsular infarct and eventually recovered from the resulting paresis. The patients were asked to touch the thumb to the different fingers of the same hand in sequence, while regional blood flow was measured. They found that in control subjects and for the unaffected hand of the patients, the contralateral motor cortex and premotor areas were active during the task. But when the previously paretic hand was used, both ipsilateral and contralateral motor areas showed increased blood flow, indicating that ipsilateral pathways were now contributing to the control of this movement (Weiller et al., 1993).

Cross-Modality Plasticity

The visual system projects to the visual cortex, and the auditory system projects to the auditory cortex. How important are the specific sensory afferents in specifying the function of a particular cortical area? Experiments by Sur et al. (1990) have shown in the ferret that retinal cells may be induced to project into the medial geniculate nucleus, which projects on to the auditory cortex. When this occurs, the primary auditory cortex also responds to visual stimulation with both orientation-selective and direction-selective neurons. Other researchers have performed similar experiments to induce visual neurons to project to somatosensory thalamus and have found somatosensory cells responding to visual stimulation. This suggests that the different primary sensory areas had many characteristics in common that allowed sensory inputs from one modality to activate cortical areas of other modalities. However, though these new connections were functional, there were many abnormalities, indicating that specification had already occurred in these primary cortical areas (Mriganka et al., 1990).

Effect of Training on Cortical Reorganization

Studies by Merzenich and colleagues have shown that the somatotopic maps in normal animals show extensive differences between individuals. But how do we know whether these differences are due to inherited genetic differences or to experience? To test for this,

Merzenich and coworkers (Jenkins et al., 1990) performed an experiment in which monkeys were able to reach for food by using a strategy that involved use of their middle fingers only. After considerable experience with this task, the monkeys' cortical map showed an area for the middle fingers that was significantly larger than normal. This reorganization in somatosensory cortex resulting from training is shown in Figure 4-9.

In a more recent experiment the same laboratory tested to see whether motor cortex, like sensory cortex, would be altered by behavioral experience. They trained monkeys to retrieve a small object from a well, which involved mainly finger movements, versus turning a key, which required mainly forearm movements. They found that as digit skills were acquired, there was little expansion of the total hand representation, but instead digit and wrist–forearm representations were redistributed within M1. Either finger representations expanded at the expense of wrist representations (digit task) or forearm areas increased at the expense of finger areas (forearm task). Repeated mapping tests made at various phases in the training revealed that the changes were progressive and reversible. However, they found that reversibility was not complete after an extinction phase, with finger representations decreasing very little, though the behavior dropped to pretraining levels. This would suggest that once a new task is learned, certain aspects of central mapping changes persist for long periods (Nudo et al., 1996).

What mechanisms contribute to the changes in receptive fields as a result of lesions or learning? The mechanisms appear to be similar to those that we have previously discussed in relation to associative learning. In further experiments with monkeys, Merzenich and his colleagues connected two fingers of the monkey so that these fingers would always be used together in the monkey's actions (Clark et al., 1988). This means that the inputs from the two areas would always be highly correlated in the cortex. This changed the mapping of area 3b in the somatosensory cortex, eliminating the sharp boundaries between the maps of these two

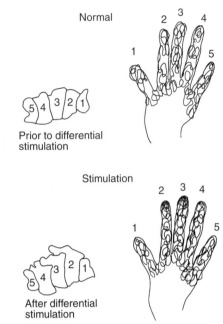

FIGURE 4-9.   Training causes an expansion of cortical representation. (Adapted with permission from Jenkins WM, Merzenich MM, Och MT, et al. Functional reorganization of primary somatosensory cortex in adult owl monkeys after behaviorally controlled tactile stimulation. J Neurophysiol 1990;63:82–104.)

fingers. Thus, the normal sharp boundaries between different parts of the body within our sensory and motor maps may depend significantly on the activity of these areas.

What do all of these studies tell us? They suggest that we have multiple pathways innervating any given part of the sensory or motor cortex, with only the dominant pathway showing functional activity. However, when a lesion occurs in one pathway, the less dominant pathway may immediately show functional connections. This leads us to the conclusion that even in adults, cortical maps are very dynamic. There appears to be use-dependent competition among neurons for synaptic connections. Thus, when one area becomes inactive, a neighboring area can take over its former targets and put them to use.

These experiments also suggest that our sensory and motor maps in the cortex are constantly changing in accordance with the amount to which they are activated by peripheral inputs. Since each one of us has been brought up in a different environment and has practiced very different types of motor skills, the map of each brain is unique and constantly changing as a result of these experiences.

Clinical Implications

What are the clinical implications of this research? First, this research can help us to understand some of the neural changes that occur following injury. For example, following the neural lesion, cortical maps will demonstrate both (*a*) immediate reorganization due to the unmasking of previously nonfunctional synaptic connections from neighboring areas and (*b*) a longer-term change in which neighboring inputs to the areas take over the parts of the map that were previously occupied by damaged or destroyed cells.

Second, it tells us that experience is important in shaping cortical maps. Thus, if we leave patients without rehabilitation training for many weeks or months, their brain will show changes in organization reflecting disuse, which will be most detrimental to these patients. However, the good news is that training appears to make a difference no matter when it is given, since the brain continues to be plastic throughout our lives.

℮ SUMMARY

The research on the neurophysiological basis for learning, memory, and recovery of function covered in this chapter suggests the following important principles:

1. The brain is incredibly plastic and has great capacity to change; this includes not just the immature brain but the mature adult brain.
2. The most important way in which the environment changes behavior in humans is through learning.
3. CNS structural changes occur because of the interaction between genetic and experiential factors.
4. A key factor in experience is the concept of active competition, and this may be summed up in the phrase "the squeaky wheel gets the oil," or in this case, it gets the new synaptic connections. This concept is applicable to simple circuits and to complex neural pathways.
5. Research suggests that short-term and long-term memory may not be separate categories but may be part of a single graded memory function involving the same synapses.
6. Short-term changes reflect relatively temporary changes in synaptic effectiveness; structural changes are the hallmark of long-term memory.
7. Scientists believe that the circuits involved in the storage of procedural and declarative learning are different, with procedural memory involving cerebellar circuitry and declarative memory involving temporal lobe circuitry.

CHAPTER 5

A Conceptual Framework for Clinical Practice

ℰ INTRODUCTION

Clinicians responsible for retraining movement in the patient with neurological impairments are faced with an overwhelming number of decisions. What is the most appropriate way to examine my patient? How much time should be spent on documenting functional ability versus evaluating underlying impairments leading to dysfunction? What criteria should I use in deciding what the priority problems are? How do I establish goals that are realistic and meaningful? What is the best approach to intervention and the most effective way to structure my therapy sessions? What are the most appropriate outcomes for evaluating the effects of intervention?

These questions reflect the critical need for a conceptual framework for clinical practice. A conceptual framework is a logical structure that helps the clinician organize clinical practices into a cohesive and comprehensive plan. It provides a context in which information is gathered and interpreted (Trombly, 1995). A conceptual framework influences clinical practice in several ways. It influences decisions about what to measure during the examination of the patient, the selection of intervention strategies, and the conclusions drawn regarding the intervention process. It provides the clinician with guidelines for how to proceed through the clinical intervention process.

The purpose of this chapter is to consider

elements that contribute to a comprehensive conceptual framework for clinical practice, and to describe a conceptual framework for retraining the patient with movement disorders, which we call a task-oriented approach. A task-oriented approach is used in later chapters as the framework for retraining posture, mobility, and upper extremity control in the patient with a neurological deficit.

☟ COMPONENTS OF A CONCEPTUAL FRAMEWORK FOR CLINICAL INTERVENTION

We suggest that four key concepts or elements contribute to a comprehensive conceptual framework for clinical practice. These include the following:

1. A model of practice, which outlines a method for gathering information and developing a plan of care consistent with the problems and needs of the patient
2. A model of disablement, which imposes an order on the effects of disease and enables the clinician to develop a hierarchical list of problems toward which intervention can be directed
3. Hypothesis-oriented clinical practice, which provides the means for systematic testing assumptions about the nature and cause of motor control problems
4. A theory of motor control from which assumptions about the cause and nature of normal and abnormal movement are derived

The following sections describe each of these important components in detail.

Model of Practice

Phoebe J. is a 67-year-old woman who had a cerebral vascular accident (CVA) approximately 7 days ago. The CVA has produced motor dyscontrol in her left side. She has a resultant left hemiparesis, decreased sensation in the left upper and lower extremities, and associated left neglect. She has good language skills but tends to be impulsive. She has just been referred to inpatient rehabilitation for management of the sequelae from her stroke.

Laurence W. is a 72-year-old man who was diagnosed with Parkinson's disease approximately 15 years ago. He lives in his own home with his wife, who is in relatively good health. He is spending more and more time sitting, and his balance and walking have become worse, as has his ability to assist in bed mobility and transfers. His wife is finding it increasingly difficult to assist him. They are referred for therapy to try to improve Laurence W.'s mobility skills, in particular to improve his independence in bed mobility and transfer abilities.

Zach C. is an 18-year-old with a recent history of a motor vehicle accident in which he suffered a closed head injury. Primary pathology was to the cerebellum, resulting in severe ataxia. In addition, Zach C. has significant cognitive impairments, including attention and memory problems. He requires moderate assistance of one person to stand and walk because of ataxia and is dependent in most of his activities of daily living (ADLs) because of dysmetria and dyscoordination. He spent 4 weeks in coma, but with the return of consciousness has been admitted to the unit to begin rehabilitation.

Sara L. is a 3-year-old child who was born with cerebral palsy and has moderate spastic diplegia. She has been in an early intervention program since she was 4 months old. She has recently moved into a new area and is referred for a continuation of her therapy to improve posture, mobility, and upper extremity skills.

This diverse group of patients is typical of those referred to therapy for motor control problems affecting their ability to move and carry out ADLs. Can the same approach used to examine motor control in an elderly man with Parkinson's disease be appropriate for an 18-year-old patient with a closed head injury? Can the same approach to intervention used with a 67-year-old woman with impaired balance following a stroke be used to habilitate mobility in a 3-year-old child with cerebral palsy?

As you will see, the answer to these questions is yes. Despite their diversity, the *process* used to gather information and design an intervention program is similar for all patients. Thus, while each patient's motor control problems and therapeutic solutions may be different, the process used to identify those problems and solutions will be consistent across patients.

APTA Model of Practice

The American Physical Therapy Association (APTA) in its publication *Guide to Physical Therapist Practice* (APTA, 1997) has described a process for managing patient/client care. The APTA's management process is composed of five elements, including examination, evaluation, diagnosis, prognosis, and intervention. These five elements are shown in Figure 5-1.

Examination

Examination is the process of obtaining data necessary to form a diagnosis, prognosis, and plan of care. The examination process has three parts: taking a history, reviewing relevant systems, and performing appropriate tests and measurements.

History. Information related to the patient's current and past health history can be gathered directly from the patient, family, caregiver, medical records, and other heath care professionals. The types of data that might be generated from a patient history include general demographics (e.g., age, race, sex), current and past history of current conditions (specific concerns expressed by patient, family, caregiver), living environment, growth and developmental history (if appropriate), family history, health status, social history (e.g., family and caregiver re-

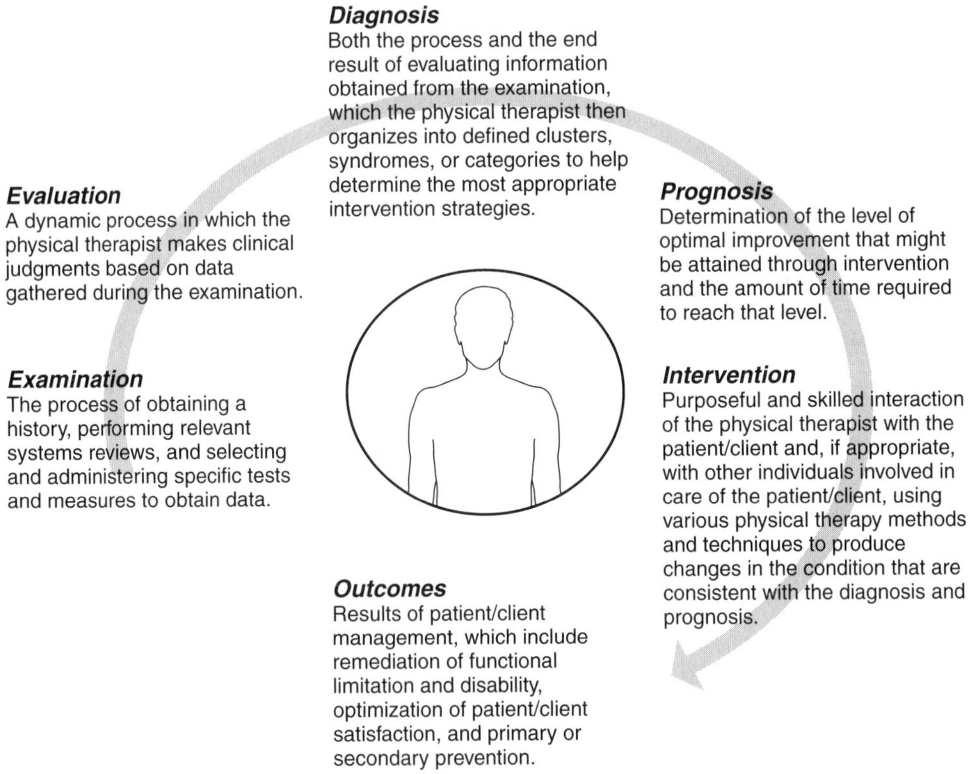

Diagnosis
Both the process and the end result of evaluating information obtained from the examination, which the physical therapist then organizes into defined clusters, syndromes, or categories to help determine the most appropriate intervention strategies.

Evaluation
A dynamic process in which the physical therapist makes clinical judgments based on data gathered during the examination.

Prognosis
Determination of the level of optimal improvement that might be attained through intervention and the amount of time required to reach that level.

Examination
The process of obtaining a history, performing relevant systems reviews, and selecting and administering specific tests and measures to obtain data.

Intervention
Purposeful and skilled interaction of the physical therapist with the patient/client and, if appropriate, with other individuals involved in care of the patient/client, using various physical therapy methods and techniques to produce changes in the condition that are consistent with the diagnosis and prognosis.

Outcomes
Results of patient/client management, which include remediation of functional limitation and disability, optimization of patient/client satisfaction, and primary or secondary prevention.

FIGURE 5-1. The patient/client management process suggested by the American Physical Therapy Association. (Adapted with permission from APTA: Guide to physical therapist practice. Phys Ther 1997:1–4).

sources, cultural beliefs, social support), occupation or employment, functional status, and activity level (current and prior level of function with respect to self-care and home management (e.g., ADLs and instrumental activities of daily living [IADLs]). Also included in the history is a list of medications and relevant lab and diagnostic tests from other medical specialties (APTA, 1997, pp. 1–6).

Interviewing the patient and/or the patient's family can be a critical part of the examination process. The interview is the first step in establishing a good rapport between the patient and the therapist. The interview can be used to gather information on the patient's goals, expectations, and motivation. The interview process also allows the therapist insight into the patient's level of understanding regarding his or her medical condition and the therapeutic process. Information on previous and current health behaviors, including exercise habits, is also critical information when planning intervention.

Systems Review. The examination also includes a brief review of the relevant systems to help direct the selection of specific tests and measurements and assist in determining diagnosis and prognosis. A review of the systems includes a brief determination of the anatomical and/or physiological status of the cardiopulmonary, integumentary, musculoskeletal, and neuromuscular systems. It also includes a brief examination of the patient's communication ability, cognition, language, and learning style.

Tests and Measurements. The last part of the examination process includes the performance of specific tests and measurements that provide the clinician with insight into specific impairments, functional limitations, and disability or other health-related conditions. This aspect of the examination process is discussed in more detail in later sections of this chapter.

Evaluation

The next step in the APTA's patient/client management process is evaluation, defined as the process of making clinical judg-

ments based on the data gathered during the examination. Factors that impact the evaluation include not just clinical findings related to tests and measurements but the extent of loss of function, social considerations, overall physical function, and health status. The evaluation reflects the severity and duration of the current problem, the presence of co-existing conditions or diseases, and the stability of the condition.

Diagnosis

The next step in the management process is determining a diagnosis. A diagnosis is a label that encompasses the signs and symptoms, syndromes, or categories of problems and is used to guide the therapist in determining the most appropriate intervention. The term diagnosis as it relates to the profession of physical therapy is distinguished from a diagnosis made by physicians. Sahrmann proposed the following definition of a physical therapy diagnosis: "Diagnosis is a term that names the primary dysfunction toward which the physical therapist directs treatment. The dysfunction is identified by the physical therapist based on information obtained from the history, signs, symptoms, examination and tests the therapist performs or requests" (Sahrmann, 1988, p. 1705). The physical therapy diagnosis allows the clinician to name and classify clusters of signs and symptoms that will potentially benefit from physical therapy treatment (Rose, 1989). Thus the purpose of a physical therapy diagnosis is to direct treatment. It allows the identification of specific problems that will likely respond successfully to a specific treatment.

Prognosis

The fourth stage in the APTA's management process is determining a patient's prognosis. A prognosis includes both the level of functional independence the patient is expected to achieve following intervention and the anticipated amount of time needed to get to that level. A part of prognosis is determining intermediate levels of function that will be accomplished during the course of therapy. At this point in the management process, the therapist establishes a plan of care to achieve established goals and outcomes. Goals relate to expected changes with respect to impairments, while outcomes relate to expectations regarding functional limitations, optimization of health status, prevention of disability, and optimization of patient satisfaction (APTA, 1997). The defined plan of care includes long- and short-term goals and outcomes, specific interventions to be used, duration and frequency of intervention required to reach goals and outcomes, and criteria for discharge.

Short-term goals are goals that are expected to be achieved in a reasonably short time, with the amount of time depending on where the patient is receiving care. For example, short-term goals in a rehabilitation patient may be defined weekly; alternatively, short-term goals in an outpatient program may be defined monthly. Short-term goals are often defined with respect to expected changes at the impairment level and their concomitant functional significance. For example, the patient will gain 30 degrees of knee flexion so he or she can climb stairs, or the patient will increase quadriceps strength by one grade on a manual muscle test so he or she can rise from a chair without the use of hands. Short-term goals may also be derived from long-term goals that are broken down into interim steps. For example, within in 1 week the patient will independently walk 10 feet, using a cane and with no loss of balance. Thus, treatment strategies geared to attaining short-term goals can focus on resolution of impairments and/or achieving interim steps on functional tasks.

Long-term goals define the patient's expected level of performance at the end of the intervention process (O'Sullivan, 1994). Long-term goals are often expressed relative to functional gains, such as (*a*) amount of independence; (*b*) supervision, or level of assistance required to carry out a task; or (*c*) in relation to the equipment or environmental adaptation needed to perform the task. These are examples of long-term goals: the patient will be able to walk 350 feet using an ankle foot orthosis with quad cane in 3 minutes with no loss of balance; the patient will need only setup assistance in all dressing ac-

tivities. Patient involvement in establishing goals is a critical determinant of compliance in therapy; thus, involving the patient and family in the planning process is essential (Payton et al., 1990).

Intervention

The last step in the APTA's management process is intervention. Intervention is the purposeful and skilled interaction of the therapist with the patient. Intervention includes (*a*) coordination, communication, and documentation; (*b*) patient/client-related instructions; and (*c*) direct interventions (APTA, 1997). Direct intervention is the heart of the plan of care and can include therapeutic exercise, functional training in self-care and home management (ADLs and IADLs), and/or functional training in community and work skills (job, school, play).

While a model of practice gives you a broad framework for proceeding through the therapeutic process, it does not provide details regarding how each step should be implemented. It does not provide answers to critical questions such as these: How shall I measure the effect of disease or injury on my patient? Toward what goals should I direct my intervention? In what order should problems be tackled? A model of disablement can help to answer these questions.

Model of Disablement

A model of disablement suggests a framework for structuring the effects of disease on the individual. The term disablement is a global term that refers to the impact of disease on human functioning at many different levels (Jette, 1994). As health care professionals, we deal with the disabling consequences of disease, injury, and congenital abnormalities (Rothstein, 1994). The goal of therapeutic intervention is to maximize function and thereby minimize disability; however, to accomplish this goal we need to understand the path from disease to disability.

A number of theoretical frameworks have been proposed to describe the path from disease to disability. These models of disability suggest a hierarchical system for categorizing patient problems and can be used as a framework for organizing and interpreting examination data and developing a comprehensive plan for intervention. Three models summarized in Figure 5-2 are reviewed in this chapter.

World Health Organization Model

The International Classification of Impairments, Disabilities and Handicaps is a model of disablement developed by Philip Wood for the World Health Organization (WHO) (WHO, 1980). The WHO model categorizes problems according to four levels of analysis: pathology, impairment, disability, and handicap. This model is shown in Figure 5-2.

The first level, disease, is a description of the pathology or injury process at the organ level. The second level, impairment, includes psychological, physiological, or anatomical problems related to structure or function, such as decreased strength or range of motion (ROM) or the presence of spastic hemiplegia. Impairments can be either the direct result of pathology, such as limited ROM in a joint associated with osteoarthritis, or indirectly associated with pathology, such as cardiopulmonary deconditioning secondary to inactivity (Jette, 1994). The third level in the WHO model, disability, is a disturbance in task-oriented or functional behaviors, such as standing, walking, climbing, transferring, lifting, or reaching. Disability is defined as any

MODELS OF DISABLEMENT

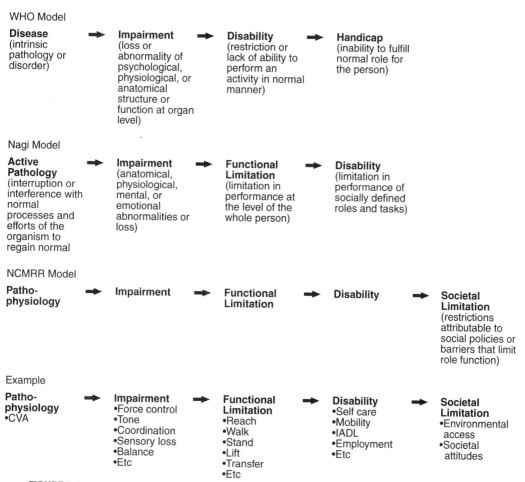

FIGURE 5-2. A summary of three models of disablement and the application of a model to the description of the effects of a CVA.

restriction or lack of ability to perform an activity in the manner or within the range considered normal for human beings (WHO, 1980). Finally, the fourth level, handicap, defines the effect of disease with respect to the society and family network of the patient. Categories of handicap include physical dependence and mobility, occupation, social integration, and economic self-sufficiency. The WHO suggests that handicap is not an attribute of the individual but rather is a social phenomenon, since it reflects the social and environmental consequences of disabilities (Jette, 1994).

Nagi Model

Saad Nagi, a sociologist, developed the Nagi model. This model, shown in Figure 5-2, also contains four levels of dysfunction (Nagi, 1965; Jette, 1989; Guccione, 1991). The first two levels, pathology and impairment, are consistent with the WHO terminology. However, in the Nagi model, the next level of disablement is functional limitation, which is the inability of the individual to perform a task or activity in the way it is usually done. Functional limitations describe a patient's problems with reference to specific tasks independent of their purpose, such as standing, walking, climbing, or reaching. Functional limitations can in turn lead to a disability, which reflects the impact of disease on the behavior of the person in desired roles and activities in society.

Nagi considers functional limitations to be attributes of the individual. In contrast, disability is not defined solely by attributes within the individual but instead is determined by looking at the individual in relation to society. Disability is expressed as a limited ability to carry out expected tasks, such as shopping and caring for children, and social roles, such as wife, mother, and therapist. It is disability, not disease per se, that determines the need for support services, long-term care, institutionalization, and ultimately the quality of a person's life (Guralnik et al., 1989). There is a clear difference between how the term disability is used in the Nagi and WHO models. The term disability in the WHO model is equivalent to functional limitations in the Nagi model, while the term disability in the Nagi model is more comparable to the term handicap in the WHO model.

Disability has been described with reference to different types of activities and/or social roles. Indicators of disability include limitations in ADLs and IADLs. ADLs include bathing, dressing, transferring from bed to chair, using the toilet, and eating (Keith et al., 1987). IADLs are complex tasks necessary for independent living in the community. IADLs include shopping, food preparation, housekeeping, doing laundry, using transportation, taking medications, handling finances, and using the telephone (Lawton, 1971).

Disability has both a personal and societal impact. Disability affects the quality of life of the individual, but the concomitant increase in health care utilization and need for long-term care makes disability a societal issue as well. Mortality rates in disabled older adults are four times greater than in nondisabled adults of the same age. Functional competence in ADLs and IADLs determines to a great extent the living situation of older adults (Kane and Kane, 1981). As severity of disability increases, the proportion of institutionalized people increases, with 59% of people dependent in five to seven ADLs residing in a nursing home. Increased disability results in increased use of health care resources, increased risk of recurrent hospitalization, greater use of outpatient care, and institutionalization. Disability also results in increased use of medical services and paid home care.

Understanding the processes leading to disability is critical to efforts aimed at prevention or postponement of disability. Efforts to prevent disability can be aimed at preventing the disease process, at preventing the development of impairments and functional limitations that result from disease, or finally, at the disability level.

NCMRR Model

A modification to the NAGI model of disablement was proposed by the National Center for Medical Rehabilitation Research (NCMRR). The NCMRR's model of disablement, shown in Figure 5-2, adds a fifth concept, that of societal limitation, to the Nagi model. Societal limitations are restrictions that arise from social policies and/or barriers that limit individuals' abilities to fulfill their expected roles (Jette, 1994). Often societal limitations reflect problems in access and attitude, that is, access within the environment and negative attitudes encountered within society.

Modifiers to the Process of Disablement

The pathway from disease to disability can be modified both positively and negatively by the presence of non–disease-related factors. Modifiers to the disablement pathway that are external to the individual include health care services, such as rehabilitation, and the availability of both physical and social support. Factors within the individual that can modify the disablement process include (*a*) lifestyle and health behaviors, such as exercise and diet; (*b*) psychosocial attributes, such as positive affect, prayer, and self-efficacy; and (*c*) the ability to adapt and accommodate to potential limitations (Verbrugge and Jette, 1994).

Recently, researchers have begun to consider the effect of the environment on the disabling process (Steinfield and Danford, 1997; Haley et al., 1994; Brandt and Pope, 1997; Patla and Shumway-Cook, 1998). Environmental factors include both the physical environment (natural and built), and the social and psychological environments (Brandt and Pope, 1997; Patla and Shumway-Cook, 1998). New models of disablement that recognize the importance of the environment suggest that physical disability cannot be determined solely by factors within the individual such as number and type of impairments or functional limitations. Instead, determination of disability must take into consideration the extent to which the environment constrains a particular potentially disabling condition. Thus, determination of physical disability cannot be made solely by factors intrinsic to

the individual; demands of the environment must be considered in the disabling process (Patla and Shumway-Cook, 1998). For example, a person who has limited walking ability may be less disabled in a flat geographical location, such as Chicago, than in a hilly location, such as San Francisco. A person with limited visual acuity may be able to function independently in daylight hours but evidence disability when light levels are low. Thus the environment and characteristics of the individual conjointly determine disability.

Posture, Balance, and Gait: Functional Limitations or Underlying Impairments?

It is often not clear where postural control, balance, and gait fit into the various levels described by models of disablement. Some clinicians place them at the functional limitation level, while others suggest they are underlying "multisystem" or composite impairments. Perhaps some of the confusion stems from the fact that models of disablement have taken a continuum of effects and broken them down into arbitrary levels, which may not have clear-cut boundaries. For example, functional limitations have been defined as limitations of tasks performed by the individual independent of the environment in which they are performed. However, as we have discussed in earlier chapters, the central nervous system (CNS) takes into consideration factors within the environment when it organizes functional behaviors. Thus, it is not possible to evaluate function independent of any environmental influence.

Posture, balance, and gait are controlled by multiple systems and thus do not easily fit into the impairment category. However, it is difficult to define balance as a functional task in the same way that standing, walking, and reaching are considered functional tasks. Rather, posture and balance are part of the many systems that contribute to the performance of these functional tasks. We suggest that the essential issue is not at what level—functional limitation or impairment—postural control is placed but rather that it be included in our understanding of the impact of disease on the individual.

Clinical Implications

How do models of disablement assist the clinician in formulating a clinical plan for intervention?

The application of this concept can be found in Lab Activity 5-1.

Figure 5-2 illustrates how a model of disablement would potentially describe the effects of a CVA at the various levels. Clinicians are involved in identifying and documenting the effects of pathology at the impairment, functional, and disability levels (Jette, 1994; Schenkman and Butler, 1989). During the examination, clinicians identify and document the sensory, motor, and cognitive impairments that potentially constrain functional abilities. These impairments can be the direct result of the neurological lesion, such as weakness, or the indirect effect of another impairment, such as the development of contractures in the weak and immobile patient. Examination also includes the identification and documentation of functional limitations, for example the ability to walk, transfer, and reach for and manipulate objects. The clinician examines the effect of functional limitations on the individual's ability to carry out the necessary activities and roles of daily life (disability level examination). Finally, a comprehensive examination includes a description of the external and internal factors that potentially modify the process of disablement in each patient.

The process of identifying functional problems and their underlying cause or causes is not always easy. Most CNS pathology affects multiple systems, resulting in a diverse set of impairments. This means that functional problems in the patient with a neurological deficit are often associated with many possible causes. How does a therapist establish a link between impairment and functional limitations? Which impairments are critical to loss of function? Which impairments should be treated, and in what order? What is the most efficacious approach to intervention? Hypothesis-driven clinical practice can assist the clinician in answering some of these questions (Rothstein and Echternach, 1986).

Hypothesis-Oriented Clinical Practice

What is a hypothesis, and how do we use it in the clinic? A hypothesis can be defined as a proposal to explain certain facts. In clinical practice, it can be considered one possible explanation of the cause(s) of a patient's problem (Rothstein and Echternach, 1986; Platt, 1964). To a great extent, the hypotheses generated reflect the theories a clinician has about the cause and nature of function and dysfunction in patients with neurological disease (Sheperd, 1991). As noted in Chapter 1, there are many theories of motor control that present varying views on the nature and cause of movement. As a result, there can be many different hypotheses about the underlying cause(s) of motor control problems in the patient with neurological dysfunction.

Clarifying the cause(s) of functional movement problems requires the clinician (*a*) to generate several alternative hypotheses about the potential cause(s); (*b*) to determine the crucial test or tests and their ex-

---

 LAB ACTIVITY 5-1

OBJECTIVE: To apply the concept of model of disablement to patients with neurological pathology.

PROCEDURE: Select one or more of the case studies presented at the beginning of this chapter. Use one of the models of disablement to describe the pathway from disease to disability.

ASSIGNMENT: Define the pathophysiology of the disease or injury. Make a list of the probable impairments associated with this disease. How will impairments change as the patient moves from an acute to a chronic condition? Given the range of impairments, what are the probable functional deficits of this patient? What disabilities might result from these functional limitations? What societal limitations will this patient encounter? What other factors will potentially affect this patient's path from disease to disability?

pected outcomes that would rule out one or more of the hypotheses; (*c*) to carry out the tests; and (*d*) to continue the process of generating and testing hypotheses, refining one's understanding of the cause(s) of the problem (Platt, 1964). Hypothesis testing is used to explain the cause(s) of functional movement problems and thus can be helpful in clarifying the relationship between the different levels of disablement.

For example, our patient Phoebe J., who has left hemiplegia secondary to a CVA, is referred for balance retraining because of recurrent falls. During the course of your evaluation, you observe that she is unable to stand safely while performing functional tasks and has a tendency to fall primarily backward (a functional level problem). Your knowledge of normal postural control suggests the importance of the ankle muscles during the recovery of stance balance. You generate three hypotheses regarding impairments that could explain why she is falling backward: (*a*) weak anterior tibialis muscle, (*b*) shortened gastrocnemius, and (*c*) a problem coordinating the anterior tibialis muscle within a postural response synergy. What clinical tests can be used to distinguish among these hypotheses? Strength testing indicates Phoebe J. can voluntarily generate force, thus weakening support for the first hypothesis. ROM tests suggest normal passive ROM at the ankle, weakening support for the second hypothesis. In response to the nudge test (a brief displacement backward), Phoebe J. does not dorsiflex the foot of the hemiplegic leg. The inability to dorsiflex the foot, even though the capacity to generate force voluntarily is present, suggests support for the third hypothesis. If it were available, surface electromyography could be used to investigate further whether the anterior tibialis muscle is activated as part of a postural synergy responding to backward instability.

The generation and testing of hypotheses are an important part of clinical practice. However, there is a difference between hypothesis testing in a research laboratory and in a clinic. In the laboratory, it is often possible to set up a carefully controlled experiment that will test the hypothesis. The outcome is a "clean result," that is, a result that accepts one hypothesis and rejects the alternative hypothesis. In contrast, in the clinic, we are often unable to get a "clean result." Clinical tests are often not sensitive and specific enough to clearly differentiate between two hypotheses. Rather, they indicate the likelihood for the origin of the problem. For example, in the case of Phoebe J., passive ROM tests may not be a valid way of predicting the active range of a muscle during dynamic activities. In addition, manual muscle testing may not be a valid way to test strength in the patient with upper motor neuron disease.

Despite the limitations of clinical tests in providing "clean results," the generation, testing, and revision of alternative hypotheses is an important part of clinical care. Hypothesis generation assists the clinician in determining the relationship between functional limitations and underlying impairments. We treat those impairments that relate directly to functional limitations and are within the scope of treatments available to us (Rothstein and Echternach, 1989).

Theories of Motor Control

The fourth element that contributes to a comprehensive conceptual framework for clinical practice is a theory of motor control. As discussed in Chapter 1, theories of motor control have led to the development of clinical practices that apply assumptions from these theories to improving the control of movement. Thus, the approach a clinician chooses when examining and treating a patient with movement disorders is based in part on both implicit and explicit assumptions associated with an underlying theory of motor control (Horak, 1991; Gordon, 1987; Woollacott and Shumway-Cook, 1990). In this book we use the systems theory of motor control as part of our framework for clinical practice. In this theory, movement results from the dynamic interplay between multiple systems that are organized around a behavioral goal and constrained by the environment. Clinical practices related to retraining the patient with motor control problems are constantly changing, in part to reflect new views on the physiological basis of motor control. As new models of motor control evolve, clinical practices are modified to reflect current concepts in how the brain controls movement. Thus, a conceptual framework for structuring clinical practice must be dynamic, changing in response to new scientific theories about motor control.

Applying the Conceptual Framework to Clinical Practice

How do these four elements work together to provide a comprehensive framework for clinical practice? A theory of motor control provides the framework of assumptions regarding the nature and control of normal movement, as well as functional movement disorders and their treatment. A model of practice identifies the steps to follow during the course of clinical intervention, including examination, identification of goals and outcomes, and the establishment of a plan for intervention to achieve them. A model of disablement provides a systematic way for examining the diverse effects of pathology on the individual. It provides a common way of thinking and communicating information regarding underlying impairments, functional limitations, and disability in patients with motor control problems. Hypothesis-oriented practice helps us to explore the relationship among these levels, including the association between impairments and functional limitations and between functional limitations and physical disability. This allows us to develop an intervention program that appropriately targets impairments and functional limitations that are critical in maximizing independence and minimizing disability.

The remaining section of this chapter discusses our task-oriented approach in more detail. In later chapters, we will show the specific application of this approach to retraining posture, mobility, and upper extremity function in the patient with neurological dysfunction.

⊘ A TASK-ORIENTED APPROACH TO EXAMINATION

A task-oriented approach to clinical practice uses a multifaceted approach to clinical management of the patient with motor control problems. Our task-oriented approach to examination looks at motor behavior at several levels, including (*a*) functional abilities, (*b*) a description of the strategies used to accomplish functional skills, and (*c*) quantification of the underlying sensory, motor, and cognitive impairments that constrain functional movement. Since no single test or measure allows one to collect information at all three levels, clinicians are required to assemble a battery of tests and measures enabling them to document problems at all levels of analysis.

Examination at the Functional Level

Examination at the functional level focuses on measuring the ability of the individual to perform essential tasks and activities. There are a number of approaches to examining function. The focus can be on quantitative measures, such as can the person do the task, how much assistance does the person need, how difficult is it for that person? Alternatively, the focus can be on qualitative measures that examine how a functional task is performed. We discuss qualitative approaches to examining functional status in the following section on examination at the strategy level, since examination at this level focuses on the strategies people use to perform functional tasks.

Performance-Based Versus Self-Report Functional Measures

Functional status can be evaluated through (*a*) interview and self-report (or by proxy report) or (*b*) by using performance-based measures. Performance-based measures examine the patient's ability to perform functional tasks, while interview measures rely on the patient's or a proxy's report of the ability to perform functional tasks. Researchers have found a high correlation between self-report and performance-based measures, suggesting that self-report can be a valid way to determine functional capacity. Self-report measures can be used when a patient is temporarily unable to perform certain activities (such as asking the patient who has had a recent hip fracture to report on premorbid independence in ADLs).

Task-Specific Tests and Measures

Some tests limit their focus to specific tasks such as balance, mobility, or upper extremity control. Examples of these types of tools include the Berg Balance Test (Berg, 1993), the Performance Oriented Mobility Assessment (Tinetti, 1986), and the Erhardt Test of Manipulatory Skills (Erhardt, 1982). These tests have been developed to provide clinicians with a clearer picture of the patient's functional skills related to a limited set of tasks the clinician will be directly involved in retraining. These task-specific tests will be covered in later chapters, which discuss retraining posture and balance, mobility, and upper extremity functions.

Age-Specific Tests and Measures

Age-specific tests and measures have also been created. There are a number of tests available for examining children, including the Gross Motor Function Measure (GMFM) (Russell et al., 1993), the Peabody Developmental Motor Scales (Folio and Fewell, 1983), the Bayley Scales of Infant Development (Bayley, 1969), and the Movement Assessment of Infants (Chandler et al., 1980). The Bruininks-Oseretsky Test is often used for examining motor function in older school-age children (Bruininks et al., 1984). At the other end of the age range are tests designed specifically for a geriatric population. Examples of these tests include the Performance Oriented Mobility Assessment (Tinetti, 1986), the Functional Reach Test (Duncan et al., 1990) and the Physical Performance and Mobility Examination (Lemsky et al., 1991).

Diagnostically Specific Tests and Measures

A number of tools have been developed to examine functional limitations and underlying impairments in specific patient populations. The most prevalent of this type of tool relates to examining function following stroke. Examples of these include the Motor Assessment Scale for Stroke Patients (Carr and Shepherd, 1983), the Fugl-Meyer Test (Fugl-Meyer et al., 1975), and the Motor Assessment in Hemiplegia by Signe Brunnstrom (1966). Several scales have been developed to evaluate the severity of symptoms associated with Parkinson's disease, including the Unified Parkinson's Disease Rating Scale (Hoehn and Yahr, 1967) and the Schwab Classification of Parkinson Progression (Schwab, 1960).

Choosing Appropriate Tests and Measures

As you can see, there are large numbers of tests and measures from which to choose. How does a clinician decide what tool to use? A number of factors can be considered when choosing an instrument. *Patient-related* factors, such as age and diagnosis, should be considered. Level of function in your patient population must also be considered to avoid floor or ceiling effects. Floor effects result when a chosen test is too difficult for the patient population; thus, scores are all uniformly too low. Alternatively, a test that is too easy will result in scores that are all uniformly too high, creating a ceiling effect.

Test-related factors should also be considered when choosing a clinical test or measure. The purpose of the examination and the ability of a test to accomplish that purpose are important factors to consider when choosing a test or measure. An examination can serve different purposes; it can be used to discriminate, evaluate, or predict (Ketelaar et al., 1998; Campbell, 1991). Discriminative measures are used to distinguish individuals who have a particular problem from those who do not. For example, the Up and Go Test (Podsiadlo and Richardson, 1991) determines the relative risk of functional dependence in older adults. Based on results from this test, an older adult could be classified as being in a low-risk or a high-risk group. Another example is the Berg Balance Test, which has been found useful in discriminating, or identifying, fall-prone elders living within the community (Shumway-Cook et al., 1997a).

An evaluative measure is used to measure change over time or after treatment. The GMFM is a standardized observational instrument developed to measure change in gross motor function over time in children with cerebral palsy (Russell et al., 1993). A predictive measure classifies people based on future status. The Bleck Scale predicts ambulation in 7-year-olds using postural and reflex activity evaluated at a preschool age (Bleck, 1975). Results from the Walk and Talk test are predictive of future falls in a population of institutionalized elders (Lundin-Olsson et al., 1997). Often therapists choose a test or measure based on personal preference rather than for theoretical reasons (Ketelaar et al., 1998). This can result in problems. For example your intention as a therapist may be to measure change following your intervention. If you select a measure designed primarily to discriminate among people you may find no significant difference in pre and post intervention scores, not because your patient has not responded to your treatment but because you have chosen a test that may not be sensitive to change.

Psychometric properties, such as reliability, validity, sensitivity and specificity, will vary from test to test. Reliability reflects the dependability or consistency of a test, that is, its ability to measure accurately and predictably without variation when no true change has occurred (Dobkin, 1996). Consistency is reflected through both intrarater and interrater reliability. Intrarater reliability indicates a high degree of correlation when performance is measured by the same therapist over repeated applications of the test; interrater reliability indicates a high degree of agreement among multiple raters. If more than one therapist is to examine a patient over time, interrater reliability is critical to accurate data collection (Guccione, 1991).

Validity of an test is a complex concept that reflects the degree to which an instrument measures what it purports to measure (Dobkin, 1996). There are many aspects to validity. **Content validity** is often determined by a panel of experts who determine whether the instrument measures all dimensions of a particular function. **Face validity** indicates the degree to which the instrument measures what it is supposed to measure. **Construct validity** indicates the degree to which the instrument behaves as hypothesized (Dobkin, 1996). **Concurrent validity** is the degree to which the instrument agrees with other instruments that are measuring the same factors. Finally, both **sensitivity** and **specificity** are important attributes of an instrument. Sensitivity is the degree to which a diagnostic test detects a disorder or dysfunction when it is present. In contrast, specificity reflects the ability of a test to rule out a disorder or dysfunction when it is not present.

Unfortunately the reliability, validity, sensitivity, and specificity of many of the tests used in the clinic are not published. This makes it difficult to judge the quality of the instrument and raises questions regarding the value of the data collected with untested instruments.

Finally, *resource-related* factors may be considered when choosing a test. Consideration must be given to the skill and level of training of the therapists giving the test. Many standardized tests require that therapists be trained to give the test with an established level of proficiency. This requires time and resources that a facility may not be willing to provide. The amount of time available for examination, as well as available space and equipment, also must be considered.

Limitations of Functional Tests and Measures

There are a number of limitations inherent in functional testing. While functional measures will allow a therapist to document functional status, such as level of independence associated with performing specific functional tasks, functional measures do not provide information as to why the patient is dependent in performing functional skills. Thus, functional tests will not allow the therapist to test hypotheses about the cause of motor dysfunction.

Therapists retraining patients with movement disorders are concerned about not just the degree to which a patient can carry out a task but how the patient performs the task as well. Functional measures in general are limited to providing information on the former but rarely the latter. Finally, functional tests are limited to evaluating performance at one instant in time under a fairly limited set of circumstances. Results from a functional-based examination do not always predict performance in less than ideal situations. For example, the fact that a patient can walk safely and independently with a cane in the clinic does not necessarily mean the patient can (or will) walk safely and independently in a cluttered, poorly lit home environment.

Despite these limitations, examination at the functional level enables the clinician to document a patient's functional status and is an important part of justifying therapy to the patient, the patient's family, and third-party insurers.

Examination at the Strategy Level: Qualitative Measures of Function

Examination at the strategy level is a qualitative approach to measuring function, since it examines the strategies used to perform functional tasks. The term strategy is not limited to the evaluation of the movement pattern used to accomplish a task but includes how the person organizes sensory and perceptual information necessary to performing a task in various environments.

Why is it important for clinicians to examine the strategies a patient uses when performing a functional task? One answer is that the strategies used to perform a task largely determine the level of performance. According to Welford (1982), a psychologist from England, performance depends on four different factors. The first relates to the demands of the task and the person's desire for particular standards of achievement. The second relates to the capacities, both mental

and physical, that a person brings to the task. The third relates to the strategies that the person uses to meet the demands of the task, while the fourth relates to the ability to choose the most efficient strategy for a given task.

Note that two of the four factors relate to strategies, emphasizing their importance in determining our level of performance. Thus, the strategies we use relate the demands of the task to our capacity to perform the task. If we choose poor strategies and the task is difficult, we may reach the limits of our capacities well before we have met the demands of the task. In contrast, inefficient strategies may still be effective in carrying out simple, less demanding tasks. As capacity to perform a task declines either because of age or disease, we may be unable to meet the demands of a task unless we use alternative strategies to maintain performance.

For example, as a young adult, you rise quickly out of a chair without the need to use your arms. You rely on the ability to generate momentum, using movements of your trunk and then your legs to rise from the sitting position. As you age, strength may slowly decline without affecting your ability to use this strategy for getting up. But at some threshold, the loss of strength no longer allows you to get up using your once-effective momentum strategy. Instead, you begin to use your arms to get up, thereby maintaining the functional ability to rise from a chair, albeit with a new strategy. Thus, in the individual with a neurological deficit, maintaining functional independence depends on the capacity of the individual to meet the demands of the task in a particular environment. When impairments limit the capacity to use well-learned strategies, the patient must learn new ways to accomplish functional tasks despite these limitations.

Limitations to a Strategy Examination of Function

Clinicians are hampered in their ability to examine sensory, motor, and cognitive strategies used to perform daily tasks because methods for examining these strategies are just being developed. There is only limited information defining sensory, motor, and cognitive strategies in neurologically intact subjects. In addition, we know very little about how compensatory strategies develop as a result of neurological impairments.

Researchers have begun to quantify movement strategies used in functional tasks, such as gait, stance, postural control, and other mobility skills, such as moving from sit to stand, supine to prone, and supine to stance. Clinical tools to examine movement strategies have grown out of these analyses. An example is the use of observational gait analysis to define the movement strategies used during ambulation.

Examination at the Impairment Level

Finally, examination at the third level focuses on identifying the impairments that potentially constrain functional movement skills. This requires examination of impairments within individual sensory, motor, and cognitive systems contributing to movement control, as well as multisystem impairments of posture, balance, and gait. Examination of the motor system includes both the neuromuscular and musculoskeletal systems. Since perception is essential to action, examination of sensory and perceptual abilities in the control of movement is necessary. Since task-specific movement is performed within the context of intention and motivation, cognitive aspects of motor control, including mental status, attention, motivation, and emotional considerations, must be examined.

In summary, a task-oriented approach to examination is directed at answering the following questions:

1. To what degree can the patient perform functional tasks?
2. What strategies does the patient use to perform the tasks, and can he or she adapt strategies to changing task and environmental conditions?
3. What is the constellation of impairments that constrains how the patient

performs the task, and can these impairments be changed through intervention?
4. Is the patient performing optimally given the current set of impairments, or can therapy improve either the strategies being used to accomplish functional tasks or the underlying impairments?

Once all three levels of examination are completed, the clinician can translate information gained through examination into a list of patient problems that reflect both functional limitations and underlying impairments. From this comprehensive list, the therapist and patient identify the most critical problems, which will become the focus for initial intervention strategies. Thus, a list of short- and long-term treatment goals is established and a specific treatment plan is formulated for each of the problems identified.

⌖ A TASK-ORIENTED APPROACH TO INTERVENTION

A task-oriented approach to establishing a comprehensive plan of care includes intervention strategies designed to achieve the following goals derived from the three-level examination:

1. Resolve, reduce or prevent impairments
2. Develop effective task-specific strategies
3. Adapt functional goal-oriented strategies to changing task and environmental conditions

These goals are not approached sequentially but rather concurrently. Thus, a clinician may use intervention strategies designed to focus on one or more of the aforementioned goals within the same therapy session. For example, when retraining mobility in a patient who has had a stroke, the clinician may use therapeutic techniques (*a*) to decrease the effect of spasticity and abnormal synergies on functional movement (impairment level intervention), (*b*) to improve weight bearing on the involved leg during the stance phase of gait to produce a more symmetrical gait pattern (strategy level intervention), and (*c*) to have the patient practice walking a distance of 100 feet on both level and uneven surfaces (quantitative oriented functional level intervention).

Recovery Versus Compensation

A question that frequently arises during the course of rehabilitating the patient with a CNS lesion is how much emphasis should be placed on promoting recovery of normal strategies versus teaching compensatory strategies for performing a task. Recovery of normal strategies for function is defined as the returning capability of the individual to perform a task using mechanisms previously used. Compensatory strategies can be defined as using alternative mechanisms to meet the requirements of the task, for example standing with the weight shifted to the nonparetic leg following a stroke. Compensatory strategies can also reflect modifications to the environment that simplify the demands of the task itself. For example, as shown in Figure 5-3, grab bars may be installed to assist a patient in transferring on and off the toilet.

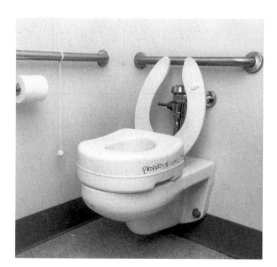

FIGURE 5-3. Changing the environment to accommodate functional limitations: bars around a toilet to facilitate transfers.

When to facilitate normal strategies versus compensatory strategies is not easy to determine and will vary from patient to patient. Often, the guideline used to determine when compensatory strategies should be taught is time. That is, in the acute patient, emphasis is on recovery of normal function, while in the chronic patient, the emphasis shifts to maximizing function through compensatory strategies.

We have found it helpful in the decision-making process to consider the nature of the impairments themselves in determining whether normal or compensatory strategies should be taught. Compensatory strategies will be needed in the case of permanent, unchanging impairments, regardless of whether the patient is acute or chronic. Examples are teaching a patient with a permanent loss of vestibular function to rely on alternative vision and somatosensory cues for maintaining balance during functional tasks and teaching a patient with a complete spinal cord lesion to become independent in ADLs using compensatory strategies. Alternatively, if impairments are temporary and changeable (either through natural recovery or in response to therapy), the emphasis is on remediating impairments and recovery of normal strategies for action.

A problem arises when it is not known whether impairments will resolve. For example, in the patient with an acute CVA whose affected extremities are flaccid, it is often not possible to predict whether the patient will remain flaccid or regain control over affected extremities. In this case, the clinician may revert to a time-based decision-making process, working toward recovery of normal strategies in the acute stage and switching to a compensatory focus in the chronic stage.

Motor Learning Principles and the Recovery of Function

Therapeutic strategies based on principles of motor learning are an important part of retraining functional movement skills. This was discussed in detail in Chapter 2. Taking a functional task and breaking it down into its component parts (whole versus part training) is frequently used when teaching tasks such as transfers, mobility, and ADLs. Systematically manipulating practice conditions is essential to retraining as well. Implementing variable practice to facilitate adaptation of skills to changing contexts requires planning and thoughtful organization of the therapeutic environment. Planning is also required if a therapist wants to retrain multiple skills under random instead of blocked conditions. Moving between skills such as transfers, bed mobility, reaching, and dressing requires that necessary equipment be gathered in advance of a therapy session. Without this type of planning, retraining will reflect what is most convenient to the situation rather than what may be in the best interests of the patient.

Consideration of the way feedback will be provided as a patient is relearning functional movement involves deciding how much feedback to give, when to give it, and what form of feedback (visual, manual, verbal) to give. Will feedback reflect knowledge of results or performance? How much emphasis will be on discovery learning versus guiding the patient toward a particular solution to the problem of performing a functional task? Can declarative learning or visualization help to facilitate learning functional movement tasks in a patient who has limited endurance?

⊘ SUMMARY

1. A comprehensive conceptual framework for clinical practice is built upon four key elements: (*a*) a model of practice that establishes the steps for intervention; (*b*) hypothesis-oriented practice, which provides a process for testing assumptions regarding the nature and cause of motor control problems; (*c*) a model of disablement that imposes a hierarchical order on the effects of disease on the individual; and (*d*) a theory of motor control that suggests essential elements to examine and treat.

2. The APTA model of practice is a five-step process, including (*a*) examination, (*b*) evaluation, (*c*) diagnosis, (*d*) prognosis, and (*e*) intervention.

3. A model of disablement provides a hierarchical system for categorizing patient problems that can be used as a framework for organizing and interpreting examination data.

4. During the course of clinical intervention, the clinician will be required to generate multiple hypotheses, proposing possible explanations regarding the problem and its cause(s), and must investigate these hypotheses through observation, tests, and measurement.

5. A systems theory of motor control contributes assumptions regarding the nature and control of movement, movement disorders and treatment.

6. These four components are combined into what we term a task-oriented approach to clinical practice. A task-oriented approach to examination measures behavior at three levels, including (*a*) quantification of functional skills, (*b*) a description of the strategies used to accomplish functional skills, and (*c*) quantification of the underlying impairments that constrain performance.

7. A task-oriented approach to intervention focuses on (*a*) resolving or preventing impairments, (*b*) developing effective task-specific strategies, and (*c*) adapting functional goal-oriented tasks to changing environmental conditions.

8. A critical aspect of retraining functional skills is helping the patient learn to adapt task-specific strategies to changing environmental contexts.

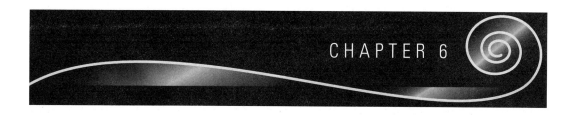

CHAPTER 6

Constraints on Motor Control: An Overview of Neurological Impairments

℮ INTRODUCTION TO IMPAIRMENTS

Clinical management of the patient with motor control problems requires both knowl-edge and skill. Part of an essential knowl-edge base in treating patients with movement problems is understanding the physiology and pathophysiology of motor control. This information enables the therapist to form initial assumptions regarding the pattern of impairments likely to be found in patients with a specific neural pathology. In addition, understanding the impairments constraining movement helps the clinician to form initial assumptions regarding the probable functional limitations that will be found. This relationship between pathophysiology, impairments, and functional limitations, shown in Figure 6-1, was described in Chapter 5 with reference to models of disablement.

The formation of initial hypotheses regarding likely impairments and functional limitations guides the selection of appropriate tests and measures that are used to examine initial assumptions relative to a specific patient. Through examination procedures, the clinician determines the impairments and functional limitations that are present in a specific patient. This leads to the selection of appropriate interventions appropriate to that patient.

Since movement arises from the interaction of multiple processes, including those related to *sensory/perception, cognitive,* and *action* or *motor systems,* pathology within any of the systems will result in impairments that potentially constrain functional movement (Fig. 6-1). A comprehensive discussion of the pathophysiology of motor control is beyond the scope of this chapter. Instead, the purpose of this chapter is to introduce the topic, presenting an **overview** of impairments within motor, sensory/perceptual, and cognitive systems resulting from central nervous system (CNS) pathology that constrain functional movement. We begin with a discussion of issues related to classifying or categorizing impairments in patients with neurological pathology. We then present an overview of impairments

that affect functional movement, with primary emphasis on problems within the motor or action systems. A discussion of each type of impairment, such as abnormal muscle tone, dyscoordination, and involuntary movement, includes a **brief** description of common approaches to clinical examination and treatment of this impairment. In later chapters we discuss in more detail the effects of these impairments on the specific functions of postural control, mobility, reach, and grasp. We conclude the chapter with a summary of the constellation of impairments likely to be found in our four case studies.

Classifying Impairments Associated With CNS Lesions

Signs Versus Symptoms

Brain pathology produces a unique pattern of behavioral signs and symptoms associated with the destruction of specific neuronal populations. Signs of neurological dysfunction are objective findings of pathology that can be determined by physical examination. For example, the presence of nystagmus suggests that a patient has a vestibular disorder. In contrast, symptoms are subjective complaints associated with pathology that are perceived by the patient but may not necessarily be objectively documented on exam. Dizziness is a common symptom associated with vestibular pathology.

Positive Versus Negative Signs and Symptoms

Hughlings Jackson described upper motor neuron lesions as damage to cortical and subcortical structures, producing motor dyscontrol because of (*a*) the release of abnormal behaviors, so-called positive symp-

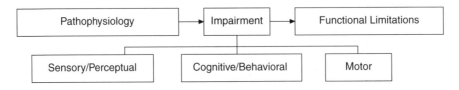

FIGURE 6-1.   Relationship between pathophysiology within the CNS and resulting impairments and functional limitations. Impairments can affect sensory/perceptual, cognitive, and/or motor systems.

toms, and/or (*b*) the loss of normal behaviors, called negative symptoms (Foerster, 1977; Walshe, 1961). Positive symptoms may include the presence of abnormal reflexes such as the extensor plantar (or Babinski) reflex or hyperactive stretch reflexes resulting in spasticity. Paresis, the loss of descending control of lower motor neurons, is an example of a negative symptom. In the rehabilitation environment, attempts to understand functional deficits in the patient with neurological pathology often emphasize positive systems, such as increased muscle tonus, at the expense of negative symptoms, such as loss of strength (Gordon, 1987; Katz and Rymer, 1989).

Primary Versus Secondary Effects

CNS lesions can result in a wide variety of primary impairments affecting motor (neuromuscular), sensory/perceptual, and/or cognitive/behavioral systems. In addition to primary impairments such as paralysis or spasticity, secondary effects contribute to motor control problems in the patient with neurological dysfunction. Secondary impairments do not result from the CNS lesion directly but rather develop as a result of the original problem (Schenkman, 1990). For example, as shown in Figure 6-2, a lesion in

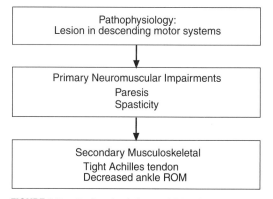

FIGURE 6-2. Pathophysiology within the CNS can result in both primary and secondary impairments. For example, a CNS lesion produces primary neuromuscular impairments, such as paresis and spasticity. These impairments, which limit movement, can result in the development of secondary musculoskeletal system impairments, which further constrain the patient's ability to move.

the descending motor system can result in primary impairments of paresis and spasticity. These impairments limit movement capabilities in the patient, and this immobility may result in the development of a secondary musculoskeletal impairment, for example tightness in the Achilles tendon, limiting ankle range of motion (ROM). Limited ROM at the ankle joint, which develops secondary to the neurological lesion, may ultimately impair function as much as the original impairments of paresis and spasticity.

✪ MOTOR SYSTEM IMPAIRMENTS

Primary Neuromuscular Impairments

Neuromuscular impairments encompass a diverse group of problems that constitute a major constraint on functional movement in the patient with neurological dysfunction.

Muscle Weakness: Paresis and Paralysis

Strength is defined as the ability to generate sufficient tension in a muscle for the purposes of posture and movement (Smidt and Rogers, 1982). Strength results from both the musculoskeletal properties of the muscle itself and the neural activation of that muscle. Neural aspects of force production reflect (*a*) the number of motor units recruited, (*b*) the type of units recruited, and (*c*) the discharge frequency (Duncan and Badke, 1987; Buchner and DeLateur, 1991; Amundsen, 1990; Rogers, 1991).

Weakness is defined as an inability to generate normal levels of force and is a major impairment of motor function in many patients with upper motor neuron lesions. Depending on the extent of the lesion, weakness in the patient with a cerebral cortex lesion can vary in severity from total or severe loss of muscle activity, called paralysis or plegia, to mild or partial loss of muscle activity, called paresis. Paresis and plegia are often referred to by their distribution: hemiplegia (or hemiparesis) is weakness affecting one side of the body; paraplegia affects the lower extremities; and tetraplegia affects all four limbs. Paresis results from a lesion within descending motor pathways, which interferes with the central excitatory drive to the motor units (Ghez, 1991c). This results in an inability to recruit and/or modulate the motor neurons leading to a loss of movement.

Many studies have documented problems in motor unit discharge behavior in patients with cerebral cortex lesions and resultant hemiparesis (Yan et al., 1998a,b; Frascarelli et al., 1998). Frascarelli et al. (1998) examined the behavior of the first and second motor units recruited during a minimal effort tonic contraction in patients with hemiplegia due to cerebrovascular lesions in the distribution of the middle cerebral artery. Results showed significant differences in the pattern of recruitment between the paretic side and the nonparetic side. The first recruited motor unit had a lower baseline firing rate, while the second recruited motor unit was activated earlier in the paretic side than the nonparetic side. In addition, motor neurons of distal muscles had a lower range of control than proximal muscle motor units. These changes were more apparent in the distal than the proximal muscles. The authors suggest that their findings are consistent with the notion that following a cerebral cortex lesion, the CNS loses its ability to modulate firing frequency during minimal voluntary movements, and this is true more in relation to distal than proximal muscles.

Prolonged paresis, a primary neuromuscular impairment, also produces peripheral changes in the muscle (a secondary musculoskeletal impairment). Several authors have documented the selective atrophy of type II (fast) and type I (slow) muscle fibers in patients with a lesion (Edstrom, 1970; Edstrom et al., 1973; Mayer and Young, 1980).

Clinical Examination of Weakness

Can strength impairments be reliably measured in a patient with a CNS lesion? Traditionally, clinicians believed that measuring strength was not appropriate. This was based on the assumption that the primary impairment affecting functional performance was not weakness but spasticity. In addition, strength training in the CNS patient was considered contraindicated, since it was believed that strength training would increase tone problems (Bobath, 1978; Davies, 1985).

In recent years there has been an increased emphasis on the examination of strength in patients with cerebral cortex lesions. In addition, researchers have begun to examine assumptions related to the positive and negative effects of strength training in the patient with a cerebral cortex lesion (Wiley and Damiano, 1998; Engart et al., 1995; Powell et al., 1999). This new research reflects the growing awareness that paresis (a negative sign) is as important a factor in impaired functional performance as spasticity (a positive sign) (Katz and Rymer, 1989; Bohannon and Walsh, 1992; Andrews and Bohannon, 2000).

Strength can be measured in three ways: isometrically, isotonically, or isokinetically (Buchner and DeLateur, 1991). However, in the clinic, the most common approach is to examine isometric or isokinetic strength during a shortening contraction (Amundsen, 1990). Manual muscle testing is the most common clinical approach to testing strength. This test assesses a subject's ability to move a body segment through its ROM against gravity or against externally applied resistance (Amundsen, 1990). An ordinal scale is used to grade strength from 0 (no contraction) to 5 (full movement against gravity and maximal resistance). A limitation of manual muscle testing is that it does not examine the ability of a muscle to participate in a functional movement pattern (Lynch, 1990).

An alternative approach to quantifying strength incorporates the use of hand-held dynamometers, which provide an objective indication of muscle group strength (Amundsen, 1990; Bohannon and Walshe, 1992). Hand-held dynamometers are used to measure the force required to break the position held by the patient against resistance applied by the examiner. Finally, muscle performance can be tested dynamically through the use of instrumented isokinetic systems.

Isokinetic testing assesses power, or the ability to generate force throughout the ROM, at different speeds and over several repetitions (Wilk, 1990).

Using these methods, researchers have begun to document the intensity and distribution of strength impairments in patients with CNS lesions. Results from these studies are beginning to challenge long-held clinical assumptions regarding strength deficits in the patient with CNS pathology. For example, Andrews and Bohannon (2000) quantified the distribution of strength impairments following stroke in 48 patients with acute stroke. The strength of eight muscles was assessed bilaterally using a hand-held dynamometer. Strength was impaired on both sides of the body, suggesting the bilateral effects of a cerebral cortex lesion. Interestingly, distal muscles were *less* impaired than proximal muscles on the nonparetic side, and extensor muscle activity was less affected than flexor activity bilaterally. The authors conclude that with few exceptions, their results do not support common clinical assumptions about the distribution of strength impairments following stroke.

Many studies are now showing the bilateral effects of ipsilateral lesions of the cerebral cortex (Marque et al., 1997; Winstein and Pohl, 1995; Hermsdorfer et al., 1999). For example, Marque et al. (1997) used a hand dynamometer, isokinetic dynamometer, finger tapping and nine-hole peg test to examine motor impairments in ipsilateral extremities in 15 patients with acute stroke. They found significant motor impairments in the side ipsilateral to the lesion at 20 days post stroke. These impairments had almost completely resolved by 90 days post stroke.

Treatment of Impaired Strength

The shift in emphasis on the functional significance of impaired strength in patients with CNS lesions has led to a growing stress on strength training in these patients. Techniques to improve strength can focus on generating force to move a body segment or alternatively, generating force to resist a movement. Progressive resistive exercises are commonly used to increase strength within individual muscles. Isokinetic equipment can also be used to improve a patient's ability to generate force throughout the ROM, at different speeds of motion, and through repeated efforts within individual and groups of muscles (Duncan and Badke, 1987).

Researchers are beginning to compare the effects of eccentric (lengthening contractions) and concentric (shortening contractions) strength training in patients with a cerebral cortex lesion. Engardt et al. (1995) examined the effects of strength training with isokinetic maximal voluntary knee extensions in patients following stroke. Half of the group of 10 patients was trained using eccentric movements exclusively, while the other patients were trained using concentric movements. Maximal voluntary strength in concentric and eccentric actions of the knee extensor and flexor muscles was recorded along with surface electromyelography (EMG) at constant velocities of 60, 120, and 180 degrees per second. The functional effects of strength training were examined in a sit-to-stand task and during gait. In the eccentric training group (but not in the concentric group), knee extensor strength increased both eccentrically and concentrically in the paretic leg compared to the nonparetic leg. The eccentrically trained group (but not the concentrically trained group) demonstrated a nearly symmetrical body weight distribution in the legs in the sit-to-stand task; there were no group differences found on the walking tasks. This suggests that the effects of strength training may depend on whether concentric or eccentric training is performed.

Biofeedback and functional electrical stimulation (ES) can also be used to assist patients in regaining volitional control over isolated muscles and joints. For example, stimulation of the peroneal nerve is commonly performed in hemiplegic patients to improve control over the anterior tibialis muscle during a voluntary contraction. A number of studies have shown that biofeedback is effective in helping the patient with a neurological impairment learn to initiate, sustain, and/or relax a voluntary muscle contraction

(Binder et al., 1981; Baker et al., 1977). There is some evidence that improved control over an isolated muscle has some carryover to gait. Thus, patients given therapy related to muscle control increased gait velocity, although this was not trained specifically (Binder et al., 1981).

Electrical stimulation has also been used as an adjunct to strength training. Neuromuscular ES has been used to enhance motor recovery, specifically improvements in strength, following stroke. Powell et al. (1999) used ES of the wrist extensors in 60 hemiparetic patients 2 to 4 weeks following stroke. Subjects were randomly assigned to a control group, who received standard treatment, or to an experimental group, who received standard treatment in addition to ES of the wrist extensors (three times a day for 30 minutes for 8 weeks). They found that the ES group had significantly greater isometric strength of the wrist extensors than the control group, suggesting that ES is a viable therapeutic intervention to improve strength in wrist extensors in patients post stroke.

Finally, researchers have begun to investigate whether strength training does in fact increase spasticity in affected muscles. Teixeira-Salmela et al. (1999) looked at the effects of muscle strengthening and conditioning in chronic (more than 9 months) stroke subjects. In their study 13 subjects underwent a 10 week (3 days per week) program consisting of warmup, aerobic exercise, lower extremity muscle strengthening, and a cool-down. Changes in peak isokinetic torque production of the major muscle groups in the paretic lower limb, quadriceps and ankle plantarflexor spasticity, gait speed, rate of stair climbing, the Human Activity Profile, and Nottingham Health Profile were examined before and after training. The researchers found a significant improvement in strength in the affected muscle groups and an increase in gait speed and rate of stair climbing post training. Improvements in strength were not associated with an increase in either quadriceps or ankle plantarflexor spasticity.

Damiano and Abel (1998) also investigated the effects of strength training in a group of adolescents with various forms of spastic cerebral palsy. They found that training significantly improved strength in the affected muscles without increasing the severity of spasticity.

In summary, research is now documenting the contribution of impaired strength to functional limitations in patients with CNS lesions. This has led to a growing awareness of the need to examine and document weakness in the patient with CNS pathology. In addition, training programs appear to be effective in improving strength; the degree to which they affect other primary impairments, such as spasticity, is not clear.

Abnormalities of Muscle Tone

Muscle tone is characterized by a muscle's resistance to passive stretch, and a certain level of muscle tone is typical of normal muscle. On the upper end of the tone spectrum, shown in Figure 6-3, is hypertonicity, manifested by spasticity or rigidity. At the other end are disorders of hypotonicity. The presence of abnormalities of muscle tone in the patient with CNS pathology is well known. However, the exact contributions of abnormalities of muscle tone to functional deficits are not well understood.

Hypertonicity
Spasticity.   Spasticity is defined as "a motor disorder characterized by a velocity-dependent increase in tonic stretch reflexes (muscle tone) with exaggerated tendon jerks, resulting from hyperexcitability of the stretch reflex, and is one component of the

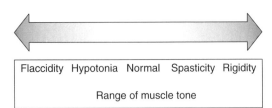

Flaccidity Hypotonia Normal Spasticity Rigidity

Range of muscle tone

FIGURE 6-3.   Continuum of muscle tone. The center illustrates the range of normal muscle tone. Decrease in muscle tone compared to normal is hypotonia. In contrast, an increase in muscle tone compared to normal is hypertonia and manifests as either spasticity or rigidity.

upper motor neuron syndrome" (Lance, 1980, p. 485).

In this chapter we typically use the term lesion in the "descending motor systems" in place of "upper motor neuron" lesion. A lesion in the descending motor systems may reflect pathology in the pyramidal tract or other nearby descending motor pathways, such as the corticoreticulospinal tract. Damage to these tracts results in increased alpha motor neuron excitability with a resulting increase in muscle tone (enhanced tonic stretch reflex activity and exaggerated tendon jerks [phasic stretch reflexes]) (Mayer, 1997).

Understanding spasticity is difficult in part because the term is used clinically to cover a wide range of abnormal behaviors. It is used to describe (*a*) hyperactive stretch reflexes, (*b*) abnormal posturing of the limbs, (*c*) excessive coactivation of antagonist muscles, (*d*) associated movements, (*e*) clonus, and (*f*) stereotyped movement synergies (Horak, 1991). Thus one word (spasticity) is used to describe many abnormal behaviors often seen in patients with CNS pathology.

A key sign of spasticity is a velocity-dependent increase in resistance of a muscle or muscle group to passive stretch. The predominant hypothesis regarding the neural mechanism underlying spasticity is that it is due to changes in descending activity that result in abnormalities within the segmental stretch reflex. Disorders in the stretch reflex mechanism may reflect alterations in the threshold and/or the gain of the stretch reflex in response to stretch. Several studies have been consistent in showing changes in the set point, or angular threshold of the stretch reflex in muscles with spastic hypertonus (Katz and Rymer, 1989; Powers et al., 1989; Thilmann et al., 1991).

Rymer and colleagues (Katz and Rymer, 1989; Powers et al., 1989) compared torque at the elbow joint during imposed elbow extension using a ramp-and-hold stimulus at a range of velocities between normal subjects and subjects with spastic hemiparesis. Their research found that patients with elbow flexor spasticity developed high levels of EMG activity at movement velocities of 112 degrees per second. Normal, healthy subjects did not exhibit substantial stretch-evoked EMG activity at this velocity. Surprisingly, stretch reflex gain was comparable between the two groups. This led the authors to conclude that enhanced EMG activity in spastic muscles in response to imposed stretch was due to a decrease in stretch reflex threshold rather than an increase in gain.

Thilmann et al. (1991) compared muscle response to passively imposed stretch in 19 patients with hemiparesis following a stroke of the middle cerebral artery. Subjects sat with their arms laterally abducted and supported, with forearm and hand lying flat within a molded plastic cast. The forearm was displaced 30 degrees (extended from 75 to 105 degrees); displacement velocity varied from 35 to 300 degrees per second. Surface EMGs were used to record velocity-dependent muscle activity in the biceps brachii. Results are summarized in Figure 6-4. Responses of the normal control subjects are shown in Figure 6-4*A*. Each trace is the rectified and averaged biceps EMG response obtained from 10 displacements at each velocity. The joint position traces are shown in the center (Fig. 6-4*B*) of the figure. Half of the 12 normal subjects showed a reflex response at 200 degrees per second. In the other 6 normal subjects, no reflex response was found even at the highest velocities. In contrast, the patients with spastic hemiparesis showed an early reflex response to displacements at velocities as low as 110 degrees per second. In addition to the early findings, a velocity-dependent increase in stretch reflex responsiveness was found in all patients with spastic paresis. This can be seen in Figure 6-4*C*. Thus, in response to imposed stretch, there was both an early activation of the muscle and a prolonged activation of the muscle that lasted as long as the displacement was applied. The results from these experiments suggest that spasticity is related to both a decrease in stretch reflex threshold and persisting reflex hyperexcitability.

What is the neural basis for abnormal stretch reflex activity? It has been proposed that enhanced stretch reflex activity can occur because the alpha motor neuron pool at the segmental level is hyperexcitable or be-

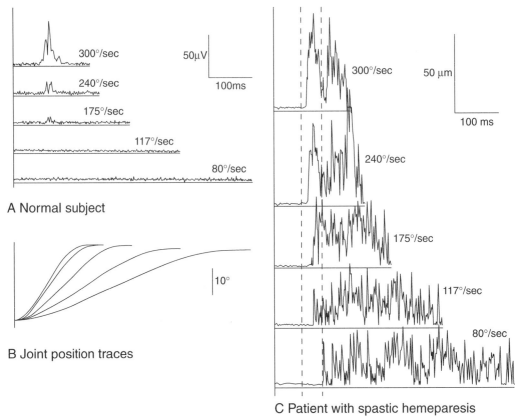

A Normal subject

B Joint position traces

C Patient with spastic hemeparesis

FIGURE 6-4. A comparison of EMG activity of the biceps brachii muscle in response to imposed elbow extension (30°) at five velocities ranging from 8 to 300°/second in a normal control subject (**A**) and a patient with spastic paresis (**B**) of the left arm due to a middle cerebral artery stroke (**C**), showing the velocity-dependent activation of muscle. (Reprinted with permission from Thilmann AF, Fellows SJ, Garms E. The mechanism of spastic muscle hypertonus. Brain 1991;114:237.)

cause the amount of excitatory afferent input elicited by muscle stretch is increased or both. Hyperexcitabilty of the alpha motor neuron pool can be due to a loss of descending inhibitory input, postsynaptic denervation supersensitivity, shortening of the motor neuron dendrites, or collateral sprouting of the dorsal root afferents (Noth, 1991; Mayer, 1997).

Spasticity also changes the physical properties of the muscle and other tissues. Stiffness and contracture reflect the plasticity and viscoelastic properties of muscle, tendons, and joints, collectively termed rheological properties (Mayer, 1997). Changes in rheological properties contribute to increased resistance of the muscle to stretch. Nerve blocks, which reduce the effect of the

reflex tension, will not impact the passive resistance due to rheological factors. Researchers analyzing gait in children with cerebral palsy have found that increased tension in the gastrocnemius muscle is not always associated with increased muscle activity in that muscle. This has led to the suggestion that in some cases, so-called spastic gait (equinus foot position at foot strike) is partly due to changes in intrinsic properties of the muscle rather than hyperexcitability of the stretch reflex mechanism (Berger et al., 1984c).

Though we have greater understanding of the neural mechanisms underlying spastic hypertonicity, there is still no agreement on the role of spasticity (a positive sign of lesions to neurons of the motor cortex) in the loss of functional performance (a negative sign) (Rymer and Katz, 1989). It has been suggested that spasticity limits a patient's ability to move quickly, since activation of the stretch reflex is velocity dependent. While excessive activation of the stretch reflex mechanism may prevent the lengthening of the antagonist muscle during shortening of the agonist, referred to as *antagonist restraint* (Bobath, 1978; Davies, 1985) or *spastic restraint* (Knutsson and Richards, 1979), a growing number of researchers are showing that inadequate recruitment of agonist motor neurons, **not** increased activity in the antagonist, is the primary basis for disorders of motor control following a CNS lesion (Gowland et al., 1992; Dietz et al., 1991; Andrews and Bohannon, 2000; Sahrmann and Norton, 1977; Tang and Rymer, 1981; McLellan, 1973; Whitley et al., 1982). Thus, other problems such as inability to recruit motor neurons (weakness), abnormalities of reciprocal inhibition between agonist and antagonist, and dyssynergia may be more disabling in relation to motor control than simple hypertonicity (Katz and Rymer, 1989).

This research has tremendous implications for clinical practice. It suggests that treatment practices directed primarily at reducing spastic hypertonicity as the major focus in regaining motor control may have limited usefulness for helping patients regain functional independence. This is because loss of functional independence is often the result of many factors that limit the recovery of motor control and is not just limited to the presence of abnormal muscle tone. Some of those factors include problems with the coordination of synergistic muscles activated in response to instability.

Rigidity.   Another form of hypertonicity is rigidity. Like spasticity, rigidity is characterized by a heightened resistance to passive movement of the limb, but it is independent of the velocity of stretch. Rigidity may be the result of hyperactivity in the fusimotor system (Noth, 1991). Rigidity tends to be predominant in flexor muscles of the trunk and limbs and results in numerous functional limitations, including difficulty with bed mobility, transfers, postural control, gait, speech, and eating. Figure 6-5 illustrates severe flexor rigidity affecting upright stance in a patient with Parkinson's disease. There are two types of rigidity, lead pipe and cogwheel. Lead pipe rigidity is characterized by a constant resistance to movement throughout the entire ROM. Cogwheel rigidity is characterized by alternative episodes of resistance and relaxation, so called catches as

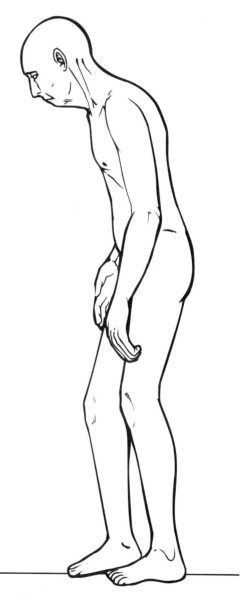

FIGURE 6-5.   An elderly man with Parkinson's disease with flexor rigidity in the trunk affecting his ability to stand with an extended posture.

the extremity is passively moved through its ROM. The pathophysiology of rigidity is poorly understood but is thought to be due to the disinhibition of cerebral structures normally inhibited by the basal ganglia.

Hypotonia

The range of muscle tone abnormalities found in patients who have CNS lesions is broad (Fig. 6-3). At the other end of the tone spectrum are flaccidity (complete loss of muscle tone) and hypotonicity, defined as a reduction in the stiffness of a muscle to lengthening. Hypotonicity is described in many different kinds of patients, including those with spinocerebellar lesions (Ghez, 1991a), and in many developmentally delayed children, such as children with Down syndrome (Shea, 1991).

Examination of Abnormal Muscle Tone

Both clinical scales and instrumented measures have been developed to measure muscle tone. Muscle tone is assessed clinically by describing a muscle's resistance to passive stretch. Subjective rating scales, such as the Modified Ashworth Scale (MAS) shown in Figure 6-6, are often used to describe alterations in muscle tone (Bohannon and Smith, 1987; Snow et al., 1990). Gregson et al. (1999) examined the reliability of the

---

0 = No increase in muscle tone.

1 = Slight increase in muscle tone, manifested by a slight catch and release or by minimal resistance at the end of the range of motion when the affected part(s) is moved in flexion or extension.

1+ = Slight increase in muscle tone, manifested by a catch, followed by minimal resistance throughout the remainder (less than half) of the range of motion (ROM).

2 = More marked increase in muscle tone through most of the ROM, but affected part(s) easily moved.

3 = Considerable increase in muscle tone, passive movement difficult.

4 = Affected part(s) rigid in flexion or extension.

FIGURE 6-6. Modified Ashworth Scale for Grading Abnormal Tone. (Reprinted with permission from Bohannon RW, Smith MB. Interrater reliability of a modified Ashworth scale of muscle spasticity. Phys Ther 1987;67:206.)

MAS in 32 patients post stroke and found both good interrater (kappa = .84) and intrarater (kappa = .83) reliability.

Behavioral indicators of spasticity can include a change in the resting position of a limb or the presence of characteristic movement patterns. Thus, careful observation of the patient at rest and while moving is essential. Table 6-1 summarizes common behavioral manifestations seen in patients with upper motor neuron dysfunction and suggests the muscles probably producing the spastic behavior (Mayer et al., 1997).

Biomechanical measures of spasticity evaluate changes in the phasic and tonic reflex activity (Dobkin, 1996). The Pendulum test was first reported by Wartenberg in the early 1950s (Wartenberg, 1951). In the Pendulum or drop test, the patient sits or lies supine with legs dangling over the edge of a table. As shown in Figure 6-7, the relaxed leg is passively straightened and released so the leg swings by gravity alone. In subjects with normal muscle tone, the leg flexes to about 70 degrees and oscillates back and forth in a pendular motion. In a patient with quadriceps or hamstring spasticity, the leg may not reach vertical and swings with fewer repetitions than an uninvolved leg. Leg motion can be quantified using isokinetic exercise equipment, an electrogoniometer, or computerized video equipment that measures leg kinematics (Stillman and McMeeken, 1995). The drop test has been shown to be a relatively simple, reliable, and practical objective measure of abnormal muscle tone (Katz et al., 1992; Brown et al., 1988). Measures of spasticity, whether clinical or instrumented, are not always good predictors of motor performance and disability, suggesting the importance of other factors.

Treatment of Abnormal Muscle Tone

A number of therapeutic interventions have been developed to manage abnormal muscle tone, including pharmacological, surgical, and physical treatments. The type of treatment chosen depends on a number of factors, including distribution, severity, and chronicity. For example, mild spasticity may be treated with a combination of thera-

TABLE 6-1.   Potentially Spastic Muscles in the Common Patterns of Upper Motor Neuron Dysfunction

Below are the common patterns of deformity seen in the upper motor neuron syndrome and the muscles that may contribute to each deformity. The weak muscles involved in each are also identified, but it should be remembered that these are unlikely to contribute to deformity even when spastic and therefore may not be candidates for chemodenervation. It must also be noted that not all listed muscles will be involved in any particular patient; strong agonists may counterbalance a spastic antagonist, and all muscles crossing a joint contribute to the net force across it.

The Upper Limbs

The Adducted/Internally Rotated Shoulder
Pectoralis major
Latissimus dorsi
Teres major
Subscapularis
The Flexed Elbow
Brachioradialis
Biceps
Brachialis
The Pronated Forearm
Pronator quadratus
Pronator teres

The Flexed Wrist
Flexor carpi radialis and brevis
Extrinsic finger flexors
The Clenched Fist
Various muscle slips of FDP
Various muscle slips of FDS
The Intrinsic Plus Hand
Dorsal interossei
The Thumb-In-Palm Deformity
Adductor pollicis
Thenar group
Flexor pollicis longus

The Lower Limbs

The Equinovarus Foot
  (with curled toes or claw toes)
Medial gastrocnemius
Lateral hamstrings
Soleus
Tibialis posterior
Tibialis anterior
Extensor hallucis longus
Long toe flexors
Peroneus longus
The Valgus Foot
Peroneus longus and brevis
Gastrocnemius
Soleus
Tibialis anterior (weak)
Long toe flexors (weak)
Striatal Toe (hitchhiker's great toe)
Extensor hallucis longus
The Stiff (extended) Knee
Gluteus maximus
Rectus femoris
Vastus lateralis
Vastus medialis
Vastus intermedius
Hamstrings
Gastrocnemius
Iliopsoas (weak)

The Flexed Knee
Medial hamstrings
Lateral hamstrings
Quadriceps
Gastrocnemius
Adducted Thighs
Adductor longus
Adductor magnus
Gracilis
Iliopsoas (weak)
Pectineus (weak)
The Flexed Hip
Rectus femoris
Iliopsoas
Pectineus
Adductors longus
Adductor brevis (weak)
Gluteus maximus (weak)

Reprinted with permission from Mayer NH, Esquenazi A, Childers MK. Common patterns of clinical motor dysfunction. Muscle and Nerve 1997;6:S21.

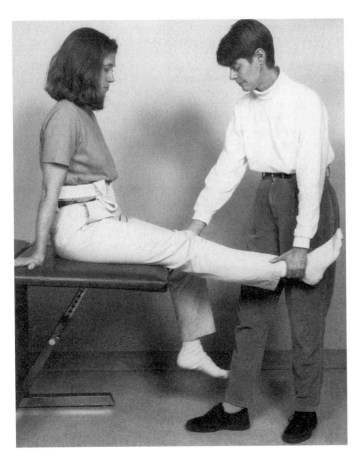

FIGURE 6-7. The Pendulum Test for spasticity in the lower extremity. The leg is passively extended, then released, so the leg swings by gravity alone. A reduction in the number of oscillations indicates spasticity.

peutic exercise, splinting, orthotics, and/oral medication. In contrast, severe spasticity may require chemodenervation (nerve blocks or injection with botulinum toxin) and/or surgery to reduce contracture and improve motor control (Gormley et al., 1997).

Pharmacological Treatments. Medications have been shown to be effective in management of spasticity, but the mechanisms and anatomical site of action of antispastic drugs are not well understood (Gracies et al., 1997a,b). Table 6-2 summarizes the efficacy of antispastic drugs in specific patient populations. Table 6-3 summarizes the potential side effects of these medications. A relatively new approach to treating severe spasticity is the continuous intrathecal application of baclofen via an implantable pump.

Surgical Management. The surgical treatment of spasticity has been aimed at

four levels: the brain, the spinal cord, peripheral nerves, and the muscle (Chambers, 1997). Because spasticity is only one symptom of lesions to motor cortex neurons, its elimination or reduction may not alleviate functional movement problems because of the continued effect of remaining impairments. Table 6-4 summarizes some of the common surgical techniques used to treat spasticity. The table summarizes the procedure and the target (brain, spinal cord, peripheral nerves, or muscle). The efficacy of surgical interventions for the treatment of spasticity and other movement disorders is beyond the scope of this chapter.

Physical Treatments. Considerable effort has been directed at developing physical therapeutic techniques to alter muscle tone in the patient with neurological impairments. One possible way to alter muscle tone is to change the background level of activity

---

TABLE 6-2.   Efficacy of Antispastic Agents in Specific Patient Populations

	MS	SCI	Stroke	TBI	CP	Comments
Dantrolene	+	+	++		+	Strength unimportant, cognitively fragile
Baclofen (oral)	++	+	+/–			
Tizanidine	++	+	+			
Diazepam	+	+	+/–		+	Night administration
Clorazepate	+		+			
Ketazolam		+		+	+	
Clonazepam	+?					Night administration
Piracetam					+	Hand function and ambulation improved
Progabide		+				
Clonidine		+?				
Cyproheptadine	+?	+?				
Thymoxamine (IV)	+	+				Preparation for PT sessions?
Orphenadrine (IV)		+				Flexor reflexes reduced
Baclofen (intrathecal)	+	+		+?	+?	

+ The antispastic efficacy and tolerance of the drug in the condition indicated have been established in a double-blind protocol.

++ The antispastic efficacy and tolerance of the drug in the condition indicated have been demonstrated to be greater than one of the standard drugs in double-blind comparative studies (e.g., baclofen ++ versus diazepam + in MS).

+/– The overall improvement was mitigated in the double-blind trials in which the drug was analyzed, usually because of bothersome side effects while the antispastic efficacy was good.

+? Open trials have been promising, but the efficacy has not been established in a double-blind protocol. An empty box means that the drug has not been investigated to our knowledge in the condition indicated in the column.

*We indicate important features of the drugs that may relate to the patient population in which they seem most appropriate (e.g., dantrolene), or to the most adequate timing of administration (e.g., diazepam, clonazepam), or to a particular feature in their efficacy (e.g., thymoxamine, orphenadrine). MS, multiple sclerosis; SCI, spinal cord injury; TBI, traumatic brain injury; CP, cerebral palsy; PT, physical therapy.

Reprinted with permission from Gracies JM, Elovic E, McGuire J, Simpson D. Traditional pharmacological treatments for spasticity II: General and regional treatments. Muscle and Nerve 1997;6:S93.

---

in the motor neuron pool of the muscle. As background level of activity in the motor neuron pool increases, so does the likelihood that the muscle will respond to any incoming stimulus, whether from the periphery or as part of a descending command. The opposite is also true; as background levels of activity decrease, the muscle is less likely to be activated. What techniques can be used to alter background activity of motor neuron pools and thereby influence muscle tone?

Sensory stimulation techniques (sensory modalities) can be used to facilitate or inhibit muscle tone, depending on the type of stimulus and how it is applied. For example, ice can facilitate muscle tone when applied quickly, as in a brief sweep over a muscle. Alternatively, prolonged icing is considered inhibitory, decreasing the level of activation.

Neutral (body) temperature is also considered inhibitory to hyperactive muscle tone.

Vibrators have also been used to facilitate or inhibit activity in a muscle. High-frequency vibration tends to facilitate muscle activity, while low frequency inhibits muscle activity levels (Bishop, 1974, 1975). In the same way, quick stretch to a muscle facilitates activation of the muscle through the stretch reflex, while prolonged stretch (manually or through the use of casts, splints, or orthoses) decreases activity levels. Brisk touch or tapping also facilitates muscle activity, while slow repetitive touching is considered inhibitory.

Techniques such as approximation, which activates joint receptors, have also been used to facilitate muscle activity in the patient with neurological impairments. Joint approximation involves compressing a joint

TABLE 6-3.   Side Effects Antispastic Agents

	Decreased Ambulation Speed	Muscle Weakness	Sedation	Others	Precautions
Dantrolene	+	+		Hepatotoxicity	Monitor liver function
Baclofen (oral)	+	+	+	Difficulty in seizure control	
Tizanidine		+/−	+	Dry mouth, liver function	Monitor liver function
Diazepam	+		++	Cognitive	
Clorazepate			+/−		
Ketazolam			+		
Clonazepam			++		
Piracetam				Nausea	
Progabide		0	+	Hepatotoxicity	Monitor liver function
Clonidine				Depression, hypotension	Blood pressure monitoring
Cyproheptadine		+	+	Dry mouth	
Thymoxamine (IV)				Risk of hypotension	
Orphenadrine (IV)		0	0		
Baclofen (intrathecal)	+	+	+	Seizure control Pump dysfunction	

+ The side effect has been demonstrated as statistically more frequent with the drug than with placebo in double-blind protocols
++ A major problem
+/− A minor problem
0 The side effect has been looked for but has not been more frequent than with placebo at the doses used in double-blind protocols.
An empty box means that the side effect has not been investigated with a double-blind protocol.

Reprinted with permission from Gracies, JM, Elovic E, McGuire J, Simpson D. Traditional pharmacological treatments for spasticity II: General and regional treatments. Muscle and Nerve 1997;6:S96.

TABLE 6-4.   Surgical Techniques Tested in the Treatment of Spasticity

Procedure	Target	Results
Stereotactic encephalotomy	Globus pallidus Ventrolateral thalamic nuclei Cerebellum	Variable to poor
Cerebellar stimulation	Cerebellum	Poor
Longitudinal myelotomy	Conus medullaris	Variable
Cervical posterior rhizotomy	C1–C3	Slight improvements Significant potential for complications
Selective posterior rhizotomy	Selected roots of L2–S2	Variable, encouraging
Neurectomy	Involved nerves	Variable, high recurrence, possibility of permanent, painful dysesthesias
Tendon lengthening, release or transfer	Contracted or spastic muscle	Variable but generally effective

Reprinted with permission from Chambers HG. The surgical treatment of spasticity. Muscle and Nerve 1997;6:S122.

either manually or through the application of weights. Manual techniques that apply traction to a joint are also used to facilitate muscle activity (Voss et al., 1985).

Altering a patient's position has also been suggested as a technique to alter both muscle tone and postural tone. The underlying assumption is that placing patients in certain positions will alter the distribution of muscle and postural tone, primarily through the changes in reflex activity. For example, it has been suggested that placing a patient supine will facilitate extensor tone, while flexor tone is facilitated when the patient is prone; this is because of the presence of released tonic labyrinthine reflexes in the patient with lesions to motor cortex neurons. The use of a side-lying position is often suggested as an approach to inhibiting the effects of the asymmetrical tonic neck reflex on muscle tone, facilitating bilateral symmetrical activities (Bobath and Bobath, 1984).

Coordination Problems

Coordinated movement involves multiple joints and muscles that are activated at the appropriate time and with the correct amount of force so that smooth, efficient, and accurate movement occurs. Thus the essence of coordination is the sequencing, timing, and grading of the activation of **multiple** muscle groups. Because of the synergistic nature of coordination, the capacity to generate force in an isolated muscle does not predict the ability of that muscle to work in concert with others in a task-specific way (Giuliani, 1991).

Movements involving more than one joint are associated with movement trajectories that are straight and smooth and that have bell-shaped velocity profiles (Hogan et al., 1987). In contrast, movement trajectories in patients with neurological pathology are often uneven and lacking a bell-shaped profile because of the loss of coordinated coupling between synergistic muscles and joints. Because coordinated functional movement emerges through the associated activity of many parts of the CNS, incoordination, defined as movements that are awkward, uneven or inaccurate, can result from pathol-

ogy in a wide variety of neural structures. For example, incoordination is commonly found following motor cortex, basal ganglia, and cerebellar lesions and in patients with proprioceptive impairments. In addition, since coordinated functional movement requires both biomechanical and neuromuscular systems, peripheral factors, including alterations in the viscoelastic properties of the muscles and tendons, can contribute to loss of coordinated functional movement (Giuliani, 1991).

Incoordination can result from a disruption of the activation, sequencing, timing, and scaling of muscle activity, resulting in functional movement abnormalities.

Activation and Sequencing Problems

Pathology within the CNS can produce problems in activating and sequencing appropriate muscles for functional tasks, which results in the production of unnecessary movements in joints and muscles not directly involved in a functional movement task. Lesions to the corticospinal centers can lead to loss of the ability to recruit a limited number of muscles controlling movement and the ability to control individual joints. The result is the emergence of mass patterns of movement, often referred to as abnormal synergies.

Abnormal Synergies.   In the rehabilitation literature, the term *synergy* has often been used to describe abnormal or disordered motor control (Bobath, 1978; Brunnstrom, 1970). Abnormal synergies are stereotyped patterns of movement that cannot be changed or adapted to changes in task or environmental demands. Abnormal synergies, also called abnormal patterns or mass patterns of movement, reflect a lack of fractionation, defined as the ability to move a single joint without simultaneously generating movements in other joints. Because muscles in an abnormal synergy are so strongly linked, movement outside of the fixed pattern is often not possible (O'Sullivan, 1994). Often synergies represent characteristic movement patterns of a specific diagnostic group, such as the patient with CVA.

A variety of abnormal synergies that impair normal movement have been described in patients with hemiplegia (Duncan and Badke, 1987; Brunnstrom, 1970). The flexion synergy of the upper extremity shown in Figure 6-8 is characterized by scapular retraction and elevation, shoulder abduction and external rotation, elbow flexion, forearm supination, and wrist and finger flexion.

The extensor synergy in the lower extremity involves hip extension, adduction, and internal rotation; knee extension; ankle plantarflexion and inversion; and toe plantarflexion. The process of recovery during stroke rehabilitation has been described as the dissolution of abnormal synergies of movement in favor of independent or selective control (Brunnstrom, 1970).

Coactivation. Inappropriate coactivation is an example of a sequencing problem. Coactivation of agonist and antagonist muscles during functional movements has been observed in many adults and children with CNS disorders (Nashner et al., 1983; Knutsson and Richards, 1979; Crenna, 1988). Crenna and Inverno (1994) suggest that excessive coactivation of agonist and antagonist muscles at a joint is one of four main factors contributing to motor control problems in children with cerebral palsy; the other factors include spasticity, muscle weakness, and increased joint stiffness.

Is coactivation a symptom of CNS impairment? Coactivation is also present in the early stages of learning a skilled movement in neurologically intact adults and children. In addition, it is found during the early stages of postural development in healthy infants and children just learning to balance. The finding that coactivation is a common characteristic of unskilled early stages of learning in healthy, neurologically intact individuals suggests that coactivation is not necessarily a result of impairment of function but a potentially primary, perhaps primitive or unrefined, form of coordination.

Impaired Interjoint Coordination. As mentioned earlier, during normally coordinated movement, joint angles at synergistic joints change smoothly and at synchronized

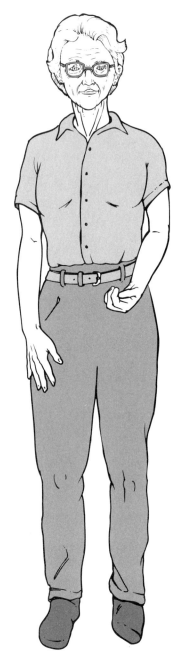

FIGURE 6-8. Flexion synergy of the upper extremity is characterized by scapular retraction and elevation, shoulder abduction and external rotation, elbow flexion, forearm supination, and wrist and finger flexion.

rates related to one another to produce a smooth movement. In contrast, many studies have reported multijoint incoordination leading to abnormal movement trajectories in patients with CNS pathology. Patients with cerebellar (CB) pathology demonstrate movement trajectories that are characterized by decomposition (moving one joint at a time) (Bastion et al., 1996). It has been suggested that in patients with CB pathology, decomposition may be a strategy used to compensate for impaired multijoint control. Since single-joint control appears to be better than multijoint control, patients with CB lesions may decompose movements into sequential movement at individual joints as a strategy to minimize the impact effect of multijoint dyscoordination.

In patients with Parkinson's disease, motor control problems seen in tasks such as handwriting are reportedly caused by a reduced capability for coordinating wrist and finger movements (Tuelings et al., 1997). In patients with spastic hemiparesis as a result of stroke, movement trajectories in the hemiparetic arm were characterized by segmented movements (movement at one joint followed by movement at a synergistic joint) rather than interjoint coordination (Levin, 1996).

Timing Problems

Incoordination can also manifest as an inability to appropriately time the activation of muscles and thus the movement itself. There are many facets to timing, including the time to initiate a movement (reaction time), the time to execute a movement (movement time) and the time needed to stop a movement.

Problems Initiating Movement: Reaction Time.   Reaction time is the time between the patient's decision to move and the actual initiation of the movement itself. Neuromuscular factors that have been proposed to affect movement initiation include (*a*) inadequate force generation (inability to overcome gravity, inertia, or antagonist muscle restraint), (*b*) decreased rate of force generation (force must be produced in a specific time period, (*c*) insufficient ROM to allow movement, (*d*)

reduced motivation to move, and (*d*) abnormal postural control, specifically the inability to stabilize the body in advance of potentially destabilizing movements.

In addition to neuromuscular factors, cognitive factors affect the initiation of movement. These include the inability to recognize a command or signal to move and difficulty recalling and selecting a movement plan or assembling and initiating a plan to move (Giuliani, 1991).

Slowed Movement Time.   Movement time is the time taken to execute a task-specific movement once it has been initiated. Delayed movement time is a commonly reported problem associated with a wide variety of neural pathologies. Longer movement times have been reported in patients with hemiparesis following stroke (Levin et al., 1993; Levin, 1996), in patients with Parkinson's disease (Teulings et al., 1997), in children with various forms of cerebral palsy (Steenbergen et al., 1998), and in patients with cerebellar dysfunction (Van Donkelaar and Lee, 1994).

Problems Terminating a Movement. Difficulty terminating a movement can manifest as inability to stop a movement or as inability to change direction of a movement. It is thought to result from an inability to control appropriate forces of the agonist at the end of a movement (Sahrman and Norton, 1977). Inability to terminate a movement can also result from inadequate timing and force generation in the antagonist muscle necessary to brake a movement. Problems terminating a movement are common in patients with cerebellar disorders and can manifest as difficulties in checking or halting a movement, resulting in a rebound phenomenon, or in the inability to perform rapidly alternating movements, referred to as dysdiadochokinesia. Rebound phenomena can be seen as involuntary movements of a limb when resistance to an isometric contraction is suddenly removed (Fredericks and Saladin, 1996).

Scaling Forces

In addition to appropriate sequencing and timing of muscle activation, coordinated functional movement requires the scaling, or grading, of forces appropriate to the metrics of the task. Dysmetria is traditionally defined as problems in judging the distance or range of a movement (Schmitz, 1994a). More recently it has been defined with reference to the ability to scale forces appropriately to task requirements (Horak et al., 1989a).

Underestimation of the required force or range of movement is hypometria, while hypermetria is overestimation of the force or range of movement needed for a specific task. Inability to scale or grade forces appropriately can be seen as undershooting or overshooting in coordination tasks such as reaching and pointing. Dysmetria is commonly found in patients with CB lesions (Hore et al., 1991; Bastion et al., 1996). However, problems scaling movements can also be seen in patients with basal ganglia disease. Patients with Parkinson's disease often demonstrate hypokinesia, defined as movements that are decreased in amplitude (Gordon et al., 1997; Horak, 1990). Thus, coordination problems in Parkinson's disease include both timing and scaling components.

Examination of Coordination

Tests of coordination have been divided into nonequilibrium and equilibrium subcategories (Schmitz, 1994; DeJong, 1970). Equilibrium tests of coordination generally reflect the coordination of multijoint movements for posture and gait and will be discussed in later chapters.

Nonequilibrium tests of coordination are important to all aspects of motor control, including posture, mobility, and upper extremity control. These tests, summarized in Table 6-5, are often used to indicate specific pathology within the cerebellum (Schmitz, 1994). They can include the following movements: finger to nose, heel to shin, finger opposition, rapid alternating movements, tapping (hand or foot), and drawing a circle (hand or foot). Performance is graded subjectively using the following scale: 5, normal; 4, minimal impairment; 3, moderate impairment; 2, severe impairment; 1, cannot perform.

Treatment of Coordination

Many therapeutic techniques are used to treat coordination problems in the patient with neurological deficits. Some techniques can be considered general approaches to dyscoordination, while others more specifically target problems in timing, sequencing, or grading synergistic muscle activity.

General Techniques. Probably the most frequently used technique to improve coordinated movement is repetition and practice of a functional task-specific movement. Since the requirement for accuracy creates increasing demands for coordination, therapists can select functional tasks with increasing demands for accuracy when training the patient. To assist the patient in recognizing errors in performance of coordinated movement, the therapist can provide feedback, either knowledge of results or knowledge of performance. Remember from Chapter 2 that intermittent feedback facilitates learning better than constant feedback.

Use of weight-bearing activities has also been recommended for improving coordinated action in the lower extremities. In addition to functional movements, therapists often have patients practice nonfunctional movements to improve coordination. Examples of nonfunctional movements are rapid alternating movements, reciprocal movements of the hands or feet, and tracing shapes and numbers, such as a figure 8, with a limb.

Timing Problems. A number of therapeutic strategies can be used to improve timing components (reaction time, movement time, and termination time) of functional movement. Practicing a functional movement under externally imposed time constraints is one approach. Having a patient perform functional movements to music or in time with a metronome is one approach to influencing timing. Timing patients while they perform a functional task and using the time taken to complete the task as external feedback (knowledge of results) is another approach. Verbal, visual, or manual feedback regarding speed of performance can also be used. Sensory stimulation such as

TABLE 6-5. Nonequilibrium Coordination Tests

1. Finger to nose — The shoulder is abducted to 90 degrees with the elbow extended. The patient is asked to bring the tip of the index finger to the tip of the nose. Alterations may be made in the initial starting position to assess performance from different planes of motion.

2. Finger to therapist's finger — The patient and therapist sit opposite each other. The therapist's index finger is held in front of the patient. The patient is asked to touch the tip of the index finger to the therapist's index finger. The position of the therapist's finger may be altered during testing to assess ability to change distance, direction, and force of movement.

3. Finger to finger — Both shoulders are abducted to 90 degrees with the elbows extended. The patient is asked to bring both hands toward the midline and approximate the index fingers from opposing hands.

4. Alternate nose to finger — The patient alternately touches the tip of the nose and the tip of the therapist's finger with the index finger. The position of the therapist's finger may be altered during testing to assess ability to change distance, direction, and force of movement.

5. Finger opposition — The patient touches the tip of the thumb to the tip of each finger in sequence. Speed may be gradually increased.

6. Mass grasp — An alternation is made between opening and closing fist (from finger flexion to full extension). Speed may be gradually increased.

7. Pronation/supination — With elbows flexed to 90 degrees and held close to body, the patient alternately turns the palms up and down. This test also may be performed with shoulders flexed to 90 degrees and elbows extended. Speed may be gradually increased. The ability to reverse movements between opposing muscle groups can be assessed in many joints. Examples include active alternation between flexion and extension of the knee, ankle, elbow, fingers, and so forth.

8. Rebound test — The patient is positioned with the elbow flexed. The therapist applies sufficient manual resistance to produce an isometric contraction of biceps. Resistance is suddenly released. Normally, the opposing muscle group (triceps) will contract and check movement of the limb. Many other muscle groups can be tested for this phenomenon, such as the shoulder abductors or flexors, elbow extensors, and so forth.

9. Tapping (hand) — With the elbow flexed and the forearm pronated, the patient is asked to tap the hand on the knee.

10. Tapping (foot) — The patient is asked to tap the ball of one foot on the floor without raising the knee; heel maintains contact with floor.

11. Pointing and past pointing — The patient and therapist are opposite each other, either sitting or standing. Both patient and therapist bring shoulders to a horizontal position of 90 degrees of flexion with elbows extended. Index fingers are touching or the patient's finger may rest lightly on the therapist's. The patient is asked to fully flex the shoulder (fingers will be pointing toward ceiling) and then return to the horizontal position such that index fingers will again approximate. Both arms should be tested, either separately or simultaneously. A normal response consists of an accurate return to the starting position. In an abnormal response, there is typically a past pointing, or movement beyond the target. Several variations to this test include movements in other directions such as toward 90 degrees of shoulder abduction or toward 0 degrees of shoulder flexion (fingers will point toward floor). Following each movement, the patient is asked to return to the initial horizontal starting position.

12. Alternate heel to knee; heel to toe — From a supine position, the patient is asked to touch the knee and big toe alternately with the heel of the opposite extremity.

13. Toe to examiner's finger — From a supine position, the patient is instructed to touch the great toe to the examiner's finger. The position of finger may be altered during testing to assess ability to change distance, direction, and force of movement.

14. Heel on shin — From a supine position, the heel of one foot is slid up and down the shin of the opposite lower extremity.

15. Drawing a circle — The patient draws an imaginary circle in the air with either upper or lower extremity (a table or the floor alone may be used). This also may be done using a figure-eight pattern. This test may be performed in the supine position for lower extremity assessment.

16. Fixation or position holding — Upper extremity: The patient holds arms horizontally in front.
    Lower extremity: The patient is asked to hold the knee in an extended position.

Tests should be performed first with eyes open and then with eyes closed. Abnormal responses include a gradual deviation from the "hold" position and/or a diminished quality of response with vision occluded. Unless otherwise indicated, tests are performed with the patient in a sitting position.

Reprinted with permission from Schmitz, TJ. Coordination Assessment. In: O'Sullivan S, Schmitz TM, eds. Physical rehabilitation: assessment and treatment. 3rd Edition, Philadelphia: FA Davis, 1994.

brisk icing or tapping to facilitate recruitment of motor neurons may improve reaction time. Again, while these are common techniques used by therapists to treat coordination problems, few if any of these techniques have been subjected to experimental testing.

Scaling Problems. Scaling problems represent an inability to grade forces appropriately to the demands of the task. Treatment focuses on having patients practice a wide variety of tasks that require precise grading of force and providing knowledge of results and/or performance. Functional movements performed quickly require less precision of force control than those performed slowly. In addition, functional tasks demanding a high degree of accuracy require more precise grading of forces than those demanding limited accuracy.

For example, moving to a large target requires less force control than moving to a small target. Picking up a paper cup full of water requires more precision than lifting an empty paper cup. Therapeutic interventions directed at remediating coordination problems during tasks related to postural control, mobility, and upper extremity functions are presented in sections of the book related to these functions.

Involuntary Movements

Involuntary movements are a common sign of CNS disorders and can take many forms.

Dystonia

The term dystonia was first used in 1911 by the neurologist Oppenheim (cited in Marsden, 1990). Dystonia is defined as a syndrome dominated by sustained muscle contractions, frequently causing twisting and repetitive movements of abnormal postures (Fahn et al., 1987). The abnormal movements associated with dystonia are diverse and range from slow athetotic to quick myoclonic dystonia (Fahn et al., 1987). Dystonic movements are often characterized by cocontraction of agonist and antagonist muscles (Hallett, 1993; Rothwell, 1995).

Types of dystonia are classified according to etiology, age at onset, and distribution of abnormal movement. Focal dystonia involves a single body region, such as torticollis (involuntary spasms of the neck) or writer's cramp. Segmental dystonia involves two or more adjoining body regions, such as neck and arm, trunk and leg. Hemidystonia involves the arm and leg on one side of the body. Multifocal dystonia involves two or more nonadjoining parts. Generalized dystonia involves the whole body (Fahn et al., 1987).

Dystonia is often divided into two categories, idiopathic (primary) dystonia, which occurs in the absence of other lesions within the CNS, and symptomatic (secondary) dystonia, which occurs in conjunction with other neurological diseases, such as multiple sclerosis, or acquired brain lesions, such as with head injury. About two-thirds of the individuals affected have idiopathic dystonia (Kramer et al., 1995).

Dystonia is thought to be a disorder of the basal ganglia, because patients with secondary dystonia often have lesions in the basal ganglia, particularly the putamen (Hallett, 1993; Marsden, 1990). However, the pathophysiology of primary idiopathic dystonia is still unclear. Animal models have identified abnormalities not only in the basal ganglia but in the thalamus, cerebellum, and brainstem. It is likely that the biochemical dysfunction varies with the subtype of dystonia (see Richter and Loscher [1998] for a review of this topic).

There is no cure for dystonia, and treatment is largely related to reducing symptoms. Relaxation exercises are often used, since dystonia is exacerbated by stressful situations. About 5% to 10% of patients with idiopathic dystonia are dopa responsive. Anticholinergic drugs have also been used successfully in the treatment of dystonia. Finally, botulinum toxin A, injected locally into the affected muscle, has been used to treat focal dystonias (Marsden, 1990; Fahn and Marsden, 1987).

Associated Movements

Associated movements are characterized by unintentional movements of one limb during the voluntary movement of another limb. Associated movements are quite often found in the presence of abnormal tone, specifically spasticity. They are commonly seen in patients with hemiplegia during forceful movements and can occur in both the paretic and nonparetic extremities. One hypothesis for the presence of associated reactions in patients with hemiplegia is the loss of supraspinal inhibitory mechanisms that normally suppress the coupling of intralimb and interlimb movements (Lasarus, 1992).

Tremor

Tremor is defined as a rhythmical, involuntary oscillatory movement of a body part (Deuschl et al., 1998). Physiological tremor is a normal phenomenon; however, pathological tremor results from disorders within the CNS (Hallet, 1998). Tremor has been classified in many ways. Because of this, the Movement Disorder Society has suggested a classification system for tremor disorder based on clinical features (Deuschl et al., 1998). Critical to this classification is an understanding of the conditions during which tremor occurs. **Resting tremor** is defined as tremor that occurs in a body part that is not voluntarily activated and is supported against gravity. The amplitude of resting tremor increases during mental stress or during movements of another body part, especially walking. It is most commonly found in Parkinson's disease. **Action tremor** is any tremor that is produced by voluntary contraction of muscle, including postural, isometric, and kinetic tremor, including intention tremor. **Postural tremor** is present when voluntarily maintaining a position against gravity. **Kinetic tremor** occurs during a voluntary movement and can vary from a simple kinetic tremor (not target related) to an intention tremor (those occurring during a target-directed movement). Intention tremors imply pathology of the cerebellum and its afferent or efferent pathways. For a complete discussion of this complex topic, refer to reviews by Deuschl et al. (1998) and Hallet (1998).

Choreiform and Athetoid Movements

Chorea or choreiform movements are involuntary, rapid, irregular, and jerky movements that result from basal ganglia lesions.

Athetosis, or athetoid movements, is slow involuntary writhing and twisting, usually involving the upper extremity more than the lower extremities; however, athetosis may also involve the neck, face, and tongue. Athetosis is a clinical feature of some forms of cerebral palsy.

Examination of Involuntary Movements

Involuntary movements are identified through systematic clinical observation describing the body parts affected and the condition under which involuntary movements are activated. For example, a clinician might observe whether a tremor is resting versus associated with activity (action tremor). The intensity of the involuntary movements can be graded on an ordinal scale. Conditions that increase or decrease the severity of involuntary movements are also noted.

Treatment of Involuntary Movements

Rehabilitation strategies for treating involuntary movement focus primarily on strategies to compensate for the movement rather than on changing the movement itself. For example, since increased effort tends to magnify involuntary movements, patients can be taught to perform functional movements with reduced effort. Patients often tend to develop compensatory strategies on their own, such as walking with hands in pockets or grasping objects to decrease resting tremor.

Weight bearing and approximation are often used by patients with choreoathetosis to increase joint stability. Distal fixation, a useful strategy in controlling involuntary movements, can be achieved by providing external hand holds on wheelchairs, lapboards, or desks (Fig. 6-9). The use of limb weighting in the management of involuntary movement is somewhat controversial. Application of a weight to the distal portion of a limb segment increases the overall mass of the limb and results in reduced motion. However, there is some evidence that limb motion is worse when the weight is removed.

In summary, neuromuscular impairments are a primary symptom of CNS pathology and represent a major constraint on the performance of efficient and effective func-

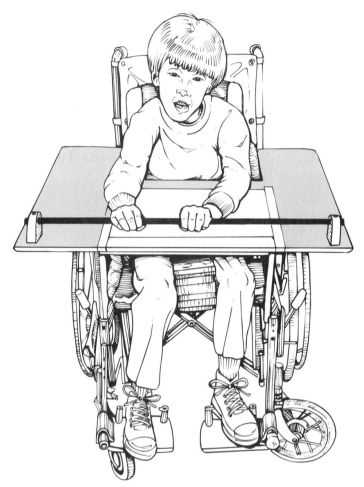

FIGURE 6-9.   A horizontal dowel on a lapboard is used for distal fixation to control athetoid movements.

tional movements in patients with neurological pathology. The examination and treatment of neuromuscular impairments depends on our understanding of the underlying pathophysiological basis, which in many cases is not known.

Secondary Musculoskeletal Impairments

In the patient with CNS lesions, musculoskeletal disorders develop most often secondary to the primary lesion. Since physical activity is necessary to the maintenance of both muscle and the bony skeleton, the absence of physical activity associated with neurological pathology can lead to a wide range of musculoskeletal problems including muscle atrophy and deconditioning, contractures, degenerative joint disease, and osteoporosis (Fredericks and Saladin, 1996).

Immobilization of a joint decreases the flexibility of the connective tissue and increases that tissue's resistance to stretch (Woo, 1975). Paralysis and subsequent immobilization also result in disuse atrophy, which affects trophic factors in the muscle itself. This can result in a reduction in sarcomere numbers, a relative increase in connective tissue, and a decreased rate of protein synthesis (Duncan and Badke, 1987). While musculoskeletal impairments develop secondary to other types of impairments, they can nonetheless be a significant constraint on functional movement in the patient with neurological pathology.

Examination and Treatment of Musculoskeletal Impairments

Examination of the musculoskeletal system includes evaluation of ROM, flexibility, strength, and alignment. This chapter does not discuss techniques for assessing the musculoskeletal system in depth; instead, the reader is urged to consult other texts (Kendall and McCreary, 1983; Saunders, 1991; Magee, 1987; Kessler and Hertling, 1983).

Musculoskeletal problems can be treated using traditional physical therapy techniques, including modalities such as heat, ultrasound, massage, and biofeedback. Passive ROM exercises are used to improve joint mobility and muscle flexibility. Manual therapies focus on regaining passive ROM and joint play. Proprioceptive neuromuscular facilitation (PNF) techniques, such as contract and relax, can be used to treat musculoskeletal problems such as contractures. Finally, plaster casts and splints are used to passively increase range and flexibility in the patient with neurological impairments. For an in-depth discussion of treatment of this important area of musculoskeletal impairments, the reader is referred to the sources cited in the previous paragraph.

@ SENSORY IMPAIRMENTS

As was discussed in Chapter 3, sensation plays multiple roles in the control of normal movement. Thus, it should not be surprising that sensory deficits are a major factor contributing to motor dyscontrol in patients with CNS lesions. The type of sensory problem depends on the location of the lesion in the sensory pathway and its size.

Somatosensory Deficits

Remember from Chapter 3 that somatic sensory information ascends to the cerebral cortex via two systems, the dorsal column–medial lemniscal (DC-ML) system and the anterolateral system. Lesions of the medial lemniscal system result in loss of discriminative touch, including light touch, and kinesthetic sense. In contrast, lesions in the lateral spinothalamic tract affect pain sensibility and the ability to detect thermal changes in addition to more coarse touch and kinesthetic discrimination. Lesions of the somatosensory cortex lead to loss of discriminative sensations such as proprioception, two-point discrimination, stereognosis, and localization of touch. Effects are contralateral to the side of the lesion.

Examination and Treatment of Somatosensation

Evaluation of somatosensation is complex, and many methods have been suggested. Sensory testing can vary from simple screening tests to complex assessment of the type and distribution of sensory function. Fess (1990) has described a hierarchy of sensory functioning. Detection, defined as the ability to distinguish a single point stimulus from background stimulation, is the lowest level of the hierarchy. Discrimination, the ability to distinguish the difference between stimulus a and stimulus b, is next. Quantification, the ability to organize tactile stimuli according to degree, such as roughness or weight, is the next level. Finally, recognition, the ability to recognize objects by touch, is at the highest level.

Sensory tests associated with these levels within the hierarchy are summarized in Table 6-6. Fess's hierarchy suggests that it may not be necessary to test every sensory modality in every patient. If the patient is able to discriminate stimuli, sensory detection tests need not be performed. In addition, researchers have shown a high correlation among sensory tests, so that results from one test, such as two-point discrimination, can be used to predict other tests, such as finger proprioception (Moberg, 1991). Thus, it may be possible to select a sample of sensory tests to predict overall somatosensory functioning.

Results from sensory testing can be interpreted in relation to established norms, expected performance based on anatomy and pathology, or in comparison to noninvolved areas. The relationship between sensory loss and function, however, is not clear. Dellon

TABLE 6-6.   A Summary of Methods for Testing Somatosensation

Sensory Modality	Stimulus	Response	Score
Discriminative Touch			
Touch awareness	Light touch to skin with cotton ball.	With vision occluded, patient says "yes" or signals when stimulus is felt.	Percent of correct responses out of total (e.g. 50% correct touches felt)
Touch localization	Lightly touch skin with cotton ball or monofilament number 4.17.	With vision occluded, patient points to location of touch.	Record error in accuracy of location.
Bilateral touch (sensory extinction)	Touch patient on one vs. both sides of the body with fingertips.	With vision occluded patient says "one" or "two" to indicate number of stimuli felt.	Record presence of sensory extinction.
Touch pressure threshold	Use range of Semmes Weinstein monofilaments.	With vision occluded, patient indicates when he or she feels stimulus.	Score the number of the thinnest filament felt (normal is perception of filament 2.83).
Two-point Discrimination	Using two paper clips, apply the two points to the skin, start 5 mm apart; gradually bring points together.	Patient responds "one," "two" or "can't tell."	Percentage of correct responses out of total.
Proprioception			
Vibration	Apply tuning fork or vibrometer to skin.	Patient indicates when he or she feels stimulus.	Percentage of correct responses out of total.
Joint position	Passively position joint in flexion or extension.	With vision occluded, patient mimics position with contralateral limb.	Percentage of correct responses out of total.
Joint motion	Passively move the joint into flexion or extension.	With vision occluded, patient reports whether joint is bending or straightening.	Percentage of correct responses out of total.
Stereognosis	Place a series of small objects in patient's hand.	Patient names object (may manipulate object first).	Percentage of correct responses out of total.
Pain			
Pain: sharp, dull	Randomly apply sharp and blunt end of safety pin to skin.	With vision occluded, patient indicates "sharp" or "dull."	Percentage of correct responses out of total.
Temperature			
Temperature	Apply cold (40 degrees) or hot (115 degrees) to patient's skin.	Patient indicates "hot" or "cold."	Percentage of correct responses out of total.

Based on material from Bentzel K. Evaluation of sensation. In: Trombly CA, ed. Occupational therapy for physical dysfunction, ed 4. Baltimore: Williams & Wilkins, 1995.

and Kallman (1983) found that tests that best predict hand function are static and moving two-point discrimination tests.

Often, clinicians tend to view sensory impairments such as loss of limb position sense or somatosensory deficits leading to decreased object recognition as being permanent or not modifiable by treatment. However, a number of interesting studies suggest that treatment can affect the patient's ability to process sensory stimuli. Based on some studies examining the reorganization of somatosensory cortex in primates (Merzenich et al., 1983a), which were previously discussed in Chapter 4, a number of researchers have developed structured sensory re-education programs to improve the patient's ability to discriminate and interpret sensory information (DeJersey, 1979; Carey et al., 1993; Dannenbaum and Dyke, 1988). The goal of these interventions is to improve a patient's ability to detect and process information in the environment and thereby improve motor performance. Suggestions for retraining sensory discrimination are presented in more detail in Chapter 19 on retraining upper extremity control.

Visual Deficits

As is true for the somatosensory system, disorders of the visual system vary according to the location of the lesion (Fig. 6-10). Impairments to vision are usually described with reference to the visual field deficit. A common visual problem following unilateral damage to the cerebral cortex is homonymous hemianopsia, or the loss of visual information for one hemifield.

Examination and Treatment of Visual Deficits

Visual testing includes information on visual acuity, including depth perception, visual fields, and oculomotor control. Visual acuity can be tested directly or determined via self-report. Depth perception is critical for such functional skills as mobility and driving. It can be tested by holding two identical ob-

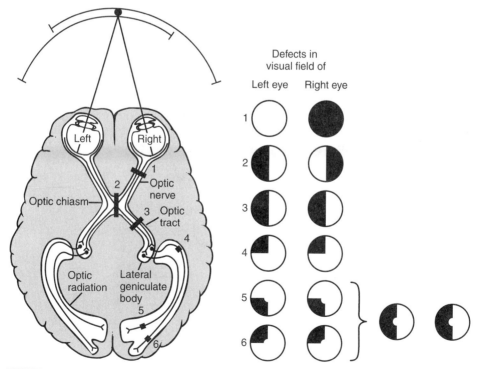

FIGURE 6-10. Visual deficits produced by lesions at various locations in the visual system. Reprinted with permission from Kandel ER, Schwartz JH, Jessell TM. Principles of Neural Science, 4th edition, New York, McGraw Hill, Page 544.

jects at eye level and moving one in relation to the other, asking the patient to indicate which is closer (Quintano, 1995). Visual acuity is tested using the confrontation test. The patient is told to look at the therapist, who sits in front of the patient. The patient is asked to indicate when he or she detects a visual stimulus in the periphery; all four visual quadrants are tested. Oculomotor tests examine the control of eye movements. These are discussed in Chapter 19, under examination of visual regard, a component of reach and grasp.

Vestibular System

The vestibular system provides sensory information regarding head movements and position with reference to gravity. Vestibular afferent information is used for gaze stabilization, posture, and balance and contributes to our conscious sense of orientation in space. Thus pathology within the vestibular system can produce problems related to (*a*) gaze stabilization, including blurred vision or oscillopsia (oscillating vision) due to the disruption of the vestibulo-ocular reflex; (*b*) posture and balance; and (*c*) vertigo or dizziness (Shumway-Cook and Horak, 1989, 1990; Herdman, 1999).

The term dizziness is often used by patients to describe a variety of sensations, including spinning (referred to as vertigo), rocking, tilting, unsteadiness, and light-headedness. The specific types of symptoms depend on the type and location of pathology within the vestibular system.

Examination and Treatment of Vestibular Function

Examination of vestibular function includes tests of gaze stabilization, posture, balance control, and dizziness. Treatment depends on the underlying cause. Specific procedures for assessing gaze stabilization are discussed in Chapter 19, while those for assessing posture and balance are presented in Chapter 11. The following section briefly overviews the examination and treatment of dizziness.

Examination begins with a careful history to determine the patient's perceptions of whether dizziness is constant or provoked and the situations or conditions that stimulate dizziness. The Vertigo Positions and Movement Test (Shumway-Cook and Horak, 1990) examines the intensity and duration of dizziness in response to movement and/or positional changes of the head while sitting, standing, and walking. The patient is asked to rate the intensity of dizziness on a scale of 0 (no dizziness) to 10 (severe dizziness). In addition, duration of symptoms is timed and recorded, as are the presence of nystagmus and autonomic nervous system symptoms, including nausea, sweating, and pallor. The Dix Hallpike maneuver, shown in Figure 6-11, is used to test for posterior semicircular canal benign paroxysmal positional vertigo (BPPV). BPPV is the most common cause of vertigo (Fetter, 2000). Most often patients describe a spinning vertigo associated with head positions involving rapid extension of the neck, such as looking up into a high shelf, or when lying down and rolling to the affected side. Key to the diagnosis of BPPV is the Dix Hallpike maneuver. In response to this rapid position change, the patient describes vertigo lasting from 30 seconds to 1 minute, and tortional nystagmus in the direction of the downward ear is present. The pathophysiology of BPPV is thought to be displacement of otoconia into the posterior semi-circular canal (SCC). For a detailed description of examination of dizziness, the reader is referred to other sources (Shumway-Cook and Horak, 1989, 1990; Herdman, 1999).

Treatment of vestibular pathology, referred to as vestibular rehabilitation, uses exercises to treat symptoms of dizziness and imbalance that result from pathology within the vestibular system. Since there are many potential causes of dizziness, including metabolic disturbances; side effects of medication; cardiovascular problems, such as orthostatic hypotension; and pathology within peripheral or central vestibular structures, it is essential that the therapist know the underlying diagnosis prior to beginning an exercise-based approach.

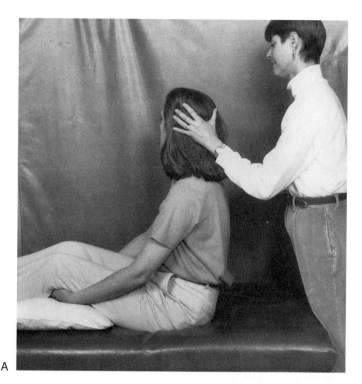

A

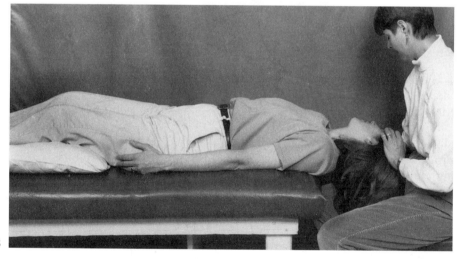

B

FIGURE 6-11. The Dix Hallpike position, a specific test for benign paroxysmal positional vertigo (BPPV). The test begins with the patient seated (**A**). The patient is quickly repositioned into a head hanging position (**B**).

The type of exercise used to treat dizziness depends on the specific type of pathology causing the dizziness. Vertigo secondary to posterior SCC BPPV is most often treated with a repositioning maneuver designed to mechanically move displaced otoconia from the semicircular canal(s) (Herdman, 1999). This procedure is shown in Figure 6-12.

In contrast to treatment of positional vertigo, dizziness associated with asymmetrical vestibular loss is treated with habituation exercises. The patient is instructed to repeat the position or movements that provoke dizziness 5 to 10 times in a row, 2 to 3 times per day. Exercises are progressive. The patient begins with fairly simple exercises, such as horizontal head movements in the seated position, and progresses to more difficult tasks, such as horizontal head movements integrated into gait. This approach is discussed

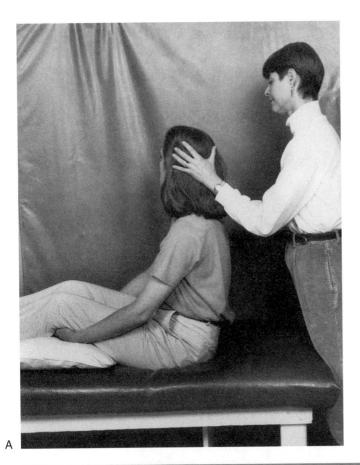

A

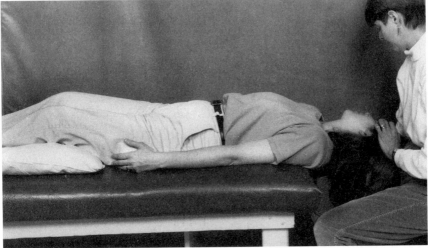

B

FIGURE 6-12.   The Canalith Repositioning Maneuver for treatment of benign parox-ysmal positional vertigo. Each position is held for 1 to 2 minutes or until nystagmus and vertigo subside. The first two positions (**A and B**) are the same as those found in the Dix Hallpike maneuver. In position 3, the head is moved into the opposite Hallpike position (**C**). In position 4, the patient rolls to the side-lying position, nose down (**D**); in position 5, the patient is brought to the sitting position, head turned to 45 degrees of midline (**E**), and finally the head is dropped into a flexed position (**F**) and held there for 2 minutes.

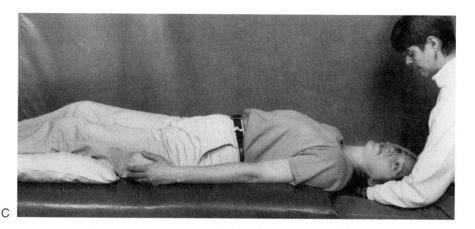

C

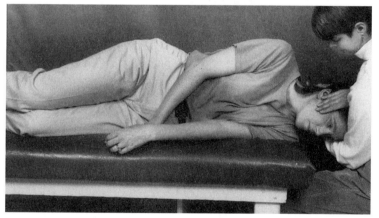

D

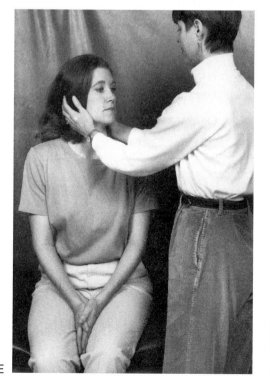

E

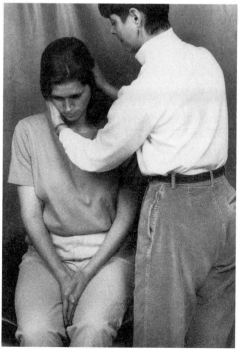

F

in more detail elsewhere (Shumway-Cook and Horak, 1989; 1990; Herdman, 1999).

℮ COGNITIVE AND PERCEPTUAL PROBLEMS

Cognition is defined as the ability to process, sort, retrieve, and manipulate information (Prigatano and Fordyce, 1986). Perception is the integration of sensory impressions into psychologically meaningful information (Lezak, 1976). Intact sensation is a necessary prerequisite for perception. Thus, patients with primary sensory impairments of necessity have some cognitive/perceptual problems.

Normally functioning cognitive/perceptual systems are critical to successful interaction with the environment. Thus, impairments in these systems affect the patient's ability to move effectively and efficiently about the environment. In addition, cognitive and perceptual deficits are a major factor in lack of progress in many patients who have sustained a neurological injury (Warburg, 1998; Bernspang et al., 1989; Sia et al., 1993).

Because of their impact on functional movement behavior, understanding cognitive/perceptual impairments is critical to therapists engaged in retraining functional movement in patients with neurological deficits. This is, however, a highly complex area of study that can only briefly be reviewed here. Table 6-7 provides a summary of cognitive/perceptual impairments. For further discussion of this subject, readers are referred to other sources (Quintana, 1995; Warburg, 1988; Perry and Hodges, 1999).

Perceptual Impairments

Body Image and Scheme Disorders

Body scheme is the awareness of body parts and their relationship to one another and the environment. Many patients with neurological dysfunction have problems with impaired body image, including somatagnosia (lack of awareness of the body structure and the relationship of body parts to one an-

other) unilateral spatial neglect, right-left discrimination, finger agnosia, and anosognosia (denial of the presence or severity of one's paralysis). Assessment of body image problems includes asking patients to identify body parts on self and others. The goal of treatment is to improve the patient's awareness of his or her own body. A number of different treatment approaches have been suggested to accomplish this, including the use of controlled tactile stimulation and developmental activities; however, there is no research to document the effectiveness of treatment strategies for improving body image and scheme disorders.

Unilateral neglect, also referred to as hemi-inattention or hemispatial neglect, is the inability to perceive and integrate stimuli on one side of the body. Assessment usually relies on observation of the patient performing functional tasks. Unilateral neglect may manifest functionally as eating food on one half of the plate, shaving one side of the face, or walking into objects on the involved side. Treatment strategies suggested for unilateral neglect include teaching patients scanning strategies, use of sensory stimulation to increase awareness, and modifying the environment to accommodate the impairment (Quintana, 1995).

Spatial Relation Disorders

Problems with spatial relations manifest as difficulty in perceiving oneself in relation to other objects or other objects in relation to oneself (Quintana, 1995). Spatial relations problems can include topographical disorientation (inability to remember the relationship of one place to another), figure ground perception problems (the inability to distinguish foreground from background), and problems with position in space, including understanding such concepts as over, under, front, and back.

Examination may be done through observation of functional skills or through more formal testing. Both adaptive and remedial strategies are used in treatment (Neistadt, 1990). An adaptive treatment approach attempts to circumvent the problem by teach-

TABLE 6-7.   Cognitive-Perceptual Deficits

Deficit	Definition	Functions Effects
Perceptual Impairments		
Body scheme	Awareness of body parts, position of body in relation to environment.	Difficulty dressing, unsafe transfers.
Right-left discrimination	Ability to understand concepts of right and left.	Difficulty with dressing, transfers, mobility, following directions that include right left.
Body part identification	Ability to identify body parts of self and others.	Incorrect response to instructions to move a body part.
Anosognosia	Unawareness or denial of deficits.	Unsafe in functional activities.
Unilateral neglect	Neglect of one side of body or extrapersonal space.	ADLs limited to half of body; transfers and mobility unsafe.
Position in space	Ability to understand concepts such as over, under, around, above, below.	Difficulty with mobility, following directions that include these terms.
Spatial relations	Ability to perceive self in relation to other objects.	Transfers and mobility unsafe.
Topographical orientation	Ability to find one's way from one place to another.	Mobility unsafe.
Figure ground perception	Ability to distinguish foreground from background.	Unable to find objects in cluttered drawing.
Limb apraxia	Inability to carry out purposeful movement in the presence of intact sensation.	ADLs affected due to difficulty in using objects.
Constructional apraxia	Deficit in constructional activities.	ADL apraxia.
Dressing apraxia	Inability to dress oneself.	Puts clothing on incorrectly.
Cognitive Impairments		
Attention	Ability to focus on a specific stimulus without being distracted.	Inability to follow directions.
Orientation	Oriented; refers to knowledge related to person, place, and time.	Disoriented.
Memory	Registration, encoding, storage, recall, and retrieval of information.	Appears disoriented; will forget names, schedules, etc.; decreased ability to learn.
Problem solving	The ability to manipulate a fund of knowledge and apply this information to new or unfamiliar situations.	Difficulty with ADLs, socially inappropriate, inability to recognize threats to safety.

Adapted with permission from Quintana LA. Evaluation of perception and cognition. In: Trombly CA, ed. Occupational therapy for physical dysfunction, ed 4. Baltimore: Williams & Wilkins, 1995.

ing the patient compensatory strategies or by changing the environment (Neistadt, 1990). An adaptive strategy for retraining topographical disorientation would be to practice using a map to find one's way around. In contrast, remedial treatment strategies are those that attempt to improve the underlying cognitive functions leading to the deficit. In the case of topographical disorientation, remedial treatment strategies would focus on having the patient practice with mazes (Borst and Peterson, 1993). A good overview of treatment of cognitive deficits may be found in a review by Quintana (1995).

Apraxia

Apraxia is the inability to carry out purposeful movement in the presence of intact sensation, movement, and coordination (Quintana, 1995). There are five types of apraxia: verbal, buccofacial, limb, constructional, and dressing. Two types of limb apraxia have been described: ideomotor and ideational apraxia. In ideomotor apraxia movement may occur automatically but cannot be performed on command. In ideational apraxia purposeful movement is not possible either automatically or on command (O'Sullivan, 1994).

Apraxia is generally found in patients with left-side brain damage. Assessment of apraxia can use either informal methods, such as observation of the patient performing functional tasks, or more formal methods using standardized tests, such as the Sensory Integration and Praxis Test (Ayres, 1972). Treatment of apraxia focuses on practicing functional tasks, such as activities of daily living, or nonfunctional tasks that are designed to improve sequencing of skills.

Cognitive Impairments

Cognitive impairments include deficits affecting memory, attention, and executive functions. Evaluation of cognitive deficits is usually carried out by a psychologist using psychometric tests. A complete discussion of this important topic is beyond the scope of this book.

Attention

Attention is the ability to focus on a specific stimulus without being distracted. Attention is multidimensional and has been subdivided into multiple factors including (*a*) focused attention (ability to respond to specific stimuli), (*b*) sustained attention (the ability to sustain attention over time), *c*) selective attention (ability to focus attention in the presence of distracting stimuli), (*d*) alternating attention (ability to shift focus of attention from one task to another) and (*e*) divided attention (ability to respond simultaneously to multiple tasks). Specific tests have

been developed to examine these different aspects of attention. For example, the Random Letter Test is used as a test of sustained attention, while the Stroop test is used for testing selective attention (Sohlberg and Mateer, 1989).

Orientation

The term orientation is used in several different contexts. In a cognitive context, it has been used to refer to an understanding of people, place, time, and situation. Used in a postural context, the term refers to the ability to maintain a position in space with reference to a specific sensory reference. In the context of cognitive function, orientation to person, place, and time is usually determined by asking the patent questions such as how old are you, what is your full name, what is today's date, what day is it today, where are you, and do you know why you are here.

A more formal measurement of mental status may be done by using either the Mini-Mental State Exam (Folstein et al., 1975) or the Short Portable Mental Status Questionnaire (Pfeiffer, 1975). The Mini-Mental State Exam is shown in Figure 6-13.

Memory

Like attention, memory is a complex concept involving many facets. Memory is the ability to process, store, and retrieve infor-

---

1. What is the date today? _____ / _____ / _____
2. What day of the week is it? _____
3. What is the name of this place? _____
4. What is your telephone number? _____
   or What is your address? _____
5. How old are you? _____
6. When were you born? _____
7. Who is the President of the US now? _____
8. Who was the President before him? _____
9. What was your mother's maiden name? _____
10. Subtract 3 from 20 and keep subtracting 3 from each new number, all the way down (20, 17, 14, 11, 8, 5, 2).

_____ Total Number of Errors

0 _____ Oriented at all times (0–2 errors on MM test)
1 _____ Mild intellectual impairment (3–4 errors)
2 _____ Moderate intellectual impairment (5–7 errors)
3 _____ Severe intellectual impairment (8–10 errors)

FIGURE 6-13. The Mini-Mental State Exam.

mation. Following brain injury, deficits in both short-term memory (STM) and long-term memory (LTM) have been reported. Assessment of STM and LTM entails asking patients to remember four words and then testing their immediate recall and their recall after 5, 10, and 30 minutes (Strub and Black, 1977).

Problem Solving

Problem solving is the ability to manipulate and apply knowledge to new or unfamiliar situations (Strub and Black, 1977). It requires the integration of many other cognitive abilities, including attention, memory, perception, and so on (Quintana, 1995). Problem solving has been divided into three steps: preparation (understanding the problem), production (generating possible solutions), and judgment (evaluating the solutions generated) (Bourne et al., 1979).

Arousal and Level of Consciousness

Alertness is a basic arousal process allowing the patient to respond to stimuli in the environment. The Rancho Los Amigos Scale is probably the best-known approach to quantifying level of consciousness in the patient with neurological impairments. This scale is shown in Figure 6-14. Assessment of level of consciousness, arousal, or state is an essential part of assessing motor control, since motor behavior is heavily dependent on arousal level (Duncan and Badke, 1987).

Treatment of Cognitive Impairments

Many patients with CNS lesions demonstrate significant cognitive impairments that affect the patient's ability to participate fully in a retraining program. With this in mind, Figure 6-15 provides a few suggestions for modifying treatment strategies when working with a patient who has cognitive problems. However, it is not within the scope of this book to discuss in detail issues related to retraining cognitive impairments affecting motor control in the patient with neurological dysfunction.

Cognitive problems are quite common in patients with CNS lesions. Cognitive prob-

I. No response: unresponsive to any stimulus.

II. Generalized response: limited, inconsistent, nonpurposeful responses, often to pain only.

III. Localized response: purposeful responses; may follow simple commands; may focus on presented object.

IV. Confused, agitated: heightened state of activity; confusion, disorientation; aggressive behavior; unable to do self-care; unaware of present events; agitation appears related to internal confusion.

V. Confused, inappropriate; nonagitated; appears alert; responds to commands; distractable; does not concentration on task; agitated responses to external stimuli; verbally inappropriate; does not learn new information.

VI. Confused, appropriate: good directed behavior, needs cueing; can relearn old skills as activities of daily living (ADLs); serious memory problems; some awareness of self and others.

VII. Automatic, appropriate: appears appropriate, oriented; frequently robot-like in daily routine; minimal or absent confusion; shallow recall; increased awareness of self, interaction in environment; lacks insight into condition; decreased judgment and problem solving; lacks realistic planning for future.

VIII. Purposeful, appropriate: alert, oriented; recalls and integrates past events; learns new activities and can continue without supervision; independent in home and living skills; capable of driving; defects in stress tolerance, judgment, abstract reasoning persist; many function at reduced levels in society.

FIGURE 6-14. Rancho Los Amigos Scale of Level of Consciousness. (Reprinted with permission from Adult Brain Injury Service, Rancho Los Amigos Medical Center, Downy, California.)

lems can include an altered level of consciousness, change in mental status, and deficits in learning, memory, attention, and information processing. Behavioral problems are also common and may include apathy, aggression, low frustration tolerance, emotional lability, and loss of behavioral inhibition resulting in impulsivity.

Ⓔ COMPOSITE IMPAIRMENTS

Composite impairments can also result from a neurological lesion. Composite impairments are those that result from an interaction of multiple systems. Impaired balance and abnormal gait are good examples of

1. Reduce confusion—make sure the task goal is clear to the patient.
2. Improve motivation—work on tasks that are relevant and important to the patient.
3. Encourage consistency of performance—be consistent in your goals and reinforce only those behaviors that are compatible with those goals.
4. Reduce confusion—use simple, clear, and concise instructions.
5. Improve attention—accentuate perceptual cues that are essential to the task, and minimize the number of irrelevant stimuli in the environment.
6. Improve problem-solving ability—begin with relatively simple tasks, and gradually increase the complexity of the task-demands.
7. Encourage declarative as well as procedural learning—have a patient verbally and/or mentally rehearse sequences when performing a task.
8. Seek a moderate level of arousal to optimize learning—moderate the sensory stimulation in the environment; agitated patients require decreased intensity of stimulation (soft voice, low lights, slow touch) to reduce arousal levels; stuporous patients require increased intensity of stimulation (use brisk, loud commands, fast movements, working in a vertical position).
9. Provide increased levels of supervision, especially during the early stages of retraining.
10. Recognize that progress may be slower when working with patients who have cognitive impairments.

FIGURE 6-15.   Strategies for modifying treatment to accommodate a cognitive impairment

composite impairments, since both result from the interaction of multiple neural and musculoskeletal systems. These will be discussed in later sections of this book.

⊘ A CASE STUDY APPROACH TO UNDERSTANDING NEUROLOGICAL IMPAIRMENTS

As therapists, we don't treat a diagnosis; we treat underlying impairments and functional problems that result from neurological pathology. Nonetheless, an important part of clinical decision making regarding the choice of appropriate tests and measures as well as therapeutic techniques is understanding what impairments are likely to manifest in patients with a certain diagnosis. The following section uses our case studies to present impairments commonly associated with specific diagnoses.

Phoebe J.: Impairments Associated With Cerebral Vascular Accident

Phoebe J. is our 67-year-old woman who has had a stroke. Stroke, or cerebral vascular accident (CVA), is defined as a sudden focal neurological deficit resulting from disruption to the blood supply in the brain that persists for at least 24 hours. Transient ischemic attacks (TIAs) result from temporary interruption of blood supply with symptoms lasting less than 24 hours. There are two main categories of brain damage: ischemia, a lack of blood flow, and hemorrhage, the release of blood into the extravascular space.

The impairments resulting from a stroke are numerous and vary with the site and extent of vascular damage. Phoebe J. has had a middle cerebral artery stroke in the right cerebral hemisphere. Her likely neuromuscular impairments include left-side weakness (paresis), abnormal muscle tone (spasticity), abnormal coordination characterized by abnormal synergies of movement, and an inability to activate muscles in isolation, so-called fractionation of movement. She is likely to have sensory and perceptual impairments, including deficits in somatosensation and proprioception. She is likely to have impaired vision, specifically homonymous hemianopsia. Cognitive/behavioral deficits depend on the side of the lesion. Patients with a left-sided CVA (resultant right hemiparesis) often have difficulty processing information and tend to be depressed, anxious, cautious, and uncertain. In contrast, patients such as Phoebe J., who have had a right-side CVA and resultant left hemiparesis, are often impulsive and unrealistic regarding their own abilities. They tend to deny problems (anosognosia), which can lead to poor judgment and safety issues. Finally, Phoebe J.'s neuromuscular impairments that restrict motion are likely to lead to the development of a variety of musculoskeletal impairments, including muscle tightness and contractures limiting ROM.

Laurence W.: Impairments Associated With Parkinson's Disease

Laurence W. has Parkinson's disease, a slowly progressing disorder of the basal ganglia resulting from degeneration of the nigrostriatal pathway. His primary neuromuscular impairments likely include cogwheel rigidity, akinesia, bradykinesia, resting tremor, and impairments of postural control and gait. Bradykinesia may manifest as decreased arm swing, slow and shuffling gait, difficulty in initiating or changing the direction of a movement, lack of facial expression, and/or difficulty in stopping a movement. Akinesia, defined as an inability to initiate movement, is likely to be associated with the assumption of fixed postures and can last for seconds to hours. Laurence W. is likely to show other common signs of Parkinson's disease, including festinating gait (small shuffling steps), stooped posture, poor balance, and a masklike facial expression. Cognitive impairments are likely to be present and may range from minimal involvement to severe depression and global dementia. Because Parkinson's disease results in a gradual and progressive loss of movement, Laurence W. is likely to develop secondary musculoskeletal impairments that will have a significant effect on functional performance.

Zach C.: Impairments Associated With Traumatic Cerebellar Injury

Zach is an 18-year-old who has suffered traumatic injury to the cerebellum following a motor vehicle accident. Because his pathology is largely limited to the cerebellum, his primary problems relate to planning and executing movements. As reported by Gordon Holmes in the 1920s and 1930s, disorders of the cerebellum result in three principal deficits: hypotonia, ataxia, and action tremor. Ataxia is a problem executing coordinated movement and is characterized by dysmetria (errors in the metrics of movement), dysdiadochokinesia (inability to sustain a regular alternating rhythmic movement), and dyssynergia (errors in the timing of multijoint movements). In general, lesions in the cerebellum result in impairments ipsilateral to the lesion; however, the specific constellation of impairments depends on what part of the cerebellum is affected.

Sara L.: Impairments Associated With Spastic Diplegia Cerebral Palsy

Sara L. is a 3-year-old child with the spastic diplegia form of cerebral palsy. Cerebral palsy is a nonprogressive disorder that results from prenatal or perinatal damage to the CNS. The site and extent of damage to the developing CNS determine the continuum of impairments seen in a patient who has cerebral palsy. Classification is based on the type of motor disorder and the extremities involved. Spastic cerebral palsy (hemiplegia, diplegia, and quadriplegia) constitute 50% to 60% of the cases and results from damage to the cerebral cortex and the corticospinal tract. Because Sara L. has spastic diplegia, her impairments affect her lower extremities more than her upper extremities. Her neuromuscular impairments likely include hypertonicity (spasticity), hyperreflexia, abnormal reflexes, weakness, and impaired coordination as well as poor postural control and gait. In addition to her primary neuromuscular impairments, she will likely develop secondary musculoskeletal impairments, particularly in the lower extremities. She is likely to have sensory deficits, particularly affecting somatosensory and proprioceptive systems.

℮ SUMMARY

1. Knowledge regarding both the physiology and pathophysiology of motor control is essential to examining and treating the patient with movement problems. This knowledge enables the therapist to form initial assumptions regarding the types of functional problems and underlying impairments likely to be present in a particular patient,

thus guiding the selection of appropriate tests, measurements, and suitable intervention methods.

2. Brain injury produces a unique pattern of behavioral signs and symptoms associated with the destruction of specific neuronal populations. Hughlings Jackson divided abnormal behaviors associated with CNS lesions into either positive signs and symptoms, that is, the presence of abnormal behaviors, or negative signs and symptoms, that is, the loss of normal behaviors. In the rehabilitation environment, emphasis is often placed on positive signs and symptoms, such as abnormalities of muscle tonus, at the expense of negative signs and symptoms, such as loss of strength, when attempting to understand performance deficits in the neurological patient.

3. CNS lesions can result in a wide variety of primary impairments, including those within the neuromuscular, sensory, perceptual, or cognitive systems.

4. Neuromuscular impairments encompass a diverse group of problems that represent a major constraint on functional movement in the patient with neurological dysfunction. Neuromuscular impairments include weakness, abnormal tone, abnormal reflexes, incoordination (including the presence of abnormal movement synergies), and the presence of involuntary movements.

5. In the patient with neurological pathology, musculoskeletal impairments develop secondary to neuromuscular impairments but can significantly constrain functional movement.

6. Sensory deficits are a major factor contributing to motor dyscontrol in patients with CNS lesions. Sensory deficits can result in a disruption of sensory information in somatosensory, visual, or vestibular systems.

7. Perceptual problems, such as impaired body image and spatial relationship disorders, also constrain functional movement in a patient with brain pathology.

8. Cognitive problems, common in patients with CNS pathology, can include altered level of consciousness, change in mental status, and deficits in learning, memory, attention, and information processing. Behavioral problems, also common, include apathy, aggression, low frustration tolerance, emotional lability, and loss of behavioral inhibition resulting in impulsivity.

9. Composite impairments, those that result from an interaction of multiple systems, are commonly the result of a neurological lesion. Impaired balance and gait are good examples of composite impairments.

10. Understanding the likely impairments associated with specific diseases of the CNS is the first step in determining appropriate assessment and treatment procedures.

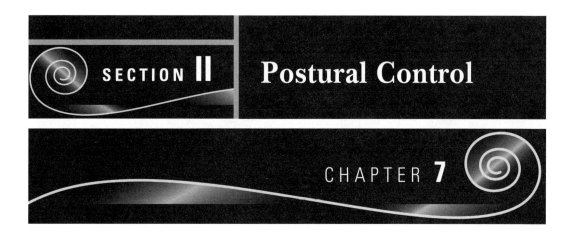

Normal Postural Control

@ INTRODUCTION

Picture yourself getting out of the car at the airport, in a hurry to catch your flight. You pick up your suitcase and run toward the terminal building. On the way, you misjudge the height of the curb and trip, but recovering, go into the terminal and check your bags. You get on the moving walkways that take you to your gate, moving quickly to avoid running into other people. Finally, you board the plane and sink gratefully into your seat.

The many tasks involved in getting from your car to your seat on the plane place heavy demands on the systems that control posture and balance. In examining some of these tasks, you can see that posture and balance involve not just the ability to recover from instability but also the ability to anticipate and move in ways that will help you avoid instability.

While few clinicians would argue the importance of posture and balance to independence in activities such as sitting, standing, and walking, there is no universal definition of posture and balance or any agreement on the neural mechanisms underlying the control of these functions.

Over the past several decades, research

into posture and balance control and their disorders has shifted and broadened. The very definitions of posture and balance have changed, as has our understanding of the underlying neural mechanisms. In rehabilitation science, there are at least two conceptual theories to describe the neural control of posture and balance: the reflex/hierarchical theory and the systems theory (Shumway-Cook, 1989; Woollacott and Shumway-Cook, 1990; Horak, 1991).

A reflex/hierarchical theory suggests that posture and balance result from hierarchically organized reflex responses triggered by independent sensory systems. According to this theory, during development there is a progressive shift from the dominance of primitive spinal reflexes to higher levels of postural reactions, until *mature* cortical responses dominate. This theory of balance control will be presented in more detail in the next chapter. This chapter discusses normal posture and balance control from a systems perspective. In this chapter we cover posture and balance related to sitting and standing. Posture and balance related to mobility, however, are covered in the next section of the book.

As noted in Chapter 1, the systems approach suggests that postural control emerges from an interaction of the individual with the task and the environment (Fig. 7-1). In addition, a systems approach implies that the ability to control the body's position in space emerges from a complex interaction of musculoskeletal and neural systems, collectively referred to as the postural control system.

Defining Postural Control

To understand postural control in the individual, we must understand the task of postural control and examine the effect of the environment on that task.

Postural control involves controlling the body's position in space for the dual purposes of stability and orientation. **Postural orientation** is defined as the ability to maintain an appropriate relationship between the body segments and between the body and

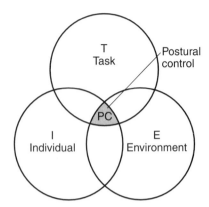

FIGURE 7-1.   Postural actions emerge from an interaction of the individual, the task with its inherent postural demands, and the environmental constraints on postural actions.

the environment for a task (Horak and Macpherson, 1996). The term *posture* is often used to describe both biomechanical alignment of the body, as well as the orientation of the body to the environment. We use the term postural orientation to include both these concepts. For most functional tasks, we maintain a vertical orientation of the body. In the process of establishing a vertical orientation, we use multiple sensory references, including gravity (the vestibular system), the support surface (somatosensory system), and the relationship of our body to objects in our environment (visual system).

Postural stability, or balance, is the ability to maintain the body in equilibrium. A body is in equilibrium either when it is at rest (static equilibrium) or when it is in steady-state motion (dynamic equilibrium). A stable system is one whose movement is not significantly altered from a desired trajectory even when it is given perturbations (Brauer, 1998). An object is considered stable when the center of mass (COM) is maintained over its base of support (BOS). The COM is defined as a point that is at the center of the total body mass, determined by finding the weighted average of the COM of each body segment. The BOS is defined as the area of the object that is in contact with the support surface. The vertical projection of the COM is often defined as the center of gravity (COG).

Postural stability, or balance, is thus defined as the ability to maintain the projected COM within the limits of the BOS, referred to as the stability limits. During quiet stance, the stability limits are defined as the area encompassed by the outer edges of the feet in contact with the ground. These are the boundaries in which the body can maintain its position without changing the base of support. **Stability limits** are not fixed boundaries but change according to the task, the individual's biomechanics, and various aspects of the environment.

The maintenance of stability is a dynamic process, involving establishing equilibrium between destabilizing and stabilizing forces (McCollum and Leen, 1989). For example, a person continually produces muscular forces to control the position of the COM. The vertical projection of these muscular forces directing COM motion is the center of pressure (COP). During quiet stance there is a separate COP point under each foot. The net COP lies between the feet and depends on the weight that each limb supports. In order to maintain a stable stance position, one can either relocate the COM through movement of the different body segments or adjust the size of the base of support, for example by taking a step (Brauer, 1998).

Stability and orientation are two distinct goals of the postural control system. Some tasks place importance on maintaining an appropriate orientation at the expense of stability. The successful blocking of a goal in soccer or catching a fly ball in baseball requires that the player always remain oriented with respect to the ball, sometimes falling to the ground in an effort to block a goal or to catch a ball. Thus, while postural control is a requirement that most tasks have in common, the demands of stability and orientation change with each task (Shumway-Cook and McCollum, 1990; Horak and Macpherson, 1996).

Throughout this chapter and this book, the term *postural control* is used broadly to cover both the control of postural orientation and stability, or balance.

Defining Systems for Postural Control

Postural control for stability and orientation requires both perception (the integration of sensory information to assess the position and motion of the body in space) and action (the ability to generate forces for controlling body position systems). Thus, postural control requires a complex interaction of musculoskeletal and neural systems, as shown in Figure 7-2. Musculoskeletal components include such things as joint range of motion, spinal flexibility, muscle properties, and biomechanical relationships among linked body segments.

Neural components essential to postural control encompass (*a*) motor processes, including neuromuscular response synergies; (*b*) sensory processes, including the visual, vestibular, and somatosensory systems; and (*c*) higher-level integrative processes essential for mapping sensation to action and ensuring anticipatory and adaptive aspects of postural control.

In this book we refer to higher-level neural processes as cognitive influences on postural control. It is important to understand, however, that the term cognitive as it is used here does not mean conscious control. Higher-level cognitive aspects of postural control are the basis for adaptive and antici-

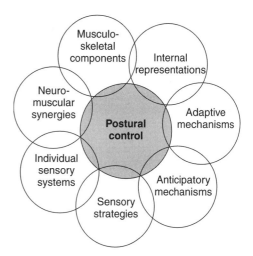

FIGURE 7-2. Conceptual model representing systems contributing to postural control.

patory aspects of postural control. **Adaptive postural control** involves modifying sensory and motor systems in response to changing task and environmental demands. Anticipatory aspects of postural control prepare sensory and motor systems for postural demands based on previous experience and learning. Other aspects of cognition that affect postural control include such processes as attention, motivation, and intent.

Thus, in a systems approach, postural control results from a complex interaction among many bodily systems that work cooperatively to control both orientation and stability of the body. The specific organization of postural systems is determined both by the functional task and the environment in which it is being performed.

Postural Control Requirements Vary With the Functional Task and Environment

The ability to control our body's position in space is fundamental to everything we do. All tasks require postural control. That is, every task has an orientation component and a stability component. However, the stability and orientation requirements vary with the task and the environment.

The task of sitting in a chair and reading has the postural orientation requirement of keeping the head and gaze stable and fixed on the reading material. The arms and hands maintain an appropriate task-specific orientation that allows the book to be held in the appropriate position in relation to the head and eyes. The stability requirements of this task are lenient. Since the contact of the body with the chair back and seat provides a fairly large base of support, the primary postural control requirement is controlling the unsupported mass of the head with respect to the mass of the trunk.

In contrast, the task of standing and reading a book has roughly the same postural orientation requirement with respect to the head, eyes, arms, and book, but the stability requirement is considerably more stringent: it involves keeping the COM within a much

smaller base of support, defined by the two feet.

Finally, a person standing on a moving bus must constantly maintain stability that is constantly threatened by the motion of the bus. The task of stability is more rigorous, reflecting the changing and unpredictable nature of the task. In this case, the task demands vary from moment to moment, requiring constant adaptation of the postural system.

Thus, you can see that while these tasks demand postural control, the specific orientation and stability requirements vary according to the task and the environment. Because of this, the sensory and motor strategies used to accomplish postural control must adapt to varying task and environmental demands.

☺ STANCE POSTURAL CONTROL

How do the sensory and motor systems work together to control a stable standing position? The task of stance postural control has stringent stability demands, requiring that the COM be kept within stability limits, defined principally by the length of the feet and the distance between them (McCollum and Leen, 1989).

Stance postural control is usually associated with the maintenance of a vertical orientation, though this is not an invariant requirement of the task. That is, one can maintain a standing position but be bent over, looking at something on the ground, or stand with the head extended, looking at a bird. In both instances, one can vary the configuration of body parts to accomplish these two standing tasks, but the stability requirements do not vary. If the center of body mass is not kept within the support base of the feet, the person will fall unless the base of support is changed by taking a step.

Over the past decade, sensory and motor strategies underlying stance postural control have been widely studied. What do we mean by strategies for postural control? A strategy is a plan for action, an approach to organizing individual elements within a system into a collective structure. Postural **motor strategies** are the organization of movements appropriate for controlling the body's position in space. **Sensory strategies** organize sensory information from visual, somatosensory, and vestibular systems for postural control. Finally, **sensorimotor strategies** reflect the rules for coordinating sensory and motor aspects of postural control (Nashner, 1989).

Research in stance postural control has focused primarily on examining strategies for controlling forward and backward sway. Why? The application of this concept can be found in Lab Activity 7-1.

As the lab exercise shows, no one stands absolutely still; instead, the body sways in small amounts, mostly forward and backward. This is why researchers have primarily concentrated on understanding how normal adults maintain stability in the sagittal plane. However, in recent years, researchers have begun to focus on mechanisms underlying lateral stability as well.

Now we can explore the underlying control mechanisms in depth, beginning with the motor mechanisms underlying postural control. In our discussion of motor mechanisms important to postural control, we first consider the role of muscle tone and postural tone in controlling small oscillations of the body during quiet stance. Then we will discuss the motor strategies and underlying muscle synergies that help us to recover stability when our balance is threatened.

Motor Mechanisms for Postural Control

Postural control requires the generation and coordination of forces that produce movements effective in controlling the body's position in space. How does the nervous system organize the motor system to ensure postural control during quiet stance? How does the organization change when stability is threatened?

Motor Control of Quiet Stance

What are the behavioral characteristics of quiet stance, and what is it that allows us to remain upright during quiet stance or sit-

 LAB ACTIVITY 7-1

OBJECTIVE: To explore the motor strategies used for stance postural control.

PROCEDURE: With a partner, observe body movement in the following conditions:
1. Stand with your feet shoulder distance apart for 1 minute.
2. Try leaning forward and backward a little, then as far as you can without taking a step. Now lean so far forward or backward that you have to take a step.
3. Come up on your toes and do the same thing.
4. Put on a pair of ski boots or other footgear constraining ankle movement and try swaying backward and forward.
5. Your partner now places three fingers on your sternum and nudges you backward, first gently and then with more force.

ASSIGNMENT: Write answers to the following questions, based on your observations of yourself and your partner's balance under the different conditions:

During quiet stance, did you stand perfectly still or did you move very slightly? In which direction did you feel yourself swaying most?

During active sway, describe the movement strategies you used to control body sway.

Describe the movement strategies you used when reacting to nudges from your partner.

Discuss how those strategies change as a function of size of base of support, speed of movement, where the center of mass was relative to the base of support (well inside, near edge, outside), when movement was constrained at the ankle.

List the muscles you think were active to control sway in these conditions. What muscles did you feel working to keep you balanced when you swayed a little? What muscles worked when you swayed farther? What happened when you leaned so far forward that your center of mass moved outside the base of support of your feet?

ting? Quiet stance is characterized by small amounts of spontaneous postural sway. A number of factors contribute to our stability in this situation. First, body alignment can minimize the effect of gravitational forces, which tend to pull us off center. Second, muscle tone keeps the body from collapsing in response to the pull of gravity. Three main factors contribute to our background muscle tone during quiet stance: (*a*) the intrinsic stiffness of the muscles themselves; (*b*) the background muscle tone, which exists normally in all muscles because of neural contributions; and (*c*) postural tone, the activation of antigravity muscles during quiet stance. Let's look at these factors (Roberts, 1979; Basmajian and De Luca, 1985; Kendall and McCreary, 1983; Schenkman and Butler, 1992).

Alignment

How does alignment contribute to postural stability? In a perfectly aligned posture,

shown in Figure 7-3, the vertical line of gravity falls in the midline between (*a*) the mastoid process, (*b*) a point just in front of the shoulder joints, (*c*) the hip joints or just behind, (*d*) a point just in front of the center of the knee joints, and (*e*) a point just in front of the ankle joints (Basmajian and De Luca, 1985). The ideal alignment in stance allows the body to be maintained in equilibrium with the least expenditure of internal energy.

Before we continue reviewing the research concerning postural control, be sure to review the information contained in the Technology Boxes, which include a discussion of techniques for movement analysis at different levels of control, including electromyography (Box 7-1), kinematics (Box 7-2), and kinetics (Box 7-3).

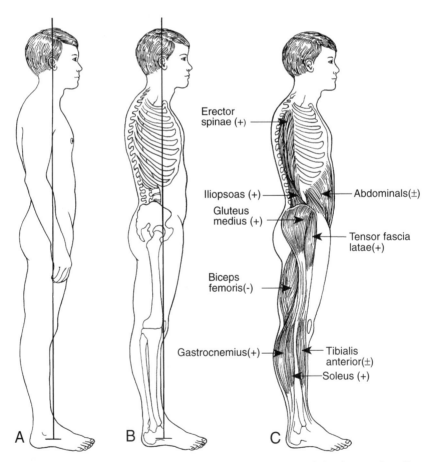

FIGURE 7-3. A, B.   The ideal alignment in stance, requiring minimal muscular effort to sustain the vertical position. **C.** The muscles that are tonically active during the control of quiet stance. (Adapted with permission from Kendell FP, McCreary EK. Muscles: testing and function. 3rd ed. Baltimore: Williams & Wilkins, 1983:280.)

TECHNOLOGY BOX 7-1

ELECTROMYOGRAPHY is a technique used for measuring the activity of muscles through electrodes placed on the surface of the skin, over the muscle to be recorded, or in the muscle itself. The output signal from the electrode (the electromyogram, or EMG) describes the output to the muscular system from the motor neuron pool. It provides the clinician with information about (*a*) the identity of the muscles that are active during a movement, (*b*) the timing and relative intensity of muscle contraction, and (*c*) whether antagonistic or synergistic muscle activity is occurring. Surface electrodes are most often used; however, the ability of these electrodes to differentiate between the activity of neighboring muscles is not very effective.

The amplitude of the EMG signal is often interpreted as a rough measure of tension generated in the muscle. However, caution must be used when interpreting EMG amplitude measurements. Many variables can affect the amplitude of EMG signals, including how rapidly the muscle is changing length, resistance associated with cutaneous tissue and subcutaneous fat, and location of the electrode. Thus, generally, it is not accurate to compare absolute amplitudes of EMG activity of a muscle across subjects or within the same subject across different days. Researchers who use EMG amplitude data to compare temporal and spatial patterns of muscle activity across subjects or within a subject on different days generally convert absolute amplitude measures to relative measures. For example, one can determine the ratio between the response amplitude (the area under the curve of EMG activity for a specified time, called integrated EMG, or IEMG) and the amplitude of a maximum voluntary contraction of that muscle. Alternatively, the ratio of IEMG for agonist and antagonist muscles at a joint can be determined. Likewise, the ratio of IEMG for synergistic muscles can be found. One can then examine how this ratio changes as a function of changing task or environmental conditions (Gronley and Perry, 1984; Winter, 1990)

Muscle Tone

What is muscle tone, and how does it help us to keep our balance? **Muscle tone** is the force with which a muscle resists being

 TECHNOLOGY BOX 7-2

KINEMATIC ANALYSIS is the description of the characteristics of an object's movement, including linear and angular displacements, velocities, and accelerations. Displacement data are usually gathered from the measurement of the position of markers placed over anatomical landmarks and reported relative either to an anatomical coordinate system, that is, relative joint angle, or to an external spatial reference system. There are various ways to measure the kinematics of body movement. Goniometers, or electrical potentiometers, can be attached to a joint to measure a joint angle (a change in joint angle produces a proportional change in voltage). Most accelerometers are force transducers that measure the reaction forces associated with acceleration of a body segment. The mass of the body is accelerated against a force transducer, producing a signal voltage proportional to the acceleration. Finally, imaging measurement techniques, including cinematography, video, or optoelectric systems, can be used to measure body movement. Optoelectric systems require the subject to wear on each anatomical landmark special infrared lights or reflective markers, which are recorded by one or more cameras. The location of the light, or marker, is expressed in terms of x and y coordinates in a two-dimensional system or x, y, and z coordinates in a three-dimensional system. Output from these systems is expressed as changes in segment displacements, joint angles, velocities, or accelerations, and the data can be used to create a reconstruction of the body's movement in space (Gronley and Perry, 1984; Winter, 1990)

lengthened, that is, its stiffness (Basmajian and De Luca, 1985). Muscle tone is often tested clinically by passively extending and flexing a relaxed patient's limbs and feeling the resistance offered by the muscles. Both nonneural and neural mechanisms contribute to muscle tone or stiffness.

A certain level of muscle tone is present in a normal, conscious, and relaxed person. However, in the relaxed state, electromyography (EMG) records no electrical activity in normal human skeletal muscle. This has led researchers to argue that nonneural con-

KINETIC ANALYSIS is the analysis of the forces that cause movement, including both internal and external forces. Internal forces come from muscle activity, ligaments, or friction in the muscles and joints; external forces come from the ground or external loads. Kinetic analysis gives us insight into the forces contributing to movement. Force-measuring devices or force transducers are used to measure force, with output signals that are proportional to the applied force. Force plates measure ground reaction forces, which are the forces under the area of the foot, from which center-of-pressure (COP) data are calculated. The center of gravity (COG) of the body is not the same as the COP. The COG of the body is the net location of the center of mass in the vertical plane. COP is the location of the vertical ground reaction force on the forceplate and is equal and opposite to all the downward acting forces (Gronley and Perry, 1984; Winter, 1990)

tributions to muscle tone are the result of small amounts of free calcium in the muscle fiber, which cause a low level of continuous recycling of cross-bridges (Hoyle, 1983).

Also, neural contributions to muscle tone or stiffness are associated with the activation of the stretch reflex, which resists lengthening of the muscle. The muscle spindles sense changes in muscle length. This afferent information goes to the motor neurons, which alter their firing to achieve the needed force to change the muscle length to the desired value. In this way, the stretch reflex loop acts continuously to keep the muscle length at a set value. For a more detailed review of the role of the muscle spindle, review Chapter 3.

The role of the stretch reflex as a contributor to normal muscle tone is fairly clear. The role of stretch reflexes in stance postural control, however, is not. According to one theory, stretch reflexes play a feedback role during the maintenance of stance posture. Thus, this theory suggests that as we sway back and forth while standing, the ankle muscles are stretched, activating the stretch reflex. This results in a reflex shortening of the muscle and control of forward and backward sway.

While some authors suggest that the stretch reflex is critical for maintaining posture, others have questioned the role of the stretch reflex in the control of quiet stance. Reports that the gain of the stretch reflex is quite low during stance has led some researchers to question its relevance to the control of sway (Gurfinkel et al., 1974).

Postural Tone

We have explained the mechanisms contributing to the generation of tone in individual muscles when a person is in a relaxed state. This background level of activity changes in certain antigravity postural muscles when we stand upright, thus counteracting the force of gravity. This increased level of activity in antigravity muscles is known as **postural tone**. What are the factors that contribute to postural tone?

A number of factors influence postural tone. Evidence from experiments showing that lesions of the dorsal (sensory) roots of the spinal cord reduced postural tone indicates that postural tone is influenced by inputs from the somatosensory system. In addition, it has long been known that activation of cutaneous inputs on the soles of the feet causes a placing reaction that results in an automatic extension of the foot toward the support surface, thus increasing postural tone in extensor muscles. Somatosensory inputs from the neck activated by changes in head orientation can also influence the distribution of postural tone in the trunk and limbs. These have been referred to as the tonic neck reflexes and are discussed further in Chapter 8, which discusses postural development (Ghez, 1991a; Roberts, 1979).

Inputs from the visual and vestibular systems also influence postural tone. Vestibular inputs, activated by a change in head orientation, alter the distribution of postural tone in the neck and limbs and have been referred to as the vestibulocollic and vestibulospinal reflexes (Massion and Woollacott, 1996).

Often, these reflex contributions to postural control are highly emphasized in the clinical literature. However, it is important to remember that there are many influences on postural control in a normal, intact, functioning individual (Anderson and Binder, 1989). It is possible that in the individual with a neurological impairment who has lost varying amounts of nonreflex influences, reflex pathways may take a more commanding role in postural control.

The clinical literature places much emphasis on the concept of postural tone as a major mechanism in supporting the body against gravity. In particular, many clinicians have suggested that postural tone in the trunk is the key element for control of normal postural stability in the erect position (Schenkman and Butler, 1992; Davies, 1985). How consistent is this assumption with EMG studies that have examined the muscles active in quiet stance?

Researchers have found that many muscles in the body are tonically active during quiet stance (Basmajian and De Luca, 1985). Some of these muscles, shown in Figure 7.3C, include (a) the soleus and gastrocnemius, since the line of gravity falls slightly in front of the knee and ankle; (b) the tibialis anterior, when the body sways backward; (c) the gluteus medius and tensor fasciae latae but not the gluteus maximus; (d) the iliopsoas, which prevents hyperextension of the hips, but not the hamstrings and quadriceps; and (e) the thoracic erector spinae in the trunk (along with intermittent activation of the abdominals), because the line of gravity falls in front of the spinal column.

These studies suggest that muscles throughout the body, not just those of the trunk, are tonically active to maintain the body in a narrowly confined vertical position during quiet stance. Once the center of mass moves outside the narrow range defined by the *ideal alignment*, more muscular effort is required to recover a stable position. In this situation, compensatory postural strategies are used to return the center of gravity to a stable position within the base of support.

Correlation of COP Measurements With Postural Control

A traditional assumption regarding COP measurements was that the effectiveness of the postural control system in maintaining balance was directly related to the amplitude of COP motion. Thus, small-amplitude

movements of the COP reflect "good" balance control; conversely, large displacements of the COP reflect "poor" balance control. This has been supported by a number of studies showing that when there is a decrease in sensory inputs contributing to postural control, with pathology or with aging, that amplitude of COP motion during quiet stance tends to increase. However, this rule has many exceptions. For example, scientists have reported a decrease in COP motion for subjects with known balance problems, such as Parkinson's disease (Panzer and Hallett, 1990; Horak, 1992). In addition, it has been reported that dancers, who have highly skilled balance abilities, show an increase in COP motion during quiet stance (Brauer, 1998).

Limits of Stability During Quiet Stance

Theoretical limits of stability in stance are traditionally considered to depend on the area of the BOS (the anteroposterior length of the foot and the mediolateral width of stance), the position of the vertical projection of the COM as it relates to the edges of the base of support, the height of the COM from the support surface (correlated with the height of the person), and the weight of the mass to be controlled (Hayes, 1982). These variables tend to show considerable covariation, so that people of varying heights show similar limits of stability (Duncan et al., 1990). Recent research suggests that actual stability limits also depend on an interaction between position and velocity of the COM. Thus, if one is very close to the edge of the BOS and the velocity of the COM is high, it is more difficult to recover stability than if one is at the center of the BOS with an equally high velocity (Pai and Patton, 1997).

Perceived limits of stability may be defined as the distance a person is willing and able to move without losing balance and taking a step. A number of studies have been performed to determine perceived limits of stability in healthy adults. As we discuss limits of stability in this section, we will be referring to perceived limits of stability. These studies (Brauer, 1998) have been summarized for both anteroposterior (Table 7-1) and mediolateral (Table 7-2) limits of stabil-

---

TABLE 7-1.   Anterior-Posterior Limits of Stability

Study	Subjects	Limits of Stability
Whitney (1962)	10 men 18–21 yr	67% of foot length
Murray et al. (1975)	24 young men	54% of foot length
Lee and Deming (1988)	40 men and women <60 yr	35%–90% of foot length
	40 men and women >60 yr	15%–60% of foot length
Blaszczyk et al. (1994)	9 men and women 22–36 yr	80% of foot length
	9 men and women 69–77 yr	50% of foot length

---

ity. It should be noted that in none of these studies was foot position standardized, and thus it probably varied between individuals. The studies show considerable variability, with means for young adults for anteroposterior stability of 54%, 67%, and 80% of foot length and for mediolateral stability of 59% and 80% of stance width. As expected, there is an interaction between stance width and mediolateral limits of stability (LOS), with LOS being greater when the feet are together than when they are at a comfortable stance width (Murray et al., 1975).

Motor Strategies During Perturbed Stance

Many research labs, including Lewis Nashner's lab in the United States and the labs of Dichgans, Dietz, and Allum in Europe, using a variety of moving platforms, such as the one shown in Figure 7-4, have studied the organization of movement strategies used to recover stability in response to brief displacements of the supporting surface (Nashner, 1976; Allum and Pfaltz, 1985; Diener et al., 1982). In addition, characteristic patterns of muscle activity, called muscle synergies, which are associated with postural movement strategies, have been described (Nashner, 1977; Nashner and Woollacott, 1979; Horak and Nashner, 1986). These movement patterns, referred to as the ankle, hip, and suspensory, or stepping, strategies are illustrated in Figure 7-5.

These postural movement strategies are used in both a feedback and feed-forward (anticipatory) manner to maintain equilibrium in a number of circumstances. Here are some examples of such situations:

1. In response to external disturbances to equilibrium, such as when the support surface moves
2. To prevent a disturbance to the system, for example prior to a voluntary movement that is potentially destabilizing
3. During gait and in response to unexpected disruptions to the gait cycle
4. During volitional center of mass movements in stance

Nashner and colleagues (Nashner, 1977; Nashner et al., 1979; Nashner and Woolla-

---

TABLE 7-2.   Mediolateral Limits of Stability

Study	Subjects	Limits of Stability
Murray et al. (1974)	24 young men	59% of stance width
Lee and Deming (1988)	40 men and women <60 yr	60%–90% of stance width
	40 men and women >60 yr	30%–65% of stance width
Blaszczyk et al. (1994)	9 men and women 22–36 yr	80% of stance width
	9 men and women 69–77 yr	68% of stance width

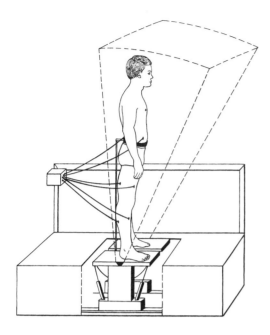

FIGURE 7-4. Moving platform posturography used to study postural control. (Adapted with permission from Woollacott MH, Shumway-Cook A, Nashner LM. Aging and posture control: changes in sensory organization and muscular coordination. Int J Aging Hum Dev 1986;22:332.)

cott, 1979; Horak and Nashner, 1986) have explored the muscle patterns that underlie movement strategies for balance. Results of postural control research in neurologically intact young adults suggest that the nervous system combines independent though related muscles into units called **muscle synergies**. A **synergy** is defined as the functional coupling of groups of muscles such that they are constrained to act together as a unit; this simplifies the control demands on the central nervous system (CNS). It is important to keep in mind that while muscle synergies are important, they are only one of many motor mechanisms that affect outputs for postural control.

What are some of the muscle synergies underlying movement strategies critical for stance postural control? How do scientists know whether these neuromuscular responses are due to neural programs (that is, synergies) or are the result of independent stretch of the individual muscles at mechanically coupled joints? Are there different

types of strategies and underlying muscle response synergies for anteroposterior stability versus mediolateral stability? In the following sections we examine strategies used for stabilization in both the anteroposterior plane and the mediolateral plane.

Anteroposterior Stability

Ankle Strategy.   The ankle strategy and its related muscle synergy were among the first patterns for controlling upright sway to be identified. The ankle strategy restores the COM to a position of stability through body movement centered primarily about the ankle joints. Figure 7-6A shows the typical synergistic muscle activity and body movements associated with corrections for loss of balance in the forward direction. In this case, motion of the platform in the backward direction causes the subject to sway forward. Muscle activity begins at about 90 to 100 msec after perturbation onset in the gastrocnemius, followed by activation of the hamstrings 20 to 30 msec later and finally by the activation of the paraspinal muscles (Nashner, 1977, 1989).

Activation of the gastrocnemius produces a plantarflexion torque that slows, then reverses the body's forward motion. Activation of the hamstrings and paraspinal muscles maintains the hip and knees in an extended position. Without the synergistic activation of the hamstrings and paraspinal muscles, the indirect effect of the gastrocnemius ankle torque on proximal body segments would result in forward motion of the trunk mass relative to the lower extremities.

Figure 7-6B shows the synergistic muscle activity and body motions used when reestablishing stability in response to backward instability. Muscle activity begins in the distal muscle, the anterior tibialis, followed by activation of the quadriceps and abdominal muscles.

How do scientists know that the ankle, knee, and hip muscles are part of a neuromuscular synergy instead of being activated in response to stretch of each individual joint? Some of the first experiments in postural control (Nashner, 1977; Nashner and Woollacott, 1979) provide some evidence for synergistic organization of muscles.

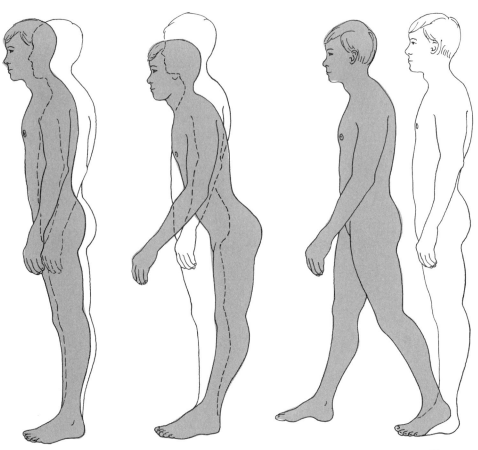

FIGURE 7-5.   Three postural movement strategies used by normal adults for controlling upright sway. (Reprinted with permission from Shumway-Cook A, Horak F. Vestibular rehabilitation: an exercise approach to managing symptoms of vestibular dysfunction. Semin Hearing 1989;10:199.)

In these early experiments the platform was rotated in a *toes-up* or *toes-down* direction. In a toes-up rotation, the platform motion provides stretch to the gastrocnemius muscle and dorsiflexion of the ankle, but these inputs are not associated with movements at the mechanically coupled knee and hip. The neuromuscular response that occurs in response to toes-up platform rotation includes activation of muscles at the ankle, knee, and hip joints despite the fact that motion has occurred only at the ankle joint. Evidence from these experiments supports the hypothesis of a neurally programmed muscle synergy (Nashner, 1976, 1977; Nashner and Woollacott, 1979), including knee and hip muscles on the same side of the body as the stretched ankle muscle.

Since these responses to rotation are desta-bilizing, to regain balance it is necessary to activate muscles on the opposite side of the body. These responses have been hypothesized to be activated in response to visual and vestibular inputs (Allum and Pfaltz, 1985) and are sometimes referred to as M3 responses as opposed to M1, or monosynaptic stretch reflex, responses and the longer-latency M2 stretch responses (Diener et al., 1982).

The ankle movement strategy described earlier appears to be used most commonly in situations in which the perturbation to equilibrium is small and the support surface is firm. Use of the ankle strategy requires intact range of motion and strength in the ankles. What happens if the perturbation to balance is large or if we are unable to generate force using ankle joint muscles?

ANKLE STRATEGY

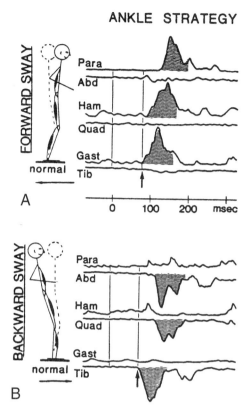

HIP STRATEGY

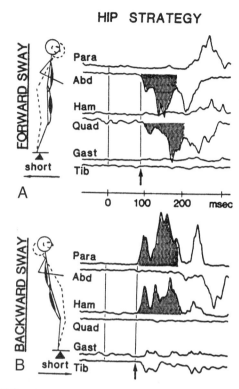

FIGURE 7-6. Muscle synergy and body motions associated with ankle strategy for controlling forward sway (**A**) and backward sway (**B**). (Reprinted with permission from Horak F, Nashner L. Central programming of postural movements: adaptation to altered support surface configurations. J Neurophysiol 1986;55:1372.)

FIGURE 7-7. Muscle synergy and body motions associated with the hip strategy for controlling A, forward sway and B, backward sway. (From Horak F, Nashner L. Central programming of postural movements: adaptation to altered support surface configurations. J Neurophysiol 1986;55: 1372.)

Hip Strategy. Scientists have identified another strategy for controlling body sway, the hip movement strategy (Horak and Nashner, 1986). This strategy controls motion of the COM by producing large and rapid motion at the hip joints with antiphase rotations of the ankles (Fig. 7-5).

Figure 7-7A shows the typical synergistic muscle activity associated with a hip strategy. Backward motion of the platform again causes the subject to sway forward. As shown in Figure 7-7A, the muscles that typically respond to forward sway when a subject is standing on a narrow beam are different from the muscles that become active in response to forward sway while standing on a flat surface. Muscle activity begins in the abdominal muscles about 90 to 100 msec after

perturbation onset, followed by activation of the quadriceps. Figure 7-7B shows the muscle pattern and body motions associated with the hip strategy, correcting for backward sway.

Horak and Nashner (1986) suggest that the hip strategy is used to restore equilibrium in response to larger, faster perturbations or when the support surface is compliant or smaller than the feet, for example when standing on a beam.

Stepping Strategy. When in-place strategies such as the ankle and hip strategy are insufficient to recover balance, a step or hop (the stepping strategy) is used to bring the support base back into alignment under the COM (Fig. 7-5). Initially, researchers believed that the stepping strategy was used solely in response to perturbations that moved the COM outside the BOS (Horak, 1991; Shumway-Cook and Horak, 1989; Nashner, 1989). More-recent research has found that in many conditions, stepping occurs even when the COM is well within the BOS (Brown et al., 1999; McIlroy and Maki, 1993).

Maki (1993) has noted that most research studies examining recovery of stability after a threat to standing balance discouraged stepping responses, with instructions to subjects to refrain from stepping unless absolutely necessary. This may encourage subjects to use other strategies, such as the hip strategy. To determine whether this is the case, McIlroy and Maki (1993) performed a study to determine the relationship between the prevalence of stepping responses and the instructions given to the subject. They noted that early automatic postural responses were recorded in ankle muscles in all trials, whether they resulted in stepping or not. They found that the frequency of stepping showed a trend to be higher in unconstrained (no specific instructions given) than constrained (keep feet in place) conditions. However, no significant effects were found (McIlroy and Maki, 1993). This raises questions as to whether instructions to the subject play a role in determining the type of movement strategy used to recover stability following perturbation.

While the ankle, hip, and stepping strategies and their associated muscular synergies are presented as discrete entities, researchers have shown that most neurologically intact individuals use various mixtures of these strategies when controlling forward and backward sway in the standing position (Horak and Nashner, 1986).

Information on the activation patterns of selected muscles and on body movement patterns can provide some information on motor control strategies used to regain balance. However, the calculation of joint torques can provide additional important information, since it provides us with information on the sum of forces provided by all the muscles acting at a given joint.

Recent experiments from two laboratories (Runge et al., 1999; Jensen et al., 1996)

have used this technique to test the hypothesis that ankle strategies are used primarily for low-velocity (COM stays well within the stability limits) perturbations, while hip strategies are used for higher velocity (COM moves closer to the limits of stability) perturbations. They have shown that as platform velocities gradually increase from 10 cm/second up to as much as 55 to 80 cm/second, subjects don't simply shift from using forces primarily at the ankles at the low velocities to forces primarily at the hip for higher velocities. Instead they continue to increase forces applied at the ankle and then begin to add forces at the hip at a certain critical threshold point. This point varies from subject to subject, with some subjects using primarily forces at the ankle for most perturbation velocities. Pure hip strategies, previously identified using EMG patterns when subjects responded to postural perturbations while standing on a narrow support surface (Horak and Nashner, 1986), were never observed. EMG records also showed that when trunk abdominal muscle activation was correlated with trunk flexion, ankle muscle activity remained (Runge et al., 1999; Jensen et al., 1996). Figure 7-8 illustrates the combination ankle and hip muscles seen in response to platform perturbations of increasing size. Muscle responses (surface EMGs) are shown in Figure 7-8*A*, and the accompanying joint torques are shown in Figure 7-8*B*.

Mediolateral Stability

Early research on postural response strategies explored stability only in the anteroposterior direction. More recent research has revealed that alternative strategies are used to recover stability in the mediolateral direction. This is due to the fact that the alignment of body segments and muscles requires the activation of forces at different joints and in different directions to recover stability. For example, in the lower limb very little mediolateral movement is possible at the ankle and knee joints; therefore, the hip joint is the primary lower limb joint that is used when recovering stability in the mediolateral direction.

A number of researchers (Kapteyn, 1973;

Rozendal, 1986; Day et al., 1993) have proposed that in contrast to anteroposterior postural control, mediolateral control of balance occurs primarily at the hip and trunk rather than at the ankle. They have noted that the primary mediolateral motion of the body is lateral movement at the pelvis, which requires adduction of one leg and abduction of the other leg. With narrow stance widths there is also motion at the ankle joint; however, this is minimal with stance widths wider than 8 cm (Day et al., 1993).

Winter et al. (1993) have examined the anteroposterior and mediolateral components of balance during quiet stance. They noted that with mediolateral sway the loading and unloading of the left and right side look like mirror images, with the weight unloaded from one side being taken up by the other. In addition, mediolateral movements that occur during quiet stance show a descending response organization, with head movements occurring first, followed by hip movements (20 msec latency) and then ankle movements (40 msec latency). Head movements occur in the opposite direction to those at the hip and ankle (Lekhel et al., 1993).

Correlated with these biomechanical changes are specific muscle responses to control lateral sway. A number of laboratories have shown that the hip abductor (gluteus medius and tensor fascia latae) and adductor muscle groups are activated in the control of the loading and unloading of the two legs with mediolateral sway (Maki et al., 1994b; Winter et al., 1993; Horak and Moore, 1989). In contrast to anteroposterior muscle response patterns, which are organized in a distal to proximal manner, mediolateral muscle patterns are organized in a proximal to distal direction, with hip muscles being activated before ankle muscles (Horak and Moore, 1989).

Similar results have been found for mediolateral perturbation studies of cats. To compare postural sway strategies in a variety of directions, Macpherson performed experiments in which she perturbed cats in 16 directions around a 360-degree continuum (Macpherson, 1988). She noted that in response to mediolateral perturbations causing a loading of one hindlimb and an unloading of the other, the hip abductors of the loaded limb were activated, while in response to anteroposterior perturbations, the hip flexors and extensors were activated (Macpherson and Craig, 1986). Despite the fact that cats were perturbed in 16 directions, they responded with force vectors in only two directions. In addition, while some muscles appeared to be functionally coupled into synergies, others appeared to be controlled independently and used to fine-tune the synergies.

More-recent work from Macpherson's lab (Jacobs and Macpherson, 1996) has shown that the muscles of the thigh can be subdivided into two distinct functional groups related to postural control. The first group includes monoarticular muscles and some biarticular muscles and contributes to the antigravity support of the body (responses were highly correlated with vertical contact forces with the support surface). For example, flexors were activated during unloading of the limb, and extensors were activated during limb loading. The second muscle group, consisting of biarticular muscles, appeared to contribute more to the horizontal stability of the body (responses were correlated with the difference between torques at the knee and the hip), helping to fine-tune the direction of the contact force. The authors state that the nervous system may thus control movement but not at the level of individual joint torques. Instead it controls posture with one channel for vertical forces (antigravity support) and a second for a combination of vertical and tangential forces that fine-tunes force vector direction (horizontal stability) (Jacobs and Macpherson, 1996).

How does this work with cats relate to human postural control experiments? Until recently, human postural research stressed the importance of a limited number of muscle synergies that are the basis for postural control. The work with cats suggests that some muscles within the synergy may be tightly coupled but other muscle activity may be highly modifiable. In addition, it

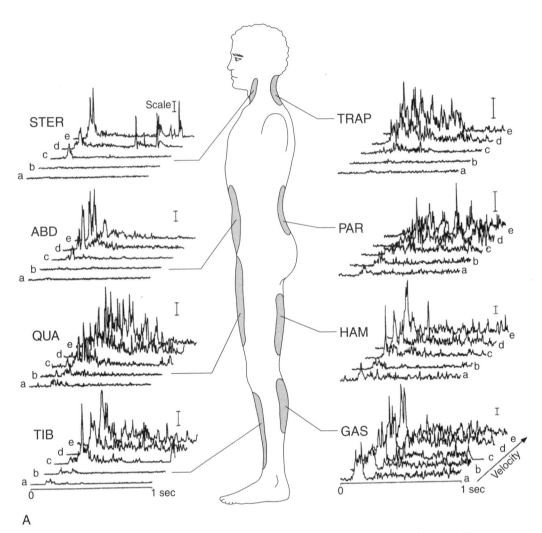

A

FIGURE 7-8.   Muscle responses **(A)** and joint torques **(B)** elicited by perturbations of increasing velocity. Muscle responses are to platform perturbations of 15 cm/s *(a)*, 20 cm/s *(b)*, 25 cm/s *(c)*, 32 cm/s *(d)*, and 40 cm/s *(e)*. STER, sternocleidomastoid; ABD, abdominals; QUA, quadriceps; TIB, tibialis anterior; TRAP, trapezius; PAR, paraspinals; HAM, hamstrings; GAS, gastrocnemius. Data are from separate subjects. (Adapted with permission from Runge CF, Shupert CL, Horak FB, Zajac FE. Postural strategies defined by joint torques. Gait Posture 1999;10:161–170.).

suggests that the CNS does not simply control posture through controlling forces at individual joints but controls more general functions, such as antigravity support and horizontal stability. Thus, the CNS may combine muscles in more ways than was originally thought. However, the way in which forces are applied may be very limited. This would change the emphasis in postural control from a limited number of muscle synergies to a limited number of force strategies.

There is some support for these hypotheses in humans from postural experiments examining muscle responses used to control sway in various directions in young adults (Moore et al., 1988). For example, experiments have shown that humans show stereotyped muscle response synergies when sway is forward or backward, but the responses are more variable in other directions. As perturbation direction is changed, activation of the recorded muscles varies continuously as a function of perturbation direction.

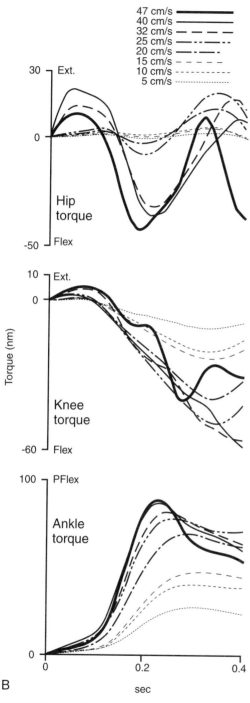

47 cm/s
40 cm/s
32 cm/s
25 cm/s
20 cm/s
15 cm/s
10 cm/s
5 cm/s

30 ┐ Ext.

0

Hip torque

-50 ┘ Flex

10 ┐ Ext.
0

Knee torque

-60 ┘ Flex

Torque (nm)

100 ┐ PFlex

Ankle torque

0 ┘

0   0.2   0.4

B

sec

FIGURE 7-8.—continued.

Adapting Motor Strategies

Studies have shown that normal subjects can shift relatively quickly from one postural movement strategy to another. For example,

when asked to stand on the narrow beam during anteroposterior platform displacements, most subjects shifted from an ankle to a hip strategy within 5 to 15 trials, and when they returned to a normal support surface, they shifted back to an ankle strategy within 6 trials. During the transition from one strategy to the next, subjects used complex movement strategies that were combinations of the pure strategies (Horak and Nashner, 1986).

Scientists theorize that the CNS may employ the different movement strategies with respect to the boundaries in space in which they can be safely used. That is, the CNS appears to map the relationship between body movements in space and the motor strategies used to control those movements. These conceptual boundaries are shown in Figure 7-9. Boundaries may be dynamic, shifting in response to the demands of the task and environment. For example, boundaries for using hip, ankle, and stepping strategies when standing on a firm, flat surface (Fig. 7-9*A*) may be different from those used when standing on a narrow beam (Fig. 7-9*B*) (Horak et al., 1989b).

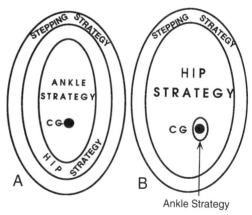

FIGURE 7-9. Boundaries for motor strategies used to control sway change as a function of the support surface. Suggested map of the relationship between body movements in space and the motor strategies used to control those movements while standing on a firm flat surface (**A**) versus crosswise on a narrow beam (**B**). (Reprinted with permission from Horak FB. Effects of neurological disorders on postural movement strategies in the elderly. In: Vellas B, Toupet M, Rubenstein L, et al., eds. Falls, balance and gait disorders in the elderly. Paris: Elsevier, 1992:147.)

This information is interesting, but is it true that we modify the amplitude of postural responses only when they are inappropriate to the task? In fact, no. Recent research has shown that we are constantly modulating the amplitudes of our postural responses, even when they are appropriate. For example, Woollacott and colleagues examined the responses of adults to repeated translational platform movements, and found that with repeated exposure to the movements, the subjects swayed less and showed smaller-amplitude postural responses (Woollacott et al., 1988). Thus, with repeated exposure to a given postural task, subjects refine their response characteristics to optimize response efficiency.

How do we modify our postural strategies to accommodate multiple task goals? For example, if we are trying to stand on a moving bus while carrying a cup of coffee, do we use a different strategy from when we are trying to read a book? To answer this question, researchers asked adults to stand on a movable platform while either keeping their arms at a fixed angle, as if they were reading a book, or keeping their finger at a fixed point in space, as if they were trying to keep a glass of water from spilling (Sveistrup et al., 1991; Moore et al., 1992b). They found that people continued to use the ankle strategy during both tasks but changed the coupling of the arm to the trunk to perform the additional upper-extremity task.

Neural Subsystems Controlling Postural Orientation and Stability

Do different neural subsystems control postural orientation and stability? Research comparing postural control in the normal and the spinal cat has contributed a partial answer to this question (Macpherson et al., 1997). It has been shown that given proper training, spinal cats are able to regain full weight support with appropriate horizontal orientation of the trunk and a semiflexed posture of the hindlimbs (Lovely et al., 1986). The ground reaction force also remains normal in orientation, though the amplitude is lower. Thus, it appears that the spinal neural circuitry by itself can tonically activate extensor muscles for antigravity support appropriately for postural orientation of the four limbs (Macpherson et al., 1997).

However, the control of postural stability in the chronic spinal cat is greatly diminished. These animals do not show lateral stability, though they can support their own weight. They also do not show the normal pattern of EMG activation, with a complete absence of flexor activation when a limb is unloaded, unlike the responses seen in the normal cat. Extensor muscles still show responses to balance perturbations but with much smaller amplitudes than normal. It is also interesting that most muscles are no longer modulated in relation to vertical force, except those tonically active for weight support. Thus it appears that postural stability is not organized at the spinal level but is controlled by higher centers, such as the brainstem (including the vestibular nuclei) and cerebellum (Macpherson et al., 1997; Macpherson and Fung, 1999).

In summary, we know that the ability to generate and apply forces in a coordinated way to control the body's position in space is an essential part of postural control. We know the CNS must activate synergistic muscles at mechanically related joints to ensure that forces generated at one joint for balance control do not produce instability elsewhere in the body. We believe the CNS internally represents the body's position in space with reference to behavioral strategies that are effective in controlling that movement; however, it is not clear whether these behavioral strategies are internally represented as muscle synergies, movement strategies, or force strategies.

Sensory Mechanisms Related to Postural Control

Effective postural control requires more than the ability to generate and apply forces for controlling the body's position in space. In order to know *when and how* to apply restoring forces, the CNS must have an accurate picture of *where* the body is in space and whether it is stationary or in motion. How does the CNS accomplish this?

Senses Contributing to Postural Control

The CNS must organize information from sensory receptors throughout the body before it can determine the body's position in space. Normally, peripheral inputs from visual, somatosensory (proprioceptive, cutaneous, and joint receptors), and vestibular systems are available to detect the body's position and movement in space with respect to gravity and the environment. Each sense provides the CNS with specific information about position and motion of the body; thus, each sense provides a different *frame of reference* for postural control (Hirschfeld, 1992; Gurfinkel and Levick, 1991).

What information does each of the senses provide for postural control? Is one sense more important than others? Does the CNS use all three senses all the time? If not, how does the CNS decide which sense to use?

Visual Inputs

Visual inputs report information regarding the position and motion of the head with respect to surrounding objects. Visual inputs provide a reference for verticality, since many things that surround us, such as windows and doors, are aligned vertically. In addition, the visual system reports motion of the head, since as your head moves forward, surrounding objects move in the opposite direction. Visual inputs include both peripheral visual information and foveal information, though there is some evidence to suggest that a peripheral (or a large visual field) stimulus is more important for controlling posture (Paillard, 1987).

Visual inputs are an important source of information for postural control, but are they absolutely necessary? No, since most of us can keep our balance when we close our eyes or are in a dark room. In addition, visual inputs are not always an accurate source of orientation information about *self-motion*. If you are sitting in your car at a stop light and the car next to you moves, what do you do? You quickly put your foot on the brake. In this situation, visual inputs signal *motion,* which the brain initially interprets as self-motion; in other words, *my car is rolling*. The brain therefore sends out signals to the mo-

tor neurons of the leg and foot, so you step on the brake and *stop* the motion. Thus, visual information may be misinterpreted by the brain. The visual system has difficulty distinguishing between object motion, referred to as exocentric motion, and self-motion, referred to as egocentric motion.

Somatosensory Inputs

The somatosensory system provides the CNS with position and motion information about the body with reference to supporting surfaces. In addition, somatosensory inputs throughout the body report information about the relationship of body segments to one another. Somatosensory receptors include muscle spindles and Golgi tendon organs (sensitive to muscle length and tension), joint receptors (sensitive to joint movement and stress), and cutaneous mechanoreceptors, including Pacinian corpuscles (sensitive to vibration), Meissner's corpuscles (sensitive to light touch and vibration), Merkel's discs (sensitive to local pressure) and Ruffini endings (sensitive to skin stretch).

Under normal circumstances, when standing on a firm, flat surface, somatosensory receptors provide information about the position and movement of your body with respect to a horizontal surface. However, if you are standing on a surface that is moving relative to you, for example a boat, or on a surface that is not horizontal, such as a ramp, it is not appropriate to establish a vertical orientation with reference to the surface. In these situations, inputs reporting the body's position with respect to the surface become less helpful in establishing a vertical orientation.

Vestibular Inputs

Information from the vestibular system is also a powerful source of information for postural control. The vestibular system provides the CNS with information about the position and movement of the head with respect to gravity and inertial forces, providing a *gravitoinertial* frame of reference for postural control.

The vestibular system has two types of receptors that sense different aspects of head position and motion. The semicircular canals (SCCs) sense angular acceleration of the head. The SCCs are particularly sensitive to fast head movements, such as those occurring during gait or during imbalance, such as slips, trips, and stumbles (Horak and Schupert, 1994).

The otoliths signal linear position and acceleration. Since gravity is detected in relation to our linear position or movement in space, the otoliths are an important source of information about head position with respect to gravity. The otoliths mostly respond to slow head movements, such as those that occur during postural sway. Thus, the vestibular system reports position and motion of the head and is important in distinguishing between exocentric and egocentric motion.

It is also interesting to note that vestibular signals alone cannot provide the CNS with a *true picture* of how the body is moving in space. For example, the CNS cannot distinguish between a simple head nod (movement of the head relative to a stable trunk) and a forward bend (movement of the head in conjunction with a moving trunk) using vestibular inputs alone (Horak and Schupert, 1994).

How does the CNS organize this sensory information for postural control? Postural demands during quiet stance, often referred to as static balance control, are different from those during perturbations to stance and during locomotion, which require more dynamic forms of control. Therefore, it is likely that information is organized differently for these tasks.

Sensory Strategies During Quiet Stance

Somatosensory inputs from all parts of the body contribute to postural control during quiet stance. Studies by the French scientist Roll and his colleagues used minivibrators to excite eye, neck, and ankle muscles and explored the contributions of proprioceptive inputs from these muscles to postural control during quiet stance (Roll and Roll, 1988). They found that vibration to the eye muscles of a standing subject with eyes closed produced body sway, with sway direction depending on the muscle vibrated. Vibration to the sternocleidomastoid muscles of the neck or the soleus muscles of the leg also produced body sway. When these muscles were vibrated simultaneously, the effects were additive, with no clear domination of one proprioceptive influence over another. This suggests that proprioception from all parts of the body plays an important role in the maintenance of postural control in quiet stance.

Other studies have shown that reduction of afferent input from the lower limb due to vascular ischemia, anesthesia, or cooling causes an increase in COP motion during quiet stance (Diener et al., 1984; Magnusson et al., 1990).

Recent work by Jeka and Lackner (1994, 1995) has shown that light touch of a fingertip to a stable surface reduces postural sway in subjects standing on one leg or in a heel-toe stance. They measured mediolateral COP under three fingertip contact conditions: no contact, light touch (up to 1 N (newton) or 100 g force), or force contact (as much force as desired). They found that sway was highest in the no-contact condition and was reduced equally in the light-contact and force contact conditions, even though fingertip contact was about 10 times higher in the force contact condition. From calculations they showed that contact forces of 0.4 N predicted a 2% to 3% reduction in sway; however, touch contact caused a 50% to 60% reduction. They showed that the additional stabilization provided by light contact is due to forces generated by muscles far from the fingertip (legs and trunk) guided by sensory information from cutaneous receptors in the fingertip and proprioceptive information about arm position (Jeka, 1997).

Many studies examining the effect of vision on quiet stance have examined the amplitude of sway with eyes open versus eyes closed and have found a significant increase in sway in normal subjects with eyes closed. Thus, it has been proposed that while vision is not absolutely necessary to the control of quiet stance, it does actively contribute to balance control during quiet stance (Edwards, 1946; Lee and

Lishman, 1975; Paulus et al., 1984). The ratio of body sway during eyes open and eyes closed has been referred to as the Romberg quotient (Romberg, 1853).

Does the way we use visual cues depend on whether we are standing quietly or responding to an unexpected threat to balance? The answer appears to be yes. Several researchers have studied sensitivity to continuous versus transient visual motion cues in people of different ages (Lee and Lishman, 1975; Butterworth and Hicks, 1977; Butterworth and Pope, 1983; Brandt et al., 1976).

The first experiments of this type were performed by David Lee and his colleagues from Edinburgh, Scotland, using a novel paradigm in which subjects stood in a room that had a fixed floor but with walls and a ceiling that could be moved forward or backward, creating the illusion of sway in the opposite direction (Lee and Lishman, 1975). The moving room can be used to create slow oscillations, simulating visual cues during quiet stance sway or an abrupt perturbation to the visual field, simulating an unexpected loss of balance. If very small continuous room oscillations are used, neurologically intact adults begin to sway with the room's oscillations, showing that visual inputs have an important influence on postural control of adults during quiet stance.

Other studies have given adults slow, continuous platform oscillations (simulating quiet stance) versus fast, transient platform perturbations (creating loss of stability). The results from these studies indicate that visual, vestibular, and somatosensory inputs all influence balance control in normal adults during slow oscillations similar to quiet stance. In contrast, somatosensory inputs appear to dominate postural control in response to transient surface perturbations (Diener et al., 1986).

Recent experiments by Dietz et al. (1994) modulated both visual flow and the support surface (a treadmill) on which the subject stood. They found that leg flexors have a higher responsiveness to visual stimuli, while leg extensors have a higher responsiveness to somatosensory input.

What can we conclude from all of these studies? They suggest that all three senses contribute to postural control during quiet stance.

Sensory Strategies During Perturbed Stance

How do visual, vestibular, and somatosensory inputs contribute to postural control during recovery from a transient perturbation to balance? Let's look at some of the research examining this question.

Moving rooms, as we just described, have also been used to examine the contribution of visual inputs to recovery from transient perturbations. When abrupt room movements are made, 1-year-old children compensate for this illusory loss of balance with motor responses designed to restore the vertical position. However, since there is no actual body sway, only the illusion of sway, motor responses have a destabilizing effect, causing the infants to stagger or fall in the direction of the room movement (Lee and Aronson, 1974; Lee and Lishman, 1975). This indicates that vision may be a dominant input in compensating for transient perturbations in infants first learning to stand.

Interestingly, older children and adults typically do not show large sway responses to these movements, indicating that in adults, vision does not appear to play an important role in compensating for transient perturbations.

Muscle response latencies to visual cues signaling perturbations to balance are quite slow, on the order of 200 msec, in contrast to the somatosensory responses that are activated at 80 to 100 msec (Nashner and Woollacott, 1979; Dietz et al., 1991). Because somatosensory responses to support surface translations appear to be much faster than those triggered by vision, researchers have suggested that the nervous system preferentially relies on somatosensory inputs for controlling body sway when imbalance is caused by rapid displacements of the supporting surface.

What is the relative contribution of the vestibular system to postural responses to support surface perturbations? Experiments by Dietz and his colleagues indicate that the contribution of the vestibular system is much smaller than that of somatosensory inputs (Dietz et al., 1991). In these experiments, the onset latency and amplitude of muscle responses were compared for two types of perturbations of stance: (*a*) the support surface was moved forward or backward, stimulating somatosensory inputs; and (*b*) a forward or backward displacement of a load (2 kg) attached to the head was given, stimulating the vestibular system (the response was absent in patients with vestibular deficits). For comparable accelerations, muscle responses to vestibular signals were about one-tenth of the magnitude of the somatosensory responses induced by the displacement of the feet. This suggests that vestibular inputs play only a minor role in recovery of postural control when the support surface is displaced horizontally.

However, under certain conditions, vestibular and visual inputs are important in controlling responses to transient perturbations. For example, when the support surface is rotated toes upward, stretching and activating the gastrocnemius muscle, this response is destabilizing, pulling the body backward. Allum, a researcher from Switzerland, has shown that the subsequent compensatory response in the tibialis anterior muscle, used to restore balance, is activated by the visual and vestibular systems when the eyes are open. When the eyes are closed, it is primarily (80%) activated by the vestibular semicircular canals (Allum and Pfaltz, 1985).

These studies, examining postural control in response to transient horizontal perturbations to stance, suggest that neurologically intact adults tend to rely on somatosensory inputs, in contrast to young children, who may rely more heavily on visual inputs.

Regardless of the task, no one sense by itself can provide the CNS with accurate information regarding the position and motion of the body in space in all circumstances. The ability of the nervous system to adapt its use of sensory information under changing task and environmental conditions is discussed in the next section.

Central Integration: Adapting Senses for Postural Control

We live in a constantly changing environment. Adapting how we use the senses for postural control is a critical aspect of maintaining stability in a wide variety of environments and has been studied by several researchers. Afferent information important to postural control is processed by many systems. One of the systems that appears to be critical for response adaptation is the cerebellum. The cerebellum receives somatosensory, visual, and vestibular inputs and thus is able to compare these inputs and adapt responses appropriately.

One approach to investigating how the CNS adapts multiple sensory inputs for postural control was developed by Nashner and coworkers. This approach uses a moving platform with a moving visual surround (Nashner 1976, 1982). A simplified version of Nashner's protocol was developed by Shumway-Cook and Horak (1986) to examine the role of sensory interaction in balance.

In Nashner's protocol, body sway is measured while the subject stands quietly under 6 conditions that alter the availability and accuracy of visual and somatosensory inputs for postural orientation. In conditions 1 to 3, the subject stands on a normal surface with eyes open (1), eyes closed (2), or the visual surround moving with body sway (3). Conditions 4 to 6 are identical to 1 to 3 except that the support surface rotates with body sway. These conditions are shown in Figure 7-10. Differences in the amount of body sway in the various conditions are used to determine a subject's ability to adapt sensory information for postural control.

Many studies have examined the performance of normal subjects when sensory inputs for postural control are varied (Nashner, 1982; Woollacott et al., 1986; Peterka and Black, 1990). Generally, these studies have shown that adults and children over age 7 easily maintain balance under all 6 conditions.

Average differences in body sway across the 6 sensory conditions within a large group of neurologically intact adults are shown in

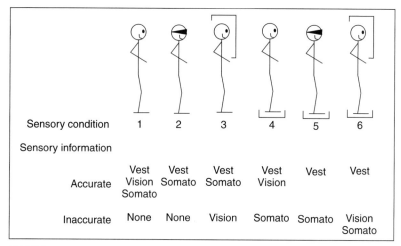

Sensory condition	1	2	3	4	5	6
Sensory information						
Accurate	Vest Vision Somato	Vest Somato	Vest Somato	Vest Vision	Vest	Vest
Inaccurate	None	None	Vision	Somato	Somato	Vision Somato

FIGURE 7-10. The six sensory conditions used to test how people adapt the senses to changing sensory conditions during the maintenance of stance. (Adapted with permission from Horak F, Shumway-Cook A, Black FO. Are vestibular deficits responsible for developmental disorders in children? Insights Otolaryngol 1988;3:2.)

Figure 7-11. Adults sway the least when support surface orientation inputs are accurately reporting the body's position in space relative to the surface regardless of the availability and accuracy of visual inputs (conditions 1, 2, and 3). When support surface information is no longer available as an accurate source of orientation information, adults begin to sway more. The greatest amount of sway is seen in conditions 5 and 6, in which only one accurate set of inputs, the vestibular inputs, is available to mediate postural control (Peterka and Black, 1990).

Similar experiments were conducted to determine the effect of cerebellar lesions on the ability to reweight postural responses under these changing task conditions. Nashner et al. (1983) showed that children with cerebellar ataxia showed significantly reduced abilities to balance under conditions of reduced or conflicting sensory input (especially conditions 5 and 6). This supports the concept that the cerebellum may be involved in processing information related to central organization and adaptation of postural responses.

The application of this concept can be found in Lab Activity 7-2.

This research suggests a number of things about how the CNS organizes and adapts

sensory information for postural control. It supports the concept of hierarchical weighting of sensory inputs for postural control based on their relative accuracy in reporting the body's position and movements in space. In environments where a sense is not providing optimal or accurate information regarding the body's position, the weight given to that sense as a source of orientation is reduced, while the weight of other more accurate senses is increased. Because of the redundancy of senses available for orientation and the ability of the CNS to modify the relative importance of any one sense for postural control, individuals are able to maintain stability in a variety of environments.

In summary, postural control includes organizing multiple sensory inputs into sensory strategies for orientation. This process appears to involve the hierarchical ordering of sensory frames of reference, thereby ensuring that the most appropriate sense is selected for the environment and the task. Sensory strategies, that is, the relative weight given to a sense, vary as a function of age, task, and environment. It appears that under normal conditions, the nervous system may weight the importance of somatosensory information for postural control more heavily than vision and vestibular inputs.

LAB ACTIVITY 7-2

OBJECTIVE: To examine central organization and adaptation of sensory inputs to stance postural control.

PROCEDURES: This lab **requires** a partner for safety. Equipment needed is a stopwatch and an 18 × 18 × 3–inch piece of medium-density foam and a meter stick mounted horizontally on the wall at shoulder height, next to your partner. You will be measuring maximum sway forward and backward during a 20-second period of quiet stance in 4 conditions. In condition 1, the subject stands on a firm surface (e.g., linoleum or wood) with feet together, hands on hips, and eyes open. Record the maximum shoulder displacement forward and backward. In condition 2, the subject stands as before but with eyes closed. Record displacement. In condition 3, the subject stands with feet together on the foam with eyes open. Record displacement. In condition 4, the subject stands on the foam with eyes closed. There is an increased risk of loss of balance in this condition, so be sure the recorder stands close and guards the subject well. Record displacement.

ASSIGNMENT: For each condition, make a list of the sensory cues that are available for postural control. Compare sway using your displacement measures across all conditions. How does sway vary as a function of available sensory cues? How do your results compare with the findings of Woollacott et al. (1986) with respect to conditions 1,2, 4, and 5 in Figure 7-11?

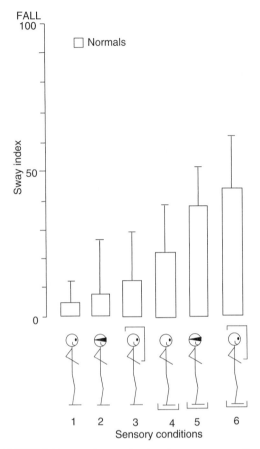

FIGURE 7-11.   Body sway in the six sensory conditions used to test sensory adaptation during stance postural control. (Adapted with permission from Woollacott MH, Shumway-Cook A, Nashner L. Aging and posture control: changes in sensory organization and muscular coordination. Int J Aging Hum Dev 1986;23:108.)

Adaptation to Rotational Support Surface Perturbations

Researchers have performed other types of experiments to explore postural adaptation. Rotational platform movements have been used to study the adaptation of postural responses to various conditions (Nashner, 1976; Keshner and Allum, 1986; Hansen et al., 1988). For example, *toes-down* rotational platform movements cause stretch to the tibialis anterior muscles, activating the T-Q-A (tibialis, quadriceps, abdominals) synergy, but when the synergy is first activated in this situation, it is inappropriate and serves to pull the subject more forward in the direction of the platform rotation. Studies indi-

cate that subjects adapt the responses by attenuating the response amplitude over a series of approximately 10 trials. It has thus been hypothesized that when subjects receive inaccurate sensory information from one sense (in this case, ankle joint inputs), they are able to compare that information with that of the other available sensory systems. They then readjust the weighting of the sensory inputs driving postural responses to shift to the remaining, accurate inputs.

Adapting Senses When Learning a New Task

Thus far, we have talked about reweighting sensory information in environments when it is not appropriate to use a particular sense for postural control. Similar reweighting of the senses appears to occur during the process of learning new motor skills. Lee and Lishman (1975) found increased weighting of visual inputs when adults were just learning a task. As the task became more automatic, there appeared to be a decrease in the relative importance of visual inputs for postural control and increased weighting given to somatosensory inputs.

It has been suggested that adults recovering from a neurological lesion also rely predominantly on vision during the early part of the recovery process. As motor skills, including postural control, are regained, patients become less reliant on vision and are better able to use somatosensory inputs (Mulder et al., 1993).

Anticipatory Postural Control

Did you ever pick up a box expecting it to be heavy and find it to be light? The fact that you lifted the box higher than you expected shows that your CNS preprogrammed the force you used according to anticipation of what the task required. Based on previous experience with lifting other boxes of similar and different shapes and weights, the CNS forms a representation of what sensorimotor processing and actions are needed to accomplish this task. It pretunes these systems for the task. Our mistakes are evidence that the CNS uses anticipatory processes in controlling action.

In the 1960s, scientists in Russia first began to explore the way we use posture in an anticipatory manner to steady the execution of our skilled movements. Belen'kii et al. (1967) noted that when a standing adult is asked to raise the arm, both postural (leg and trunk) and prime mover (arm) muscles were activated. They observed that the postural muscle activation patterns could be divided into two parts. The first part was a preparatory phase, in which postural muscles were activated more than 50 msec in advance of the prime mover muscles to compensate in advance for the destabilizing effects of the movement. The second part

was a compensatory phase, in which the postural muscles were again activated after the prime movers, in a feedback manner, to stabilize the body further. They found that the sequence of postural muscles activated, hence the manner of preparing for the movement, was specific to the task.

After it was discovered that postural responses involved in feedback control of posture were organized into distinct synergies (Nashner, 1977), an important question was raised: Are the synergies used in feedback postural control the same synergies that are used in anticipatory postural control? To answer this question, Cordo and Nashner (1982) performed experiments in which they asked standing subjects to forcefully push or pull on a handle, in a reaction-time task. They found that the same postural response synergies used in standing balance control were activated in an anticipatory fashion before the arm movements. For example, when a person is asked to pull on a handle, first the gastrocnemius, hamstrings, and trunk extensors are activated, and then the prime mover, the biceps of the arm.

One feature of postural adjustments associated with movement is their adaptability to the conditions of the task. In the experiment of Cordo and Nashner (1982), when the subjects leaned forward against a horizontal bar at chest height, the leg postural adjustments were reduced or disappeared. Thus, there is an immediate preselection of the postural muscles as a function of their ability to contribute appropriate support.

A number of factors contribute to the timing of postural versus prime mover muscle activity during voluntary tasks. First, the muscle studied and its role in the task is important. For example, activation of lower limb muscles tends to precede that of prime mover muscles in tasks requiring an arm raise or a pull–push. Trunk muscles are typically activated simultaneously with the prime mover muscles in arm-raising tasks (Cordo and Nashner, 1982; Belen'kii et al., 1967; Brauer, 1998). Second, there may be a change in timing of postural muscle activity when moving in different directions, such as pushing versus pulling. Third, the support that is given during the task and the initial posture also influence activation of postural muscles. For example, when pulling a lever while steadying yourself with your other arm, the first muscles activated are in the arm used to steady yourself. However, when doing the same task with no upper limb support, leg muscles are activated first (Marsden et al., 1977). Fourth, preparedness for the task results in a shortening of the onset time for both postural and prime mover muscles (Brown and Frank, 1987; Inglin and Woollacott, 1988). Fifth, behavioral context and speed of the focal movement affect anticipatory aspects of postural control. For example, when subjects are told to move as fast as possible versus at a comfortable speed, postural responses tend to be earlier and more reliably activated (Horak et al., 1984; Lee et al., 1987). Sixth, the mass of the limb or of the load to be moved may influence the amplitude of the postural muscle activity (Horak et al., 1984; Bouisset and Zattara, 1981). Finally, degree of practice and complexity of task influence postural response latency. It has been shown that the more complex the task, the more the anticipatory adjustments are delayed (Inglin and Woollacott, 1988). In addition, dancers have been shown to activate anticipatory postural adjustments in a leg-lifting task significantly earlier than nondancers (Mouchnino et al., 1992; Brauer, 1998).

Though we usually think of anticipatory adjustments in terms of activating postural muscles in advance of a skilled movement, we also use anticipation when scaling the amplitude of postural adjustments to perturbations to balance. The amplitude of the muscle response is related to our expectations regarding the size or amplitude of the upcoming perturbation.

Horak et al. (1989a) examined the influence of prior experience and central set on the characteristics of postural adjustments by giving subjects platform perturbations under the following conditions: (*a*) serial versus random conditions, (*b*) expected versus unexpected conditions, and (*c*) practiced versus unpracticed conditions. They found that expectation played a large factor in modulating the amplitude of postural responses. For example, subjects overresponded when they expected a larger perturbation than they received and underresponded when they expected a smaller one.

Practice also caused a reduction in the magnitude of postural response and in the amplitude of antagonist muscle responses. However, central set did not affect EMG onset latencies. The authors noted that when different perturbations were presented in random order, all scaling disappeared. Evidently, scaling of postural responses is based on our anticipation of what is needed in a given situation.

It is important to realize that anticipatory postural adjustments are not isolated to tasks we perform while standing. The application of this concept can be found in Lab Activity 7-3.

 LAB ACTIVITY 7-3

OBJECTIVE: To explore the use of anticipatory postural adjustments in a lifting task.

PROCEDURE: Work with a partner. Tape a ruler vertically to the wall near where you are standing. Stand with your arm outstretched at about waist height, palm up. Place a heavy book on your outstretched palm and have your partner note the vertical position of your hand on the ruler. Now have your partner lift the book off that hand and note the movement of your hand when your partner lifts the book. Reposition the book. Now lift the book off your own hand with your opposite hand. Have your partner note the movement of your hand in this condition.

ASSIGNMENT: Answer the following questions: What did the hand holding the book do when your partner lifted the book? Was it steady, or did it move upward as the book was lifted? How much did it move? What happened when you lifted the book yourself? Was it steady? How much did it move? In which of these two conditions is there evidence for anticipatory postural adjustments? What was necessary for the anticipatory postural adjustment to occur? How do your results compare with those of Hugon et al. (1982), explained next?

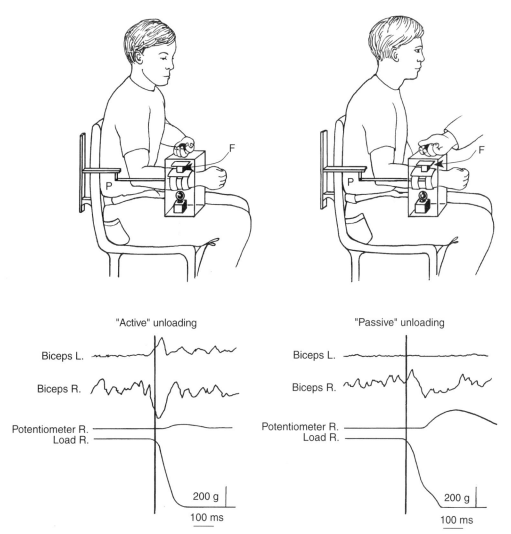

FIGURE 7-12. Experiments examining anticipatory postural activity associated with lifting a weight from a subject's arm. (Adapted with permission from Hugon M, Massion J, Wiesendanger M. Anticipatory postural changes induced by active unloading and comparison with passive unloading in man. Pflugers Arch 1982;393:292-296.)

What you may have noticed through this lab activity is that you are able to use anticipatory postural adjustments when you are lifting the book out of your own hand, so that your hand does not involuntarily move upward, while you cannot use these adjustments when someone else is lifting the same book from your hand.

Scientists from France and Switzerland, Hugon et al., (1982), first made this discovery in experiments in which they measured the EMGs of the biceps of the left and right arms during a modification of the task just

mentioned. In this case, either the subject or the experimenter lifted a 1-kg weight from the subject's forearm (Fig. 7-12). They found that in the active unloading of the arm by the subject, there was preparatory biceps muscle inhibition to keep the arm from moving upward when it was unloaded. The anticipatory reduction in the biceps EMG of the arm holding the load was time-locked with the onset of the activation of the biceps of the lifting arm. This reduction was not observed during passive unloading.

How are these anticipatory postural adjustments associated with movements centrally organized? Massion and his colleagues performed animal experiments to address this question in more detail (Massion, 1979). They trained animals to perform a leg-lifting task that required the animal to activate postural muscles in the other three legs as it lifted the prime mover leg. They found that they could also directly stimulate the motor cortex or the red nucleus in the area of the forelimb flexors and produce the leg-lifting movement. When they did this, the movement was always accompanied by a postural adjustment in the other limbs, initiated in a feed-forward manner. They hypothesized that the postural adjustments are organized at the bulbospinal level and that the pyramidal tract activates these pathways as it sends descending commands to the prime mover. Massion suggests that while the basic mechanisms for postural adjustments may be organized at this level, they appear to be modulated by several other parts of the nervous system, including the cerebellum.

SEATED POSTURAL CONTROL

The maintenance of postural control in the seated position has not been studied to the extent of stance postural control. However, many scientists believe that concepts important for stance postural control will be shown to be equally valid for understanding postural control in sitting.

A study was performed to compare the postural responses elicited by platform translations versus rotations of subjects seated with the legs extended forward (Forssberg and Hirschfeld, 1994). The authors noted that forward platform movements causing the body to sway backward elicited well-organized, consistent responses in the quadriceps, abdominal, and neck flexor muscles at 63 ± 12 msec, 74 ± 21 msec, and 77 ± 10 msec, respectively. Similar responses were elicited by legs-up rotations. However, in response to backward platform perturbations, causing forward sway, smaller and more variable responses were elicited in the trunk and neck extensor muscles. These differences reflect the asymmetry of the stability limits during sitting.

The authors suggest that the postural control system sets a threshold for activation of postural responses according to an internal representation of the body, including the relationship between the COG and the support surface. Since the rotational and translational perturbations caused very different head movements but very similar muscle response patterns, the authors conclude that somatosensory inputs from the backward rotation of the pelvis trigger the postural response synergies in sitting.

Experiments have also been performed to examine the characteristics of anticipatory postural adjustments used in reaching for an object while sitting (Moore et al., 1992a). Researchers found that increased reach distance and decreased support were associated with earlier, larger postural adjustments. It has also been shown that leg muscles are consistently active during anticipatory postural adjustments in advance of voluntary reaching while sitting (Shepherd et al., 1993).

SUMMARY

1. The task of postural control involves controlling the body's position in space for (*a*) stability, defined as controlling the center of body mass within the base of support, and (*b*) orientation, defined as the ability to maintain an appropriate relationship between the body segments and between the body and the environment for a task.

2. A number of factors contribute to postural control during quiet stance (so-called static balance), including (*a*) body alignment, which minimizes the effect of gravitational forces; (*b*) muscle tone; and (*c*) postural tone, which keeps the body from collapsing in response to the pull of gravity.

3. When quiet stance is perturbed, the recovery of stability requires movement strategies that are effective in controlling the center of mass relative to the base of support.

4. Movement patterns used to recover stance balance from sagittal plane instability are referred to as ankle, hip, and suspensory, or stepping, strategies. Normal subjects can shift relatively quickly from one postural movement strategy to another.

5. The CNS activates synergistic muscles at mechanically related joints, possibly to ensure that forces generated at one joint for balance control do not produce instability elsewhere in the body.

6. Inputs from visual, somatosensory (proprioceptive, cutaneous, and joint receptors), and vestibular systems are important sources of information about the body's position and movement in space with respect to gravity and the environment. Each sense provides the CNS with a different kind of information about position and motion of the body; thus, each sense provides a different frame of reference for postural control.

7. In adults, all three senses contribute to postural control during quiet stance; in contrast, in response to transient perturbations, adults tend to rely on somatosensory inputs, while young children rely more heavily on visual inputs.

8. Because of the redundancy of senses available for orientation and the ability of the CNS to modify the importance of any one sense for postural control, individuals are able to maintain stability in a variety of environments.

9. Postural adjustments are also activated before voluntary movements to minimize potential disturbances to balance that the movement may cause. This is called anticipatory postural control.

10. The maintenance of postural control in the seated position has not been studied in depth. However, many scientists believe that concepts important for stance postural control will be shown to be equally valid for postural control in sitting.

CHAPTER **8**

Development of Postural Control

℮ INTRODUCTION

During the early years of life, the child develops an incredible repertoire of skills, including crawling, independent walking and running, climbing, eye–hand coordination, and the manipulation of objects in a variety of ways. The emergence of all of these skills requires the development of postural activity to support the primary movement.

To understand the emergence of mobility and manipulatory skills in children, therapists need to understand the postural substrate for these skills. Similarly, understanding the best therapeutic approach for children with difficulties in walking or reaching skills requires the knowledge of any limitations in their postural abilities. Understanding the basis for postural development, then, is the first step in determining the best

therapeutic approach for improving related skills.

This chapter discusses the research on the development of postural control and how it contributes to the emergence of stability and mobility skills. Later chapters consider the implications of this research when assessing postural control.

Postural Control and Development

Let's first look at some of the evidence showing that postural control is a critical part of motor development. Research on early development has shown that the simultaneous development of the postural, locomotor, and manipulative systems is essential to the emergence and refinement of skills in all of these areas. In the neonate, when the chaotic movements of the head that regularly disturb the infant's seated balance are stabilized, movements and behaviors normally seen in more mature infants emerge (Amiel-Tison and Grenier, 1980). For example, as shown in Figure 8-1, when the clinician stabilizes the head of the newborn, the babies may begin to attend to the clinician, reach for objects, and maintain their arms at their sides, with the fingers open, suggesting inhibition of the grasp and Moro reflexes.

These results support the concept that an immature postural system is a limiting factor or a constraint on the emergence of other behaviors, such as coordinated arm and hand movements, as well as the inhibition of reflexes. It has also been suggested that delayed or abnormal development of the postural system may constrain a child's ability to develop independence in mobility and manipulatory skills.

Motor Milestones and Emerging Postural Control

The development of postural control traditionally has been associated with a predictable sequence of motor behaviors re-ferred to as motor milestones. Some of the major motor milestones in development are shown in Figure 8-2. They include crawling, sitting, creeping, pull-to-stand, independent stance, and walking. The sequence and timing of the emergence of these motor milestones has been well described by several developmental researchers.

In 1946, Arnold Gesell, a pediatrician, described the emergence of general patterns of behavior in the first few years of life. He noted the general direction of behavioral development as moving from head to foot and proximally to distally within segments. Thus, he formulated the law of developmental direction (Gesell, 1946).

In addition, Gesell portrayed development as a spiraling hierarchy. He suggested that the development of skilled behavior does not follow a strict linear sequence, always advancing, constantly improving with time and maturity. Instead, Gesell believed that development is much more dynamic in nature and seems to be characterized by alternating advancement and regression in ability to perform skills.

Gesell gave the example of children learn-

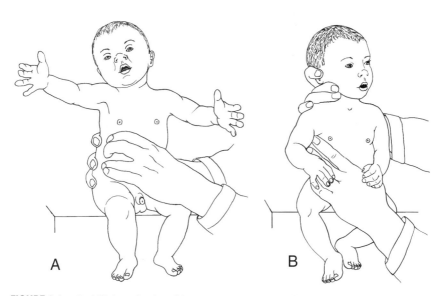

FIGURE 8-1.   Stabilizing the head in a neonate can produce dramatic changes in behavior. **A.** Uncontrolled movements of the head produce a Moro response. **B.** External support to the child's head and trunk results in more mature behaviors, including attending to people and objects and even reaching. (Adapted with permission from Amiel-Tison C, Grenier A. Neurological evaluation of the human infant. New York: Masson, 1980:82.)

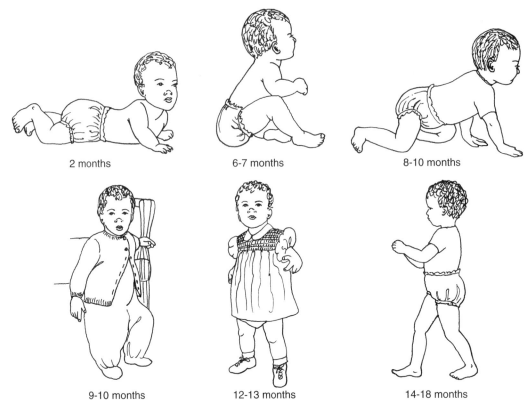

2 months   6-7 months   8-10 months

9-10 months   12-13 months   14-18 months

FIGURE 8-2. Motor milestones that emerge with the development of postural control. They include crawling (2 months), sitting (6 to 7 months), creeping (8 to 10 months), pull-to-stand (9 to 10 months), independent stance (12 to 13 months) and walking (14 to 18 months) (Adapted with permission from Shumway-Cook A, Woollacott M. Theoretical issues in assessing postural control. In: Wilhelm I, ed. Physical therapy assessment in early infancy. NY: Churchill Livingstone, 1993:163.)

ing to crawl and then creep. Initially, in learning to crawl, the child uses a primarily symmetrical arm pattern, eventually switching to a more complex alternating arm pattern as the skill of crawling is perfected. When the child first begins to creep, there is a return to the symmetrical arm pattern. Eventually, as creeping becomes perfected, the emergence of an alternating arm pattern occurs.

Thus, as children progress to each new stage in the development of a skill, they may appear to regress to an earlier form of the behavior as new, more mature and adaptive versions of these skills emerge.

Most of the traditional assessment scales created to evaluate the emergence of motor behaviors use developmental norms estab-lished by McGraw (1932) and Gesell. Using these scales, the therapist evaluates the performance of the infant or child on functional skills that require postural control. These skills include sitting, standing, walking unsupported, reaching forward, and moving from sitting to standing position. Examples of developmental tests and measures include the Gross Motor Function Measure (Russell et al., 1993), the Peabody Developmental Motor Scales (Folio and Fewell, 1983), the Bayley Scales of Infant Development (Bayley, 1969), and the Movement Assessment of Infants (Chandler et al., 1980). These and other tests follow normal development and are used to identify children at risk for developmental problems.

THEORIES OF DEVELOPING POSTURAL CONTROL

What is the basis for the development of postural control underlying this predictable sequence of motor behaviors? Several theories of child development try to relate neural structure and behavior in developing infants. Classical theories of child development place great importance on a reflex substrate for the emergence of mature human behavior patterns. This means that in the normal child the emergence of posture and movement control is dependent on the appearance and subsequent integration of reflexes. According to these theories, the appearance and disappearance of these reflexes reflect the increasing maturity of cortical structures that inhibit and integrate reflexes controlled at lower levels within the central nervous system (CNS) into more functional postural and voluntary motor responses (see Fig. 1.6). This theory has been referred to as a reflex–hierarchy theory (Woollacott and Shumway-Cook, 1990; Horak and Shumway-Cook, 1990).

Alternatively, more recent theories of motor control, such as the systems, ecological, and dynamical action theories, have suggested that postural control emerges from a complex interaction of musculoskeletal and neural systems collectively referred to as the postural control system. The organization of elements within the postural control system is determined by both the task and the environment. Systems theory does not deny the existence of reflexes but considers them as only one of many influences on the control of posture and movement.

Let's briefly review the reflexes that have been associated with the emergence of postural control.

Reflex-Hierarchical Theory of Postural Control

Postural reflexes were studied in the early part of this century by investigators such as Magnus (1926), DeKleijn (1923), Rademaker (1924), and Schaltenbrand (1928). In this early work, researchers selectively lesioned different parts of the CNS and examined an animal's capacity to orient. Magnus and associates took the animal down to what they referred to as the zero condition, a condition in which no postural reflex activity could be elicited. Subsequent animals underwent selective lesions, leaving systematically greater and greater amounts of the CNS intact. In this way, Magnus identified individually and collectively all of the reflexes that worked cooperatively to maintain postural orientation in various types of animals.

Postural reflexes in animals were classified by Magnus as local static reactions, segmental static reactions, general static reactions, and righting reactions. **Local static reactions** stiffen the animal's limb for support of body weight against gravity. **Segmental static reactions** involve more than one body segment and include the flexor withdrawal reflex and the crossed extensor reflex. **General static reactions**, called attitudinal reflexes, involve changes in position of the whole body in response to changes in head position. Finally, Magnus described a series of five **righting reactions**, which allowed the animal to assume or resume a species-specific orientation of the body with respect to its environment.

Postural Reflexes in Human Development

Examination of reflexes has become an essential part of the study of motor development. Many researchers have tried to document accurately the time frame for appearance and disappearance of these reflexes in normal children, with widely varying results. There is little agreement on the presence and time course of these reflexes or on the significance of these reflexes to normal and abnormal development (Claverie et al., 1973).

Figure 8-3 summarizes the results from a number of studies examining the presence and time course of the asymmetrical tonic neck reflex in normal development. This

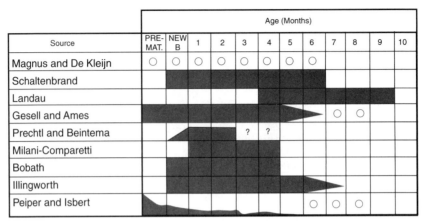

FIGURE 8-3. A summary of various studies that examined the presence and time course of the asymmetrical tonic neck reflex in normal development. O, reflex not present. (Adapted with permission from Capute AJ, Accardo PJ, Vining EPG, et al. Primitive reflex profile. Baltimore: University Park Press, 1978:36.)

chart shows obvious disagreement over whether the reflex is present in infancy and regarding the time course for its appearance and disappearance.

Attitudinal Reflexes

According to the reflex theory of postural control, tonic attitudinal reflexes produce persisting changes in body posture that result from a change in head position. These reflexes are not obligatory in normal children but have been reported in children with various types of neural pathology. These reflexes include (*a*) the **asymmetrical tonic neck reflex** (ATNR), (b) the **symmetrical tonic neck reflex** (STNR), and (c) the **tonic labyrinthine reflex** (TLR) (Milani-Comparetti and Gidoni, 1967). The behaviors attributed to these reflexes are shown in Figure 8-4, along with the time course for emergence and disappearance. The ATNR (Fig. 8-4*A*) produces extension in the face arm and flexion in the skull arm when the head is turned. The STNR (Fig. 8-4*B*) results in flexion in the upper extremities and extension in the lower extremities when the head is flexed (upper part of Fig. 8-4*B*); however, when the head is extended (lower part of Fig. 8-4*B*), the upper extremities extend while the lower extremities flex. The TLR (Fig. 8-4*C*) produces an increase in extensor tone when the body is supine and flexion when the body is prone.

Righting Reactions

According to a reflex-hierarchical model, the interaction of five righting reactions produces orientation of the head in space and orientation of the body in relation to the head and ground. Righting reactions are considered automatic reactions that enable a person to assume the normal standing position and maintain stability when changing positions (Barnes et al., 1978).

The three righting reactions that orient the head in space include (*a*) the **optical righting reaction** (Fig. 8-5*A*), which contributes to the reflex orientation of the head using visual inputs; (*b*) the **labyrinthine righting reaction** (Fig. 8-5*B*), which orients the head to an upright vertical position in response to vestibular signals (Peiper, 1963; Ornitz, 1983); and (*c*) the **body-on-head righting reaction** (Fig. 8-5*C*), which orients the head in response to proprioceptive and tactile signals from the body in contact with a supporting surface. The **Landau reaction**, shown in Figure 8-6, combines the effects of all three head-righting reactions (Cupps et al., 1976).

Two reflexes interact to keep the body oriented with respect to the head and the surface. The **neck-on-body righting reaction** orients the body in response to cervical afferents, which report changes in the position of the head and neck. Two forms of this

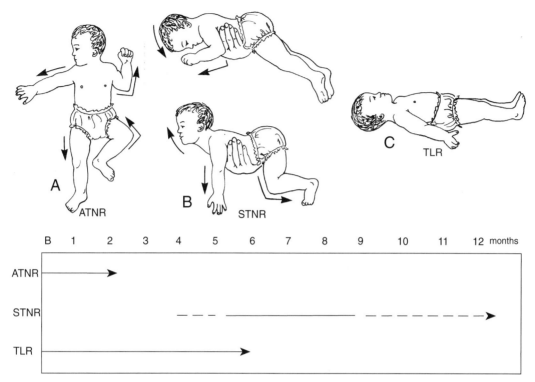

FIGURE 8-4.   The attitudinal reflexes. **A.** The ATNR reflex: extension in the *face* arm and flexion in the *skull* arm when the head is turned. **B.** The STNR reflex: head flexion causes flexion of the upper extremities and extension of the lower extremities; head extension causes extension in the upper extremities and flexion in the lower extremities. **C.** The tonic labyrinthine reflex produces an increase in extensor tone when the body is supine and (not shown) flexion when prone. Also shown is the time course for these reflexes. (Adapted with permission from Barnes MR, Crutchfield CA, Heriza CB. The neurophysiological basis of patient treatment. Morgantown, WV: Stokesville, 1978:222.)

reflex have been reported: an immature form, resulting in log rolling, which is present at birth, and a mature form, shown in Figure 8-7A, producing segmental rotation of the body (Paine, 1964). The **body-on-body righting reaction**, shown in Figure 8-7B, keeps the body oriented with respect to the ground regardless of the position of the head.

Balance and Protective Reactions

According to reflex-hierarchical theory, balance emerges in association with a sequentially organized series of equilibrium reactions. Balance reactions are often separated into three categories. The **tilting reactions** and their time course for emergence are shown in Figure 8-8A–C. Tilting re-

actions are used for controlling the center of gravity in response to a tilting surface. They are reported to emerge in sequence beginning in the prone position. **Postural fixation reactions** and their time course for emergence are shown in Figure 8-9A–C. These reactions are used to recover from forces applied to the other parts of the body, and like the tilting reactions, they are purported to emerge in a developmental sequence beginning in prone (Martin, 1967). **Parachute or protective responses** protect the body from injury during a fall and are shown in Figure 8-10A–C. Parachute reactions are also reported in the legs in response to downward movements of the infant in space. Finally staggering reactions (sideways stepping) are reported in response to instability in the lat-

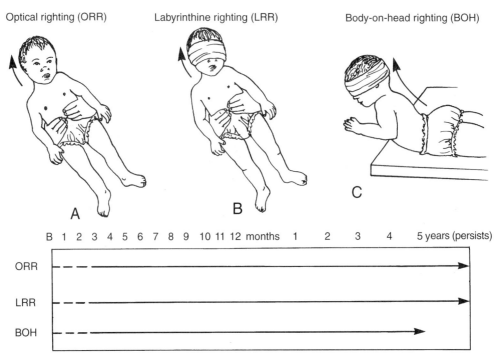

Optical righting (ORR)   Labyrinthine righting (LRR)   Body-on-head righting (BOH)

FIGURE 8-5. The righting reactions that orient the head. **A.** The optical righting reaction orients the head to visual vertical. **B.** The labyrinthine righting reaction orients the head in response to vestibular signals signaling vertical. **C.** The body-on-head righting reaction uses tactile and neck proprioceptive information to orient the head to vertical. Also shown is the time course for these reflexes. (Adapted with permission from Barnes MR, Crutchfield CA, Heriza CB. The neurophysiological basis of patient treatment. Morgantown, WV: Stokesville, 1978: 222.)

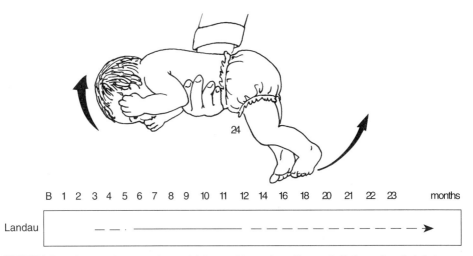

FIGURE 8-6. The Landau reaction, which combines the effects of all three head-righting reactions, and its time course during development. (Adapted with permission from Barnes MR, Crutchfield CA, Heriza CB. The neurophysiological basis of patient treatment. Morgantown, WV: Stokesville, 1978: 222.)

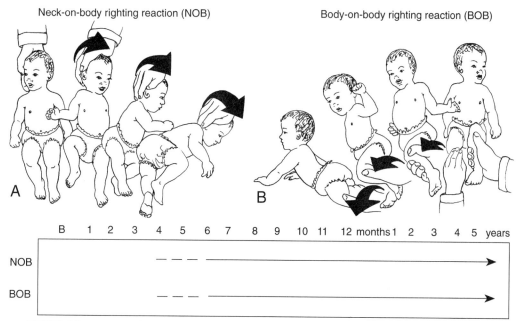

FIGURE 8-7. The righting reactions of the body. Shown are the mature form of the NOB righting reaction (**A**) and the BOB righting reaction (**B**), and their time course for emergence. NOB, neck on body; BOB, body on body. (Adapted with permission from Barnes MR, Crutchfield CA, Heriza CB. The neurophysiological basis of patient treatment. Morgantown, WV: Stokesville, 1978:222.)

eral direction. Parachute responses, like other types of balance reactions, emerge sequentially, with forward reactions preceding sideways and backward reactions (Barnes et al., 1978).

Many investigators have suggested that emerging balance reactions are necessary precursors to the acquisition of associated developmental milestones (Bobath and Bobath, 1976; Capute et al., 1982; Haley, 1986). Figure 8-11 summarizes the times of appearance of postural reflexes purported to underlie the emergence of postural control in children.

Role of Reflexes in Development

What is the role of reflexes in motor development? Scientists do not know for sure; as a result, the role of reflexes in motor control is controversial. Many theorists believe that reflexes form the substrate for normal motor control. For example, it has been suggested that the asymmetrical tonic neck reflex is part of the developmental process of

eye–hand coordination, since movement of the head and eyes brings the hand within view (Gesell, 1954; Coryell and Henderson, 1979). However, another study showed no relationship between reaching behavior and the presence or absence of this reflex in a 2- to 4-month-old group of infants (Larson et al., 1990). Various researchers have intimated that the asymmetrical tonic neck reflex contributes to movements in adults, since there is facilitation of extension in the extremities when the head is rotated (Fukuda, 1961; Hellebrandt et al., 1962; Hirt, 1967; Tokizane et al., 1951).

The neck-on-body and body-on-body righting reactions are reported to be the basis for rolling in infants. The persistence of the immature form of rolling at 4 months of age is purported to be predictive of CNS pathology, including cerebral palsy (Campbell and Wilhelm, 1985) and developmental delay (Molnar, 1978). The role of these reflexes in more mature rolling patterns has recently been questioned (VanSant, 1990).

Clearly, there is considerable uncertainty

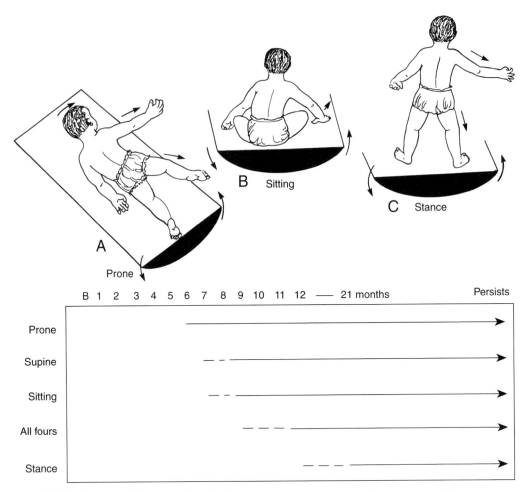

FIGURE 8-8.   The tilting reactions. Tilting responses are purported to emerge first in prone **(A)**, then supine (not shown), then sitting **(B)**, in all fours (not shown), and finally standing **(C)**. Also shown is the time course for these reflexes. (Adapted with permission from Barnes MR, Crutchfield CA, Heriza CB. The neurophysiological basis of patient treatment. Morgantown, WV: Stokesville, 1978:222.)

about the contribution of reflex testing in clarifying the basis for normal and abnormal development in children.

New Models of Development

Many of the newer theories of motor control presented in Chapter 1 have associated theories of motor development. These newer theories are consistent in suggesting that development involves much more than the maturation of reflexes within the CNS. Development is a complex process, with new behaviors and skills emerging from an interaction of the child and its maturing nervous

and musculoskeletal system with the environment.

With this framework, the emergence of postural control is likewise ascribed to complex interactions between neural and musculoskeletal systems. These include the following (see Fig. 7.2):

1. Changes in the musculoskeletal system, including development of muscle strength and changes in relative mass of the different body segments
2. Development or construction of the coordinative structures or neuromuscular response synergies used in maintaining balance

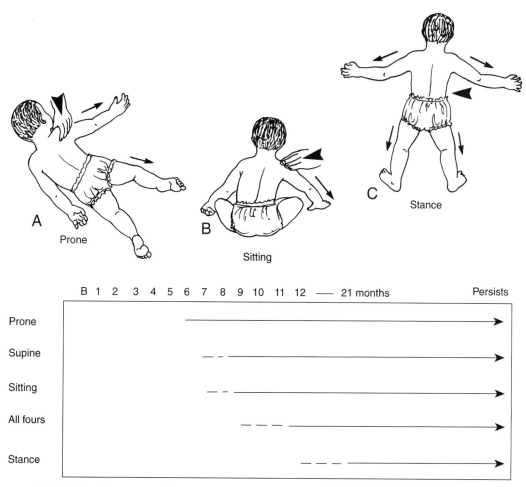

FIGURE 8-9.   The postural fixation reactions. Fixation reactions stabilize the body in response to destabilizing forces applied to the body from anywhere but the supporting surface and emerge in parallel to the tilting reactions. Shown are reactions in prone (**A**), sitting (**B**), and stance (**C**). Also shown is the time course for these reflexes. (Adapted with permission from Barnes MR, Crutchfield CA, Heriza CB. The neurophysiological basis of patient treatment. Morgantown, WV: Stokesville, 1978:222.)

3. Development of individual sensory systems including somatosensory, visual, or vestibular systems
4. Development of sensory strategies for organizing these multiple inputs
5. Development of internal representations important in the mapping of perception to action
6. Development of adaptive and anticipatory mechanisms that allow children to modify the way they sense and move for postural control (Woollacott et al., 1989)

An important part of interpreting senses and coordinating actions for postural control is the presence of an internal representation, or body schema, providing a postural frame of reference. It has been hypothesized that this postural frame of reference is used as a comparison for incoming sensory inputs, as an essential part of interpreting self-motion, and to calibrate motor actions (Gurfinkel and Levik, 1978).

Development of sensory and motor aspects of postural control has been hypothesized to involve the capacity to build up appropriate internal postural representations that reflect the rules for organizing sensory inputs and coordinating them with motor actions. For example, as the child gains experi-

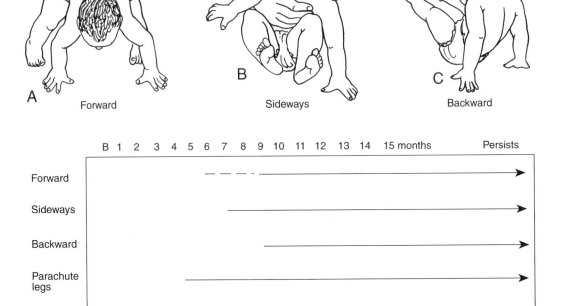

FIGURE 8-10. The protective reactions, which protect the body from injury resulting from a fall. They develop first in the forward direction (**A**), then sideways (**B**), then backward (**C**). Also shown is the time course for these reflexes. (Adapted with permission from Barnes MR, Crutchfield CA, Heriza CB. The neurophysiological basis of patient treatment. Morgantown, WVA: Stokesville, 1978:222.)

ence moving in a gravity environment, sensory-motor maps develop. These maps relate actions to incoming sensory inputs from vision, somatosensory, and vestibular systems. In this way, rules for moving develop and are reflected in altered synaptic relationships. Thus, researchers argue, the path from sensation to motor actions proceeds via an internal representational structure or body schema (Gurfinkel and Levik, 1978; Hirschfeld, 1992).

Examination Based on Newer Models

According to these newer theories, examination of early motor development is directed at both emerging behavioral motor milestones and the supporting systems, such as postural control, for that behavior. In addi-

tion, examination must occur within the context of various tasks and environments. The child's capacity to anticipate and adapt to a changing environment, as evidenced by variability of performance, is also included in an analysis of development. The ability to adapt how we sense and how we move is a critical part of normal development. As a result, it is as important to assess as the acquisition of stereotyped motor milestones.

Since different systems affecting postural control develop at different rates, it is important to understand which components are rate limiting at each developmental stage and conversely, which ones push the system to a new level of function when they have matured. According to newer models of development, finding the connection between critical postural components and develop-

Reflex Model of Postural Development

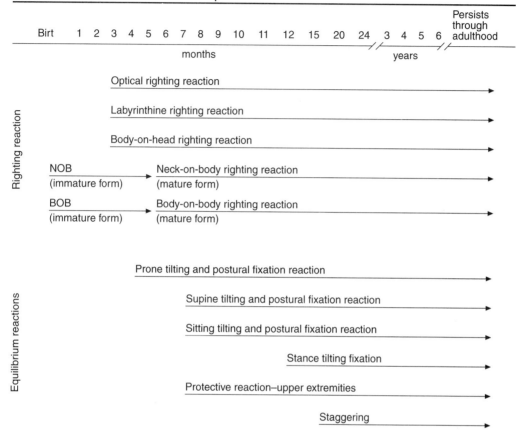

FIGURE 8-11. A reflex model of postural development showing the emergence of righting and equilibrium reactions purported to underlie the emergence of postural stability.

ment ultimately guides the clinician in determining which systems should be examined and how the contribution of these systems changes at various developmental stages. It also allows the clinician to determine appropriate interventions specific to the system that is dysfunctional.

⦿ DEVELOPMENT OF POSTURAL CONTROL: A SYSTEMS PERSPECTIVE

Since Gesell's original studies in 1946 describing the cephalocaudal nature of development, many researchers have found exceptions to some of his general developmental rules. For example, recent stud-

ies have found that infants show control of the legs in kicking and supported walking behaviors well before they can control their head and trunk in space (Thelen et al., 1989; Forssberg, 1985). However, in the area of balance and postural control, it does appear that development follows a cephalocaudal sequence.

Emerging Head Control

Motor Coordination

Heinz Prechtl (1986), a researcher and physician from the Netherlands, used ultrasound techniques to study the spontaneous postural behavior of infants during prenatal development. He observed spontaneous postural changes and described several motor patterns responsible for these changes. Positional changes occurred as often as 20 times per hour in the first half of pregnancy but decreased in later pregnancy, perhaps due to space restriction.

Prechtl (1986) also attempted to test responses to perturbations and noted that he was unable to activate vestibular reflexes in utero. He reported that the vestibulo-ocular reflex and the Moro response were absent prenatally but were present at birth and suggested that these reflexes were inhibited until the umbilical cord was broken, which prevented the fetus from moving every time the mother turned.

Prechtl and colleagues also observed spontaneous head control in neonates and noted that infants had very poor postural or antigravity control at birth. They hypothesized that this could be due either to lack of muscle strength (a musculoskeletal constraint) or alternatively to lack of maturity of the motor processes controlling posture of the head and neck at this age (motor coordination constraint). To test this, they examined spontaneous head movements using both electromyographic (EMG) recordings and video recordings to determine whether coordinated muscle activity was present. They found no organized patterns of muscle activity that appeared to counteract the force of gravity on any consistent basis. This finding suggests that the lack of head control in newborns is not solely the result of a lack of strength but also results from a lack of organized muscle activity (Schloon et al., 1976).

To examine infants' responses to perturbations of balance, they placed infants on a rocking table that could be tipped up or down, noting any antigravity responses. Newborns and infants up to 8 to 10 weeks did not respond either to head-downward or head-upward tilts. However, by 8 to 10 weeks, with the onset of spontaneous head control, infants showed clear EMG patterns in response to the tilting surface, and this response became consistent at about the third month of age.

This research suggests that the emergence of coordinated postural responses in neck muscles, underlying both spontaneous

head control and responses to perturbations, occurs at about 2 months of age. However, it does not give us specific information about the ability of individual sensory systems to drive postural responses in the neck.

Sensory Contributions

Babies as young as 60 hours old are able to orient themselves toward a source of visual stimulation and can follow a moving object by correctly orienting the head (Bullinger, 1981; Bullinger and Jouen, 1983). These orientation movements appear to be part of a global form of postural control involving the head and entire body.

When do visually controlled postural adjustments become available to the infant? To examine visual contributions to spontaneous control of head movements, Jouen and colleagues (Jouen, 1993) performed a study with preterm infants (32 to 34 weeks of gestation), examining head alignment both with and without visual feedback (goggles were worn). They kept the infant's head initially in a midline position, then released it and measured the movements of the head. They found that without vision, there was a significant tendency to turn the head to the right, but with vision, the neonate oriented to midline. Thus, at least from 32 to 34 weeks of gestation, infants show a simple type of head postural control that uses vision to keep the head at midline.

A second study examined the capability of neonates to make responses to visual stimuli giving the illusion of a postural perturbation (Jouen, 1993). Infants were placed between two video screens showing patterns of stripes that moved either forward or backward. Postural responses were measured with a pressure-sensitive pillow behind the infant's head. The neonates made postural adjustments of the head in response to the optical flow; for example, when the visual patterns moved backward, the infants appeared to perceive forward sway of the head, because they moved the head backward as if to compensate.

Research has also examined the early development of sensory contributions to antigravity responses in infants. In these experiments, infants of 2.5 or 5 months were placed in a chair that could be tilted to the right or left 25 degrees. During some trials, a red wool ball was placed in the visual field to catch the infant's attention (Jouen, 1984, 1990). The infants showed an antigravity response (keeping the head from falling to the side to which the baby was tilted), that improved with developmental level, with the older infants dropping the head less than the younger infants. Interestingly, when the wool ball was placed in the visual field, both age groups tilted the head less, with the effect being stronger in the younger group. The authors conclude that vision has a significant effect on the vestibular antigravity response in infants and that the response improves with age. However, in this paradigm it is difficult to determine whether the improvement is due to enhanced neck muscle strength, somatosensory-motor processing in neck muscles, or vestibular-motor processing.

Relating Reflex to Systems Theory

How consistent are systems and reflex theories in describing the development of head control? Reflex-hierarchical theory suggests that visual-motor coordination appears at approximately 2 months of age and is the result of maturation of the optical righting reaction. Systems theory suggests that certain basic visual-postural mapping is present at birth and that with experience in moving, the child develops more refined rules for mapping visual information to action.

Reflex theory suggests that since body-righting reactions acting on the head and labyrinthine-righting reactions also emerge between birth and 2 months, this type of sensory-motor mapping is occurring in these sensory systems as well.

According to a reflex model, the Landau reflex, which requires the integration of all three righting reactions, does not emerge until 4 to 6 months. This finding is consistent with Jouen's findings, which suggest that mapping between vision and vestibular systems for postural action is present at 2.5 to 5

months of age. Thus, both theories are consistent in suggesting that mapping of individual senses to action may precede the mapping of multiple senses to action. This type of sensory-to-sensory and sensory-to-motor mapping may represent the beginning of internal neural representations necessary for coordinated postural abilities.

Emergence of Independent Sitting

As infants begin to sit independently and thus develop trunk control, they must learn to master the control of both spontaneous background sway of the head and trunk and to respond to perturbations of balance. This requires the coordination of sensory-motor information relating two body segments (the head and the trunk) in the control of posture. To accomplish this, they must extend to the new set of muscles controlling the trunk the rules they learned regarding sensory-motor relationships for head postural control. It is possible that once these rules have been established for the neck muscles, they can readily be extended to the control of the trunk muscles.

Motor Coordination

The emergence of independent sitting is characterized by the infant's ability to control spontaneous sway sufficiently to remain upright. This occurs at approximately 6 to 8 months of age (Butterworth and Cicchetti 1978).

The ability to respond to postural perturbations with organized postural adjustments appears to develop simultaneously. How do the muscles that coordinate sway responses develop in the neck and trunk? Both cross-sectional and longitudinal studies have been used to explore the development of muscle coordination underlying neck and trunk control in infants 2 to 8 months of age (Woollacott et al., 1987; Hirschfeld and Forssberg, 1994; Harbourne et al., 1993). In a study by Woollacott and colleagues, EMGs were used to record postural muscle responses in the neck and trunk in infants who were either seated in an infant seat or sitting

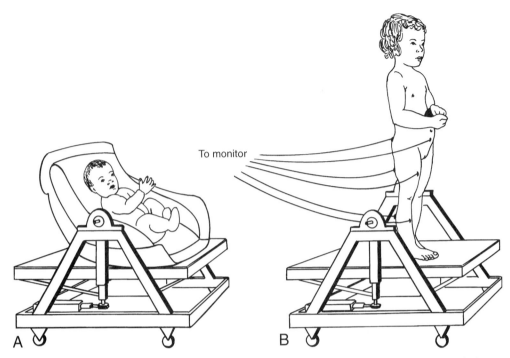

To monitor

A   B

FIGURE 8-12.   Moving platform posturography used to study postural response patterns in infants in response to a moving surface in sitting (**A**) and standing (**B**).

independently on a movable platform, shown in Figure 8-12*A*. Motion of the platform forward or backward caused a disturbance of the infant's head and trunk posture, requiring a subsequent compensatory adjustment to regain balance.

At 2 months, infants did not show consistent, directionally appropriate responses to the platform perturbations. By 3 to 4 months, infants showed directionally specific responses in the neck muscles 40% to 60% of the time. By 5 months, coordinated postural activity in the trunk muscles in response to platform motion was occurring approximately 40% of the time. By 8 months of age, when infants had mastered independent sitting, muscles in the neck and trunk were coordinated into effective patterns for controlling forward and backward sway in the seated position.

A more recent study (Hirschfeld and Forssberg, 1994) showed that platform movements causing backward sway give much stronger and less variable postural muscle response synergies than those causing forward sway. This may be caused by the larger base of postural support in the for-

ward direction in seated infants (Hirschfeld and Forssberg, 1994). In this study presitting infants (5 to 7 months) responded with only one or two muscles for most forward perturbations, with all three anterior muscles (NF, RA, RF [neck flexors, rectus abdominis, rectus femoris, respectively]) being activated in 25% of the trials. By the time infants were independent sitters (7 to 8 months) all three muscles were activated in 100% of the trials. These results suggest that response synergies are being shaped during the months prior to the emergence of independent sitting and are organized appropriately in all trials by the time infants are able to sit independently.

Sensory Contributions

Early research investigated the role of vision in seated postural control by examining the response to visual stimuli giving the illusion of a postural perturbation (the moving room paradigm) of infants at different stages in the development of independent sitting (Butterworth and Hicks, 1977; Butterworth and Pope, 1983). Infants with relatively little experience in sitting independently showed a complete loss of balance in response to the visual stimulation (a single-ramp stimulus); with increasing experience in sitting, they showed a decline in the response amplitude. This implies that newly sitting infants rely heavily on visual inputs when controlling sway and decrease this dependence with increasing experience in independent sitting, as they rely more on somatosensory inputs.

Recent experiments by Bertenthal et al. (1997) have also examined responses of infants to visual cues using continuous oscillations as they mastered independent sitting. In this study infants of 5 to 13 months sat on a child's bicycle seat (with back) in a room that continuously oscillated at a variety of speeds and amplitudes. The postural responses were measured with a force plate under the bicycle seat. They noted that even 5-month-old infants who were presitters showed some entrainment to the driving frequency of the moving visual stimuli; however, this response became more consistent with age and experience. They concluded that during the process of learning to sit independently, infants are learning to scale or map visual sensory information to their postural activity.

Other studies have examined sensory contributions to the emergence of independent sitting balance using support-surface perturbations that activate all three senses rather than just vision alone. Woollacott and coworkers studied muscle patterns in the head and trunk in response to platform perturbations in seated infants with and without vision. They found that taking away visual stimuli did not change the muscle activation patterns in response to a moving platform. They concluded that somatosensory and vestibular systems are capable of eliciting postural actions in isolation from vision in infants first learning to sit (Woollacott et al., 1987).

In an effort to understand the relationship among vestibular and visual inputs reporting head motion and proprioceptive inputs from the trunk, experiments were performed in which head orientation was systematically varied in seated infants undergoing platform perturbations (Hirschfeld and Forssberg, 1994). Coordinated muscle activity stabilizing the trunk did not change no matter how the head was oriented. This suggests that when the infant is in the seated position, postural responses to perturbations are largely controlled by somatosensory inputs at the hip joints, not by vestibular or visual stimulation.

These studies suggest that coordinated postural activity in the neck and trunk develops gradually about the same time the infant is developing independent head control and the ability to sit independently. First, infants appear to map relationships between sensory inputs and the neck muscles for postural control; this is later extended to include the trunk musculature with the onset of independent sitting. Different laboratories interpret the development of these response synergies in alternative ways. They are either described as being constructed gradually, with a resulting reduction in nonorganized tonic background activity in nonparticipating muscles (Woollacott et al., 1987; Sveistrup and Woollacott, 1996) or as being selected from a wide variety of response patterns (Hadders-Algra et al., 1996a). These studies do not tell us whether it is nervous system maturation or experience that allows neck and trunk muscle responses to emerge, since maturation and the refinement of synergies through experience are both gradual, and they seem to occur synchronously.

Modifiability of Postural Responses

What is the effect of practice on the emergence of postural responses? A study examining the effect of training on the development of postural adjustments in presitting infants (Hadders-Algra et al., 1996b) used parents to train the infants at home (5 minutes 3 times per day for 3 months). The training consisted of toy presentation to the side or semibackward at their limits of stability. When comparing EMG responses to platform perturbations before and after training, they found that the trained infants (compared to untrained controls) showed a higher probability of complete responses to perturbations and increased response modulation at higher perturbation velocities, along with decreased pelvic displacement. There were no changes in muscle response onset latencies.

These data give support for the development of similar types of postural training programs in children with motor delays. Studies are being conducted in our own labs to determine whether postural training programs are effective in children with cerebral palsy.

Relating Reflex to Systems Theory

The research we just reviewed suggests that the child's ability to orient the trunk with respect to the head and the support surface occurs at approximately 6 to 8 months of age, coincident with the emergence of independent sitting. These results are quite similar to findings from studies using a reflex-hierarchical approach. In those studies, orientation of the body reportedly emerges at about 6 months of age with the emergence of the mature neck-on-body and body-on-body righting reactions.

While the neck-on-body and body-on-body righting reactions have traditionally been used to describe the emergence of rolling patterns, we have chosen to describe their actions as Magnus did, as they affect body orientation to the head and neck (neck on body) and supporting surface (body on body). Thus, there appears to be agreement between the two theories concerning the emergence of trunk control but a difference in the underlying explanation for these emerging behaviors.

Transition to Independent Stance

During the process of learning to stand independently, infants must learn (*a*) to balance within significantly reduced stability limits compared to those used during sitting and (*b*) to control many additional degrees of freedom as they add the coordination of the leg and thigh segments to those of the trunk and head.

Motor Coordination

The following sections examine the emergence of this control during both quiet stance and in response to perturbations of balance.

Role of Strength

Several researchers have suggested that a primary rate-limiting factor for the emergence of independent walking is the development of sufficient muscle strength to support the body during static balance and walking (Thelen and Fisher, 1982). Can leg muscle strength be tested in the infant to determine whether this is the case?

Researchers have shown that by 6 months of age infants are producing forces well beyond their own body weight (Roncesvalles and Jensen, 1993). These experiments suggest that the ability to support weight against the force of gravity in the standing position occurs well before the emergence of independent stance and so is probably not the major constraint to emerging stance postural control in infants.

Development of Muscle Synergies

How do postural response synergies compensating for perturbations to balance begin to emerge in the newly standing infant? Longitudinal studies have explored the emergence of postural response synergies in infants aged 2 to 18 months, during the transition to independent stance (Woollacott and Sveistrup, 1992; Sveistrup and Woollacott, 1996). As shown in Figure 8-12*B*, infants stood with varying degrees of support on the moving platform while EMGs were used to record muscle activity in the leg and trunk in response to loss of balance.

Figure 8-13 shows EMG responses from one child during the emergence of coordinated muscle activity in the leg and trunk muscles in response to a backward fall. Infants tested at 2 to 6 months of age, before the onset of pull-to-stand behavior and often during the beginning of pull-to-stand behavior, did not show coordinated muscle response organization in response to threats to balance (Fig. 8-13*A*). As pull-to-stand behavior progressed (7 to 9 months), the infants began to show directionally appropriate responses in their ankle muscles (Fig. 8-13*B*). As pull-to-stand skills improved, muscles in the thigh segment were added and a consis-

Early pull-to-

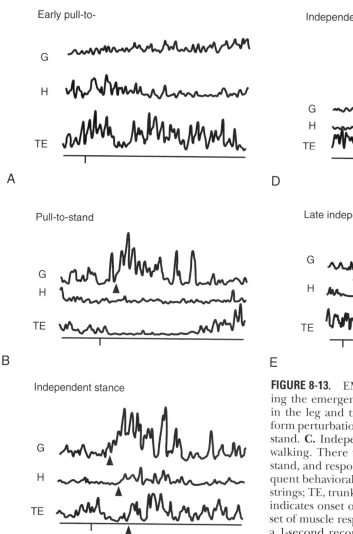

A

Pull-to-stand

B

Independent stance

C

Independent walking

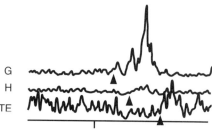

D

Late independent walking

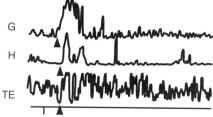

E

FIGURE 8-13.   EMG responses from one child during the emergence of coordinated muscle activity in the leg and trunk muscles in response to platform perturbations: **A.** Early pull to stand. **B.** Pull to stand. **C.** Independent stance. **D–E.** Independent walking. There was no response in early pull-to-stand, and responses gradually developed at subsequent behavioral levels. G, gastrocnemius; H, hamstrings; TE, trunk extensors. Vertical line under TE indicates onset of platform movement. *Arrows,* onset of muscle responses. Each trace corresponds to a 1-second recording. (Adapted with permission from Sveistrup H, Woollacott MH. Longitudinal development of the automatic postural response in infants. J Motor Behav 1996;28:63.)

tent distal-to-proximal sequence began to emerge during late pull-to-stand, independent stance, and walking (9 to 11 months) (Fig. 8-13*C–E*); trunk muscles were consistently activated, resulting in a complete synergy. Figure 8-14 shows the gradual shift in percentage of trials in which a one-muscle response versus a three-muscle response was found as children moved from early pull-to-stand to independent walking. Note the gradual addition of muscles to the synergy with experience and development.

Sensory Contributions

Once an infant learns how to organize synergistic muscles for controlling stance in association with one sense, will this automatically transfer to other senses reporting sway? This may not always be the case. It appears that vision maps to muscles controlling stance posture at 5 to 6 months, prior to somatosensory system mapping and long before the infant has much experience with standing (Foster et al., 1996). This suggests

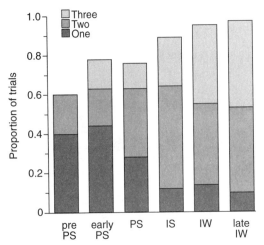

that the infant has to reassemble the synergies when somatosensory inputs are mapped for stance postural control.

EMG responses and sway patterns in response to visual flow created by a moving room were examined in infants and children of varying ages and abilities and compared to those of young adults (Foster et al., 1996). Figure 8-15 shows an example of an infant positioned in a moving room. The child's sway was recorded through a one-way mirror with a video camera mounted outside the room, and muscle responses were recorded from the legs and hips. Infants who were unable to stand independently were supported by their parents at the hip.

Children as young as 5 months of age swayed in response to room movements; sway amplitudes increased in the pull-to-stand stage, peaking in the independent walkers, and dropped to low levels of sway in experienced walkers (Foster et al., 1996).

FIGURE 8-14. Proportion of trials with responses recorded in one, two, or three muscles following the platform perturbation in each stage of stance development. PS, pull to stand; IS, independent stance; IW, independent walking. (Adapted with permission from Sveistrup H, Woollacott MH. Longitudinal development of the automatic postural response in infants. J Motor Behav 1996;28 : 67.)

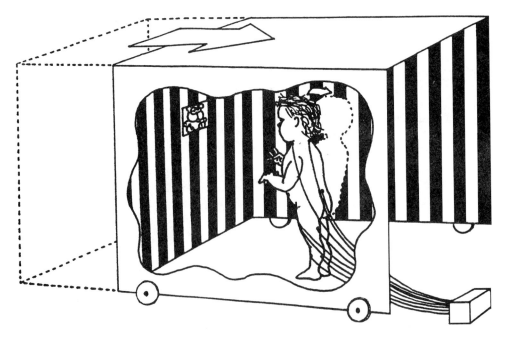

FIGURE 8-15. The moving room paradigm used to examine the development of visual contributions to postural control. When the room moves toward the child, the child perceives forward sway and responds by swaying backward. (Reprinted with permission from Sveistrup H, Woollacott MH. Systems contributing to the emergence and maturation of stability in postnatal development. In: Savelsbergh GJP, ed. The development of coordination in infancy. Amsterdam: Elsevier, 1993:324.)

Sway responses were associated with clear patterns of muscle responses that pulled the child toward the visual stimulus.

These experiments suggest that the visual system will elicit organized postural responses in standing infants at an earlier time than the somatosensory system and that the somatosensory system develops postural synergies separately in association with somatosensory inputs signaling sway.

Development of Adaptive Capability

To determine if higher level adaptive processes are available to the infant during pull-to-stand behavior, independent stance, and early walking, the ability of the infants to attenuate postural responses to the visual flow created by the moving room was monitored (Foster et al., 1996). None of the infants in any of these behavioral categories was able to adapt inappropriate postural responses to low levels over a period of five trials. The researchers concluded that higher-level adaptive processes related to postural control have not yet matured by the emergence of independent walking.

When does the ability to adapt responses to changes in support surface characteristics emerge? A recent study examined the ability of infants during their first year of walking (13 to 14 months old) to adapt to altered support surface conditions, including high friction (high-friction plastic), low friction (Formica coated with baby oil), and foam surfaces, as well as standing crosswise on a narrow beam (Stoffregen et al., 1997). The children had two poles available to hold if necessary to help with balance. It is interesting to note that the highest amount of time spent in free standing was on the high-friction surface, with minimal hand support used. As the surfaces became more compliant (foam) or low friction (baby oil), pole holding increased substantially, with a concomitant drop in free standing. Finally, it was impossible for the infants to stand crosswise on the beam while standing independently. Since standing crosswise on a beam requires active control of the hips rather than purely control of ankle movements, this suggests

that this adaptive ability to use the hips in balance is not mastered in infants during their first year of walking.

Previous research on adults has shown that increasing the size of a balance threat will often elicit a hip strategy (activated by abdominal muscle activity) rather than an ankle strategy as the center of mass nears the edges of the base of support. To determine when the ability to control the hips during balance recovery emerges Woollacott et al. (1998) gave new walkers (10 to 17 months) through hoppers (2 to 3 years), gallopers (4 to 6 years) and skippers (7 to 10 years of age) increasing magnitudes of balance threats to elicit a hip strategy if it was available in these children. They found that hip-dominated responses were present in the walkers with only 3 to 6 months of walking experience. However, these responses were passively activated, with minimal abdominal activity used. It was not until the children reached 7 to 10 years of age (skippers) that they began to show consistent active control of the strategy with high levels of abdominal muscle activity.

The Effect of Practice: Modifiability of Postural Responses

To determine if experience is important in the development of postural response characteristics in infants learning to stand, postural responses were compared in two groups of infants in the pull-to-stand stage of balance development (Sveistrup and Woollacott, 1997). One group of infants was given extensive experience with platform perturbations, receiving 300 perturbations over 3 days. The second (control) group of infants did not receive this training.

Infants who had extensive experience on the platform were more likely to activate postural muscle responses, and these responses were better organized. Figure 8-16 shows the probability of seeing a response in tibialis anterior, quadriceps, and abdominal muscles in response to platform movements causing backward sway, both before and after training. Note that probability of seeing a response in all three muscles was significantly increased. However, onset latencies of postural responses did not change.

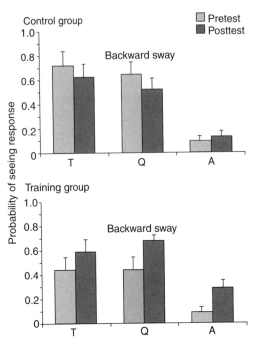

FIGURE 8-16. The probability of seeing a response in tibialis anterior (T), quadriceps (Q) and abdominal muscles (A) in response to platform movements causing backward sway, both before and after 3 days of balance training. Probability of seeing a response in all three muscles was significantly increased by balance training. (Adapted with permission from Sveistrup H, Woollacott M. Can practice modify the developing automatic postural response? Exp Brain Res 1997;114:36.)

These results suggest that experience can influence the strength of connections between the sensory and motor pathways controlling balance, thus increasing the probability of producing postural responses. However, the lack of a training effect on muscle response latency suggests that neural maturation may be a rate-limiting factor in latency reduction with development. It is probable that the myelination of nervous system pathways responsible for reducing latencies of postural responses during development is not affected by training.

Relating Reflex to Systems Theory

Differences in focus between reflex-hierarchical and systems models make it difficult to relate findings examining the emergence of independent stance. Reflex-hierarchical theory distinguishes the righting reactions underlying orientation from the tilting and postural fixation reactions essential to the emergence of balance, suggesting that different neural mechanisms are involved in these two functions. Researchers studying tilting and postural fixation reactions have not examined the importance of individual sensory systems to these reactions or their capability for adaptation.

Systems-based research suggests that the time course for emerging stability behaviors is different in each of the sensory systems. Visual inputs relating the body's position in space map to muscular actions controlling the body's position during stance earlier than do inputs from the somatosensory system. It is not known yet how early vestibular inputs map to stance postural actions. Results from systems-based studies suggest that for the most part, experience within a specific posture is important for sensory information signaling the body's position in space to be mapped to muscular actions, which control the body's position in space.

Refinement of Stance Control

Up until now, we have examined changes within the postural control system in the first 12 months of life that contribute to the emergence of sitting and stance. Researchers have found that postural control is essentially adultlike by 7 to 10 years of age. What are the key changes that contribute to this refinement of postural control? It appears that the emergence of adult levels of control occurs at different times for different aspects of postural control.

Musculoskeletal System: Changes in Body Morphology

Are children inherently more stable than adults? Children are shorter and therefore closer to the ground. Does their height make balancing an easier task? Anyone who has watched a fearless young child ski down a steep slope with relative ease, falling and bouncing back up, might assume that their task is easier. They don't have as far to fall! It turns out that while children are shorter than adults, they are proportioned differently. Children are top-heavy. The relative size of the head in comparison to lower extremities places the center of mass at about T12 in the child, compared to L5-S1 in the adult. Because of their shortness and the difference in the location of their center of mass, children sway at a faster rate than adults. Thus, the task of static balance is slightly more difficult, since the body is moving at a faster rate during imbalance (Zeller, 1964).

Motor Coordination

Quiet Stance

How does the control of spontaneous sway during quiet stance change as children develop? A number of studies have examined changes in spontaneous sway with development (Taguchi and Tada, 1988; Hayes and Riach, 1989). One study examining children 2 to 14 years of age showed that the amplitude of sway decreased with age. There was considerable variation in sway amplitude in the young children. This variance systematically lowered with age and with the children's improved balance. Effects of eye closure were represented by the Romberg quotient (eyes-closed sway expressed as a percentage of eyes-open sway), giving an indication of the contributions of vision to balance during quiet stance. Very low Romberg quotients were recorded for the youngest children who completed the task (4-year-olds) with values of less than 100%. This indicates that these children were swaying more with eyes open than with eyes closed (Hayes and Riach, 1989). Spontaneous sway in children reaches adult levels by 9 to 12 years of age for eyes-open conditions and at 12 to 15 years of age for eyes-closed conditions. Sway velocity also decreased with age, reaching adult levels at 12 to 15 years of age (Taguchi and Tada, 1988).

Compensatory Postural Control

Refinement of compensatory balance adjustments in children 15 months to 10 years of age has been studied by several re-

searchers using a movable platform to examine changes in postural control (Forssberg and Nashner, 1982; Shumway-Cook and Woollacott, 1985a; Berger et al., 1985; Hass et al., 1986). Research has shown that compensatory postural responses of children 15 months of age are more variable and slower than those of adults (Forssberg and Nashner, 1982). These slower muscle responses and the more rapid rates of sway acceleration observed in young children cause sway amplitudes in response to balance threats that are bigger and often more oscillatory than those of older children and adults.

Even children 1.5 to 3 years of age generally produce well-organized muscle responses to postural perturbations while standing (Shumway-Cook and Woollacott, 1985a). However, the amplitudes of these responses are larger, and the latencies and durations of these responses are longer than those of adults. Other studies have also found a longer duration of postural responses in young children and have noted the activation of monosynaptic stretch reflexes in young children in response to platform perturbations. These responses disappear as the children mature (Berger et al., 1985; Hass et al., 1986).

Surprisingly, postural responses in children 4 to 6 years of age are in general slower and more variable than those found in the 15-month- to 3-year-olds, 7- to-10-year-olds, or adults, suggesting an apparent regression in the postural response organization. Figure 8-17 compares EMG responses in the four age groups.

In these studies, by 7 to 10 years of age, postural responses were essentially like those of the adult. There were no significant differences in onset latency, variability, or temporal coordination between muscles within the leg synergy between this age group and adults (Shumway-Cook and Woollacott, 1985a).

Why are postural actions so much more variable in the 4- to 6-year-old child? It may be significant that the variability in response parameters of 4- to 6-year-old children occurs during a period of disproportionate growth with respect to critical changes in

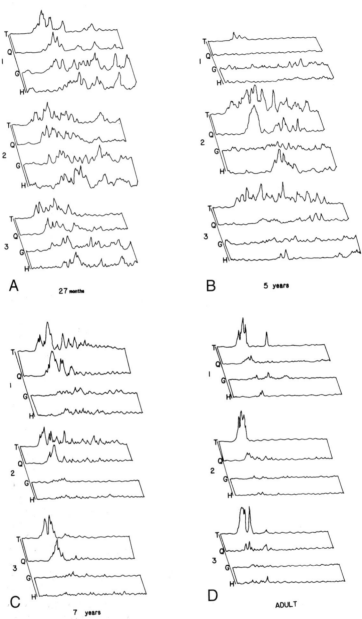

FIGURE 8-17.   A comparison of muscle activation patterns in leg and trunk muscles in response to forward platform perturbations causing backward sway in children from four age groups. Three successive responses to platform perturbations are shown for each child. Platform perturbation started at the onset of the electromyogram recording. Recording is 600 msec. T, tibialis anterior; Q, quadriceps; G, gastrocnemius; H, hamstring muscles. (Reprinted with permission from Shumway-Cook A, Woollacott M. The growth of stability: postural control from a developmental perspective. J Motor Behav 1985;17:136.)

body form. It has been suggested that discontinuous changes seen in the development of many skills, including postural control, may be the result of critical dimension changes in the body of the growing child (Kugler et al., 1982). The system would remain in a state of stability until dimensional changes reached a point where previous motor programs were no longer highly effective. At that point, the system would undergo a period of transition marked by instability and variability and then a new plateau of stability.

Research analyzing the movements of different segments of the body in response to platform perturbations in both children and adults (Woollacott et al., 1988) has shown that the kinematics of passive body movements caused by platform translations are very similar in the 4- to 6-year-old, 7- to 9-year-old, and adult. Thus, it is more probable that changes in response latencies and variability seen in 4- to 6-year-olds represent developmental changes in the nervous system itself.

In addition to looking at the development of reactive balance control from a neurophysiological perspective, one can examine it from a biomechanical perspective, examining the development of forces used to recover from balance threats. Recent work has used kinetics to examine the refinement in the development of force capabilities in infants 9 months to 10 years of age as they recover from balance threats (Roncesvalles et al., in press). In examining center of pressure (COP) trajectories used to recover from balance threats, it was noted that children just learning to stand and walk were the slowest to recover stability (about 2 seconds), with COP trajectories more than twice as large as those of the older children (7- to 10-year-olds, at 1.1 second). Why was this the case? Examination of the torque profiles at the ankle, knee, and hip showed that in contrast to older children and adults, who rapidly generated large torques, the younger children (standers and walkers 9 to 23 months of age) used multiple torque adjustments before regaining control. Figure 8-18 shows torque profiles of children 9 to 13

months (new standers), 14 to 23 months (advanced walkers), 2 to 3 years (runners, jumpers), 4 to 6 years (gallopers) and 7 to 10 years (skippers). Note that there are at least three bursts of torque production at the ankle, knee, and hip in the stander and walker, while this is reduced to two and then one burst in the older groups. The youngest groups tended to overshoot and undershoot torque requirements, with many torque reversals.

These data support the previous work on refinement of balance strategies using neurophysiological and kinematic measures (Forssberg and Nashner, 1982; Shumway-Cook and Woollacott, 1985a) that showed that children 1 to 3 years exhibited large and oscillatory sway excursions, while response patterns were gradually refined and became similar to those of adults by 7 to 10 years of age.

Development of Sensory Adaptation

Postural control is characterized by the ability to adapt the ways we use sensory information about the position and movement of the body in space to changing task and environmental conditions. How does the CNS learn to interpret information from vision, vestibular, and somatosensory receptors and relate it to postural actions?

We have already described evidence from moving-room experiments suggesting that the visual system plays a predominant role in the development of postural actions. That is, visual inputs reporting the body's position in space appear to be mapped to muscular actions earlier than inputs from other sensory systems. In young children, the invariant use of visual inputs for postural control can sometimes mask the capability of other senses to activate postural actions. Results from the experiments in which children balanced without visual inputs suggest that in certain age groups, postural actions activated by other sensory inputs can be better organized than those associated with vision!

Moving platform posturography in conjunction with a moving visual surround has also been used to examine the development

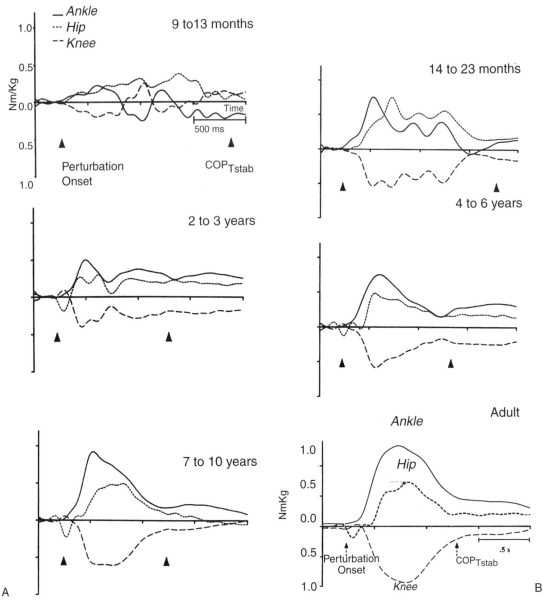

FIGURE 8-18.   Torque profiles of children 9 to 13 months (new standers), 14 to 23 months (advanced walkers), 2 to 3 years (runners, jumpers), 4 to 6 years (gallopers) and 7 to 10 years (skippers) in response to backward platform movements causing forward sway. There are at least three bursts of torque production at the ankle, knee, and hip in the stander and walker, while this is reduced to two and then one burst in the older children. *Arrows,* The onset of perturbation and recovery of balance. The ankle and hip torques are extensor (positive) and responsible for returning the center of mass to its resting range. Knee torque was flexor, counterbalancing the extensor torques generated at ankle and hip. Muscle torques were normalized to body mass and all graphs plotted on the same scale. Time scale is 500 msec.

of intersensory integration for postural control. The platform protocols used to study the organization and selection of senses for postural control are described in detail in Chapter 7.

The development of sensory adaptation in children aged 2 to 10 was studied using a modification of this protocol (Shumway-Cook and Woollacott, 1985a). Children 4 to 6 years old swayed more than older children and adults, even when all three sensory inputs were present (condition 1). With eyes closed (condition 2), their stability decreased further, but they did not fall.

Reducing the accuracy of somatosensory information for postural control by rotating the platform surface (condition 3) further reduced the stability of 4- to 6-year-olds, and half of them lost balance. When children 4 to 6 years of age had to maintain balance using primarily vestibular information for

postural control, all but one fell. In contrast, none of the children 7 to 10 years of age lost balance. Figure 8-19 compares body sway in children of various ages and adults in these four sensory conditions (Shumway-Cook and Woollacott, 1985a).

These results suggest that children under 7 years are unable to balance efficiently when both somatosensory and visual cues are removed, leaving only vestibular cues to control stability. In addition, children under

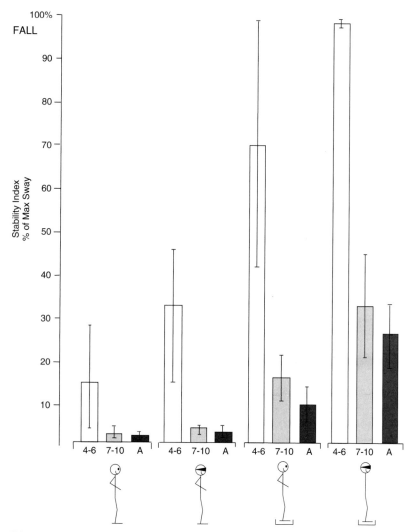

FIGURE 8-19.   A comparison of body sway in 4- to 6-year-olds, 7- to 10-year-olds, and adults in four sensory conditions. *Left to right*: Eyes open, firm support surface; eyes closed, firm support surface; eyes open, sway-referenced surface; eyes closed, sway-referenced surface. (Adapted with permission from Shumway-Cook A, Woollacott M. The growth of stability: postural control from a developmental perspective. J Motor Behav 1985;17:141.)

7 show a reduced ability to adapt senses for postural control appropriately when one or more of these senses is inaccurately reporting body orientation.

A study by Foudriat et al. (1993) examined the ability of children 3 to 6 years of age to balance under the six sensory conditions of the Sensory Organization Test (firm versus sway-referenced surface and eyes open, closed, and sway-referenced visual conditions). They noted that the ability to ignore misleading visual sensory inputs was present in 76% of the 3-year-olds. In addition, postural stability was greater when visual inputs were sway-referenced than in conditions that manipulated support surface compliance. They concluded that the predominance of visual control of balance gives way to a somatosensory control of balance by age 3 but

that adultlike responses are not apparent until past age 6.

Refinement of Anticipatory Postural Control

Skilled movement has both postural and voluntary components; the postural component establishes a stabilizing framework that supports the second component, the primary movement (Gahery and Massion, 1981). Without this supporting postural framework, skilled action deteriorates, as seen in patients with a variety of motor problems. The development of reaching in seated infants shows changes that parallel postural development. Later sections of this book detail the development of manipulatory function.

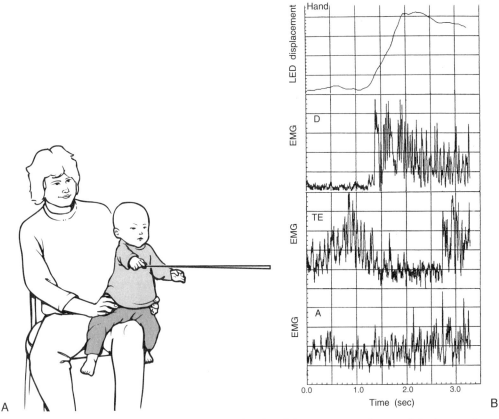

FIGURE 8-20.   A. Experimental setup for study of anticipatory postural control during reaching movements. The infant was balanced on the thigh of the parent with support only at the hip while toys were presented (Hofsten and Woollacott, 1989). **B.** EMG response of the postural muscle, the TE, and the arm muscle, the AD, during a forward reach. The TE is activated in advance of the AD. TE, trunk extensor; AD, anterior deltoid.

Infants as young as 9 months show activation of the postural muscles of the trunk in advance of most but not all reaching movements. In one study infants of 9 months of age were balanced on the thigh of their parent with support only at the hip while toys were presented to them, as in Figure 8-20*A* (Hofsten and Woollacott, 1989). By 9 months of age, when infants were able to sit independently and were showing relatively mature reaching movements, they were also showing advance activation of postural muscles to stabilize voluntary movements in the seated position. Figure 8-20*B* shows the activation of trunk muscles before the anterior deltoid during a forward reach.

In standing, children as young as 12 to 15 months are able to activate postural muscles in advance of arm movements (Forssberg and Nashner, 1982). By 4 to 6 years, anticipatory postural adjustments preceding arm movements while standing are essentially mature (Nashner et al., 1983; Woollacott and Shumway-Cook, 1986).

Thus, this research has described some of the critical refinements in the components of the postural control system that occur between 12 months and 10 years. Changes in the motor components involve changes in body morphology as well as refinement of the muscular response synergies, including (*a*) a decrease in onset latencies, (*b*) improvement in the timing and amplitude of muscle responses, and (*c*) a decrease in variability of muscle responses. Refinements in postural motor behavior are associated with a decrease in sway velocity and a reduction of oscillatory sway behavior.

Refinements in the sensory aspects of postural control include a shift from predomi-

Systems Model of Postural Development

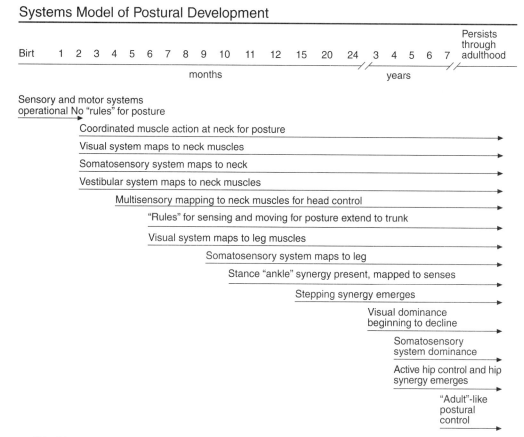

FIGURE 8-21. A systems model of postural development showing the emergence of critical stages in the development of postural control

LAB ACTIVITY 8-1

OBJECTIVE: To explore both reflex-hierarchical and systems methods for evaluating balance development

PROCEDURE: Test one or two infants of the following ages: 1 to 2 months, 4 to 6 months, 8 to 9 months, 18 months.
- A. Motor milestones
  1. Make a list of the major motor milestones observed in each child at the varying ages.
- B. Reflex–hierarchy: Test for the presence of the following reflexes in each infant:
  1. ATNR
  2. STNR
  3. Optical righting
  4. Landau
  5. Tilting reactions (prone, sitting, stance, when possible)
  6. Postural fixation reactions (prone, sitting, stance, when possible)
  7. Protective reactions (forward, sideways, backward)
- C. Systems: Test each infant under the following postural conditions
  1. Steady-state postural control
     a. Vertical suspension: Hold the infants vertically with feet in contact with the supporting system. You will have to provide varying amounts of support to the infants depending on their age. For infants able to stand, observe spontaneous sway in standing.
     b. Sitting: With the infants sitting quietly (supported as needed) check spontaneous sway of head and trunk.
  2. Reactive balance
     a. Vertical suspension: Tip the children gently to the right, to the left, forward, and backward. Observe their ability to right their head, bringing it back to vertical.
     b. Sitting: For infants able to sit with minimal support, give a gentle nudge on the sternum while they are sitting. Note their responses. Could they control the neck? Trunk?
     c. Standing: Repeat the gentle nudge and again observe the response. Could they control and recover stability?
- D. Sensory dominance: Twirl a large cardboard wheel in front of the infants. How do they respond posturally to this visual stimulus?

ASSIGNMENT: Write answers to the following questions based on your observations of the infants' responses:
  1. Reflexes: In which children (what ages) were each of the reflexes present? Did your observations coincide with those of Figure 8-11?
  2. Systems: What were the differences in control of quiet stance and reactive sway in the children? What postural responses to a visual stimulus did you detect? Did your observations coincide with those of Figure 8-21? For example, when did you see coordinated muscle action at the neck for posture? When did the visual system begin to map to neck muscles? At what age were they able to respond to sternum nudges when sitting? (When did rules for sensory-motor mapping extend to trunk?) At what age were they able to respond to sternum nudges when standing? (When did rules for sensory-motor mapping extend to leg posture control?)

nance of visual control of balance to a somatosensory control of balance by age 3. The ability to adapt senses for postural control appropriately when one or more of these senses is inaccurately reporting body orientation information is reduced in children under 7.

Figure 8-21 summarizes the emergence of postural control from a systems perspective. By comparing Figures 8-11 and 8-21, you can see the similarities and differences between this model and the reflex-hierarchical model in describing the emergence of posture control in neurologically intact children. The application of this concept can be found in Lab Activity 8-1.

☙ SUMMARY

1. The development of postural control is an essential aspect of the development of skilled actions, such as locomotion and manipulation.

2. Consistent with Gesell's developmental principles, postural development appears to be characterized by a cephalo-caudal progression of control.

3. The emergence of postural control can be characterized by the development of rules that relate sensory inputs about the body's position with respect to the environment to motor actions controlling the body's position.

   a. Control begins in the head segment. The first sense that is mapped to head control appears to be vision.

   b. As infants begin to sit independently, they learn to coordinate sensory-motor information relating the head and trunk segments, extending the sensory-motor rules for head postural control to trunk muscles.

   c. The mapping of individual senses to action may precede the mapping of multiple senses to action, thus creating internal neural representations necessary for coordinated postural abilities.

4. Anticipatory, or proactive, postural control, which provides a supportive framework for skilled movements, develops in parallel with reactive postural control.

5. Adaptive capabilities that allow the child to modify sensory and motor strategies to changing task and environmental conditions develops later. Experience in using sensory and motor strategies for posture may play a role in the development of adaptive capacities.

6. The development of postural control is best characterized as the continuous development of multiple sensory and motor systems, which manifests behaviorally in a discontinuous steplike progression of motor milestones. New strategies for sensing and moving can be associated with seeming regression in behavior as children incorporate new strategies into their repertoire for postural control.

7. Not all systems contributing to the emergence of postural control develop at the same rate. Rate-limiting components limit the pace at which an independent behavior emerges. Thus, the emergence of postural control must await the development of the slowest critical component.

8. Much debate has occurred in recent years over the relative merits of the reflex-hierarchical versus systems models in explaining postural development. In many respects, the two models are consistent. Their differences include these factors: (*a*) The reflex-hierarchical model views balance control from a reactive perspective, while the systems model stresses the importance of proactive, reactive, and adaptive aspects of the system. (*b*) The reflex-hierarchical model tends to weight the role of CNS maturation more heavily than experience, while the systems model does not emphasize the role of one over the other.

Aging and Postural Control

⊘ INTRODUCTION

Why is it that George M. at age 90 is able to run marathons, while Lew N. at age 78 is in a nursing home, confined to a wheelchair, and unable to walk to the bathroom without assistance? Clearly, the answer to this question is complex. Many factors affect outcomes with respect to health and mobility. These factors contribute to the tremendous differences in abilities found among older adults.

This chapter does not describe all aspects of aging. Rather, the focus is on age-related changes occurring in systems critical to postural control. We review the research examining age-related changes in systems whose dysfunction may contribute to instability among older adults and recent studies that look at the effects of training on improving balance function in these systems. Some introductory comments about research examining changes in older adults are important to keep in mind.

Models of Aging

Though many studies have examined the process of aging and have shown a decline in a number of sensory and motor processes in many older adults, scientists do not agree on how and why we age (Aniansson et al., 1978; Tinetti and Ginter, 1988; Kosnik et al., 1988; Sloane et al., 1989; Lewis and Bottomley, 1990; Duncan et al., 1993). This has led to a number of models of aging (Birren and Cunningham, 1985; Davies, 1987; Woollacott, 1989). They can be divided into two general categories. The first category includes theories that focus on the internal causes of aging and the concept that the life span is genetically determined. According to this point of view, one might expect that the organism begins life with all systems functioning at optimal levels. However, with time, the cells in the system are slowly reduced in number until failure of the system results at a specific point in time. Included in this category are theories predicting that specific genetic programs lead to breakdown in the immune system or the neuroendocrine system, and this leads to death. This type of aging can be considered *primary aging*, since it is specific to the organism.

The second category of theories suggests that aging is due primarily to external causes. In this theory the life span would be indefinite without the insults and damage caused by environmental factors, such as radiation, pollutants, bacteria, viruses, foods, toxins, and catastrophic insults, that cause damage to the system. Thus, according to this type of theory, functions of specific systems may remain high until death unless specific pathologies or catastrophes occur to cause a more rapid decline in system function. This type of aging can be considered *secondary aging*, since it is a result of interaction with the environment.

Models of aging representing these two categories are shown in Figure 9-1. The first model (Fig. 9-1*A*) describes the process of aging within the nervous system as a linear decline in neuron function across all levels of the central nervous system (CNS). It predicts that as the number of neurons declines in a specific part of the CNS, various disease states become evident. Alternatively, the second model of aging (Fig. 9-1*B*) suggests that the CNS continues to function at a relatively high level until death unless there is a catastrophe or disease that affects a specific part of the CNS. Thus, pathology within individual parts of the CNS may result in a rapid decline in a specific neural function (Woollacott, 1989).

These models lead to very different conclusions regarding the inevitability of functional decline with aging. The first model, focusing on mechanisms associated with primary aging as the main determinant of nervous system function with age, offers a rather pessimistic view of aging, since it suggests that neuronal loss is inevitable and thus functional loss is an invariant part of growing old. This type of reasoning can lead to self-limiting perceptions on the part of older individuals regarding what they can do (Tinetti et al., 1990). These self-limiting perceptions can be inadvertently reinforced by the medical professional, who may hold a

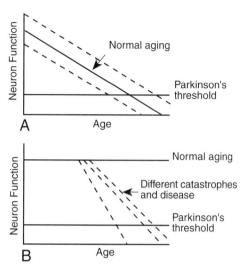

FIGURE 9-1.   Two models of aging. **A.** The first model suggests that aging is associated with an inevitable decline in neuronal function in all systems. Thus, at a particular age, neuron function will be reduced sufficiently in areas such as the basal ganglia for symptoms such as those of Parkinson's disease to appear. **B.** The second model suggests that neuronal function remains optimal with aging unless specific catastrophe or disease affects specific parts of the system. (Reprinted with permission from Woollacott M. Aging, posture control, and movement preparation. In: Woollacott MH, Shumway-Cook A, eds. Development of posture and gait across the life span. Columbia, SC: University of South Carolina Press, 1989:156.)

limited view regarding what older adults can accomplish. For example, when assessing an older adult, a therapist may perceive that the patient's strength is good considering the patient's age. As a result, a strength grade of 3 of 5, which would never be accepted in a 30-year-old, is often accepted in a 70-year-old as normal.

In contrast, the second model of aging, which focuses predominantly on secondary aging processes as the reason for loss of function with age, leads to a more optimistic view (Woollacott, 1989). In this model, one expects optimal function from the CNS unless unexpected pathology occurs and if optimal experiential factors are present. Optimal experiential factors involve leading a healthy and active life. Thus, when therapists with this perspective on aging evaluate an older person, they anticipate that function will be optimal. If a decline is detected in any area of the nervous system, this perspective will allow the therapist to work on rehabilitation strategies aimed at returning function toward that of a normal young adult.

Interactions Between Primary and Secondary Factors

Primary and secondary factors may interact in the aging process. For example, genetic factors can include a genetic predisposition to a specific disease process. An example of a genetic predisposition to a condition is a person who carries the genes for degeneration of auditory neurons and suffers hearing loss in old age. This genetic predisposition could interact with environmental factors in the following way. A person who comes from a family with a tendency towards hearing loss and who works in a noisy environment may experience accelerated hearing loss because of a combination of genetic and environmental influences. Primary factors do not necessarily lead to a generalized decline in function but rather to a loss of function within specific systems (Birren and Cunningham, 1985).

Research is beginning to suggest that secondary factors have a profound effect on aging (Tinetti et al., 1990; Rowe and Kahn, 1998). Secondary, or experiential, factors are more or less under our control. Some of these include nutrition, exercise, insults, and pathologies that affect our mind and body. Environmental factors, such as air pollution and carcinogens in our drinking water, also fall into this category, though you may not agree that these factors are under your control!

Scientists have shown that proper nutrition results in prolonged and healthier lives (Lee et al., 1993). Further, animal studies have shown that dietary restriction increases the life span (Yu et al., 1985; McCarter and Kelly, 1993). In addition, exercise programs have been shown to improve cardiovascular health, control obesity, and increase physical and mental function. The resultant gains in aerobic power, muscle strength, and flexibility can improve biological age by 10 to 20 years. This can result in delaying the age of

dependency and increasing the quality of the remaining years of life (McCarter and Kelly, 1993; Shephard, 1993). This knowledge that how we age is largely determined by how we live leads to an emphasis on preventative health care measures. It also has implications for rehabilitation. Therapists work to assist older patients who have experienced pathology to return to optimal lifestyles (Tinetti, 1986).

Thus, the factors that determine the health and mobility of George M. versus Lew N. are a combination of primary aging factors, primarily genetics, over which they have limited control, and secondary aging, primarily experiential factors, over which they have considerable control.

It appears that neural aging, whether it is primary or secondary, may not necessarily be characterized by an overall decline in all functions. Rather, decline may be limited to specific neural structures and functions. This is consistent with a major theme in this book, that function and dysfunction are not generalized but emerge through the interaction of the capacities of the individual carrying out particular tasks within specific environmental contexts.

Heterogeneity of Aging

A review of the literature on aging shows that some studies report no change in function of the neural subsystems controlling posture and locomotion with age (Gabell and Nayak, 1984), while others show a severe decline in function in the older adult (Imms and Edholm, 1981). How can there be such a discrepancy in studies reporting age-related changes in systems for posture and gait? This may be due to fundamental differences in the definition that researchers use in classifying an individual as elderly.

For example, some researchers have classified the elderly adult as anyone over 60 years of age. When no exclusionary criteria are used in the study of older adults, results can be very different from when researchers use restrictive criteria for including subjects for study. For example, a study on the effects of aging on walking ability selected a group of 71 subjects ranging in age from 60 to 99 years, using no exclusion criteria for possible pathology (Imms and Edholm, 1981). These researchers noted that the mean walking velocities for their older adults were slower than any previous studies reported.

In contrast, another study examined walking in healthy older adults. In this study, 1,187 individuals 65 years and over were screened to find 32 who were free of pathology, that is, had no disorders of the musculoskeletal, neurological, or cardiovascular systems or any history of falls (Gabell and Nayak, 1984). Interestingly, this study found no significant differences between their younger and older adult groups when comparing four parameters measuring the variability of gait. They thus concluded that an increase in variability in the gait cycle among older adults was not normal but always due to some pathology.

These types of results suggest that there is much heterogeneity among older adults.

This amazing variability reminds us that it is important not to assume that declining physical capabilities occur in all older adults.

This continuum of function among older adults has been nicely described by Spirduso (1995) who has illustrated the continuum of function found among older adults. This continuum is illustrated in Figure 9-2. At the highest end of the continuum are older adults who are physically elite, who engage in competitive sports and are considered to undergo optimal aging. Moving down the continuum are older adults who are physically fit, that is, who engage in sports, games, and hobbies and who are capable of moderate physical work. Physically independent adults are also active but engage in less physically demanding activities, such as golf or social dancing. Independence in all basic activities of daily life (BADLs) and instrumental activities of daily life (IADLs) is characteristic of this group. Most adults in the physically frail group are independent in

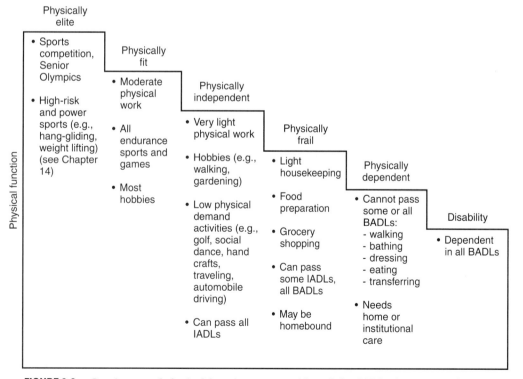

FIGURE 9-2.   Continuum of physical function among older adults. IADLs, instrumental activities of daily life; BADLs, basic activities of daily life. (Adapted from Spirduso W. *Physical Dimensions of Aging.* Champaign Ill. Human Kinetics, 1995: Figure 12.9, p339.)

BADLs but dependent in many IADLs. They are capable of light housekeeping but often require assistance to continue living independently. Physically dependent adults are disabled; they are dependent in both BADLs and IADLs. They require full time assistance or institutional care. Using this continuum, you can see that George M. falls at the upper end, in the physically elite group, while Lew N. falls at the lower end of the continuum.

ℯ BEHAVIORAL INDICATORS OF INSTABILITY

Defining Falls

Before we can discuss falls and their causes in more detail, it is important to have a clear understanding of the definition of a fall and the different categories of falls. This knowledge allows the therapist to question patients more effectively regarding the frequency and nature of their falls and provides a better understanding of the type of rehabilitative strategies appropriate for situations with a variety of types of balance risk. Falls are often defined differently in the clinic than in the research environment. For example, in the clinic, a fall is often defined as a situation in which the older adult falls to the ground or is found lying on the ground. In addition, it is often defined as any unintended contact with nearby surfaces, such as a chair or a counter, to recover balance.

In the research environment, the safety of older adults is considered of utmost importance, and thus balance testing is typically done with a safety harness protecting the older adult from actual falls. In the laboratory, balance threats are often simulated by moving the support surface under the older adult varying distances. In the presence of small platform perturbations, a fall or loss of balance may be defined by movement of the center of mass outside the limits of the base of support, since this could result in a fall if a safety harness were not being used. However, it is important to remember that this definition may also include any situation in which the participant simply stepped in re-sponse to the balance threat and still recovered stability, although with a different strategy than might be used by a young adult.

Since the term fall is used in a variety of contexts, it is important for clinicians to define their own meaning of the term when talking to patients about falls. One clinical definition used to define a fall is an unplanned, unexpected contact with a supporting surface. In this definition, a supporting surface is not defined solely by the floor, but could be a chair (as when a person begins to arise and falls back unexpectedly into the chair) or a wall (as when a person loses balance and staggers into a wall).

Risk Factors for Falls

Statistics on injuries and accidents in the older adult indicate that falls are the seventh leading cause of death in people over 75 years of age (Ochs et al., 1985). In addition, fall rates in persons 65 years of age and older are at least 33% per year in community-dwelling older adults, with women being found to fall more frequently than men (Campbell et al., 1981; Nevitt et al., 1989). What are the factors that contribute to these losses of balance? Many early studies on balance loss in the elderly expected to isolate a single cause of falls for a given older adult, such as vertigo, sensory neuropathy, or postural hypotension. In contrast, more current research indicates that many falls in the elderly have multiple contributing factors, including extrinsic environmental factors and intrinsic factors such as physiological, musculoskeletal, and psychosocial factors (Tinetti et al., 1986; Campbell et al., 1989; Lipsitz et al., 1991). The application of this concept can be found in Lab Activity 9-1.

You may have discovered that both the activity level and the risk of falls for the activity in which the person is engaged are critical to know when attempting to determine fall risk. Falls are not determined solely by factors within the individual, such as poor balance; falls emerge from an interaction of the individual performing specific tasks in certain environments. In fact, research shows that adults older than 75 years tend to fall at

LAB ACTIVITY 9-1

OBJECTIVE: To explore issues related to determining fall risk.

PROCEDURE: Take a moment and ask yourself how many times you have fallen in the past 12 months. Think about the activities and list the activities you were performing at the time you fell. What were the environmental conditions like when you fell? What were the consequences of your falls? Were you injured? Since the fall, have you been afraid or reluctant to return to those activities? Now, find an older adult living within the community or within a residential facility, such as an assisted-living retirement center or skilled nursing facility. Ask this older adult the same set of questions. What is his or her fall rate? What activities was the person performing when he or she fell? What was the environment like? Was the person injured, and what was the psychological consequence of the fall? Was the person more fearful and reluctant to return to his or her prior level of activity?

ASSIGNMENT: Write answers to these questions and compare your responses to those of the older adult. What is the difference between your falls and those you would expect to see in a 70- to 80-year-old? What were the consequences?

home, while younger old adults (70 to 75 years) fall more frequently away from home and are more seriously injured (Tinetti et al., 1988; Speechley and Tinetti, 1991).

Let's look at some of the risk factors contributing to falls. Individual characteristics, such as age and sex, increase the risk of falling, with the risk of falling rising with increasing age over 64 and with women being at a higher risk than men. Psychosocial factors include being depressed or anxious, having a fear of falling, and circumstances of social isolation, such as living alone or making fewer than one trip away from home per week (Nevitt et al., 1989). Environmental factors that increase fall risk include the presence of stairs, throw rugs, slippery surfaces, and poor lighting (Rubenstein, 1988; Sheldon, 1960).

Many studies have examined the physiological factors that contribute to a risk of falls (Nevitt et al., 1989; Campbell et al., 1989; Lipsitz et al., 1991; Lord et al., 1993; Tinetti et al., 1988; Maki et al., 1994a). For example, Lipsitz and his colleagues followed a group of community-dwelling older adults over 70 years of age for a year and identified all falls that occurred. They found that a number of factors were associated with an increased risk of falling, including reduced physical activity, reduced proximal muscle strength, and reduced stability while standing. Other significant factors included arthritis of the knees, stroke, impairment of gait, hypotension, and the use of psychotropic drugs. The conclusions of this study were that most falls in older adults involve multiple risk factors and that many of these factors may be remediated. Thus, it was suggested that the clinician who is working with an older adult should determine both intrinsic and extrinsic factors associated with a particular fall and reduce or correct as many of these as possible (Lipsitz et al., 1991).

Studies examining intrinsic factors leading to falls have included examining the role of balance control. Several researchers, including Tinetti from the United States, Berg from Canada, and Mathias and colleagues from England, have measured functional skills related to balance to identify people at high risk for falls (Tinetti et al., 1986; Mathias et al., 1986; Berg et al., 1989; Speechley and Tinetti, 1990). Functional skills include sitting, standing, and walking unsupported, standing and reaching forward, performing a 360-degree turn, and moving from sit to stand position.

A more recent approach to understanding balance function in the elderly examines specific variables relating to normal postural control and determines the extent to which deterioration in their function contributes to loss of stability and mobility in the elderly.

In the remaining sections of this chapter we examine the intrinsic factors related to balance problems in the older adult from a systems perspective. We discuss changes in the motor system, the sensory systems, and higher-level adaptive systems, as well as the use of anticipatory postural responses before making a voluntary movement. Studies on the ability of older adults to integrate balance adjustments into the step cycle are covered in the mobility section of this book.

℮ AGE-RELATED CHANGES IN THE SYSTEMS OF POSTURAL CONTROL

In previous chapters, we discussed the many systems that contribute to postural control (see Fig. 7.2). What have researchers learned about how changes in these systems contribute to an increased likelihood of falls in the elderly?

Musculoskeletal System

Muscle Strength

Several researchers have reported changes in the musculoskeletal system in many older adults, including Buchner's and Wolfson's labs in the United States and Aniansson's lab in Scandinavia (Buchner and deLateur, 1991; Aniansson et al., 1986; Whipple et al., 1987). Strength, or the amount of force a muscle produces, declines with age. Lower extremity muscle strength can be reduced by as much as 40% between ages 30 and 80 years (Aniansson et al., 1986). This condition is more severe in older nursing home residents with a history of falls (Whipple et al., 1987). In these subjects, the mean knee and ankle muscle strengths were one-half and one-quarter, respectively, that of nonfallers.

Endurance, which is the capacity of the muscle to contract continuously at submaximal levels, also decreases with age. However, endurance is better preserved with age than is strength. As muscles age, they become smaller in size, and this reduction in muscle mass is greater in the lower extremities than in the upper extremities (Medina, 1996). As muscle cells die, they are replaced with connective tissue and fat. A number of studies have examined the preferential loss of muscle fiber types with aging, with mixed results.

There appears to be an age-related loss of both fiber types; however type II fast twitch fibers may be lost at a faster rate than type I (Timiras, 1994). Researchers have also shown that the number of motor units declines with age; there is a reduction in both large and small myelinated fibers. In addition, there are age-related changes at the neuromuscular junction (Medina, 1996).

Changes in skeletal muscle affect the functional capacity of the muscles. Maximum isometric force decreases, the muscles fatigue more rapidly, and the rate of tension development is slower. It appears that concentric contractions are more affected by age related changes in the neuromuscular system than are eccentric contractions. Rapid-velocity contractions are more affected than slow-velocity contractions.

Researchers have shown that the association between strength and physical function is large, with more than 20% of the variance in functional status explained by relative strength (Buchner and deLateur, 1991). However, the amount of strength needed for physical function depends on the task. For example, it has been suggested that the typical healthy 80-year-old woman is very near if not at the threshold value for quadriceps strength necessary to rise from a chair (Young, 1986). When strength falls below the threshold needed for a task, functional disability occurs.

Range of Motion

Decreased range of motion and loss of spinal flexibility in many older adults can lead to a characteristic flexed or stooped posture (Fig. 9-3) (Studenski et al., 1991; Lewis and Bottomley, 1990). This can be associated with other changes in postural alignment, including a compensatory shift in the vertical displacement of the center of body mass back toward the heels. Other conditions, such as arthritis, can lead to decreased range of motion in many joints throughout the body. In addition, pain may limit the functional range of motion of a particular joint (Horak et al., 1989c).

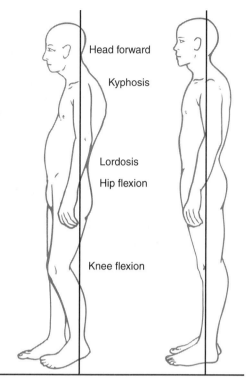

FIGURE 9-3. A comparison of postural alignment in a young versus an older adult. Changes in spinal flexibility can lead to a stooped or flexed posture in many elderly people. (Adapted with permission from Lewis C, Bottomley J. Musculoskeletal changes with age. In: Lewis C, ed. Aging: health care's challenge. 2nd ed. Philadelphia: FA Davis, 1990:146.)

Neuromuscular System

The neuromuscular system contributes to postural control through the coordination of forces effective in controlling the body's position in space.

Changes in Quiet Stance

Traditional methods for assessing balance function in the older adult have used global indicators of balance control, such as determination of spontaneous sway during quiet stance (Sheldon, 1963). One of the earliest studies examined the extent to which subjects in age groups from 6 years through 80 years swayed during quiet stance. Subjects at both ends of the age spectrum (ages 6 to 14 and 50 to 80) had greater difficulty in mini-

mizing spontaneous sway during quiet stance than the other age groups tested (Sheldon, 1963). This study tested a great variety of older adults and did not try to limit subjects in the older groups to those who were free of pathology.

More recent studies have measured spontaneous sway in different age groups using stabilometry, or static force plates. One study examined 500 adults aged 40 to 80 years who were free of pathology and found that postural sway increased with each decade of life. Thus, the greatest amount of spontaneous sway was seen in the 80-year-olds (Toupet et al., 1992). Similarly, a study examining spontaneous sway in older adults with and without a history of falls found a significant increase in sway in even healthy older adults compared to young adults, with the greatest amount of sway found in older people with a history of recent falls (Shumway-Cook et al., 1997a). A number of studies that have examined spontaneous sway have found only small differences between young and older adults. For example Wolfson et al. (1992) found only a 3% (nonsignificant) difference between young adults (35 plus or minus 12 years) and healthy older adults (76 plus or minus 5 years) who were relatively free of neurological disease.

Another study by Fernie and colleagues examined both sway amplitude and velocity in a population of institutionalized elderly and determined that sway velocity (but not amplitude) was significantly greater for those who fell one or more times in a year than for those who had not fallen (Fernie et al., 1982). This implies that in certain populations, velocity of sway may be more sensitive to balance problems than absolute sway.

If total magnitude or velocity of spontaneous sway or center of pressure (COP) displacement during a given period is seen as a clear measure of balance control, then according to a number of the studies cited earlier, one might conclude that there is a small decline in balance function in the older adult. However, Patla et al. (1990) and others make the point that measures of spontaneous sway during normal quiet stance are not necessarily appropriate measures of balance dyscontrol, since older adults are not challenged by normal quiet stance balance and are thus typically well within their balance capacity. Patla notes that larger excursions of COP are generally interpreted as a reflection of a poor balance control system but that some older adults may use larger and higher-frequency excursions of COP to obtain more information about their posture from their sensory systems while remaining well within their limits of stability (Patla et al., 1990). They suggest that static balance be assessed under challenging conditions, such as tandem stance with eyes open versus closed.

Horak (1992) also reminds us that a variety of patients with neurological disorders, such as Parkinson's disease, have normal or even reduced sway in quiet stance. This may be because they show increased stiffness or rigidity and this limits sway to a smaller area during quiet stance. This is one reason that clinical measures of sway with eyes open during normal quiet stance may not be the best way to evaluate balance dysfunction in the older adult.

Changes in Motor Strategies During Perturbed Stance

Is the older adult capable of activating muscle response synergies with appropriate timing, force, and muscle response organization when balance is threatened? Most research addresses this question by using a moving platform to provide an external threat to balance. Measures of balance control have included (*a*) EMG: postural muscle response characteristics (onset latency, duration, magnitude); (*b*) kinematics: changes in center of mass (COM) and joint angle during the balance threat and the recovery; and (*c*) kinetics: the forces (for example, COP) applied by the older adult to respond to the balance threat and recover stability. In the following pages we summarize the studies examining changes in these variables that are correlated with aging and with falls.

Woollacott et al. (1986) performed one of the first studies to examine age-related changes in postural muscle response characteristics elicited when balance was threatened. They found that the muscle response organization of adults 61 to 78 years old and adults 19 to 38 years old was generally similar, with responses being activated first in the stretched ankle muscle and radiating upward to the muscles of the thigh.

However, there were also differences between the two groups in certain response characteristics. The older adults showed significantly slower onset latencies in the ankle dorsiflexors in response to anterior platform movements, causing backward sway. This has been observed in other laboratories as well (Studenski et al., 1991). In addition, in some older adults, the muscle response organization was disrupted, with proximal muscles being activated before distal muscles. This response organization has also been seen in patients with CNS dysfunction (Nashner et al., 1983).

The older group also tended to coactivate the antagonist muscles along with the agonist muscles at a given joint significantly more often than the younger adults. Thus, many of the elderly people studied tended to stiffen the joints to a greater degree than young adults when compensating for sway perturbations.

Several labs have found that many older adults generally used a strategy involving hip movements rather than ankle movements significantly more often than young adults (Horak et al., 1989c; Manchester et al., 1989). Hip movements are typically used by young adults when balancing on a short support surface that doesn't allow them to use ankle torque in compensating for sway. It has been hypothesized that this shift toward use of a hip strategy for balance control in older adults may be related to pathological conditions such as ankle muscle weakness or loss of peripheral sensory function. Horak et al. (1989c) have suggested that in older adults some falls, particularly those associated with slipping, may be the result of using a hip strategy when the surface cannot resist the sheer forces associated with the use of this strategy, for example on ice.

More recent studies have extended this

research and have compared young adults to stable older adults and to older adults with balance problems (Lin, 1998; Woollacott et al., 1999; Studenski et al., 1991). Figure 9-4 summarizes some of the effects found in these studies. Figure 9-4*A* shows examples of responses (from individual trials) to anterior platform movements causing posterior sway in a young adult, a healthy older adult, and an older adult who had problems with balance and falls. Note that the onset latencies for the tibialis anterior and quadriceps postural muscles become progressively later for the stable and then the unstable older adults. Figure 9-4*B* shows the mean muscle onset latencies for all individuals in each group.

Adapting Movements to Changing Tasks and Environments

These early research studies provided information on age-related changes in responses to balance threats of a single size. It is possible that these changes in postural response characteristics in the older adult are simply indications of deterioration in postural muscle response efficiency, as implied in the previous literature. However, it is also possible that some of these changes may be due to the older adults using a different response strategy than that seen in young adults, as a way of adapting to certain constraints associated with aging, such as muscle weakness, reduced ankle joint sensation, or joint stiffness. For example, it is possible that a shift toward the use of hip movements in balance control may be due to ankle muscle weakness and the inability to generate large amounts of force at the ankle joint (Horak et al., 1989c; Manchester et al., 1989). This may be seen more clearly as an older adult is subjected to larger balance threats that exceed his or her muscle response capacity at the ankle. In addition, older adults with balance problems may show more severe constraints within their neural and musculoskeletal systems and therefore show more limited response capacity.

In order to explore this question further, recent studies have examined the response

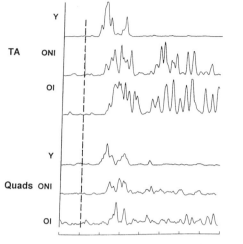

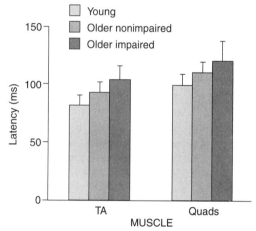

FIGURE 9-4. Changes in timing of muscle response synergies in the elderly. **A.** Examples of muscle responses to an anterior platform movement causing posterior sway in a young adult, a healthy older adult, and an older adult who had problems with balance and falls. The onset latencies for the tibialis anterior and quadriceps postural muscles become progressively later for the stable and then the unstable older adults. **B.** Graphs showing mean response onset latencies for tibialis anterior (TA) and quads (quadriceps) in each subject group. Y, young; ONI, older nonimpaired; OI, older impaired. (Woollacott and Moore, unpublished data.)

characteristics of both well-balanced and less stable older adults during balance threats of increasing magnitude and velocity, to simulate environmental situations with changing balance conditions (Lin, 1998; Woollacott et al., 1999). Young (aged 25 ± 4 years) and older adults were recruited from the community for the study. Older adults were divided into stable and unstable groups according to their scores on three tests, the Berg functional balance test, the Dynamic Gait Index test, and a test of self-perceived balance ability. Stable older adults (aged 74 ± 4) were defined as those with scores from at least two tests that fell within the upper quartile for all subjects, while unstable older adults (aged 76 ± 5) were defined as scores from at least two tests falling within the low quartile. A comparison of the fall history of the three groups revealed that the unstable older adults showed a mean of 0.63 falls in the past 6 months, while stable older adults showed only 0.06 in the last six months, and young adults showed no falls.

As one might expect, there were variations in the ability of older stable and older unstable adults in their ability to respond effectively to balance threats of different magnitudes and velocities. For example, in response to small or slow forward perturbations, onset latencies across the three muscles tested (tibialis anterior [TA], quadriceps [Q], and abdominals [A]) were significantly delayed in both the stable and unstable older adults compared to the young adults, but for the large and fast perturbations, only the unstable older adults showed significant delays compared to the young. Figure 9-5 shows these changes in latency across perturbation sizes for the three groups when averaging across all muscles. This effect was most apparent in the Q and A muscles. This suggests that the stable older adults had difficulty in sensing the onset of small or slow perturbations but were able to compensate adequately for large scaling factors.

A comparison of the ability of the three groups to activate increased amplitudes of muscle responses to larger balance threats showed that the TA response of the unstable older adults was significantly lower than that of the stable and young adults for even smaller perturbations. In response to larger perturbations both the stable older adults and unstable older adults showed significantly smaller responses than the young adults. This suggests that both older stable

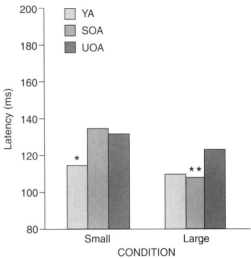

FIGURE 9-5. Ability of young adults (YA), stable older adults (SOA), and unstable older adults (UOA) to use effective muscle response timing when responding to forward balance threats of different magnitudes and velocities (10 cm at 10 cm/second and 15 cm at 40 cm/second). The graph shows changes in latency across perturbation sizes for the three groups when averaged across all muscles (tibialis anterior, quadriceps, abdominals). Onset latencies were significantly slower in both the stable and unstable older adults than in the young adults for small or slow perturbations, but for the large or fast perturbations, only the unstable older adults showed significant delays compared to the young. This suggests that the stable older adults had difficulty in sensing the onset of small or slow perturbations but were able to compensate adequately for large scaling factors. *P < .05 between YA and the other two groups. **P < .05 between UOA and the other two groups. (Reprinted with permission from Lin SI. Adapting to dynamically changing balance threats: differentiating young, healthy older adults and unstable older adults. Doctoral dissertation, University of Oregon, 1998.)

and older unstable adults show a limited response capacity, compared to young adults, in dealing with perturbation threats but the limitations of the stable older adults do not become apparent until balance threats are large.

In order to determine the percent of maximal voluntary capacity that older adults were using when responding to balance threats of different sizes and velocities, Lin (1998) and Woollacott (1989) asked subjects to stand maximally on toes to determine their maximal gastrocnemius capacity. They then compared their postural response amplitudes for similar time intervals to those of their on-toes responses. Figure 9-6 shows that for small perturbations the young and stable older adults used similar amounts of maximum capacity (about 20%), but the unstable older adults used significantly more (almost 40%). As perturbation velocity increased to 40 cm/second, the stable older adults as well showed significantly larger amounts of maximum capacity utilization than the young.

In order to determine if these changes in muscle response characteristics were associated with behavioral changes in the stable and unstable older adults, the behaviors of the three groups were coded by analyzing videotapes of the responses. It was interesting to see that for even very small or slow perturbation conditions that did not require a step, there were clear differences in strategies used by the three groups. Both stable and unstable older adults used significantly less ankle-dominated responses and more hip-dominated responses than young adults. In addition, unstable older adults used other strategies, such as bending at the knee and using the arms to balance. These differences were increased with faster perturbations, with older adults showing a significant percentage of stepping responses when young adults were still using in-place (ankle or hip) responses.

These differences can also be seen in the quantitative data showing COP changes in response to platform perturbations for young adults, stable older adults, and unstable older adults. Figure 9-7 shows that when young adults were given a platform perturbation, they efficiently returned the center of pressure to a stable position, whereas the stable and unstable older adults each showed more COP oscillation before coming to a stable position, with the unstable group showing the largest excursion of the COP. This was accompanied by an increased time for the COP to come to stabilization. It is interesting that in spite of the increases in these variables, there were no differences in peak COM displacements between the groups.

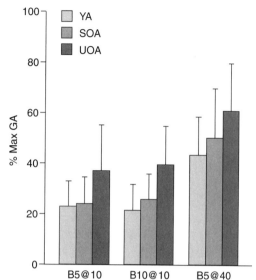

FIGURE 9-6. Comparison of postural response amplitudes of young adults (YA), stable older adults (SOA), and unstable older adults (UOA) for similar intervals when standing maximally on toes (maximum gastrocnemius capacity) versus when responding to balance threats of different sizes and velocities. For small perturbations, the young adults and stable older adults used similar amounts of maximum capacity (about 20%), but the unstable older adults used significantly more (almost 40%). As perturbation velocity increased to 40 cm/second, the stable older adults also showed significantly larger amounts of maximum capacity use than the young. GA, gastrocnemius. (Reprinted with permission from Lin SI. Adapting to dynamically changing balance threats: differentiating young, healthy older adults and unstable older adults. Doctoral dissertation, University of Oregon, 1998.)

This suggests that each group aims at keeping a fairly low COM displacement, and when it goes beyond this point, the older adults simply shift strategies and take a step.

What might be the causes of these age-related changes in postural response characteristics to perturbations? Clinical tests showed that muscle strength was significantly lower for the unstable older adults than for the young and stable older adults for most muscles tested. In addition, the strength of the muscles tested was found to be significantly correlated with the scores of the three functional balance tests for almost all muscles tested. Scores for vibration and proprioceptive sense were also significantly

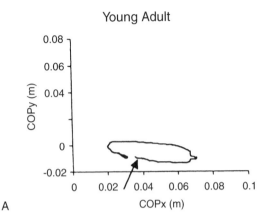

Young Adult

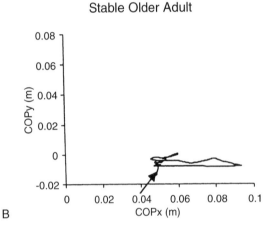

Stable Older Adult

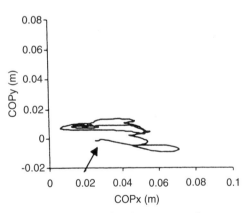

Unstable Older Adult

FIGURE 9-7. Graphs showing center of pressure (COP) trajectory (in x and y coordinates) from perturbation onset to 2 seconds after the perturbations. *Arrows,* perturbation onset. The COP trajectory shows much more movement within the 2-second period for the unstable older adult. (Reprinted with permission from Lin SI. Adapting to dynamically changing balance threats: differentiating young, healthy older adults and unstable older adults. Doctoral dissertation, University of Oregon, 1998.)

lower for the unstable older adults than for the young adults and stable older adults. There were also significant correlations between these scores and those of the Berg Functional Balance Test, the Dynamic Gait Index and the Self-Perceived Balance Test. In addition, there was a significant correlation between poor cutaneous vibration scores and high peak hip angular displacements in response to perturbations, suggesting that older adults with peripheral neuropathy tend to use a hip strategy.

In summary, these data suggest that both stable and unstable older adults show changes in the motor systems affecting postural control and that these can contribute significantly to an inability to maintain balance. Some of these motor system changes include (*a*) muscle weakness, (*b*) impaired timing and organization among synergistic muscles activated in response to instability, and (*c*) limitations in the ability to adapt movements for balance in response to changing task and environmental demands.

Sensory Systems

How do changes in the sensory systems important for posture and balance control contribute to declining stability as people age? The following sections review changes within individual sensory systems and then examine how these changes affect stability in quiet stance, as well as our ability to recover from loss of balance.

Changes In Individual Sensory Systems

Somatosensory

Studies have shown that *vibratory* sensation threshold at the great toe increases threefold by the age of 90 (Kenshalo, 1979). Vibratory thresholds in general increase more in the lower extremity than the upper extremities. In fact, in some cases researchers reported an inability to record vibratory responses from the ankle, because many of the older subjects were not able to perceive sensation there (Whanger and Wang, 1974).

Many studies have shown that *tactile* sensitivity decreases with age as measured by threshold to touch stimuli (Bruce, 1980). Researchers have documented a decline in fine touch, pressure, and vibration sensation mediated by Meissner end organs and Pacinian corpuscles. Aging affects both the quantity and the quality of the Meissner and Pacinian corpuscles; however, it is thought that functional effects are primarily determined by the number of receptors lost. In addition to receptor loss, there is a decline of up to 30% of the sensory fibers innervating the peripheral receptors, causing peripheral neuropathy.

This peripheral neuropathy will cause increased reliance on other sensory systems, such as the visual and vestibular systems. Studies examining postural responses in patients with somatosensory deficits due to peripheral neuropathy have shown significant delays in muscle response onset latencies in response to platform perturbations and an inability to modulate response amplitudes in relation to stimulus size. Figure 9-8A shows electromyographs (EMGs) from a patient with peripheral neuropathy and a normal

subject in response to a platform perturbation. Figure 9-8B compares the onset latencies of muscles in the normal versus the subjects with neuropathy. Note that EMGs from all recorded muscles slow equally (Inglis et al., 1994). Patients with multiple sclerosis show similar problems to those with peripheral neuropathy (Nelson et al., 1995; Jackson et al., 1995).

Vision

Studies on the visual system show similar declines in function. Because of multiple changes within the structure of the eye itself, less light is transmitted to the retina; thus visual threshold (the minimum light needed to see an object) increases with age. In addition, there is typically a loss of visual field, decline in visual acuity, and visual contrast sensitivity, which causes problems in contour and depth perception. Loss of visual acuity can result from cataracts, macular degeneration, and loss of peripheral vision due to ischemic retinal or brain disease. These age-related changes in the visual system affect a

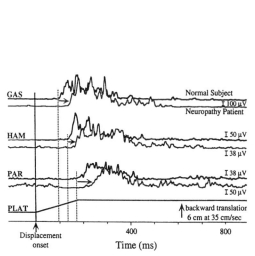

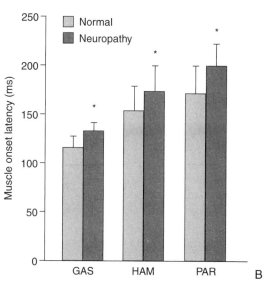

FIGURE 9-8.   A. EMGs from the leg and trunk muscles of a patient with peripheral neuropathy and from a normal subject in response to a platform perturbation. EMGs from all recorded muscles slow equally. **B.** Mean onset latencies for muscles in control (normal) subjects versus patients with peripheral neuropathy. GAS, gastrocnemius; HAM, hamstrings; PAR, paraspinal muscles; PLAT, platform displacement. (Reprinted with permission from Inglis JT, Horak FB, Shupert CL, Rycewicz C. The importance of somatosensory information in triggering and scaling automatic postural responses in humans. Exp. Brain Res 1994;101: 161.)

broad range of functional skills, including postural control (Pitts, 1982; Pastalan et al., 1973). For example, a number of studies have indicated that age-related increases in sway during quiet stance become larger when vision is removed (Sheldon, 1963; Patla et al., 1990; Wolfson, 1992; Schultz et al., 1993).

As mentioned in Chapter 8, one can test the influence of vision on balance control by creating the illusion of postural sway through visual flow generated by an experimental moving room. Normally, young adults show small amounts of sway in response to visual flow–simulating sway. A study by Wade et al. (1995) comparing the effects of visual flow on postural responses (COP measurements) in older adults indicated that healthy older adults show more sway than young adults under these conditions. The authors suggest that this may be due to decreased somatosensory information available to older subjects compared to younger ones.

A second study by Sundermier et al. (1996) compared the effects of visual flow on postural responses of young adults, stable older adults, and unstable older adults. Figure 9-9A (left) shows the paradigm used. As the room moves forward (a), the subjects perceive that they are swaying backward (b) and sway forward (c) to compensate. Figure 9-9A (right) shows the center of pressure (COP) responses of individuals in each group. As you can see, the unstable older adults showed significantly more reliance on the visual flow than the young or stable adults as measured by COP. In addition, they showed continuing COP oscillations after the room movements had stopped. They also noted that the unstable older adults used higher levels of sheer forces when compensating for the simulated postural sway, which suggests more use of hip strategies even in response to visual perturbations to posture. When analyzing characteristics of muscle response to these room movements, they found that when the room moved away from the subjects, the unstable older adults used larger ankle dorsiflexor (TA) responses, which caused high amounts of for-

ward sway (Fig. 9-9B) (Woollacott and Sundermier, in press).

In a similar study Ring et al. (1988) used a visual image on a screen in front of subjects to create the illusion of movement toward the subject. In these visual push experiments, they noted that recent fallers (within 2 weeks), and remote fallers (within the past year) swayed significantly more than nonfaller older adults (ages 65 to 86). They thus concluded that the visual push test might be capable of pointing out older adults who are at risk for falls.

Vestibular

The vestibular system also shows a reduction in function, with a loss of 40% of the vestibular hair and nerve cells by 70 years of age (Rosenhall and Rubin, 1975). One of the functions of the vestibular system is as an absolute reference system to which the other systems (visual and somatosensory) may be compared and calibrated (Black and Nashner, 1985). The vestibular system is especially important for balance control during visual and somatosensory system conflict. A decline in vestibular function with age causes this absolute reference system to be less reliable, and thus the nervous system has difficulty dealing with conflicting information coming from the visual and somatosensory systems. This may be the reason that older adults with vestibular deficits have problems with dizziness and unsteadiness when they are in environments with conflicting visual and somatosensory inputs.

In addition to its function as an absolute reference system, vestibular inputs contribute to the amplitude of automatic postural adjustments to balance threats. Thus older adults with vestibular deficits show postural responses that are inappropriately small (Allum et al., 1994).

Dizziness, an additional consequence of some types of vestibular dysfunction, can also contribute to instability among older adults. Dizziness is a term used to describe the illusion of movement. It can encompass feelings of unsteadiness and imbalance and feelings of faintness or the sense of being light-headed. Dizziness can be a symptom of

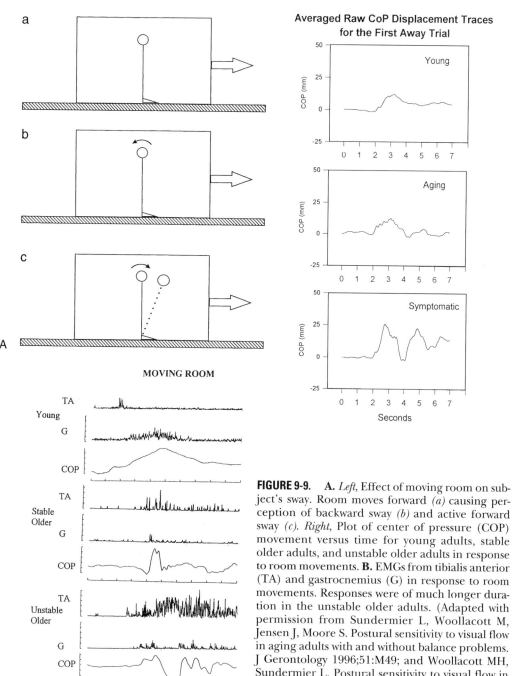

FIGURE 9-9.   A. *Left,* Effect of moving room on subject's sway. Room moves forward *(a)* causing perception of backward sway *(b)* and active forward sway *(c)*. *Right,* Plot of center of pressure (COP) movement versus time for young adults, stable older adults, and unstable older adults in response to room movements. **B.** EMGs from tibialis anterior (TA) and gastrocnemius (G) in response to room movements. Responses were of much longer duration in the unstable older adults. (Adapted with permission from Sundermier L, Woollacott M, Jensen J, Moore S. Postural sensitivity to visual flow in aging adults with and without balance problems. J Gerontology 1996;51:M49; and Woollacott MH, Sundermier L. Postural sensitivity to visual flow in older adults: Electromyographic responses. J Gerontology. In press.)

a variety of diseases, including those of the inner ear. Partial loss of vestibular function can lead to complaints of dizziness, which can be a significant factor contributing to imbalance in the elderly. Degenerative processes within the otoliths of the vestibular system can produce positional vertigo and imbalance during walking.

Multisensory Deficit

Multisensory deficit is loss of more than one sense important for balance and mobility (Brandt and Daroff, 1979). In many older people with multisensory deficits, compensation for loss of one sense with alternative senses is not possible because of numerous impairments in all of the sensory systems important for postural control.

Adapting Senses for Postural Control

In addition to showing declines in function within specific sensory systems, research from many labs has indicated that some older adults have more difficulty than younger adults in maintaining steadiness when sensory information for postural control is severely reduced (Brandt and Daroff, 1979; Woollacott et al., 1986; Horak et al., 1989c; Toupet et al., 1992; Wolfson et al., 1985; Peterka and Black, 1990; Teasdale et al., 1991).

To understand the contribution of vision to the control of sway during quiet stance in older adults, researchers examined sway under altered visual conditions. When young people close their eyes, they show a slight increase in body sway, and this is also true for healthy older adults (Woollacott et al., 1986; Teasdale et al., 1991).

In addition, when their eyes are open, healthy older adults are often as steady as young adults when standing on a compliant surface, such as foam, a condition that reduces the effectiveness of somatosensory inputs reporting body sway. However, when healthy older adults stand with their eyes closed on a compliant surface, thus using vestibular inputs alone for controlling posture, sway significantly increases compared to young adults (Teasdale et al., 1991).

Several studies have examined the ability of healthy older adults to adapt senses to changing conditions during quiet stance using posturography testing (Wolfson et al., 1985; Woollacott et al., 1986; Horak et al., 1989c; Peterka and Black, 1990). These studies found that healthy active older adults did not show significant differences from young adults in amount of body sway (Fig. 9-10) except when both ankle joint inputs and visual inputs were distorted or absent (conditions 5 and 6).

When both visual and somatosensory inputs for postural control were reduced (conditions 5 and 6), half of the older adults lost balance on the first trial for these conditions and needed the aid of an assistant. However, most of the older adults were able to maintain balance on the second trial within these two conditions. Thus, they were able to adapt senses for postural control, but only with practice in the condition (Woollacott et al., 1986).

These results suggest that healthy older adults do not sway significantly more than young people when there is a reduction in the availability or accuracy of a single sense

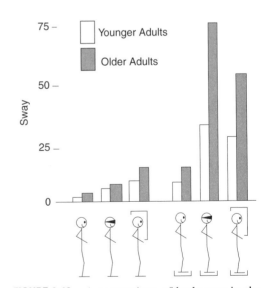

FIGURE 9-10. A comparison of body sway in the six sensory conditions between young and a group of active healthy elderly. (Adapted from Woollacott MH, Shumway-Cook A, Nashner LM. Aging and posture control: changes in sensory organization and muscular coordination. Int J Aging Hum Dev 1986;23:340.)

for postural control. However, in contrast to young adults, reducing the availability of two senses appears to have a significant effect on postural steadiness in even apparently healthy older adults.

Are these changes the result of an inevitable decline in nervous system function, or are they the result of borderline pathology in specific subsystems contributing to postural function?

To determine if evidence of borderline pathology existed in subjects who participated in a postural study and who considered themselves fit, active older adults, researchers gave each subject a neurological exam and then correlated the existence of borderline pathology with performance on the balance tasks. Although all of the older adults considered themselves to be healthy, a neurologist participating in the study found neural impairment, such as diminished deep tendon reflexes, mild peripheral nerve deficits, distal weakness in TA and gastrocnemius, and abnormal nystagmus in many adults in the population. Loss of balance in two subjects accounted for 58% of total losses of balance (Manchester et al., 1989).

These subjects had no history of neurological impairment, but the neurologist diagnosed them as having borderline pathology of CNS origin. These results again suggest the importance of pathologies within specific subsystems as contributing to imbalance in the older adult, rather than a generalized decline in performance.

Other researchers have also studied the adaptation to changing sensory information during quiet stance in older adults (Horak et al., 1989c). One group of older adults was active and healthy and had no history of falls (labeled asymptomatic). The second group was symptomatic for falling. Figure 9-11 illustrates some of the results of their study, showing that more than 20% of the elderly (both symptomatic and asymptomatic) lost balance when visual information was inaccurate for balance (condition 3); none of the subjects aged 20 to 39 lost balance in the same situation. Of the asymptomatic elderly, 40% lost balance in condition 6, when both visual and somatosensory information were

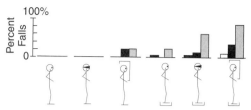

FIGURE 9-11. A comparison of number of falls in the six sensory conditions in young, elderly nonfallers, and elderly fallers. Open box, 20 to 39 years; black box, more than 70 years nonfallers; shaded box, more than 70 years fallers.) (Reprinted with permission from Horak F, Shupert C, Mirka A. Components of postural dyscontrol in the elderly: a review. Neurobiol Aging 1989;10:732).

inaccurately reporting body sway. By contrast, fewer than 10% of the normal young adults fell in this condition. The symptomatic elderly had a larger percentage of falls in any condition that was sway-referenced, that is, with misleading somatosensory cues (conditions 4, 5, and 6).

This led researchers to conclude that the ability to select and weight alternative orientation references adaptively is a crucial factor contributing to postural dyscontrol in many older adults. This is true especially for those who are symptomatic for balance problems (Horak et al., 1989c).

Another approach to studying adaptation of sensory systems involves the use of rotational movements of a platform. These experiments were described in more detail in earlier chapters. Results from platform rotation studies with older adults found that 50% of the healthy older subjects lost balance on the first trial. However, all but one of the subjects were able to maintain balance on subsequent trials (Woollacott et al., 1986). This finding could suggest a slower ability to adapt postural control in this population.

A propensity for falls in the first trial of a new condition is a finding in many studies examining postural control in older adults (Woollacott et al., 1986; Horak et al., 1989c; Peterka and Black, 1990; Teasdale et al., 1991). Perhaps this means that a slowing, rather than a total lack of adaptability, occurs in many elderly people. A propensity to fall in new or novel situations may also be the result of impaired anticipatory mechanisms. Anticipatory processes related to postural control enable the selection of appropriate sensory and motor strategies needed for a particular task or environment.

Anticipatory Postural Abilities

Postural adjustments are often used in a proactive manner, to stabilize the body before making a voluntary movement. Adults in their 70s and 80s may begin to have more difficulty maneuvering in the world because they have lost some of their ability to integrate balance adjustments into ongoing voluntary movements, such as lifting or carrying objects. Thus, it is important to study the effects of age on the ability to use postural responses proactively within the context of voluntary movements. It is in these dynamic conditions, including walking, lifting, and carrying objects, that most falls occur.

One of the first researchers to study age-related changes in anticipatory postural adjustments was the Russian Man'kokii (1980). He compared the characteristics of anticipatory postural responses and prime mover (voluntary) responses for young (aged 19 to 29), medium-old (aged 60 to 69), and very old (aged 90 to 99) adults who were asked to do the simple task of flexing one leg at the knee (prime mover response) while using the other leg for support (postural response), both at a comfortable and at a fast speed. Both the medium-old adults and very old adults showed a slowing in both the postural (contralateral rectus femoris) and prime mover (ipsilateral biceps femoris) muscle response latencies for the movements at a comfortable speed, but this slowing did not result in an increased probability of losing balance. However, at the fast speeds, for both medium-old and very old adults, (*a*) the correlation between the postural and prime mover muscles decreased and (*b*) there was a decrease in the period between the onset of postural and prime mover muscles. In the very old, postural and prime mover muscles were activated almost simultaneously. This inability to activate postural muscles soon enough before the prime

mover caused a loss of balance on many trials (Man'kokii et al., 1980).

In a previous chapter we mentioned that in the normal young adult, the same postural response synergies that are activated during stance balance control are activated in an anticipatory manner before making a voluntary movement while standing. Thus, when a young adult pulls on a handle, first the gastrocnemius is activated, followed by the hamstrings, trunk extensor, and then the prime mover muscle, the biceps of the arm.

A slowing in onset latency or a disruption of the sequence of activation of these postural synergies could affect the ability of an older adult to make such movements as lifting objects.

Experiments were performed to explore age-related changes in the ability of older adults to activate postural muscle response synergies in an anticipatory manner (Inglin and Woollacott, 1988; Frank et al., 1987). In one study, in response to a visual stimulus, standing young (mean age 26 years) and older (mean age 71 years) adults pushed or pulled on a handle that was adjusted to shoulder level. Results of the study showed that the onset latencies of the postural muscles were significantly longer in the older adults than in the younger adults when they were activated in a complex reaction time task. There were also large age-related increases in onset times for voluntary muscles. According to a systems perspective, this slowing in voluntary reaction time in the older adult may be caused either by the need for advanced stabilization by the already delayed and weaker postural muscles or by slowing in the voluntary control system itself. Since the absolute differences in onset times between the young and the older adults were larger for the voluntary muscles than the postural muscles, there may be a slowing in both systems in the older adult (Inglin and Woollacott, 1988).

These results suggest that many older adults have problems making anticipatory postural adjustments quickly and efficiently. This inability to stabilize the body in association with voluntary movement tasks such as lifting or carrying may be a major contributor to falls in many elderly people.

Cognitive Issues and Posture Control

Eulalia H., who is 80 years old, normally has no problems with falls. She is walking down a busy sidewalk in the city, talking to a friend while carrying a fragile piece of crystal she just bought at the department store. Suddenly, a dog runs in front of her. Will she be able to balance in this situation as well as she does when she is walking down a quiet street by herself?

Eulalia H.'s friend, Shelby L., has within the past 6 months recovered from a series of serious falls. These falls have led to a loss of confidence and fear of falling, which resulted in a reduction in his overall activity level and an unwillingness to leave the safety of his own home. Can fear of falling significantly affect how we perceive and move in relation to balance control? Determining the answer to these and other questions related to the complex role of cognitive issues in postural control may be a key to understanding loss of balance in some older adults.

As we mentioned in the first part of this chapter, the capacity of an individual, the demands of a task, and the strategies the person uses to accomplish a task are important factors that contribute to the ability of a person to function in different environments. As individuals get older, their capacities to perform certain tasks such as balance control may be less than their abilities at age 20, but they will still be able to function in normal situations when they can focus on the task. However, when they are required to perform multiple tasks at once, such as the one just described, they may not have the capacity to perform both tasks.

Researchers are beginning to explore how our attentional capacities affect our balance abilities in different environments. If postural control does require attentional processing, one might ask whether decreasing sensory information demands more attention and whether older adults have more difficulty than young adults under these circumstances.

Teasdale et al. (1993) studied the balance (COP measurements) of eight young (mean age 24 years) and nine older (mean age 71

years) adults who were sitting (control condition) versus standing with eyes open versus closed on a normal surface versus a foam surface. The foam surface was used to decrease sway-related somatosensory information available for balance control. They also measured reaction time (RT) on a secondary task in which the subject pressed a button at the sound of an auditory cue. Figure 9-12 shows the RTs for the young and older adults under the four conditions. Note that as sensory information decreased, RT became significantly longer for both younger and older adults, but the effect was exaggerated in the older adults. This implies that the amount of attention is dependent on the degree of instability inherent in the task and that older adults require more attention to perform the postural task.

How does performing an attentionally demanding task affect postural sway in healthy older adults versus fallers? Shumway-Cook et

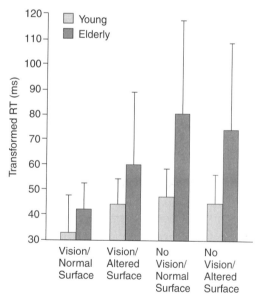

FIGURE 9-12.   Reaction time scores of young versus older adults for four sensory conditions. As sensory information decreased, reaction time (RT) became significantly longer for older adults than young adults. This implies that the amount of attention depends on the degree of instability inherent in the task. (Adapted with permission from Teasdale N, Bard C, LaRue J, Fleury M. On the cognitive penetrability of postural control. Exper Aging Res 1993;19:8.)

al., (1997c) examined the ability of young adults, healthy older adults, and older adults with a history of falls or recent recurrent falls to perform postural tasks of varying difficulty (standing on a normal surface versus foam) while performing cognitively demanding secondary tasks. They found that during the simultaneous performance of a postural and cognitive task, there were decrements in performance in the postural stability measures rather than the cognitive measures for young adults, healthy older adults, and balance-impaired older adults. It is interesting that differences between the young and healthy older adults became apparent only when task complexity was increased, either by adding the secondary task or by adding the more challenging postural condition. However, balance-impaired older adults showed problems even in less complex task conditions.

These experiments examined attentional constraints on older adults in quiet stance situations, but it is also important to know if recovery from perturbations to stance requires more attention for the older adult than the young, contributing to increased likelihood for falls among older adults. To explore this situation Brown et al. (1999) asked older and younger subjects to respond to unexpected platform displacements either with no secondary task or while performing a math task (count backward by threes). They found that attentional requirements for the recovery of balance are higher for older adults than young adults. Performing a secondary task caused subjects to step earlier when using a stepping strategy. It is interesting to note that the postural muscle responses of the older adults were smaller when performing the secondary cognitive task. This may have been the reason the subjects were required to step earlier; their muscle responses were too small to use an in-place strategy (Rankin et al., 2000).

Although many studies have explored the differences in postural performance between fallers and nonfallers, very few have explored the effect of fear of falling on the control of balance. There is now experimental evidence that anxiety and fear of falling

affect the performance of older adults on tests of balance control (Tinetti et al., 1990; Maki et al., 1991). As a result, older adults probably modulate strategies for postural control based on their perception of the level of postural threat. Thus, older adults who have a great deal of anxiety about falling because of poor perceptions regarding their level of balance skills move in ways that reflect these perceptions. More work is needed to clarify the relationship between fear of falling and postural control.

✑ BALANCE RETRAINING

Our review of research has shown that there is a significant loss of balance function in many older adults and that there are specific decreases in function of the various neural and musculoskeletal systems contributing to postural control. Can these losses of balance function be reversed with training? It is widely accepted that exercise is an important factor in maintaining health and fitness. It is also clear that a portion of the lost reserve accompanying aging is due to disuse and deconditioning and can be reversed with training. In recent years, many research labs have begun to design and test training programs with the specific goal of improvement on functional tests, including those of standing balance. These training programs may be classified into four categories: strengthening, aerobic, balance, and combined (Chandler and Hadley, 1996). In the next sections we review the results of these studies to determine their effectiveness in improving function.

Strength Training

A number of studies have shown that a decline in muscle strength is partially reversible with exercise. For example, it has been shown that resistance exercise programs that are performed two to three times per week for 6 weeks or more result in consistent strength gains. How effective is strength training in the older adult? It depends. A study by Aniansson et al. (1984) included women 63 to 84 years and men 74 to 86 years in an intervention involving low-intensity strength training twice a week for 10 months. They found only a 6% to 13% increase in **isometric** knee extensor strength and fast twitch fiber area.

On the other hand, a study by Frontera et al. (1988) included men 60 to 72 years in an intervention involving high-intensity resistance training of knee flexors and extensors at 80% of 1 repetition max 3 times per week for 12 weeks. They found that knee strength (1 rep max) increased to a much greater degree (107% to 226%) (p < .0001). Do these results translate to improved skills, such as balance control and gait? It depends. In healthy older adults changes are minimal if present at all. In one study, resistance training improved strength but failed to increase gait velocity or decrease chair rise time in comparison to a control group (Judge et al., 1994). In a second study, resistance training improved single-leg stance time but not other balance measures (Wolfson et al., 1996; Chandler and Hadley, 1996).

Similar results have been observed in frailer community-dwelling populations; however, the changes are larger. For example Fiatarone and colleagues (Fiatarone et al., 1990; Fiatarone, 1994) performed an intervention that focused on strengthening the leg muscles of frail nursing home residents in their 90s. They used high-resistance strength training of the quadriceps, hamstrings, and adductor muscles three times per week for 8 weeks and found significant gains in muscle strength (174% for 1 rep max). They noted that performance on functional measures also increased. For example, tandem gait speed increased 48%, and two subjects no longer used canes to walk.

In summary, high-resistance strength training appears to be more efficient at improving muscle strength than low-resistance training, and functional effects are most pronounced in frail older adults.

Aerobic Conditioning

Aerobic conditioning improves resting heart rate and VO_{2max} and other dimensions of well-being (sleep, productivity, and so on). However, it is not clear if it improves balance function (Chandler and Hadley, 1996).

Balance Training

A number of recent studies have examined the effects of different types of balance training on improved balance function in older adults (Province et al., 1995; Wolf et al., 1993, 1996). Wolf et al. (1993, 1996) compared the effects of three types of training programs on balance function in community-dwelling older adults (76 ± 5 years) in a randomized control trial. The groups tested were involved in static balance training (balance recovery on a balance platform), dynamic balance (t'ai chi) training versus wellness discussions, with training sessions once or twice per week for 15 weeks. Wolf and colleagues found that the risk ratio for falls was reduced to .63 in the t'ai chi group (significantly less than controls) but not the static balance group. There were no effects of training on lower extremity range of motion, strength, or cardiovascular endurance.

In a second study (Judge et al., 1994), community-dwelling men and women 75 years and older were given 45 minutes of balance training three times per week for 3 months. Sessions included training on a computerized balance platform and floor-based exercises (single leg standing on foam, tandem walking on foam, walking a narrow beam, and sitting balance on a rubber ball). The authors found significant improvement in single-leg stance, functional base of support, and the sensory organization test of balance function, but no change in strength. There was actually a decrease in gait velocity. Balance improvements were maintained for 6 months with a follow-up t'ai chi program.

Combined Exercise Programs

Do exercise programs that affect multiple systems improve balance function? Most combined exercise programs have included strengthening, aerobics, and balance coordination. Judge et al. (1993) studied community-dwelling adults 62 to 75 years of age in a training program that combined lower extremity resistance training, brisk walking, and t'ai chi training versus flexibility training alone (three times per week for 6 months). They found that balance did improve in the first group but not the flexibility group. Single-leg stance center of force displacement decreased by 18% in the first group (p = .02).

Shumway-Cook et al. (1997b) also examined the effects of multidimensional exercise on balance, mobility, and fall risk in community-dwelling older adults. A total of 105 community-dwelling adults above 65 years of age with documented balance and

mobility impairments leading to recurrent falls or near falls participated in a multidimensional exercise program addressing impairments and functional limitations identified during assessment. This group was subsequently divided into two groups, a fully compliant exercise group (exercised 5 to 7 days per week) and a partially compliant group (exercised 4 days or fewer per week). A control group of 21 older adults were assessed but not treated.

Multidimensional exercises included combinations of lower extremity strength and flexibility exercises, static and dynamic balance exercises, and participation in an

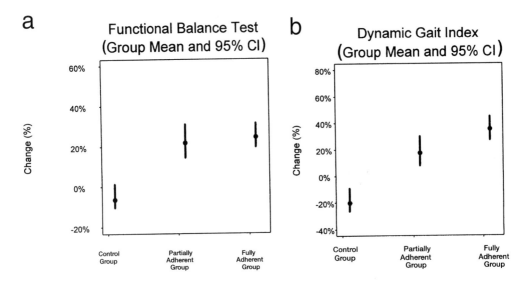

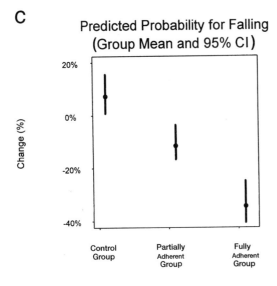

FIGURE 9-13. Percentage change in performance on two clinical tests, the Functional Balance Test (**A**) and the Dynamic Gait Index (**B**). **C.** A measure of predicted probability for falling following 12 weeks of exercise. Data from three groups of community-dwelling balance-impaired older adults, *left to right:* a control group of nonexercising, balance-impaired older adults; a partially adherent group; and a fully adherent exercise group. (Adapted with permission from Shumway-Cook A, Gruber W, Baldwin M, Liao S. The effect of multidimensional exercises on balance, mobility and fall risk in community-dwelling older adults. Phys Ther 1997;77:46–57.)

aerobic activity (usually walking). The exercise subjects participated in twice weekly physical therapy sessions for 8 to 12 weeks and exercised 5 to 7 days a week at home. Changes in performance on five clinical tests of balance and mobility as well as fall risk were compared in the three groups.

Figure 9-13 compares percentage change in performance on two of the clinical tests, the Functional Balance Test and Dynamic Gait Index, and a measure examining predicted probability for falling after 12 weeks. The exercise groups performed significantly better than did the controls in all three measures. The fully adherent exercise group outperformed the partially adherent group in most tests as well. This study suggests that multidimensional exercises can improve balance and mobility function and reduce the likelihood of falls among community-dwelling older adults with a history of falling. How much exercise is needed to accomplish these goals and how long the results last are not yet clear.

Sensory Orientation Training

A study from our own laboratory (Hu and Woollacott, 1994a,b) used a balance training protocol that focused on the use of different sensory inputs and the integration of these inputs under conditions in which sensory inputs were reduced or altered. Subjects 65 to 87 years participated in training five times per week for 2 weeks in 1-hour sessions. The training conditions consisted of standing on a force plate under the following sensory conditions: normal support surface, eyes open, head neutral; normal surface, eyes closed, head neutral; normal support surface, eyes open, head extended; normal surface, eyes closed, head extended; then all trials were repeated on the foam surface. We found significant improvements in the sway of the training group between the first and last day of training in five of the eight training conditions (all foam surface conditions; eyes closed, head extended on the normal surface). Figure 9-14 shows the

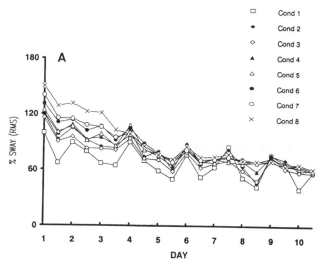

FIGURE 9-14. Reduction in sway across 10 days of training for a single older adult standing under eight sensory conditions. *Condition 1.* Normal support surface, eyes open, head neutral. *Condition 2.* Normal surface, eyes closed, head neutral. *Condition 3.* Normal support surface, eyes open, head extended. *Condition 4.* Normal surface, eyes closed, head extended. *Condition 5.* Foam support surface, eyes open, head neutral. *Condition 6.* Foam support surface, eyes closed, head neutral. *Condition 7.* Foam support surface, eyes open, head extended. *Condition 8.* Foam support surface, eyes closed, head extended. (Redrawn from Woollacott MH, Moore S, Hu, MH. Improvements in balance in the elderly through training in sensory organization abilities. In: GE Stelmach, V Homberg, eds. Sensorimotor impairment in the elderly. Dordrecht: Kluwer, 1993:384.)

reduction in sway across the 10 days for one of the subjects in the training group.

Can sensory organization training transfer to other balance tasks? Yes; the sensory training effect transferred to the sensory organization test used in many clinics and to the one-legged stance test and was associated with changes in muscle response patterns during platform perturbations (less coactivation of antagonist muscles). Subjects in the control group retained these effects over a 4-week follow-up period. These experiments suggest that a sensory training program in balance control may result in significant improvements in balance under altered sensory conditions and that this improvement may transfer to other balance tasks. The application of this concept can be found in Lab Activity 9-2.

 LAB ACTIVITY 9-2

OBJECTIVE: Through the interview process, to explore the balance abilities of a healthy versus a balance-impaired older adult and define possible events that lead up to their current functional status.

PROCEDURE: Find two older adults in your community whom you can interview, one who is very active and well-balanced and the other with balance problems and falls. In your interview ask the following questions:
1. What is your age?
2. Do you exercise regularly? If so, how much?
3. Have you had any medical problems that have affected your balance abilities?
4. Ask your subjects to try standing in a tandem Rhomberg position (one foot in front of the other) for 20 seconds. Time their attempts.
5. Ask them to get up out of a chair, walk 10 feet, turn around, walk back, , and sit down again in the chair. Using a watch with a second hand, determine the time taken for the task (Timed Up and Go test).

ASSIGNMENT: Write up an evaluation of each of the older adults based on the following information:
1. Where do you think each of the people you interviewed would fit on Spirduso's (1995) scale:
   Physically Elite
   Physically Fit
   Physically Independent
   Physically Frail
   Physically Dependent
2. What do you think is their physiological age as compared to their chronological age?
3. Compare their performance on the static balance task and on the Up and Go task. How did each of them do when getting up out of the chair during the Up and Go test?
4. What do you think are factors contributing to reasons for their current balance status?

⊘ SUMMARY

1. Two models of aging include (*a*) the concept that aging involves a linear decline in neuron function across all levels of the CNS and (*b*) the concept that during aging, the CNS continues to function well until death unless there is a catastrophe or disease that affects a specific part of the CNS.

2. Many scientists believe that factors contributing to aging can be considered either primary or secondary. Primary factors, such as genetics, contribute to the inevitable decline of neuronal function in a system. Secondary factors are experiential and include nutrition, exercise, insults, and pathologies.

3. Researchers in all areas find much heterogeneity among older adults, suggesting that assumptions about declining physical capabilities cannot be generalized to all older adults.

4. Falls are the seventh leading cause of death in people over 75 years of age. Falls in the elderly have multiple contributing factors, including intrinsic physiological and musculoskeletal factors and extrinsic environmental factors. Understanding the role of declining postural and balance abilities is a critical concern in helping to prevent falls among older adults.

5. Many factors can contribute to declining balance control in older adults who are at risk for imbalance and falls. Researchers have documented impairments in all of the systems contributing to balance control; however, no one predictable pattern is characteristic of all elderly fallers.

6. On a positive note, many older adults have balance function equivalent to that of young people, suggesting that balance decline is not necessarily an inevitable result of aging. Experiential factors such as exercise can aid in the maintenance of good balance and decrease the likelihood for falls as people age.

CHAPTER **10**

Abnormal Postural Control

℮ INTRODUCTION

The recovery of functional independence following a neurological insult is a complex process requiring the reacquisition of many skills. Since controlling the body's position in space is an essential part of functional skills, restoring postural control is a critical part of recovery of function. In the therapeutic environment, the ability to retrain postural control requires a conceptual framework that incorporates information on the physiological basis for normal postural control, as well as knowledge regarding the basis for instability.

Our understanding of the sensory and motor basis for instability comes from research examining postural control in differ-

ent categories of patients with specific neurological lesions such as post-CVA (cerebral vascular accident) hemiparesis, traumatic brain injury, Parkinson's disease, Multiple Sclerosis, cerebellar disorders, and developmental disorders such as Down syndrome and cerebral palsy. This has led to an understanding of the different types of sensory and motor problems that contribute to instability. As we shall see, often the same type of postural control problem can manifest in a wide variety of neurological disorders. For example, delayed onset of postural responses has been found in patients with traumatic brain injury, patients with hemiplegia following CVA, and children with various types of cerebral palsy.

In this chapter we first explore studies

that have examined problems in the motor components of postural control in patients with neurological deficits. Next, we examine studies that have investigated problems within the sensory components of postural control. Finally we summarize the types of postural control problems in our case study patients to provide an understanding of the types of problems found in patients with various types of neurological diagnoses.

✑ PROBLEMS IN THE MOTOR COMPONENTS OF POSTURAL CONTROL

Motor components of postural control include both musculoskeletal and neuromuscular systems. Within the neuromuscular system the ability to coordinate multiple muscles into postural muscle synergies is a critical aspect of the maintenance of stability.

Motor Coordination Problems

A number of researchers have begun to explore how neurological deficits influence the coordination of muscles into postural synergies. In discussing this research, we divide coordination problems that manifest within postural movement strategies into (*a*) sequencing problems, (*b*) problems with the timely activation of postural responses, (*c*) disorders related to the scaling of postural muscle activity, and (*d*) problems adapting motor responses to changing task conditions.

Sequencing Problems
*Reversals in the Orderly
Recruitment of Muscles*
One of the earliest studies that reported information on motor coordination problems affecting stance postural control was a study by Nashner and colleagues that examined postural control in children with different types of cerebral palsy (Nashner et al., 1983). Ambulatory children (7 to 10 years of age) with various types of cerebral palsy stood on a platform that perturbed stance

balance in the forward or backward direction. Electromyelography (EMG) and ground reaction forces were used to examine the coordination of leg muscles responding to this induced sway. Figure 10-1 is an example of the EMG records from one of the children with spastic hemiplegia. Shown is muscle activity (gastrocnemius, hamstrings, anterior tibialis, and quadriceps) in both the spastic hemiplegic and nonhemiplegic legs in response to a backward platform perturbation producing forward sway. The sequencing of muscle activity in the nonhemiplegic leg (labeled less involved) began in the gastrocnemius muscle at approximately 100 msec, followed 30 msec later by activation of the hamstring muscle. In contrast, muscle activity in the spastic leg began first in the hamstrings, followed 30 to 50 msec later by activation of the gastrocnemius.

What is the consequence of changing the sequence in which muscles are activated when responding to a loss of balance? This can be seen in Figure 10-2, which presents the average torque, weight, and sway records for 10 forward sway trials from this child. As you can see, abnormal sequencing of muscle activity in the hemiplegic leg (also labeled the left leg) resulted in significantly less torque than the right leg. In addition, this pattern of muscle activity resulted in large lateral shifts of the body's center of mass, shown as the large oscillatory shifts in the weight record.

The delay in the activation of the gastrocnemius in the spastic leg was surprising for a number of reasons. On clinical examination, this child showed positive signs of spasticity in the gastrocnemius muscle, including increased stiffness in response to passive stretch, clonus, equinus gait, and lack of dorsiflexion at the ankle, in response to a backward displacement.

Given these clinical findings, one might predict a hyperactive stretch response in the gastrocnemius when the child stood on the platform and swayed in the forward direction, since during forward sway the first muscle to be stretched is the gastrocnemius. But during forward sway, imposing a stretch on the hyperactive gastrocnemius, the first mus-

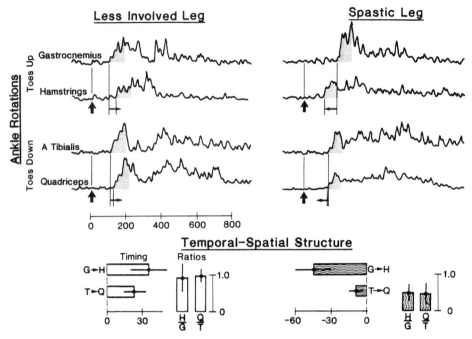

FIGURE 10-1. Abnormal sequencing of muscles in a child with hemiplegia responding to a backward translation of a moving platform. EMG records show an inappropriate activation of muscles responding to forward sway, with proximal muscles (hamstrings) activated in advance of the so-called spastic distal muscles (gastrocnemius). *Upward arrow,* platform movement onset. *Horizontal arrows,* onset of muscle activity. (Reprinted with permission from Nashner LM, Shumway-Cook A, Marin D. Stance posture control in select groups of children with cerebral palsy: deficits in sensory organization and muscular coordination. Exp Brain Res 1983;49:399.)

cles to respond were the hamstrings. The gastrocnemius muscle was slow to become active, and the amplitude of the muscle activity was low compared to that of the uninvolved side. The finding of delayed activation of "spastic" muscle is consistent with other authors' reports of an inability to recruit and regulate the firing frequency of motor neurons in patients with spastic hypertonia (Badke and DiFabio, 1990; Sahrmann and Norton, 1977).

The lack of an ascending (distal to proximal) pattern of muscle recruitment in response to perturbations to stance balance has also been reported in young children with spastic diplegia and limited walking experience (Burtner et al., 1999). In addition, these children, many of whom stand and walk on their toes, activated the antagonist tibialis anterior (TA) muscle before the gastrocnemius muscle in many trials. It is inter-

esting that this is also the activation pattern seen in bipedal animals that stand on toes. Thus, this pattern of activating the TA in response to backward displacements, causing forward sway, may be due to the varying stimulus characteristics created from an on-toes stance.

Brogren and colleagues also reported a disruption in the recruitment order of muscles responding to loss of balance in the seated position in children with the spastic diplegia form of cerebral palsy (Brogren et al., 1998). Neurologically intact children recruit muscles in a distal-to-proximal sequence, beginning with the muscles closest to the support surface. In contrast, as can be seen in Figure 10-3, children with spastic diplegia tended to recruit muscles in a proximal-to-distal sequence, that is, beginning at the neck and progressing downward. In addition, the children with spastic diplegia showed significant coactivation of muscles in the neck and hip, with antagonists being activated before agonists, similar to what Burtner et al. (1999) found for standing children.

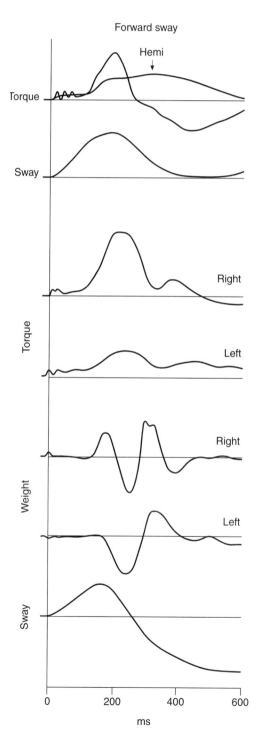

Delayed Recruitment of Proximal Synergistic Muscles

Patients with neurological deficits sometimes have abnormally long delays in the recruitment of proximal muscle synergists. This type of timing problem has been reported in children with Down syndrome (Shumway-Cook and Woollacott, 1985b) and in adults with traumatic brain injury causing focal cortical contusions (Shumway-Cook and Olmscheid, 1990). Delayed activation of proximal muscles following platform perturbations can be seen in Figure 10-4, which compares EMG responses in a child with Down syndrome to an age-matched normal child. In the normal child proximal muscle delays were on the order of 36 msec compared to 60 to 80 msec in the child with Down syndrome (Shumway-Cook and Woollacott, 1985b). The biomechanical consequences of delayed activation of proximal muscles compared to the distal muscles include excessive motion at the knee and hip. This is because the timing of synergistic muscles is not efficient in controlling the indirect effects of forces generated at the ankle on more proximal joints.

Coactivation of Antagonist Muscles

Coactivation is a common postural coordination problem reported in both very young healthy children and a wide variety of patients with neurological deficits, including cerebral palsy (Nashner et al., 1983; Woollacott et al., 1998; Crenna and Inverno, 1994), cerebral vascular accident (Duncan and Badke, 1987), traumatic brain injury (Shumway-Cook and Olmscheid, 1990),

FIGURE 10-2.   Illustration of the average torque, weight, and sway records for 10 forward-sway trials from a child with spastic hemiplegia. Abnormal sequencing of muscle activity in the left hemiplegic leg (*Hemi*) resulted in significantly less torque than the right leg. In addition, this pattern of muscle activity resulted in large lateral shifts of the body's center of mass, shown as the large oscillatory shifts in the weight record. (Adapted with permission from Nashner LM, Shumway-Cook A, Marin D. Stance posture control in select groups of children with cerebral palsy: deficits in sensory organization and muscular coordination. Exp Brain Res 1983;49:401.)

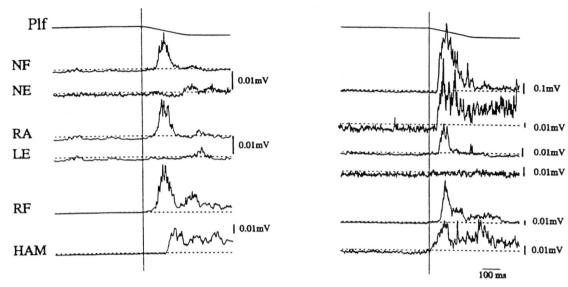

FIGURE 10-3.   A comparison of EMG records from a normal control child (**A**) and a child with spastic diplegia (**B**). The sequencing of muscles in a child with spastic diplegia responding to a backward translation of a moving platform (Plf) while seated is abnormal compared to those of the control child. EMG records show an inappropriate activation of muscles responding to forward sway, with proximal neck flexors and extensors (NF and NE) firing simultaneously with distal trunk (RA and LE) and leg (RF and HAM) muscles. (Reprinted with permission from Brogren E, Hadders-Algra M, Forssberg H. Postural control in children with spastic diplegia: Muscle activity during perturbations in sitting. Dev Med Child Neuro 1998:38:381.)

Down syndrome (Shumway-Cook and Wool-lacott, 1985b), and Parkinson's disease (Horak et al., 1992). Coactivation is characterized by the simultaneous contraction of muscles on anterior and posterior aspects of the body.

Coactivation in patients with Parkinson's disease can been seen in Figure 10-5, which compares EMG responses in an elderly subject to one with Parkinson's disease. This activation of muscles on both sides of the body results in a stiffening of the body and is a very inefficient strategy for the recovery of balance (Horak et al., 1992).

These results are not consistent with the classic work on Parkinson's patients by Purdue Martin, who reported absence of equilibrium and righting reactions in Parkinson's patients (Martin, 1967). The rigidity and loss of balance found in patients during tilt tests imply that equilibrium reactions were absent. EMGs of the muscles of Parkinson's disease patients have allowed researchers to see that these patients do indeed respond to disequilibrium, but the

pattern of muscular activity used is ineffective in recovering balance.

Since appropriate sequencing of multiple muscles is critical to the recovery of balance, a loss of normal sequencing can be a significant contribution to instability in patients with neurological problems.

Delayed Activation of Postural Responses

Researchers have also found that significant delays in the onset of postural responses can contribute to instability in patients with neurological deficits. Muscle activity in response to platform perturbations (both horizontal translations and rotations) has been studied in patients with hemiplegia resulting from a cerebral vascular accident (Diener et al., 1984; DiFabio et al., 1986). Researchers have reported deficits in sequencing, timing, and amplitude of postural muscle activity in the paretic limb. Figure 10-6 shows the EMG responses in the paretic and nonparetic legs of

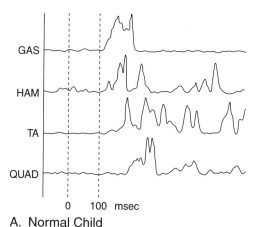

A. Normal Child

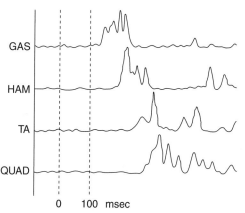

B. Child with Down Syndrome

FIGURE 10-4.   A comparison of EMG responses in a normal child (**A**) and an age-matched child with Down syndrome (**B**) illustrating the delay in proximal muscle activation during recovery of balance. In the normal child, proximal muscle delays were on the order of 36 msec, compared to 60 to 80 msec in the child with Down syndrome. GAS, gastrocnemius; HAM, hamstrings; TA, tibialis anterior; QUAD, quadriceps. (Adapted with permission from Shumway-Cook A, Woollacott M. Postural control in the Down's syndrome child. Phys Ther 1985;9:1317).

a subject with hemiplegia in response to a forward sway perturbation (DiFabio et al., 1986). Onset latencies in the paretic distal muscles were significantly longer than in the nonparetic side. Delays in the activation of distal muscles in the paretic limb were compensated for by early activation of proximal muscles in the nonparetic limb.

Significant delays in the onset of postural activity have been reported in developmental abnormalities, including Down syndrome (Shumway-Cook and Woollacott, 1985b) and some forms of cerebral palsy (Nashner et al., 1983). This can be seen in Figure 10-7, which compares onset latencies to forward sway in healthy control children, children with Down syndrome, and children with cerebral palsy (spastic hemiplegia and ataxia).

Problems Scaling the Amplitude of Muscle Responses

Maintaining balance requires that forces generated to control the body's position in space be appropriately scaled to the degree of instability. This means that a small perturbation to stability is met with an appropriately sized muscle response. Thus, force output must be appropriate to the amplitude of instability. Researchers are beginning to examine the physiological mechanisms underlying the scaling of postural responses in neurologically intact subjects. In addition, researchers are looking at the effects of lesions in the cerebellum or basal ganglia on the ability to scale the amplitude of postural responses to different-sized perturbations to balance (Horak et al., 1989a, 1990; Horak and Diener, 1994).

Results from these studies have shown that neurologically intact subjects use a combination of feed-forward, or anticipatory, and feedback control mechanisms to scale forces needed for postural stability. Grading or scaling force output probably involves anterior portions of the cerebellum, since patients with anterior cerebellar lesions were found to be unable to anticipate and scale forces appropriate to changes in the size of a postural perturbation (Horak, 1990; Horak and Diener, 1994).

Postural responses that are too large have been called hypermetric and are associated with excessive compensatory body sway in the direction opposite the initial direction of instability. For example, patients with unilateral cerebellar pathology affecting the anterior lobe can show hypermetric responses on the involved side of the body. An example of

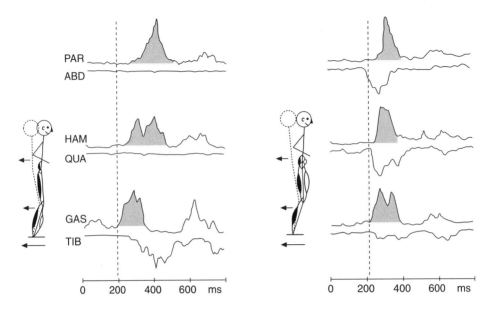

A. Elderly Subject   B. Parkinsonian Subject

FIGURE 10-5.   A comparison of muscle activation patterns in an elderly subject **(A)** and a subject with Parkinson's disease **(B)** illustrating muscle activation patterns in response to forward sway. The subject with Parkinson's disease coactivates antagonistic muscles around the hip and knee, while the elderly subject does not. Shown are the EMG response and a schematic representation of the responses. GAS, gastrocnemius; TIB, tibialis anterior, QUA, quadriceps, HAM, hamstring; ABD, abdominals; PAR, paraspinals. (Adapted with permission from Horak FB, Nutt JG, Nashner LM. Postural inflexibility in Parkinsonian subjects. J Neurol Sci 1992:111:46-58:49.)

hypermetric postural responses found in patients with anterior lobe cerebellar damage is shown in Figure 10-8. EMG responses in cerebellar patients are larger in amplitude and longer in duration than those found in healthy normal subjects. An examination of the sway and torque records shown in Figure 10-8 shows that hypermetric muscle activity resulted in both excess torque and an overcorrection in sway during the recovery of stability (Horak and Diener, 1994).

Motor Adaptation Problems

Normal postural control requires the ability to adapt responses to changing tasks and environmental demands. This flexibility requires the availability of multiple movement strategies and the ability to select the appropriate strategy for the task and environment. The inability to adapt movements to changing task demands is a characteristic of many patients with neurological disorders.

Patients become fixed in stereotyped patterns of movement, showing a loss of movement flexibility and adaptablity. The fixed movement synergies seen in the patient with hemiparesis are an example of impairments related to loss of flexibility and adaptability of movements. Infants with cerebral palsy who have trouble dissociating movements of their legs are constrained to kick symmetrically because of these obligatory movement patterns in the legs (Kamm et al., 1991).

Inability to adapt movement strategies to changes in support has been found in patients with Parkinson's disease (Horak et al., 1992). In this study, normal controls and a group of patients with Parkinson's disease were asked to maintain stance balance in a variety of situations, including standing on a flat surface, standing across a narrow beam, and sitting on a stool with the feet unsupported. Normal subjects were able to adapt muscle responses used for

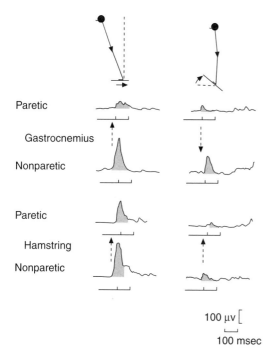

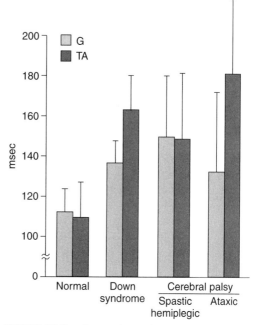

FIGURE 10-6. The EMG responses in the gastrocnemius and hamstring muscles in paretic and nonparetic limbs in a patient with hemiplegia following a cerebrovascular accident in response to a forward sway perturbation and a toes-up rotational perturbation. Muscle responses in the paretic limb are slow and reduced in amplitude. (Adapted with permission from DiFabio RP, Badke MB, Duncan PW. Adapting human postural reflexes localized cerebrovascular lesion: analysis of bilateral long latency responses. Brain Res 1986;363:259.)

FIGURE 10-7. Onset latencies of postural responses to platform perturbations in normal children, children with Down syndrome, and children with cerebral palsy (spastic hemiplegic and ataxic). Onset latencies in the children with neurological deficits are significantly slower than those of the normal age matched peers. G, gastrocnemius; TA, tibialis anterior.

postural control in response to changing task demands (Fig. 10-9A). In contrast, Parkinson's disease patients were unable to modify the complex movement strategy used in recovering balance while standing on a flat surface, on the beam, or seated, showing inability to modify how they moved in response to changes in environmental and task demands (Fig. 10-9B).

Musculoskeletal Contributions to Coordination Problems

In the patient with a CNS lesion, musculoskeletal disorders most often develop secondary to immobility and restricted movement (Schenkman, 1990). Yet musculoskeletal problems can be a significant fac-

tor in motor coordination problems affecting postural control.

Alignment

Alignment of the body refers to the arrangement of body segments to one another, as well as the position of the body with reference to gravity and the base of support (Shumway-Cook and Horak, 1992). Alignment of body segments over the base of support determines to a great extent the effort required to support the body against gravity. In addition, alignment determines the constellation of movement strategies that will be effective in controlling posture. Changes in initial position or alignment are often characteristic of the patient with a neurological deficit. Abnormalities in alignment can reflect changes in the alignment of one body part to another or in alignment of the center of mass relative to the base of support.

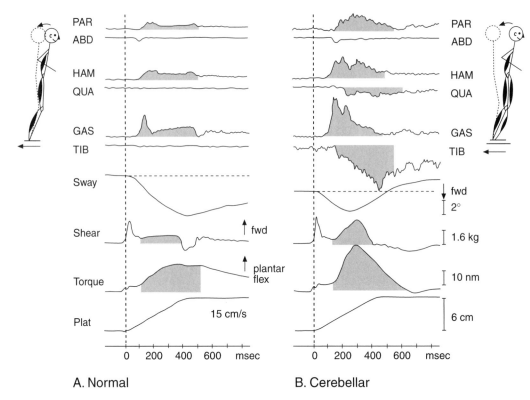

A. Normal   **B. Cerebellar**

FIGURE 10-8.   A comparison of EMG activity in normal subjects versus subjects with anterior lobe cerebellar degeneration. Muscle responses are hypermetric, that is, significantly larger in amplitude and longer in duration than in normals. (Adapted with permission from Horak FB. Diener HC. Cerebellar control of postural scaling and central set in stance. J Neurophysiol 1994;72:483.)

Children with cerebral palsy frequently show restricted range of motion in many joints, including the ankle, knee, and hip. Contractures of the hip, knee, and ankle muscles result in atypical postures in sitting (Figure 10-10A) and standing (Figure 10-10, B and C).

Habitual postures influence how muscles are recruited and coordinated for recovery of stability. For example, in their study on postural control in children with spastic diplegia, Burtner and colleagues found that the children with spastic diplegia who stood in a habitual crouched posture showed a marked increase in the coactivation of muscles responding to loss of balance. Interestingly, healthy children standing in a crouched position, mimicking the posture of the children with diplegia, used antagonistic muscles more often in response to platform perturbations, suggesting that the muscu-

loskeletal constraints associated with standing in a crouched posture may play a significant role in the atypical postural muscle response patterns seen in children with spastic diplegia (Burtner et al., 1999; Woollacott, et al., 1998).

Abnormal alignment can also be expressed as a change in the position of the body with reference to gravity and the base of support. For example, asymmetrical alignment in sitting and standing is often characteristic of patients with a unilateral neural lesion such as is produced by a CVA (Duncan and Badke, 1987; Shumway-Cook et al., 1988). Patients with this type of lesion tend to stand with weight displaced toward the uninvolved side. Other patients, most notably patients with cerebellar lesions, tend to stand with a wide base of support (Ghez, 1991a).

Finally, many patients stand with the cen-

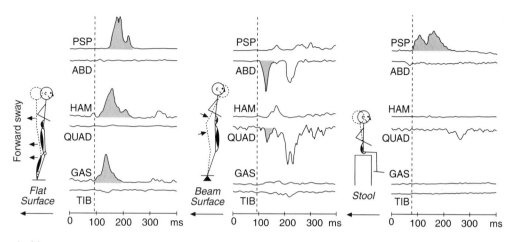

A. Young subject

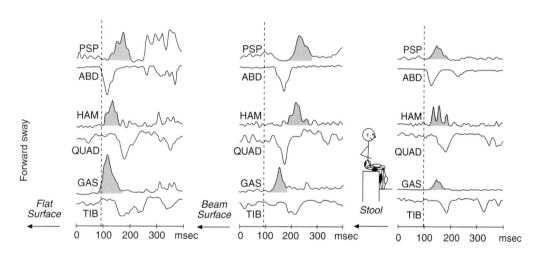

B. Parkinsonian subject

FIGURE 10-9.   Normal and abnormal adaptation. **A.** Normal adaptation of muscle activity in response to perturbations producing forward sway under three task conditions: standing on a flat surface, on a beam surface, and sitting on a stool. In contrast to a normal young subject, EMG patterns in a subject with Parkinson's disease **(B)** revealed a complex strategy of muscle activity that did not adapt to changes in task demands. (Adapted with permission from Horak FB, Nutt JG, Nashner LM. Postural inflexibility in Parkinsonian subjects. J Neurol Sci 1992: 111:52.)

ter of mass displaced either forward or backward. For example, it has been reported that elderly patients with a fear of falling tend to stand in a forward lean posture with the center of mass displaced anteriorly (Maki et al., 1991). However, other types of patients stand with the center of mass displaced posteriorly (Shumway-Cook and Horak, 1992).

Changes in alignment can be viewed as ei-

ther a musculoskeletal impairment or as a strategy compensating for other impairments. For example, in the elderly person, alignment that is often characterized by a prominent kyphosis and forward-flexed head represents a musculoskeletal impairment that constrains movements necessary for posture and balance (Lewis and Phillipi, 1993). In contrast, the asymmetrical alignment com-

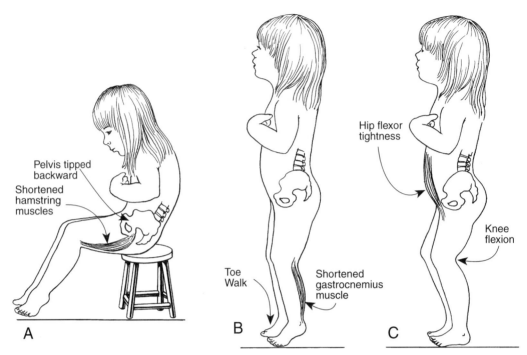

Pelvis tipped
backward

Shortened
hamstring
muscles

Hip flexor
tightness

Knee
flexion

Toe
Walk

Shortened
gastrocnemius
muscle

A

B

C

FIGURE 10-10. Atypical postures due to musculoskeletal impairments. **A.** Excessive posterior tilt of pelvis in sitting accommodates shortened hamstrings. **B.** Shortening of the gastrocnemius muscle results in toe walk. **C.** Hip flexor tightness can result in tilting of the pelvis and flexion of the knee. (Adapted with permission from Reimers J. Clinically based decision making for surgery. In: Sussman M, ed. The diplegic child. Rosemont, IL: American Academy of Orthopedic Surgeons, 1992:155,156,158.)

monly seen in the patient with hemiplegia, who stands with weight shifted to the non-hemiplegic side, is a strategy that often develops to compensate for other impairments, such as weakness in the hemiparetic leg (Shumway-Cook and Horak, 1992). Understanding these differences is important, since achieving a symmetrically aligned position may not be a reasonable goal for the patient with hemiplegia until underlying impairments have resolved sufficiently to ensure that the hemiparetic leg will not collapse under the weight of the body.

Constraining Movement at a Joint

Ankle-foot orthoses (AFOs) are often used by clinicians to control spasticity and prevent excessive plantarflexion. A variety of orthoses are used, including both solid AFOs, which do not allow movement at the ankle joint, and spiral or hinged AFOs, which allow a degree of ankle joint movement. What are the effects of the use of AFOs on the coordi-

nation of muscles for postural control? In order to answer this question experiments were performed to compare balance response characteristics in both children with spastic diplegia and typically developing children when using no AFO as compared to solid and spiral AFOs (Burtner et al., 1999). The study showed that in both typically developing children and children with spastic diplegia the percent of trials in which the ankle strategy was used was significantly reduced when balancing with the solid AFO (no responses) as compared to balancing with no AFO and with a dynamic AFO. This was associated with a significant delay in onset latency and reduction in the probability of recording a response in the gastrocnemius muscle in response to backward perturbations causing forward sway. In addition, the frequency of observing the normal distal-to-proximal muscle response sequence was also reduced in both typically developing children and those with spastic diplegia, in the solid AFO condition, as compared to the no AFO and dynamic AFO conditions. These results are shown in Figure 10-11, *A* and *B*. Note that there is typically a reduction in both percent use of ankle strategy and in distal-to-proximal response sequencing in the dynamic AFO condition, but it is significantly less than that seen for the solid AFO condition. These results suggest that the types of devices we use to control position and motion at the ankles can have a significant impact on the sequencing and timing of muscles used for recovery of balance. AFOs that restrict motion at the ankle will reduce the participation of ankle joint muscles in the control of stability. This will result in an increase in the use of hip and trunk muscles for balance control. This increased motion at the hips and trunk during recovery of balance is not the result of proximal weakness but rather the consequence of constraining motion at the ankles.

Changes in Muscle Structure and Function

What is the effect of abnormal postures and movements on the structure and function of skeletal muscles in patients with neurological deficits? Berger et al. (1984c) found that tension development in spastic muscles in adult patients with hemiparesis could be only partially explained by hyperactive reflex responses to stretch. They examined EMG activity in the gastrocnemius and soleus in spastic and nonspastic muscles in response to perturbations to gait in three patients with spastic hemiparesis. In addition, a goniometer was used to measure ankle joint changes, and tension in the Achilles tendon was measured using a force-measuring strain gauge. Figure 10-12 compares muscle activity (TA and gastrocnemius), changes in ankle joint motion, and force in the Achilles tendon in both the normal and spastic leg. In the normal leg, peak tension in the Achilles tendon was associated with maximal EMG activity in the gastrocnemius. In contrast, in the spastic leg, despite the fact that EMG activity in the gastrocnemius was very small, tension development in the Achilles tendon was comparable with that found in the normal leg. The authors suggest that spasticity changes the properties of the muscle fibers themselves and that this is a contributing factor to coordination deficits found in patients with spasticity.

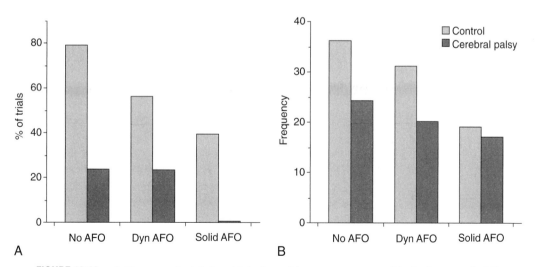

FIGURE 10-11. **A.** Percent of trials in which the ankle strategy was used in both control children and in children with cerebral palsy when wearing no ankle-foot orthoses (AFO), a dynamic AFO, or a solid AFO. **B.** Frequency of observing the normal distal-to-proximal muscle response in both control children and those with cerebral palsy in the no AFO condition as compared to the dynamic and solid AFO conditions. Solid AFOs cause a reduction in both use of the ankle strategy and in distal-to-proximal response sequencing.

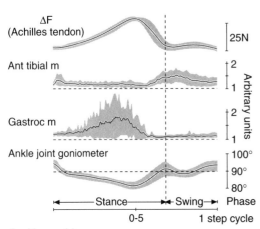

A. Normal leg

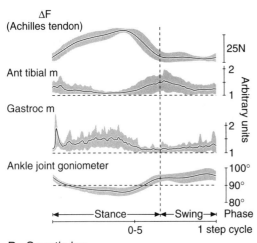

B. Spastic leg

FIGURE 10-12. Changes in structure and function in spastic muscles. The response to stretch of the gastrocnemius during gait (EMG trace, joint angle changes and change in force) is compared in a normal and a spastic leg in a patient with hemiplegia. Tension in the Achilles tendon (*F*) is comparable in both the normal (**A**) and spastic (**B**) leg despite a lower EMG output from the spastic gastrocnemius (gastroc m), suggesting that changes in muscle structure in spastic muscles may contribute to the tension development when the muscle is stretched (Reprinted with permission from Berger W, Horstmann GA, Dietz VL. Tension development and muscle activation in the leg during gait in spastic hemiparesis: the independence of muscle hypertonia and exaggerated stretch reflexes. J Neurol Neurosurg Psychiatry 1984;47:1031.)

Researchers have performed biopsies to examine changes in the structure of skeletal muscle in children with cerebral palsy (Rose et al., 1994; Castle et al., 1979). Children with cerebral palsy who routinely have excessive and prolonged contraction of certain muscles show abnormal variation in the size of muscle fibers and altered distribution of fiber types. There was a significant difference between the mean area of type 1 and type 2 fibers between spastic and normal muscles, with spastic muscles showing increased type 1 area. In addition, the degree of muscle pathology was correlated with gait abnormalities, including an increase in energy expenditure and prolonged EMG activity during walking (Rose et al., 1994).

Changes in Strength

There is growing evidence that weakness, the inability to recruit agonist motor neurons, is a significant problem in patients with neurological pathology. Wiley and Damiano (1998) compared strength profiles in lower extremity muscles in 30 children with cerebral palsy (15 children with spastic diplegia and 15 with spastic hemiplegia) with 16 age-matched normal peers. Using a hand-held dynamometer, they quantified isometric strength in major lower extremity muscle groups bilaterally. The results of this study are summarized in Figure 10-13, *A* and *B*, which compares strength values normalized by body weight in the three groups of children across a variety of muscles, as shown along the x-axis. Significant results from the study included these findings: (*a*) Children with cerebral palsy were weaker than age-matched peers in all muscles tested. (*b*) the children with hemiplegia showed significant weakness on both the involved and noninvolved limbs. (*c*) Weakness was greater in the distal muscles than in the proximal muscles. (*d*) Hip flexors and ankle plantar flexors were stronger than their antagonist muscles. In trying to explain the basis for weakness in these children, the authors collected EMG data during strength testing on several of their subjects. These data are shown in Figure 10-14, *A* and *B*. Shown are the rectified EMG recordings of

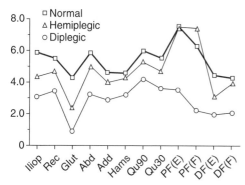

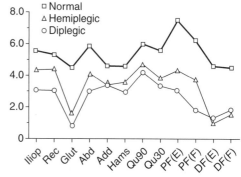

A Dominant Side   B Nondominant Side

FIGURE 10-13.   A comparison of strength profiles in lower extremity muscles (normalized to body weight) in children with spastic hemiplegia and diplegia and age-matched peers (labeled normal). Strength is shown in the muscles of the dominant side (**A**) and the nondominant side (**B**). (Adapted with permission from Wiley ME, Damiano DL. Lower-extremity strength profiles in spastic cerebral palsy. Dev Med Child Neurol 1998;40:104.)

the agonist and antagonist muscles during a strength test in a normally developing 8-year-old (Fig. 10-14*A*) and a child with cerebral palsy. When asked to contract the hamstrings maximally, the normally developing child shows a phasic burst of activity in the left hamstrings with no activation of the antagonist quadriceps. Similarly, a maximal contraction of the quadriceps (Fig 10-14*B*) is not associated with activation of the antagonist hamstrings. In contrast, when the child with cerebral palsy is asked to activate the quadriceps (10-14*D*), there is a concomitant activation of the antagonist hamstrings. Interestingly, there is poor activation of the hamstring muscle when this child is trying to activate it for a maximal contraction (Fig 10-14*C*). Thus, the previous studies suggest that weakness in children with cerebral palsy may have both a neurophysiological and biomechanical basis.

In summary, musculoskeletal problems, while often not a primary result of a neurological lesion, present a major constraint to normal posture and movement control in many patients. Loss of range of motion and flexibility can limit the ways in which a patient can move for postural control. For example, loss of ankle range or strength limits a patient's ability to use an ankle strategy for postural control. Therapeutic interventions that constrain motion at the ankle, such as

the use of an AFO, may also limit the patient who has adequate ankle range of motion from using it effectively in controlling body sway. Finally, musculoskeletal problems can contribute to the inability to sustain an ideal alignment of body segments in the upright position, requiring excessive force to counter the effects of gravity and sustain a vertical posture.

Loss of Anticipatory Postural Control

We have seen that inability to adapt how we move in response to changing task and environmental conditions can be a source of instability in many patients with neurological impairments. Another source of postural dyscontrol is the loss of anticipatory processes that activate postural adjustments in advance of potentially destabilizing voluntary movements. Anticipatory postural activity is heavily dependent on previous experience and learning.

Inability to activate postural muscles in anticipation of voluntary arm movements has been described in many patients who are neurologically impaired, including stroke patients (Horak et al., 1984), children with cerebral palsy (Nashner et al., 1983), children with Down syndrome (Shumway-Cook and Woollacott, 1985b), and people with Parkinson's disease (Rogers, 1990, 1991).

Normal Child

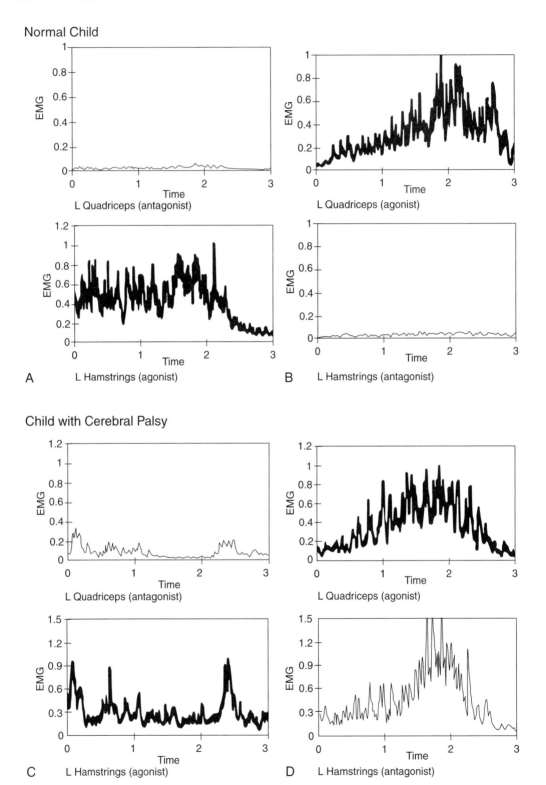

FIGURE 10-14.   Rectified integrated EMG activity of the agonist and antagonist muscles in a normally developing 8-year-old child during isometric strength test of the left hamstrings (**A**) and quadriceps (**B**). EMG activity in the same set of muscles in an 8-year-old child with spastic cerebral palsy (**C, D**). (Adapted with permission from Wiley ME, Damiano DL. Lower-extremity strength profiles in spastic cerebral palsy. Dev Med Child Neurol 1998;40:105.)

Problems in initiating postural muscle activity prior to voluntary muscle activity have been seen in two studies examining children with spastic hemiplegia secondary to cerebral palsy and adults with hemiparesis secondary to CVA. In both studies EMG onset in postural muscles in the trunk and leg of the intact side preceded activity in the prime movers of the arm. In contrast, in the hemiparetic side, muscle activity in the arm preceded that of the postural muscles (Nashner et al., 1983; Horak et al., 1984). Figure 10-15 shows this lack of preparatory postural activity for the hemiparetic side compared to the normal side in the children with cerebral palsy when they were asked to push or pull on a handle while standing.

℮ SENSORY DISORDERS

As we mentioned earlier, normal postural control requires (*a*) the organization of sensory information from visual, somatosensory,

and vestibular systems, which provide information about the body's position and movement with respect to the environment, and (*b*) the coordination of sensory information with motor actions.

Sensory problems can disrupt postural control by: (*a*) affecting a patient's ability to adapt sensory inputs to changes in task and environmental demands and (*b*) preventing the development of accurate internal models of the body for postural control (Horak and Shupert, 1994).

Problems With Sensory Adaptation

Researchers examining the effect of neurological injury on patients' ability to adapt sensory information for postural control have primarily focused on the use of computerized force platforms in conjunction with moving visual surrounds, first developed by Nashner and colleagues (Black et al., 1988; Horak et al., 1990; Shumway-Cook et al., 1988). This approach, described in de-

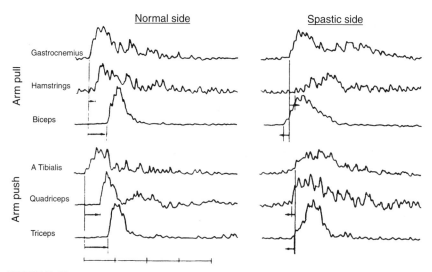

FIGURE 10-15. Normal and abnormal anticipatory postural control. EMG responses in arm (biceps, triceps) and leg (gastrocnemius, hamstrings, tibialis, quadriceps) muscles during a push or pull task in the normal versus spastic side of a child with spastic hemiplegia. Muscle responses on the normal side show the activation of postural muscles in the leg in advance of the prime mover in the arm. In contrast, on the spastic side, muscle activity in the arm precedes postural activity in the legs, resulting in instability. (Reprinted with permission from Nashner LM, Shumway-Cook A, Marin O. Stance posture control in select groups of children with cerebral palsy: deficits in sensory organization and muscular coordination. Exp Brain Res 1983;49: 401.)

tail in the chapters on normal postural control, measures changes in body sway during stance when sensory information is reduced or made inaccurate for postural control. Alternatively, therapists have used compliant foam surfaces in conjunction with a visual dome to examine sensory adaptation in the clinic. This test, referred to as either the Clinical Test for Sensory Interaction in Balance or the Sensory Organization Test, measures the number of seconds (30 seconds maximum) a person can stand in six different sensory conditions (Shumway-Cook and Horak, 1986; Horak, 1987).

Loss of One Sense

What is the effect of loss of a sensory input on postural control? It depends! Some important factors include (*a*) the availability of other senses to detect position of the body in space, (*b*) the availability of accurate orientation cues in the environment, and (*c*) correct interpretation and selection of sensory information for orientation (Shumway-Cook and Horak, 1992).

As shown in Figure 10-16, patients with loss of vestibular information for postural control may be stable under most conditions as long as alternative sensory information from vision or the somatosensory systems is available for orientation. If vision and somatosensory inputs are reduced, leaving mainly vestibular inputs (the last two conditions in Fig. 10-16) for postural control, the patient may suddenly fall, as indicated by the score of 100 on the sway index (Horak et al., 1990).

Functionally, patients with this type of postural dyscontrol may perform normally on most tests of balance as long as they are performed in a well-lit environment and on a firm, flat surface. However, performance on balance tasks under ideal sensory conditions does not necessarily predict the patient's risk of falling when getting up to go to the bathroom at night and negotiating a carpeted surface in the dark.

How does disruption of somatosensory information affect postural control? One might expect that a patient with sudden loss

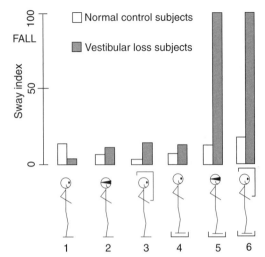

FIGURE 10-16.   A comparison of body sway in the six sensory conditions between neurologically intact adults and patients with loss of vestibular function. Results show that instability in patients with loss of vestibular function occurs only in conditions 5 and 6, when vision and somatosensory inputs are not available for postural control. (Adapted from Horak F, Nashner LM, Diener HC. Postural strategies associated with somatosensory and vestibular loss. Exp Brain Res 1990:418.)

of somatosensory information could maintain stability as long as alternative information from vision and vestibular senses was available. Horak et al. (1990) examined this question by applying pressure cuffs to the ankles of normal subjects and inflating them until cutaneous sensation in the feet and ankles was lost. As can be seen in Figure 10-17, neurologically intact subjects were able to maintain balance on all sensory conditions despite the loss of somatosensory cues from the feet and ankles, since they always had an alternative sense (either vision or vestibular) available for orientation.

Loss of Sensory Redundancy

In some cases, the loss of multiple sensory inputs can result in instability. DiFabio and Badke (1991) used the clinical sensory organization test to examine sensory adaptation in patients with hemiplegia following stroke. As can be seen in Figure 10-18, patients were able to maintain good stability, scoring 150

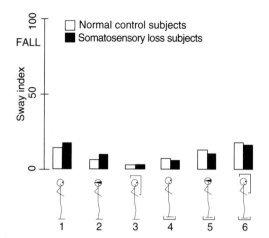

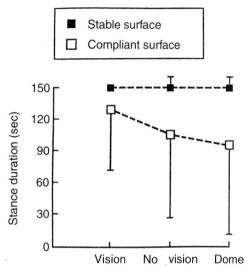

FIGURE 10-17. Body sway in the six sensory conditions in normal subjects before use of pressure cuffs at the ankle and after subsequent temporary loss of cutaneous sensation with use of pressure cuffs. Loss of somatosensory inputs did not affect the ability of these neurologically intact subjects to maintain balance, due to the availability of alternative senses and the capacity to adapt remaining senses to the changing demands. (Adapted from Horak F, Nashner LM, Diener HC. Postural strategies associated with somatosensory and vestibular loss. Exp Brain Res 1990:418.)

FIGURE 10-18. Mean stance duration scores for 10 subjects with hemiplegia standing under six sensory conditions. Stability declines (as indicated by a decrease in seconds able to stand) as sensory redundancy decreases. (Reprinted with permission from DiFabio RP, Badke MB. Stance duration under sensory conflict conditions in patients with hemiplegia. Arch Phys Med Rehab 1991;72:294.)

(30 seconds × 5 trials) when standing on a firm surface with eyes open. Changing the availability of visual information (no vision or dome) did not significantly impair stance balance as long as patients had at least two sensory inputs (somatosensory and vestibular) to rely on. However, changing the availability of visual cues significantly affected stability when somatosensory inputs were reduced (patients stood on a compliant foam surface). This suggests that following a CVA, the ability to maintain balance is significantly reduced when sensory redundancy is lost. Patients can maintain stability in the absence of useful visual cues as long as somatosensory inputs from the surface are readily available. However, when both somatosensory and visual cues are reduced, significant instability results.

Inflexible Weighting of Sensory Information

Sensory adaptation problems can also manifest as an inflexible weighting of sensory information for orientation. This means that a patient may depend heavily on one particular sense for postural control, for example, either vision dependent or somatosensory dependent. When that sense is either not available or not accurately reporting self-motion, patients continue to rely on the preferred sense even though instability may be a consequence.

Patterns of sway associated with this type of sensory inflexibility are summarized in Figure 10-19. Patients who are dependent on visual information for postural control (visually dependent in Fig. 10-19) tend to show abnormally increased sway in any condition of reduced visual cues, such as standing with eyes closed, or inaccurate visual cues, such as standing in the presence of visual motion in the environment (Black and Nashner, 1985).

Patients who demonstrate an inflexible use of somatosensory inputs for postural control (surface dependent) become unstable when surface inputs do not allow patients to establish and maintain a vertical orientation (Horak and Shupert, 1994). This can be seen as

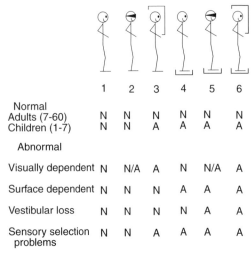

	1	2	3	4	5	6
Normal						
Adults (7-60)	N	N	N	N	N	N
Children (1-7)	N	N	A	A	A	A
Abnormal						
Visually dependent	N	N/A	A	N	N/A	A
Surface dependent	N	N	N	A	A	A
Vestibular loss	N	N	N	N	A	A
Sensory selection problems	N	N	A	A	A	A

FIGURE 10-19. A classification scheme for identifying different problems related to organizing sensory information for stance postural control based on patterns of normal and abnormal sway in six sensory conditions used during dynamic posturography testing. N, normal sway; A, abnormal sway; N/A, may be normal or abnormal.

excessive amounts of body sway in conditions 4, 5, and 6 (Fig. 10-19). Thus, when standing on a compliant surface, such as sand or thick carpet; on a tilted surface, such as a ramp; or on a moving surface, such as a boat, the position of the ankle joint and other somatosensory and proprioceptive information from the feet and legs does not correlate well with the orientation of the rest of the body (Horak and Shupert, 1994). Overreliance on somatosensory inputs for postural control in these environments will result in instability.

Inability to select an appropriate sense for postural control in environments where one or more orientation cues inaccurately report the body's position in space has been referred to as a sensory selection problem (Shumway-Cook et al., 1988b; Horak et al., 1988b). Patients with a sensory selection problem are often able to maintain balance in environments where sensory information for postural control is consistent; however, they are unable to maintain stability when there is incongruence among the senses. Patients with a sensory selection problem do not necessarily show a pattern of overreliance on any one sense but rather appear to be unable to select an accurate orientation

reference; therefore, they are unstable in any environment in which a sensory orientation reference is not accurate. This is shown in Figure 10-19, in which abnormal sway is seen in conditions 3, 4, 5, and 6.

Sensory selection problems have been reported in stroke patients (DiFabio and Badke, 1990), traumatic brain injury patients (Shumway-Cook and Olmscheid, 1990), and children with developmental disorders, including cerebral palsy (Nashner et al., 1983), Down syndrome (Shumway-Cook and Woollacott, 1985b), and learning disabilities (Shumway-Cook et al., 1988b).

Since sensory information varies with the environment, maintaining stability requires the ability to adapt how sensory information is used for postural control. Results from research studies examining sensory adaptation in patients with neurological deficits suggest that to maintain stability, some patients with balance impairments may be restricted to a limited set of environmental conditions in which sensory conditions are optimal. A critical part of retraining balance in these patients is learning to adapt how the senses are used in response to changing environmental conditions.

Misrepresentation of Stability Limits

An important part of interpreting senses and coordinating actions that control the body's position in space appears to be the presence of an internal representation or body schema providing an accurate representation or postural frame of reference. Figure 10-20 provides an example of this concept. Illustrated are the proposed stability limits for the task of independent stance on a firm, flat surface in a neurologically intact adult with normal postural control (Fig. 10-20*A*) (McCollum and Leen, 1989). Figure 10-20*B* depicts modified stability limits for a patient with hemiplegia who requires a cane for support because of unilateral weakness. Stability limits now exclude the left leg, which cannot support the body because of weakness, but include the cane, which serves as an addition to the base of support (Shumway-Cook and McCollum, 1990).

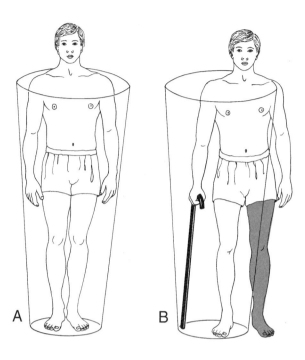

FIGURE 10-20.   Proposed stability limits for the task of independent stance on a firm, flat surface in a neurologically intact adult with normal postural control **(A)** versus modified stability limits for a patient with hemiplegia **(B)** who requires a cane for support because of unilateral weakness. Stability limits exclude the left leg, which cannot support the body because of weakness, but include the cane, which serves as an addition to the base of support. (Adapted with permission from Shumway-Cook A, McCollum G. Assessment and treatment of balance deficits. In: Montgomery P, Connolly B, eds. Motor control and physical therapy. Hixson, TN: Chattanooga Group, 1990:129.)

It has been suggested that an accurate representation, or model, of stability limits is essential to the recovery of postural control. This allows the development of new sensory and motor strategies while the patient remains within his or her new stability limits, regardless of the impairments resulting from the neurological lesion (Shumway-Cook and McCollum, 1990). Thus, the process of recovering postural control after a lesion includes the development of accurate new representations of the body's capability as it relates to postural control. Usually the individual's model of stability limits is consistent with actual stability limits. In many patients, however, perceived stability limits may be inconsistent with actual stability limits, which have changed as a result of sensory and motor limitations following a neurological lesion.

A discrepancy between actual and internal representations of limits of stability can result in instability and the risk of falls (Shumway-Cook and McCollum, 1990). In the drawing in Figure 10-20*B*, the patient's actual stability limits exclude the hemiparetic leg, which is incapable of generating sufficient force to control the body in the up-right position. If the patient's internal model of stability limits includes the affected leg as part of the base of support, the patient will have a tendency to fall to that side when the center of mass shifts to that side.

On the other hand, inaccurate representations of the body with respect to postural control can limit the patient's ability to use new skills for postural control (Shumway-Cook and McCollum, 1990). For example, in the case of the patient with hemiplegia, if during the course of recovery the internal model of stability limits fails to change to reflect new abilities to control the left leg for purposes of support, the patient may continue to stand and walk asymmetrically.

Many patients with neurological disorders fail to develop accurate models of their body related to the dynamics of moving and sensing for postural control (Shumway-Cook and McCollum, 1990; Shumway-Cook and Horak, 1989, 1990). Inaccurate internal models result in patterns of moving and sensing that seem inconsistent with the patient's apparent abilities. This aspect of disordered postural control is just beginning to be explored, and much research is needed in this area.

@ A CASE STUDY APPROACH TO UNDERSTANDING POSTURAL DYSCONTROL

Until now, our discussion of postural dyscontrol following neurological impairment has focused on presenting a wide variety of sensory and motor problems leading to instability. You can see that the range of problems is great, and this reflects the complexity of problems that affect the CNS. In the last section of this chapter we use our case studies to summarize postural control problems by diagnosis. Several warnings must be stated prior to beginning this section. Remember that even patients with the same diagnosis can be very different. Differences in postural control problems can result from variations in type, location, and extent of neural lesions. Other factors, such as age, premorbid status, and degree of compensation, also have a profound influence on the behavior seen.

Phoebe J.: Postural Problems Following Cerebral Vascular Accident

Motor Components of Postural Control

Phoebe J., our 67-year-old woman who has left hemiparesis following a stroke, is likely to have significant postural control problems affecting her ability to function independently. Her postural responses may be delayed in the paretic left limb. The synergistic organization of muscles in the paretic limb may also be disrupted. During recovery from challenges to balance, proximal muscles in the hemiparetic limb may fire either in advance of distal muscles or quite late in relation to distal muscles.

She is also likely to have lost anticipatory activation of postural muscles during voluntary movements. This will make her unsteady when she carries out functional activities such as lifting, reaching, and carrying physical loads. She may have difficulty modifying and adapting postural movements to changing task demands. This may make it difficult for her to maintain stability in response to a change in the base of support or to respond appropriately to challenges to balance that vary in speed and amplitude.

Neuromuscular problems resulting from her stroke are likely to produce secondary musculoskeletal problems that can affect postural control. Phoebe J. may develop a shortening of the gastrocnemius and soleus muscle groups and loss of ankle range of motion. Her static alignment is likely to be characterized by displacement of the center of body mass away from the paretic limb.

Sensory Components of Postural Control

In addition to her motor changes, Phoebe J. is likely to have sensory problems that are contributing to her impaired postural control. She may have reduced sensory information from her visual system (hemianopsia), as well as reduced somatosensation in her hemiparetic limbs. She may also have difficulty in adapting sensory information to changing environmental demands. This will affect her ability to maintain stability in certain environments, such as in low light or when the surface is soft or unsteady. Inability to maintain balance when there is a loss of sensory redundancy will probably be a critical factor in Phoebe J.'s balance problems.

Laurence W.: Postural Problems in Parkinson's Disease

Motor Components of Postural Control

Laurence W. is our 72-year-old man with Parkinson's disease. He is having increasing difficulty with mobility skills, including bed mobility, transfers, and gait. Postural problems affecting orientation and stability are likely to be a significant factor in his declining independence. Interestingly, despite the fact that he has significant bradykinesia, or slowed voluntary movement, common in Parkinson's patients, the onset latencies of his automatic postural responses are likely to be normal (Horak et al., 1988a). If we were to do an EMG study of his postural muscle responses, we would likely find that he uses a complex pattern of muscle activity involving muscles on both sides of the body when responding to instability. This coactivation of muscles on both sides of his body will result in a rigid body and an inability to recover adequate stability (Horak et al., 1988a). In addition, he may be unable to modify movement patterns in response to changing task demands. That is, he may use the same pattern of muscle activity when responding to perturbations to balance while sitting or standing. Finally, like Phoebe J.'s, his anticipatory postural activity will be disrupted, making him unsteady when carrying out functional tasks that are potentially destabilizing, such as lifting or reaching for objects (Rogers, 1990, 1991).

Sensory Components of Postural Control

Laurence W., like many patients with Parkinson's disease, is likely to have sensory organization problems. One of the categories of sensory organization abilities is the task of suppressing postural muscle responses when they are no longer useful. For example, when responding to horizontal support surface displacements in the backward direction, a response in the stretched gastrocnemius muscle serves to return the center of gravity to resting position. However, when responding to a toes-up rotation of the support surface, activation of the gastrocnemius serves to pull the center of gravity further in the direction of the perturbation and increases instability. Thus, under these conditions, healthy subjects suppress gastrocnemius activity to maintain stability. In contrast, Laurence W. is likely to be significantly slower than age-matched healthy adults in suppressing gastrocnemius activity under these changing support surface conditions (Chong et al., 2000).

Zach C.: Postural Problems in Cerebellar Disorders

Motor Components of Postural Control

Zach C. is our 18-year-old who received a closed head injury and traumatic injury to the cerebellum resulting in severe ataxia. Much of the research on postural control in cerebellar disorders has been with patients who have anterior lobe cerebellar degeneration. Thus, findings from these studies may not necessarily completely apply to Zach C., who has more generalized damage to the cerebellum, or other patients with specific lateral hemisphere lesions or vestibulo-cerebellar lesions. Certainly impaired postural control, however, is a hallmark of cerebellar disorders.

Onset latencies in Zach C. are likely to be normal (Horak, 1990), although in children with ataxic forms of cerebral palsy, onset latencies are often reported as delayed (Nashner et al., 1983). Zach C. will probably have difficulty in scaling postural activity, resulting in hypermetric postural responses (Horak, 1990; Nashner et al., 1983). This means that if you stand in front of Zach C. and give him a small perturbation to balance in the backward direction when he is standing, he may well fall forward onto you. The amplitude of his muscle responses may be hypermetric, that is, too large for the size of the challenge. Thus, he overshoots when trying to return to a stable position.

Sensory Components of Postural Control

Zach C. may also have problems with adapting how sensory information is used for postural control in response to changing environmental demands. He may have difficulty maintaining balance in conditions in which he must adapt sensory information for postural control (Horak, 1990; Nashner et al., 1983).

Sara L.: Postural Problems in Cerebral Palsy

Motor Components of Postural Control

Sara L. is a 3-year-old girl with the spastic diplegia form of cerebral palsy. She is likely to have both neuromuscular and musculoskeletal problems affecting postural control. The onset latencies of her postural muscle activity are likely to be quite delayed despite her having hyperactive stretch reflexes in spastic muscles (Nashner et al., 1983). An EMG analysis of responses in stretched spastic muscles will show that muscle activity is slow and reduced in amplitude. In addition to delayed onset of spastic muscles, she is likely to show a disruption of the normal sequencing of muscle activation patterns. Other factors contributing to muscle sequencing problems are changes in postural alignment (specifically the crouched stance posture) and changes in the structure and function of skeletal muscles. She is likely to have anticipatory postural control problems that also affect her stability during performance of voluntary motor acts (Nashner et al., 1983).

Sensory Components of Postural Control

Problems in sensory adaptation do not appear to affect all children with spastic forms of cerebral palsy. There is, however, very little research in this area.

⊚ SUMMARY

1. An enormous range of problems can contribute to postural dyscontrol in the patient with a neurological deficit. In the therapeutic environment, the ability to retrain postural control requires a conceptual framework that incorporates information on the physiological basis for normal postural control, as well as knowledge regarding the basis for instability.

2. Coordination problems that manifest within postural movement strategies include (*a*) sequencing problems, (*b*) problems with the timely activation of muscle response synergies, (*c*) disorders related to the scaling of postural muscle activity, and (*d*) problems adapting motor responses to changing task conditions.

3. In the patient with a neurological deficit, musculoskeletal disorders most often are secondary to the neurological lesion. Yet musculoskeletal problems can be a major limitation to normal postural function in the neurologically impaired patient.

4. Sensory problems can disrupt postural control by (*a*) affecting a patient's ability to adapt sensory inputs to changes in task and environmental demands and (*b*) preventing the development of accurate internal models of the body for postural control.

5. Differences in postural control problems can result from variability in type, location, and extent of neural lesion. Other factors, such as age, premorbid status, and degree of compensation, also have a profound influence on postural behavior.

CHAPTER **11**

Clinical Management of the Patient With a Postural Control Disorder

INTRODUCTION

This chapter discusses a task-oriented approach to examination and treatment of postural control disorders in the patient with neurological dysfunction. In Chapter 5, we introduced a conceptual framework for clinical practice that incorporated four key elements: the patient management process, hypothesis-oriented clinical practice, a model of disablement, and a theory of motor control. We referred to this framework as a task-oriented approach. In previous chapters in this section, we reviewed the research on normal and abnormal postural control. This research provides a logical structure from which to develop clinical methods used to treat patients with postural disorders.

Where it is available, we will examine research evidence that supports the effectiveness of specific therapeutic methods used to

treat postural disorders, including those related to orientation and balance. However, it is important to remember that the development of clinical methods based on current theories of motor control is just beginning. Thus, there is a scarcity of research examining the efficacy of new therapeutic methods that can serve as evidence for our practice. As our understanding of normal and abnormal postural control increases, new methods for examining and treating these disorders will emerge, as will research investigating the effectiveness of new therapeutic approaches to managing the patient with postural disorders.

EXAMINATION

A task-oriented approach examines postural control on three levels: (*a*) functional skills requiring postural control, (*b*) the sensory and motor strategies used to maintain postural control in various contexts and tasks, and (*c*) the underlying sensory, motor, and cognitive impairments that constrain the control of posture. The information gained through examination is used to develop a comprehensive list of problems, establish short- and long-term goals, and formulate a plan of care designed to optimize postural control.

Safety: The First Concern

During the examination of postural control, patients are asked to perform a number of tasks that are likely to destabilize them. Safety is of paramount importance. All patients should wear an ambulation belt during testing and be closely guarded at all times. In determining what tasks and activities cause loss of balance, the patient must be allowed to experience instability. However, the therapist should protect the patient at all times to prevent a fall.

Functional Tests and Measures

Examination from a functional perspective uses tests and measures that examine how well a patient can perform a variety of functional tasks that require postural control. Tasks may reflect the need for (*a*) steady state postural control, such as maintaining a safe independent sitting or standing position; (*b*) anticipatory postural control, such as reaching, leaning, and lifting; and (*3*) reactive postural control, such as recovery from a small nudge or perturbation.

In addition to the tests and measures performed by the patient, gathering self-report information on the number of recent falls and the circumstances leading to the fall(s) or loss of balance is very important. Self-report information on conditions of instability can shed light on what aspects of postural control may be impaired. For example, a patient who reports instability when leaning over to pick something up from the ground may have difficulty with anticipatory aspects of postural control. A patient who loses bal-

ance when shampooing in the shower suggests problems in the sensory components of balance control, specifically difficulty in maintaining balance when visual cues are removed.

Examination of postural control from a functional perspective can provide the clinician with information about the patient's level of performance compared with standards established for normal individuals. Results can indicate the need for therapy, serve as a baseline level of performance, and when repeated at regular intervals, provide both the therapist and patient with objective documentation of change in functional status. A number of tests measure functional skills related to postural control.

Get Up and Go Test

The Get Up and Go test (Mathias et al., 1986) was developed as a quick screening tool for detecting balance problems affecting daily mobility skills in elderly patients. The test requires that subjects stand up from a chair, walk 3 meters, turn around, and return. Performance is scored according to the following scale: 1, normal; 2, very slightly abnormal; 3, mildly abnormal; 4, moderately abnormal; 5, severely abnormal. An increased risk of falls was found among older adults who scored 3 or higher on this test.

The Up and Go (TUG) test modifies the original test by adding a timing component to performance (Podsiadlo and Richardson, 1991). Neurologically intact adults who are independent in balance and mobility skills are able to perform the test in less than 10 seconds. This test correlates well to functional capacity as measured by the Barthel Index. Adults who took more than 30 seconds to complete the test were dependent in most activities of daily living and mobility skills.

A more recent study investigated the sensitivity and specificity of the TUG in single versus dual task (either a cognitive or manual task) conditions in identifying fall-prone older adults living in the community (Shumway-Cook et al., in press). Older adults with and without a history of falls were asked to complete the TUG in three conditions. In the first condition, the TUG alone was performed. In the TUG$_{cognitive}$, subjects were asked to complete the TUG while counting backward by threes. Finally in the TUG$_{manual}$, subjects were asked to complete the TUG while carrying a cup of water. Because so many older adults have difficulty maintaining stability while performing multiple tasks, it was hypothesized that performing the TUG under dual task conditions would be a particularly sensitive way to identify fall prone elders. Table 11-1 compares the sensitivity and specificity of the TUG for identifying fall-prone elders in the three conditions. While the time taken to complete the TUG was significantly longer in the dual task condition, the study found that the TUG alone was a sensitive and specific indicator of fall status in community-dwelling older adults. Thus this relatively simple screening test, which takes only minutes, appears to be a valid method for screening for both level of functional mobility and risk of falls in community-dwelling elders.

Functional Reach Test

The Functional Reach Test (Duncan et al., 1990) is another single-item test developed as a quick screen for balance problems in older adults. As shown in Figure 11-1A, subjects stand with feet a shoulder distance apart and with the arm raised to 90 degrees of flexion. Without moving their feet, subjects reach as far forward as they can while still maintaining their balance (Fig. 11-2B). The distance reached is measured and compared to age-related norms, shown in Table 11-2. The Functional Reach Test has good interrater reliability and is shown to be highly predictive of falls among older adults (Duncan et al., 1990).

The Functional Reach Test examines the limits of stability in the forward direction. The Lateral Reach Test was developed to look at mediolateral postural control (Brauer, 1999). It examines the ability to control the body in a sideways direction at the limits of stability. In the Lateral Reach Test subjects stand near a wall with their arm abducted to 90 degrees, with weight equal between both feet. They are asked to reach directly sideways as far as possible without overbalancing, taking a step, or touching a wall. Both feet are required to remain in contact with the surface, no knee flexion is permitted, and the trunk may not rotate. The maximum hand excursion is measured. In a study of 60 community-dwelling women aged 72.5 ± 5 years, the mean lateral reach was 20.06 cm ± 4.88, range 10 to 36 cm. The test–retest reliability was quite high (ICC = .943) and was correlated with mediolateral center of pressure (COP) excursion (r, .331). These results suggest that the clinical lateral reach test is an accurate test of lateral reach ability. Lateral reach, like anterior reach, decreases with age and decreasing height and arm length. Brauer (1999) recommends that reach measures be normalized to subject height.

TABLE 11-1. **A Comparison of the Sensitivity and Specificity for Identifying Fall Status in Older Adults**

	Sensitivity (% fallers)	Specificity (% nonfallers)	Overall Prediction
TUG	13/15 (87%)	13/15 (87%)	26/30 (87%)
TUG$_{manual}$	12/15 (80%)	14/15 (93%)	26/30 (87%)
TUG$_{cognitive}$	12/15 (80%)	14/15 (93%)	26/30 (87%)

TUG, the up and go.
Reprinted with permission from Shumway-Cook A et al., Phys Ther, in press.

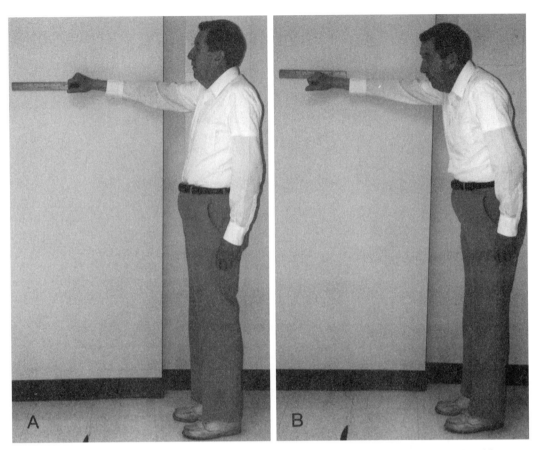

FIGURE 11-1. The Functional Reach Test. **A.** Subjects begin by standing with feet a shoulder distance apart, arm raised to 90 degrees of flexion. **B.** Subjects reach as far forward as they can while maintaining their balance.

Performance Oriented Mobility Test

Mary Tinetti, a physician researcher at Yale University, has published a test to screen for balance and mobility skills in older adults and to determine the likelihood of falls (Tinetti, 1986; Tinetti and Ginter, 1988).

TABLE 11-2.	Functional Reach Norms	

Norms	Men (inches)	Women (inches)
20–40 yr	16.7 ± 1.9	14.6 ± 2.2
41–69	14.9 ± 2.2	13.8 ± 2.2
70–87	13.2 ± 1.6	10.5 ± 3.5

Reprinted with permission from Duncan PW, Weiner DK, Chandler J, Studenski S. Functional reach: a new clinical measure of balance. J Gerontol 1990;45:M195.

Table 11-3 presents Tinetti's balance and mobility scale, which rates performance on a three-point scale. The maximum score is 28 points. In general, patients who score less than 19 are considered at high risk for falls. Those who score in the range of 19 to 24 are at a moderate risk for falls. The test takes about 10 to 15 minutes to administer, and the interrater reliability is good (Tinetti and Ginter, 1988).

Berg Balance Scale

Kathy Berg, a Canadian physical therapist, developed The Berg Balance Scale (Berg, 1993). This test, shown in Table 11-4, uses 14 items rated 0 to 4. The test is reported to have good test-retest and interrater reliability, and it can discriminate older adults at risk for falls. The Berg Balance Scale has

TABLE 11-3.   Performance Oriented Mobility Assessment

I. Balance Tests
    Initial instructions: Subject is seated in a hard, armless chair. The following maneuvers are tested.

    1. Sitting balance_____
        Leans or slides in chair = 0
        Steady, safe = 1

    2. Arises_____
        Unable without help = 0
        Able, uses arms to help = 1
        Able without using arms = 2

    3. Attempts to arise_____
        Unable without help = 0
        Able, requires more than 1 attempt = 1
        Able to rise, 1 attempt = 2

    4. Immediate standing balance (first 5 seconds)_____
        Unsteady (staggers, moves feet, trunk sway) = 0
        Steady, but uses walker or other support = 1
        Steady without walker or other support = 2

    5. Standing balance_____
        Unsteady = 0
        Steady but wide stance (medial heels more than 4 inches apart) and uses cane or other support = 1
        Narrow stance without support = 2

    6. Nudged (subject at maximum position with feet as close together as possible; examiner pushes lightly on
        subject's sternum with palm of hand 3 times)_____
        Begins to fall = 0
        Staggers, grabs, catches self = 1
        Steady = 2

    7. Eyes closed (at maximum position no. 6)_____
        Unsteady = 0
        Steady = 1

    8. Turning 360 degrees_____
        Continuous steps = 0
        Discontinuous steps = 1
        Unsteady steps (grabs, staggers) = 2

    9. Sitting down_____
        Unsafe (misjudges distance, falls into chair) = 0
        Uses arms or not a smooth motion = 1
        Safe, smooth motion = 2
        Balance score:_____/16

II. Gait Tests
    Initial instructions: Subject stands with the examiner, walks down hallway or across room, first at usual pace,
    then back at rapid but safe pace (usual walking aids)

    10. Initiation of gait (immediately after told to go)_____
        Any hesitancy or multiple attempts to start = 0
        No hesitancy = 1

11. Step length and height_____
   a. Right swing foot
      Does not pass left stance foot with step = 0
      Passes left stance foot = 1
      Right foot does not clear floor completely with step = 0
      Right foot completely clears floor = 1
   b. Left swing foot
      Does not pass right stance foot with step = 0
      Passes right stance foot = 1
      Left foot does not clear floor completely with step = 0
      Left foot completely clears floor = 1

12. Step symmetry_____
   Right and left step length not equal (estimate) = 0
   Right and left step appear equal = 1

13. Step continuity_____
   Stopping or discontinuity between steps = 0
   Steps appear continuous = 1

14. Path (estimated in relation to floor tiles, 12-inch diameter; observe excursion of 1 foot over about 10 feet of
      the course)_____
   Marked deviation = 0
   Mild/moderate deviation or uses walking aid = 1
   Straight without walking aid = 2

15. Trunk_____
   Marked sway or uses walking aid = 0
   No sway, but flexion of knees or back pain or spreads arms out while walking = 1
   No sway, no flexion, no use of arms, and no use of walking aid = 2

16. Step width_____
   Heel apart = 0
   Heels almost touching while walking = 1

Gait score: _____ /12
  Balance and gait score: _____ /28

_____

Reprinted with permission from Tinetti M. Performance-oriented assessment of mobility problems in elderly patients. J Am Geriatr Soc 1986;34:119–126.

been shown to have excellent interrater and test–retest reliability (ICC, .98) and good internal consistency (Cronbach's Alpha, .96) (Berg et al., 1989). It has been shown to be correlated with other tests of balance and mobility, including the Tinetti mobility index (r, −.91) and the Get Up and Go test (r, −.76) (Berg et al., 1992).

Shumway-Cook et al. (1997a) reported that the Berg Balance Test was the best single predictor of fall status in community-dwelling older adults. Declining Berg Balance scores were associated with increased fall risk, but as can be seen in Figure 11-2, this relationship was nonlinear. In the range of 56 to 54, each 1 point drop in the Berg was associated with a 3% to 4% increase in fall risk. However, in the range of 54 to 46, a 1-point change in the Berg was associated with a 6% to 8% increase in fall risk. Below 36, fall risk was close to 100%. Thus a 1-point change in the Berg can lead to a much different predicted probability of a fall, depending on where the baseline score is in the scale.

Limitations of Functional Tests and Measures

How well do functional tasks capture postural control from a systems perspective? The application of this concept can be found in Lab Activity 10-1.

As you can see, the Berg Balance Test is heavily weighted toward tasks requiring steady-state and anticipatory postural con-

TABLE 11-4.   Berg Balance Test

1. Sitting to standing

Instruction: Use a chair with arms. Ask the patient to please stand up. If the patient stands up using the arms of the chair, ask the patient to stand up without using the hands if possible.

Grading: Please mark the lowest category that applies.

(4) Able to stand, no hands and stabilize independently

(3) Able to stand independently using hands

(2) Able to stand using hands after several tries

(1) Needs minimal assist to stand or to stabilize

(0) Needs moderate or maximal assist to stand

2. Standing unsupported

Instruction: Stand for 2 minutes without holding on to any external support.

Grading: Please mark the lowest category that applies.

(4) Able to stand safely 2 minutes

(3) Able to stand 2 minutes with supervision

(2) Able to stand 30 seconds unsupported

(1) Needs several tries to stand 30 seconds unsupported

(0) Unable to stand 30 seconds unassisted

IF SUBJECT IS ABLE TO STAND 2 MINUTES SAFELY, SCORE FULL MARKS FOR SITTING UNSUPPORTED. PROCEED TO POSITION CHANGE STANDING TO SITTING.

3. Sitting unsupported, feet on floor

Instruction: Sit with arms folded for 2 minutes.

Grading: Please mark the lowest category that applies.

(4) Able to sit safely and securely 2 minutes

(3) Able to sit 2 minutes under supervision

(2) Able to sit 30 seconds

(1) Able to sit 10 seconds

(0) Unable to sit without support 10 seconds

4. Standing to sitting

Instruction: Please sit down.

Grading: Please mark the lowest category that applies.

(4) Sits safely with minimal use of hands

(3) Controls descent by using hands

(2) Uses back of legs against chair to control descent

(1) Sits independently but has uncontrolled descent

(0) Needs assistance to sit

5. Transfers

Instruction: Please move from this chair (chair with arm rests) to this chair (chair without arm rests) and back again.

Grading: Please mark the lowest category that applies.

(4) Able to transfer safely with only minor use of hands

(3) Able to transfer safely with definite need of hands

(2) Able to transfer with verbal cueing and/or supervision

(1) Needs one person to assist

(0) Needs two people to assist or supervise to be safe

6. Standing unsupported with eyes closed

Instruction: Close your eyes and stand still for 10 seconds.

Grading: Please mark the lowest category that applies.

(4) Able to stand 10 seconds safely

(3) Able to stand 10 seconds with supervision

(2) Able to stand 3 seconds

(1) Unable to keep eyes closed 3 seconds but stays steady

(0) Needs help to keep from falling

7. **Standing unsupported with feet together**

   Instruction: Place your feet together and stand without holding on to any external support.

   Grading: Please mark the lowest category that applies.

   (4) Able to place feet together independently and stand 1 minute safely

   (3) Able to place feet together independently and stand 1 minute with supervision

   (2) Able to place feet together independently but unable to hold for 30 seconds

   (1) Needs help to attain position but able to stand 15 seconds with feet together

   (0) Needs help to attain position and unable to hold for 15 seconds

THE FOLLOWING ITEMS ARE TO BE PERFORMED WHILE STANDING UNSUPPORTED

8. **Reaching forward with outstretched arm**

   Instruction: Lift arm to 90 degrees. Stretch out your fingers and reach forward as far as you can. Examiner places a ruler at end of fingertips when arm is at 90 degrees. Fingers should not touch the ruler while reaching forward. The recorded measure is the distance forward that the fingers reach while the subject is in the most forward leaning position.

   Grading: Please mark the lowest category that applies.

   (4) Can reach forward confidently more than 10 inches

   (3) Can reach forward more than 5 inches safely

   (2) Can reach forward more than 2 inches safely

   (1) Reaches forward but needs supervision

   (0) Needs help to keep from falling

9. **Pick up object from the floor**

   Instruction: Pick up the shoe/slipper that is placed in front of your feet

   Grading: Please mark the lowest category that applies.

   (4) Able to pick up slipper safely and easily

   (3) Able to pick up slipper but need supervision

   (2) Unable to pick up but reaches 1 to 2 inches from slipper and keeps balance independently

   (1) Unable to pick up and needs supervision while trying

   (0) Unable to try; needs assist to keep from falling

10. **Turning to look behind over left and right shoulders**

    Instruction: Turn to look behind you over your left shoulder. Repeat to the right.

    Grading: Please mark the lowest category that applies.

    (4) Looks behind from both sides and weight shifts well

    (3) Looks behind one side only, other side shows less weight shift

    (2) Turns sideways only but maintains balance

    (1) Needs supervision when turning

    (0) Needs assist to keep from falling

11. **Turn 360 degrees**

    Instruction: Turn around in a full circle. Pause. Then turn a full circle in the other direction.

    Grading: Please mark the lowest category that applies.

    (4) Able to turn 360 degrees safely in less than 4 seconds each side

    (3) Able to turn 360 degrees safely one side only in less than 4 seconds

    (2) Able to turn 360 degrees safely but slowly

    (1) Needs close supervision or verbal cueing

    (0) Needs assistance while turning

12. **Count number of times step stool is touched**

    Instruction: Place each foot alternately on the stool. Continue until each foot has touched the stool four times for a total of eight steps.

    Grading: Please mark the lowest category that applies.

    (4) Able to stand independently and safely and complete 8 steps in 20 seconds

    (3) Able to stand independently and complete 8 steps in less than 20 seconds

    (2) Able to complete 4 steps without aid with supervision

    (1) Able to complete fewer than 2 steps, needs minimal assist

    (0) Needs assistance to keep from falling/unable to try

13. **Standing unsupported, one foot in front**

   Instruction: (Demonstrate to subject) Place one foot directly in front of the other. If you feel that you cannot place your foot directly in front, try to step far enough ahead that the heel of your forward foot is ahead of the toes of the other foot.

   Grading: Please mark the lowest category that applies.

   (4) Able to place foot tandem independently and hold 30 seconds
   (3) Able to place foot ahead of other independently and hold 30 seconds
   (2) Able to take small step independently and hold 30 seconds
   (1) Needs help to step but can hold 15 seconds
   (0) Loses balance while stepping or standing

14. **Standing on one leg**

   Instruction: Stand on one leg as long as you can without holding on to an external support.

   Grading: Please mark the lowest category that applies.

   (4) Able to lift leg independently and hold more than 10 seconds
   (3) Able to lift leg independently and hold 5 to 10 seconds
   (2) Able to lift leg independently and hold up to 3 seconds
   (1) Tries to lift leg, unable to hold 3 seconds, but remains standing independently
   (0) Unable to try or needs assist to prevent fall

Reprinted with permission from Berg K. Measuring balance in the elderly: validation of an instrument. Dissertation. Montreal, Canada: McGill University, 1993.

trol. No task (such as the Nudge test in Tinetti's POMA test) on it requires reactive postural control. In addition, the test does not look at performance under altered environmental conditions. This does not mean that the Berg Balance Test is a poor test; it just indicates the limitations of the test with respect to the systems conceptual framework.

 LAB ACTIVITY 11-1

OBJECTIVE: To examine the relationship between a clinical test of balance and certain aspects of the systems framework of postural control, specifically the range of tasks and environments examined.

PROCEDURES: Examine Table 11-4, which outlines the Berg Balance Test. By each test item, indicate whether the task requires steady-state, reactive, or proactive postural control. Examine the environmental condition for each item.

ASSIGNMENT: How many items test steady-state balance control? How many test anticipatory balance control? How many test reactive balance control? Do any of the items examine the same task under different conditions?

Like the Berg Balance Test, most functional measures have limitations. First a patient's performance is examined under a limited set of environmental conditions; thus, it may not always predict actual performance in more complex environments. In addition, few tests examine all three aspects of postural control, including steady-state, reactive, and anticipatory postural control. Finally, most functional tests provide little insight into the quality of movement used to accomplish the task and provide no way to identify specific neuronal or musculoskeletal subsystems responsible for a decline in performance. Additional tests are necessary to gain insight into the quality of movement used to accomplish balance and the underlying system impairments.

Examination at the Strategy Level

The next level of examination identifies the motor and sensory strategies used to control the body's position in space under a variety of conditions.

Motor Strategies

Examination of motor strategies for postural control determines both the alignment of body segments during unperturbed sitting

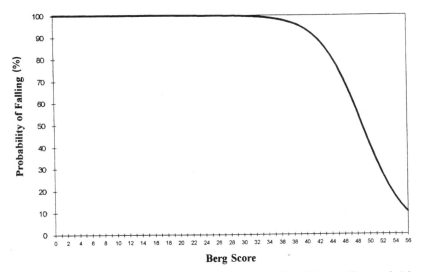

FIGURE 11-2. The relationship between scores on the Berg Balance Test and risk of falls. On the y-axis is the predicted probability for being a faller; scores from the Berg Balance Test are on the x-axis. (Reprinted with permission from Shumway-Cook A, Baldwin M, Pollisar N, Gruber W. Predicting the probability of falls in community-dwelling older adults. Phys Ther 1997;77:817.)

and standing and the patient's ability to generate multijoint movements, or strategies, that effectively control motion of the center of mass relative to the base of support (Shumway-Cook and McCollum, 1990; Shumway-Cook and Horak, 1990; Woollacott and Shumway-Cook, 1990).

Alignment in Sitting and Standing

Examination of postural control includes observation of the patient's alignment in sitting and standing. Is the patient vertical? Is weight symmetrically distributed right to left and front to back? A plumb line in conjunction with a grid can be used to quantify changes in alignment at the head, shoulders, trunk, pelvis, hips, knees, and ankles. In addition, the width of the patient's base of support upon standing can be measured and recorded using a tape to measure the distance between the medial malleoli or alternatively, the metatarsal heads.

Alternative ways to quantify placement of the center of mass of a standing person include the use of static force plates to measure placement of the COP and the use of two standard weight scales to determine whether there is weight discrepancy between the two sides (Fig. 11-3).

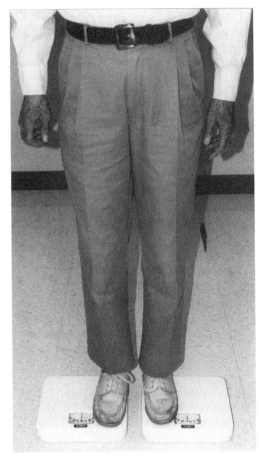

FIGURE 11-3. Two standard scales can be used to quantify static asymmetrical standing alignment.

Movement Strategies

Movement strategies used for postural control in sitting and standing are observed under various task conditions, including during self-initiated sway, in response to externally induced sway, and anticipatory to a potentially destabilizing upper extremity movement. In addition, the ability to adapt movement strategies to changes in task and environmental demands, such as standing with a reduced base of support or on a moving surface, is examined.

Movements used to control self-initiated body sway are observed while the patient voluntarily shifts the weight forward, then backward, then side to side. The patient is tested both sitting and standing. Figure 11-4 illustrates the range of movement patterns seen in a seated neurologically intact individual as she shifts the trunk further and further laterally while seated. As weight is transferred to one side of the body, the trunk begins to curve toward the unweighted side, resulting in elongation of the weight-bearing side and shortening of the trunk on the unweighted

side (Fig. 11-4A). As weight continues to shift laterally, maintaining stability requires the subject to abduct the arm and leg to keep the trunk mass within the base of support (Fig. 11-4B). Finally, when stability can no longer be maintained within the current base of support, the arm is extended, changing the base of support and preventing a fall (Fig. 11-4C).

Figure 11-5 illustrates two types of movement strategies being used to control voluntary sway in standing. Two patients have been asked to sway forward as far as they can without taking a step. Patient A (Fig. 11-5A) is swaying forward primarily about the ankles, using an ankle strategy to control center of mass motion. In contrast, patient B (Fig. 11-5B) is moving primarily the trunk and hips (a hip strategy), which minimizes forward motion of the center of mass.

The presence of coordinated movement strategies can also be examined during recovery from an external perturbation. Figure 11-6 illustrates one approach to assessing movement patterns used to recover stability

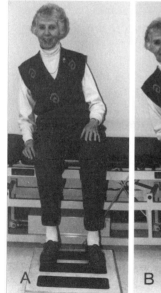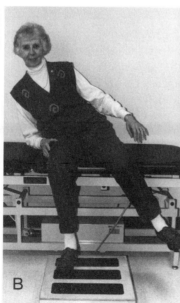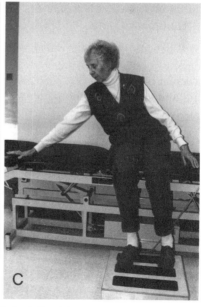

FIGURE 11-4. Maintaining stability during self-initiated weight shifts with trunk movements in sitting. **A.** Small movements produce adjustments at the head and trunk. **B.** Larger movements require counterbalancing with the arms and legs. **C.** When movements of the head and trunk can no longer control stability with the base of support, the arm reaches out to change the base of support and prevent a fall.

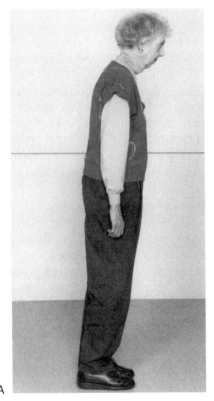
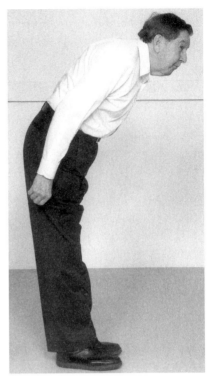

A   B

FIGURE 11-5.   Controlling stability during voluntary sway in stance. Two types of
movement strategies to control self-initiated voluntary sway in standing: the ankle
strategy (**A**) and the hip strategy (**B**).

in response to an external displacement at the hips (Shumway-Cook and Horak, 1992; Carr and Sheperd, 1998). Holding the patient about the hips, the therapist displaces the patient forward, backward, right, and left. As shown in Figure 11-6, *A* and *B*, in-place strategies (ankle or hip) are used to recover from small displacements, while a step (Figure 11-6*C*) may be used to maintain stability in response to larger displacements or when subjects do not perceive they can maintain stability using in-place movement strategies.

Movement strategies used to minimize instability in anticipation of potentially destabilizing movements can be assessed by asking a patient to lift a heavy object as rapidly as possible (Figure 11-7) or to place one foot on a stool. Both of these tasks require subtle shifts of the center of mass prior to the voluntary movement (of the arms in the lifting task, the leg in the stepping task). An absence of anticipatory adjustments results in

instability and loss of balance (Shumway-Cook and Horak, 1992).

Finally, observing movements made to maintain stability in response to changing task demands can provide insight into the range of coordinated movement strategies available for postural control. Commonly used balance tasks, such as standing on one foot (Figure 11-8*A*) or in a tandem Romberg (heel–toe) position (Figure 11-8*B*) can increase the likelihood that a subject will use a hip or stepping strategy to maintain stability and prevent a fall.

The most common clinical approach to evaluating multijoint dyscoordination within movement strategies used for postural control is through observation and description during tests such as the Nudge Test (Tinetti, 1986). Following a small perturbation in the backward direction, the clinician may note that during recovery of stance balance the patient demonstrates excessive flexion of the

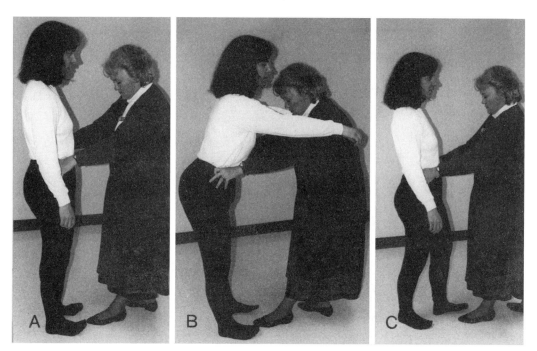

FIGURE 11-6. Movement strategies used to recover from an external perturbation to balance. An ankle strategy (**A**) is used to recover from a small displacement at the hips. A larger displacement produces a hip strategy (**B**). When in-place strategies can no longer control the center of mass (COM) with respect to the existing base of support, a step is used to change the base of support and prevent a fall (**C**).

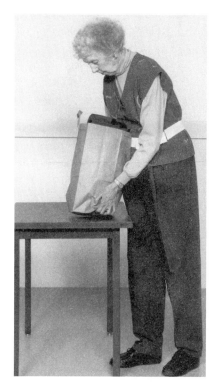

knees or excessive flexion or rotation of the trunk. Differences in onset of muscle responses in the two sides can often be noted by testing for symmetry in when the toes come up in response to a backward perturbation (Figure 11-9). However, determination of the underlying nature of the dyscoordination, that is, specific timing and/or amplitude errors in synergistic muscles responding to instability, most often requires the use of technical apparatus such as electromyography (Shumway-Cook and McCollum, 1990).

Sensory Strategies

Shumway-Cook and Horak suggested a method for clinically assessing the influence

FIGURE 11-7. Movement strategies examined during anticipatory postural control. Activities such as lifting a heavy bag require subtle shifts of the COM prior to the voluntary movement to prevent loss of balance.

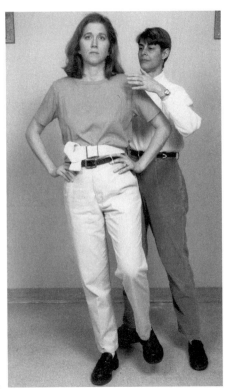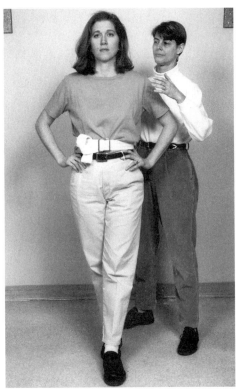

FIGURE 11-8. Adapting movement strategies to changes in the base of support either through one-foot stand (**A**) or tandem Romberg (**B**) position.

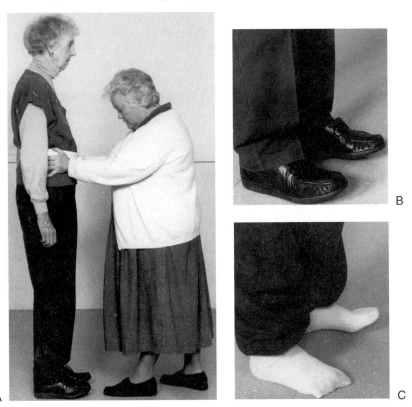

FIGURE 11-9. Symmetry of muscle responses at the ankle can be observed in response to backward displacement. Neurologically intact subjects show a symmetrical toes-up pattern (**A, B**), while subjects with asymmetrical movement pathology, such as stroke, show asymmetry (**C**).

of sensory interaction on postural stability in the standing position (Shumway-Cook and Horak, 1986; Horak, 1987). The Clinical Test for Sensory Interaction in Balance (CT-SIB) uses a 24 × 24–inch piece of medium-density Temper foam in conjunction with a modified Japanese lantern. A large Japanese lantern is cut down the back and attached to a headband. Vertical stripes are placed inside the lantern, and the top and bottom of the lantern are covered with white paper (Fig. 11-10).

The CTSIB is based on concepts developed by Nashner (1982) and requires the subject to maintain standing balance for 30 seconds under six sensory conditions that either eliminate input or produce inaccurate visual and surface orientation inputs. These six conditions are shown in Figure 11-11. Patients are tested in the feet-together position with hands on the hips. Using condition 1 as a baseline reference, the therapist observes the patient for changes in the amount and direction of sway over the subsequent five conditions. If the patient is unable to stand for 30 seconds, a second trial is given (Horak et al., 1992).

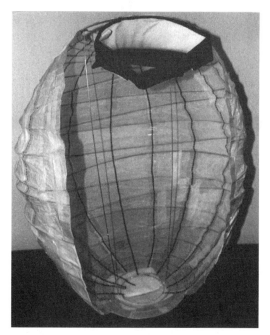

FIGURE 11-10. A modified Japanese lantern used to change the accuracy of visual input for postural orientation.

Neurologically intact young adults are able to maintain balance for 30 seconds in all six conditions with minimal amounts of body sway. As was true for the computerized sensory organization testing, normal adults sway on the average 40% more in conditions 5 and 6 than in condition 1 (Horak et al., 1992).

Results from a number of research studies that have used either a moving platform or the CTSIB suggest the following scoring criteria (Peterka and Black, 1990; DeFabio and Badke, 1990; Cohen et al., 1993a; Horak et al., 1992). A single fall, regardless of the condition, is not considered abnormal. However, two or more falls indicate difficulties adapting sensory information for postural control.

A proposed model for interpreting results is summarized in Figure 11-12. Patients who show increased amounts of sway or lose balance in conditions 2, 3, and 6 are thought to be visually dependent, that is, highly dependent on vision for postural control. Patients who have problems in conditions 4, 5, and 6 are thought to be surface-dependent, that is, dependent primarily on somatosensory information from the feet in contact with the surface, for postural control (Shumway-Cook and Horak, 1990). Patients who sway more or fall in conditions 5 and 6 demonstrate a vestibular loss pattern, suggesting an inability to select vestibular inputs for postural control in the absence of useful visual and somatosensory cues. Finally, patients who lose balance in conditions 3, 4, 5, and 6 are said to have a sensory selection problem. This is defined as inability to adapt sensory information for postural control (Shumway-Cook and Horak, 1992).

It is important to remember the following caution when interpreting results showing increased sway on a compliant surface. While we suppose that the primary effect of standing on a foam surface relates to altering the availability of incoming sensory information for postural orientation, additional factors can affect performance in this condition. Standing on foam changes the dynamics of force production with respect to the surface, and this may be a significant factor affecting performance in this condition.

VISUAL CONDITIONS

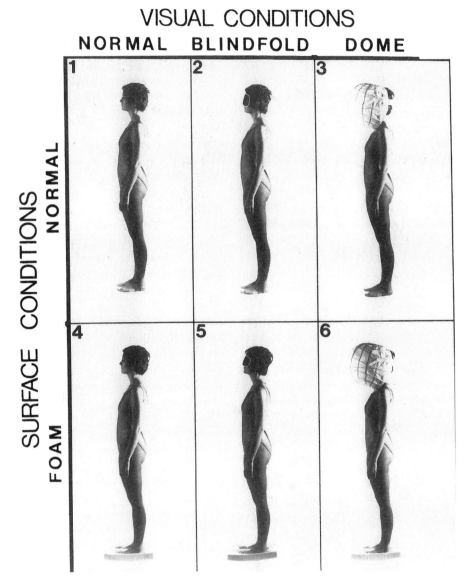

FIGURE 11-11. Six sensory conditions used to examine postural orientation under altered sensory contexts, testing the ability to adapt the use of senses to maintain orientation. (Reprinted with permission from Shumway-Cook A, Horak F. Assessing the influence of sensory interaction on balance. Phys Ther 1986;66:1549.)

There has been no research examining the dynamics of standing on foam; therefore, clinicians should be careful in interpreting results when using the foam condition.

Examination of Underlying Impairments

The final step in a task-oriented approach is examining the sensory, motor (neural and musculoskeletal), and cognitive subsystems that contribute to postural control. During this portion of the examination, the emphasis is on examining impairments that most directly affect postural control. Thus, examination of strength may focus on examining lower extremity muscle strength, with particular attention to ankle muscles, such as anterior tibialis, gastrocnemius, and soleus, because of their role in control of upright

Patterns	1	2 A	3	4	5	6
Visually Dependent	N	N/A	A	N	N/A	A
Surface Dependent	N	N	N	A	A	A
Vestibular Loss	N	N	N	N	A	A
Sensory Selection	N	N	A	A		A

N= Body sway within normal limits
A= Body sway abnormal

FIGURE 11-12.   A proposed model for interpreting the CTSIB test based on information gained through dynamic posturography testing.

stance. For that same reason, examining range of motion at the ankle is also considered critical. Understanding the integrity of sensory inputs critical to postural control, such as vision and somatosensation in the feet and ankles, is also an important part of examination at the impairment level. For a discussion of methods for examining impairments, refer to Chapter 6.

⊘ EVALUATION: INTERPRETING THE RESULTS OF THE EXAMINATION

Following completion of the examination, the clinician must interpret results, identify the problems at the levels of both function and impairments, and establish goals and a plan of care. The application of this concept can be found in Lab Activity 10-2.

Before we establish goals and a plan of care for Phoebe J., let's review a task-oriented approach to treating the patient with postural control problems.

⊘ INTERVENTION

The goals of a task-oriented approach to treating the patient with postural control

---

▦ LAB ACTIVITY 11-2

OBJECTIVE: To apply to a patient with hemiplegia a task-oriented approach to examining postural control and to establish goals and a plan of care for improving posture and balance based on assessment information.

PROCEDURES: Read the case study of Phoebe J. in Table 11-5, or use a real case study if you have access to a patient with a neurological diagnosis.

ASSIGNMENT: Based on the information you have, answer the following questions:

1. What are the patient's functional limitations?
2. Based on the patient's Berg Test score, what is the current fall risk (Fig. 11-2)?
3. Does the patient have steady-state balance problems? anticipatory control problems? reactive control problems?
4. What movement strategies does the patient use for control of balance? What impairments are contributing to the choice of movement strategy?
5. How well is the patient able to organize sensory information for postural control? Based on the results from the CTSIB test, in what environments would you expect the patient to have difficulty maintaining balance?

TABLE 11-5.   Assessment Case Study

Phoebe J. is a 67-year-old woman with left-sided hemiplegia, referred for evaluation of balance 4 weeks following her stroke.

Prior medical history: Positive for hypertension. Following her 5-day acute hospital stay for a middle cerebral artery infarct, she spent 2 weeks in rehabilitation and was discharged to her home.

Social history: She lives with her husband and college-age son in a two-story house. She was a full-time legal assistant.

Reason for referral: Continued problems with balance

On examination:

Self-report fall/balance history: She reports two falls since her return home. One occurred while she was walking to the bathroom at night and one, while she was walking outside. She indicates she loses her balance several times a day, often when arising, turning, and walking.

Tests and Measures:

A. Function: Berg Balance Test (performed without her single-point cane)

Test Item		Test Item	
1. Sit to stand	3	8. Functional reach	3
2. Stand to sit	3	9. Look over shoulder	3
3. Transfers	3	10. Slipper reach	2
4. Standing 2 minutes	4	11. 360° turn	2
5. Sitting	4	12. Stool touch	0
6. Standing feet together	2	13. One-foot stand	0
7. Standing eyes closed	3	14. Tandem stand	0

B. Strategy Assessment
  1. Motor
     Alignment in sitting and standing: shifted to the left
     Voluntary sway: tends to bend at the hips when leaning forward or backward, has difficulty shifting weight laterally to the right.
     Nudge test: small perturbations; tends to bend at the hips; does not show a toes-up response to backward displacement in the right foot. Large perturbations: can step with the right foot (but slowly), cannot step with the left
  2. Sensory to CTSIB (feet a shoulder distance apart, no cane)

Surface, visual condition	Trial 1	Trial 2	Surface, visual condition	Trial 1	Trial 2
Firm, open	30		Foam, open	0	5
Firm, closed	30		Foam, closed	0	0
Firm, dome	10	20	Foam, dome	0	0

C. Underlying impairments
  1. Decreased cognitive status; specific problems with judgment, and safety issues
  2. Musculoskeletal impairments, including 5 degrees of ankle dorsiflexion in the right leg
  3. Neuromuscular impairments, including reduced ability to generate force voluntarily (2/5 manual muscle testing in right lower extremity muscles), decreased ability to recruit ankle muscles in the right leg for postural control, moderate increase in muscle tone in the right elbow flexor and ankle extensors
  4. Sensory/perceptual problems, including decreased sensory discrimination (somatosensation) in the right arm and leg; right hemianopsia

problems include therapeutic strategies (*a*) to resolve, reduce, or prevent impairments that contribute to imbalance; (*b*) to develop effective task-specific sensory and motor strategies for maintaining postural control; and (*c*) to retrain functional tasks with varying postural control demands (steady state, reactive, and anticipatory control), under changing environmental contexts.

Intervention at the Impairment Level

The goal of intervention aimed at the impairment level is to correct impairments that can be changed and to prevent the development of secondary impairments. Alleviating underlying impairments enables the patient to resume use of previously developed strategies for postural control. When permanent impairments make resumption of previously used strategies impossible, it is necessary to develop new strategies that are effective in meeting task requirements in the face of persisting impairments.

The focus of intervention at the impairment level is to ameliorate impairments that have the greatest effect on postural control. For example, in our case study of Phoebe J., improving range of motion and strength at the ankle would be a critical part of working on recovery of stance balance control. Treatment of impairments associated with central nervous system disorders was presented in Chapter 6 and thus will not be reviewed here.

Will intervention aimed solely at remediating underlying sensory and motor impairments result in improved balance? As mentioned in Chapter 6, the evidence for improving functional outcomes and level of disability using interventions aimed at the impairment level is mixed. Many of the research studies focusing on improving balance and mobility have used a combination of treatments aimed at improving the systems essential to balance, such as strength and range of motion, as well as treatments that more directly affect postural control (orientation and balance). The results of some of these studies are summarized at the end of this chapter.

Intervention at the Strategy Level

The goal of interventions aimed at the strategy level is to facilitate the development of sensory and motor strategies that are effective in meeting postural control demands associated with a variety of functional tasks. Movement strategies must successfully control the center of mass relative to the base of support. This includes the development of both (*a*) strategies that move the center of mass relative to a stationary base of support, such as in standing, the ankle and hip strategy, and in sitting, the appropriate lengthening and shortening of the trunk as the COM is moved laterally, and (*b*) strategies that change the base of support to contain the COM, such as taking a step to recover stability or reaching for support with an arm.

Development of sensory strategies includes learning to organize and select the most appropriate sensory input(s) for postural control. Perceptual strategies reflect changing patients' conscious and unconscious perceptions related to stability: How well am I able to control my balance? How safe is it to move? How likely am I to fall?

Tasks for Retraining Strategies

Recovery of postural control can be facilitated through the use of tasks and therapeutic activities that shape postural behaviors needed for more complex movement tasks. The tasks chosen can be a powerful tool in facilitating the recovery of postural control. Thus, during initial stages of balance retraining, when the patient has minimal ability to control the center of mass, tasks with minimal demands for postural control may be used. As the patient is successful in controlling orientation and stability in less challenging tasks, tasks with increasing postural demands are introduced. For example, postural demands involved in maintaining an upright seated posture while in a supported or semisupported seated position are relatively light. As support is decreased, as for example when sitting unsupported on the edge of the mat or bed, the number of degrees of freedom increases, as does the need for active postural control. Degrees of freedom requiring active postural control increase as support decreases, as when moving from the seated position (a relatively large base of support) to the standing position (a relatively small base of support). Another way to increase the challenge for postural control is to increase the number of tasks being performed, as for example sitting or standing on compliant foam while holding a cup of water.

In addition to sequencing tasks based on degree of postural demand, therapeutic strategies that facilitate the coordination of sensory and motor activity for postural control may be useful when retraining the patient with postural control problems. The following sections discuss some of these ideas. Many of the methods are based on current theory and research that provide a logical foundation for the approach. However, controlled clinical research is needed to prove the efficacy of these methods.

Alignment

The goal when retraining alignment is to help the patient develop an initial position that (*a*) is appropriate for the task; (*b*) is efficient with respect to gravity, that is, with minimal muscle activity requirements for maintaining the position; and (*c*) maximizes stability, that is, places the vertical line of gravity well within the patient's stability limits; this allows the greatest range of movements for postural control. Many tasks are done in a symmetrical vertical position, but this is not always a realistic goal (Shumway-Cook and McCollum, 1990).

A number of approaches can be used to help patients develop a symmetrically vertical posture. Commonly, the clinician uses verbal and manual cues to assist a patient in finding and maintaining an appropriate vertical posture. Patients practice with eyes open and closed, learning to maintain a vertical position in the absence of visual cues.

Mirrors can also be used to provide patients with visual feedback about their position in space. The effect of a mirror can be enhanced by having the patient wear a white T-shirt with a vertical stripe down the center and asking him or her to try to match the stripe on the T-shirt to a vertical stripe on the mirror (Fig. 11-13). The patient can use the mirror and T-shirt approach when performing a variety of tasks, such as reaching for an object, which require that the body be moved away from the vertical line and then reestablish a vertical position. Given the results from motor learning research on frequency of knowledge of results (KR) summarized in Chapter 2, learning might be better if visual feedback regarding midline alignment is given intermittently rather than during every trial. For example, the therapist could turn or cover the mirror and ask the patient to repeat the task in the absence of visual feedback.

Another approach to retraining vertical alignment, shown in Figure 11-14, uses flashlights attached to the patient's body in conjunction with targets on the wall (Shumway-

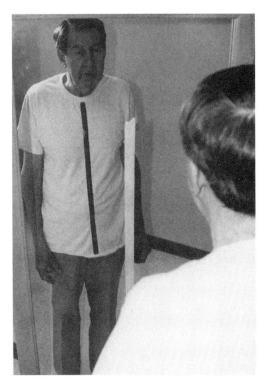

FIGURE 11-13. Using a mirror when retraining alignment. The patient is asked to line up the vertical stripe on his T-shirt with a vertical stripe on the mirror.

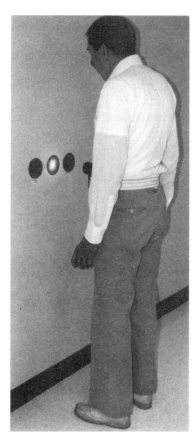

FIGURE 11-14.   Use of a flashlight in conjunction with targets on a wall to help a patient learn to control COM movements.

Cook and Horak, 1992). In this task, the patient is asked to bring the light or lights in line with the target(s). Again, lights can be turned on and off during the task so that visual feedback is intermittent.

Another approach to retraining vertical posture involves having patients stand or sit back against the wall, which provides enhanced somatosensory feedback about their position in space. This feedback can be further increased by placing a yardstick or small roll vertically on the wall (Fig. 11-15) and having the patient lean against it. Somatosensory feedback can be made intermittent by having the patient lean away from the wall, only occasionally leaning back to get KR.

Kinetic or force feedback devices are often used to provide patients with information about postural alignment and weight-

bearing status (Herman, 1973; Shumway-Cook et al., 1988a). Kinetic feedback can be provided with devices as simple as bathroom scales (Fig. 11-3). Alternatively, kinetic feedback can be given through load-limb monitors (Herman, 1973), feedback canes (Baker et al., 1979) or force plate biofeedback systems such as the one shown in Figure 11-16.

What evidence do we have that use of force plate biofeedback helps patients reestablish symmetrical postural alignment? Shumway-Cook et al. (1988a) compared the effect of postural sway biofeedback to usual-care physical therapy in reestablishing symmetrical weight bearing while standing in patients with hemiparesis. The researchers randomly assigned 16 patients, 6 months post cerebral vascular accident, to feedback

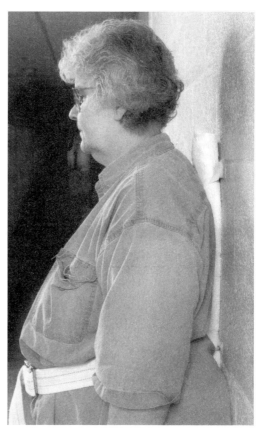

FIGURE 11-15.   Enhancing somatosensation regarding verticality when retraining vertical posture by having the patient lean against a small roll placed vertically on the wall.

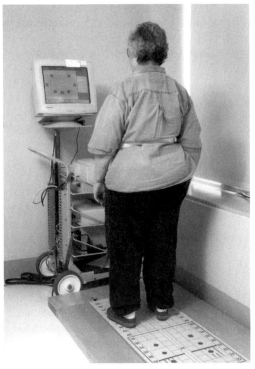

FIGURE 11-16. Use of a force-plate biofeedback system to provide visual feedback regarding alignment and weight-bearing status.

or usual-care groups. Prior to treatment all patients were shown to carry about 70% of total body weight on the uninvolved leg. The feedback group received 15 minutes of stance biofeedback twice a day for 2 weeks. The usual-care group received 15 minutes of balance retraining for the same amount of time. Balance retraining included use of verbal, manual, and visual (mirror) cues to stand symmetrically. Following two weeks of training, the experimental group had significantly less lateral displacement (Fig. 11-17) than did the patients in the control group, 6 of whom were more asymmetrical at the end of 2 weeks of therapy.

Winstein et al. (1989) also examined the effects of providing visual feedback about relative weight distribution over paretic and nonparetic limbs on standing balance and locomotor performance in patients with hemiplegia. They provided visual feedback through a standing feedback trainer to 21 patients randomly assigned to the experimental treatment. Another 21 patients served as controls and received conventional therapy. Consistent with the previous study, results

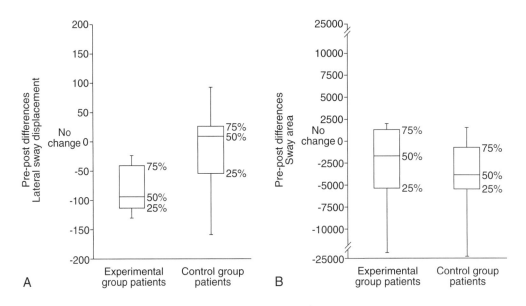

FIGURE 11-17. A comparison of differences (median, quartile, and range scores) for lateral sway displacement **(A)** and total sway area **(B)** between stroke patients receiving biofeedback and control patients receiving conventional therapy. Lateral sway displacement was significantly reduced in the experimental group. (Reprinted with permission from Shumway-Cook A, Anson D, Haller S. Postural sway biofeedback, its effect on reestablishing stance stability in hemiplegic patients. Arch Phys Med Rehabil 1988;69:398).

showed that stance symmetry significantly improved with the visual feedback therapy; however, there was no change in the asymmetrical locomotor pattern. These authors remind us that while control mechanisms for balance and locomotion may be highly interrelated, a reduction in standing asymmetry does not necessarily lead to a reduction in asymmetrical locomotion patterns.

Clinicians routinely provide the unsteady patient with assistive devices, such as canes and walkers. What effect does external support, such as a cane, have on postural alignment and stability? Such assistive devices increase the base of support. Since stability requires keeping the center of gravity within the base of support, increasing the base of support makes maintenance of stability easier. Milezarek et al. (1993) studied the effects of a cane on standing balance in patients with hemiparesis, using a force plate to record changes in COP under various conditions of support. As illustrated in Figure 11-18, they found that using a cane resulted in a significant shift in the COP toward the cane side and a decrease in both anteroposterior and mediolateral postural sway. Thus, al-

though using a cane reduced postural sway, it increased the asymmetrical alignment of patients toward the side holding the cane (Milezarek et al., 1993).

Movement Strategies

The goal when retraining movement strategies is to help the patient develop multijoint coordinated movements that are effective in meeting the demands for postural control in sitting and in standing. This includes movements that move the center of mass relative to a stationary base of support (in-place strategies) and movements that change the base of support relative to the center of mass (changing base-of-support strategies).

Developing Coordinated In-Place Strategies

Before one retrains the use of an ankle strategy for postural control, it is essential to remember that this strategy requires the patient to have adequate range of motion and strength at the ankle (Shumway-Cook and McCollum, 1990; Shumway-Cook and Horak, 1992). In the face of persisting impairments that preclude the use of an ankle strat-

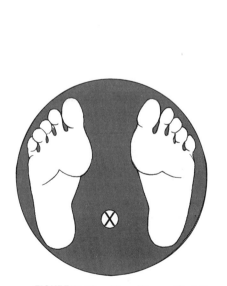 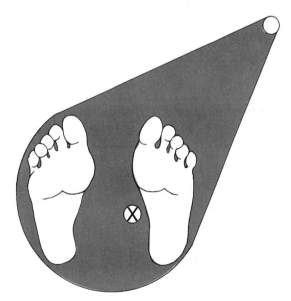

FIGURE 11-18.   The effects of holding a cane while standing: widening the base of support and shifting the mean position of the COP laterally toward the cane side. The x shows COP position. (Adapted with permission from Milezarek JJ, Kirby LM, Harrison ER, MacLeod DA. Standard and four-footed canes: Their effect on the standing balance of patients with hemiparesis. Arch Phys Med Rehabil 1993;74:283.)

egy, patients should be encouraged to develop alternative strategies, such as the hip or step, when controlling body sway. In addition, as we saw in Chapter 10, the use of a fixed ankle–foot orthosis also results in a shift away from ankle strategy to alternative movement strategies for controlling stability.

When retraining the use of an ankle strategy during self-initiated sway, patients are asked to practice swaying back and forth and side to side within small ranges, keeping the body straight and not bending at the hips or knees. KR regarding how far the center of mass is moving during self-initiated sway can be facilitated using static force plate retraining systems. Flashlights attached to the patient in conjunction with targets on the wall can also be used to encourage patients to move from side to side (Fig. 11-11).

Patients who are very unsteady or extremely fearful of falling can practice movement in the parallel bars, standing close to a wall, or in a corner with a chair or table in front of them (Fig. 11-19). Modifying the environment, either home or clinic, in this manner allows a patient to continue practicing movement strategies for balance control safely and without the continuous supervision of a therapist.

Use of perturbations at the hips or shoulders is an effective way to help patients develop strategies for recovery of balance. Small perturbations can facilitate the use of in-place strategies for balance control, while larger perturbations encourage the use of a hip or step.

Finally, patients can be asked to carry out a variety of manipulation tasks, such as reaching, lifting, and throwing, which helps them to develop strategies for anticipatory postural control. A hierarchy of tasks reflecting increasing anticipatory postural demands can be helpful when retraining patients in this important area. The magnitude of anticipatory postural activity is directly related to the potential for instability inherent in a task. Potential instability relates to speed, effort, degree of external support, and task complexity. Thus, lifting a light load slowly while externally supported by the therapist requires minimal anticipatory pos-

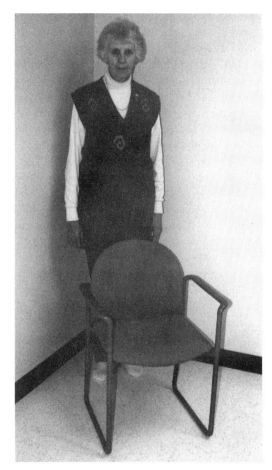

FIGURE 11-19.   Placing a patient near a wall with a chair in front of her increases safety when retraining standing balance in a fearful or unstable patient.

tural activity. Conversely, an unsupported patient who must lift a heavy load quickly must use a substantial amount of anticipatory postural activity to remain stable.

Treatment of Timing Problems.   How can a clinician help a patient recover an ankle strategy in the face of coordination problems that affect the timing and scaling of postural movement strategies? When a patient is unable to activate distal muscles quickly enough to recover stability during a postural task, we have used a variety of techniques to facilitate muscle activation, including icing, tapping, and vibration to the distal muscles while the patient is standing, immediately prior to and during perturbations to standing balance or self-initiated sway

(Shumway-Cook, unpublished data). This is shown in Figure 11-20.

Biofeedback and electrical stimulation can also be used to improve the automatic recruitment and control of muscles during task-specific movement strategies for recovery of stance stability (Shumway-Cook, unpublished data). For example, we have used electrical stimulation in conjunction with a foot switch to decrease onset latencies of postural responses. As shown in Figure 11-21, we placed a foot switch under the heel so that increased weight on the switch triggered a tetanic stimulation of the anterior tibialis muscle. Electrical stimulation to recruit a muscle within a postural movement strategy was used at home during both self-initiated backward sway and in response to backward perturbations to balance.

Several clinicians have combined the use of biofeedback and functional electrical stimulation (FES) during retraining motor control and found that the combined use of

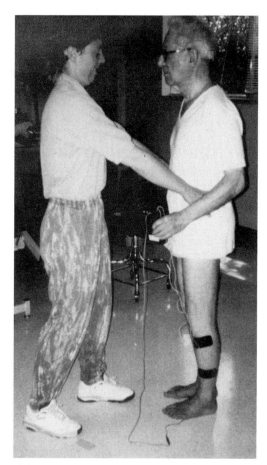

FIGURE 11-21.   Use of electrical stimulation of the distal muscle in conjunction with a foot switch to facilitate activation of the anterior tibialis muscle during stance balance retraining.

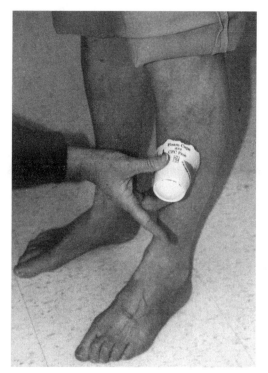

FIGURE 11-20.   The use of ice on the anterior tibialis muscle just prior to a small backward displacement to facilitate its activation during recovery of balance.

biofeedback and FES was superior to either in isolation (Cozean et al., 1988). Another approach we have tried successfully is to use electromyographic biofeedback on the tibialis anterior muscle and to link the biofeedback with a functional electrical stimulator whose electrodes were placed on the quadriceps muscle of the same leg (FES). The two units were set up such that a minimal level of tibialis activation was sufficient to trigger stimulation of the quadriceps. This setup was used in conjunction with external perturbations to balance and was successful in changing the timing of quadriceps activation within the postural response synergy responding to loss of balance in the backward direction (Shumway-Cook, unpublished data).

There is no established research that provides guidelines to the clinician regarding the optimal frequency and duration of stimulation techniques during postural retraining. Further research is needed in this area.

Treatment of Scaling Problems.   To produce effective movements of the center of body mass during postural control, the level of muscle activation must be appropriately scaled, or graded, to the amplitude of body sway. Normal subjects use a combination of feed-forward and feedback control mechanisms to scale forces for postural control (Horak et al., 1989a). To improve amplitude scaling of postural synergies, patients may practice responding to perturbations of various amplitudes. The clinician provides feedback regarding the appropriateness of their response. Interestingly, we have found that it is often easier for many cerebellar patients, who consistently overrespond to small pushes, to scale postural movements to large perturbations initially and progress to smaller perturbations. In contrast, patients with paresis may find it easier to begin with small-amplitude perturbations and progress to larger-amplitude perturbations requiring the generation of more force during recovery of balance.

Static force plate retraining systems are being used by many clinics to retrain postural control in patients with scaling problems. Patients are asked to move the center of mass voluntarily to different targets displayed on a screen. Targets are made progressively smaller and are placed closed together, requiring greater precision in force control. KR is given with respect to movements that overshoot the target, indicating an error in amplitude scaling.

Finally, another approach to treating scaling problems in patients with cerebellar pathology producing ataxia is to add weights to the trunk or limbs. Two rationales are proposed to explain the possible benefits of weighting. The first is that joint compression associated with weights may facilitate coactivation of muscles around a joint, increasing stiffness. The other explanation is mechanical; adding weights increases the mass of the system. In this way, the increased forces generated in the cerebellar patient match the increased mass of the system. Researchers have found that adding weights to cerebellar patients has inconsistent effects. Some patients become more stable, while others are destabilized (Morgan, 1975; Lucy and Hayes, 1985).

Developing Changing Base of Support Strategies

Strategies that change the base of support, either by stepping or reaching for a support surface, are important for postural control. In sitting, helping a patient learn to reach for support as a method for controlling stability is as important as learning to maintain stability using movements of the trunk and head.

Stepping to avoid a fall requires the capacity to maintain the body's weight on a single limb momentarily, without collapse of that limb. Stepping is normally used to prevent a fall when in-place strategies are insufficient to regain stability. Traditionally, stepping is taught within the context of step initiation during gait retraining. Unexpected stepping is often viewed by the clinician as the patient's failure to maintain balance. However, learning to step as a strategy for controlling stability is an essential part of postural retraining.

The clinician can manually facilitate stepping by shifting the patient's weight to one side and quickly bringing the center of mass toward the unweighted leg (Fig. 11-22). The clinician can further assist the patient with a step by manually lifting the foot and placing it during the maneuver. To ensure a patient's safety, stepping can be done within the parallel bars or near a wall. When the clinician is helping a patient develop the ability to step for postural control, it is important to tell the patient that the goal of the exercise is to take a step to prevent a fall.

Sensory Strategies

The goal when retraining sensory strategies is to help the patient learn to coordinate and select appropriate sensory information for

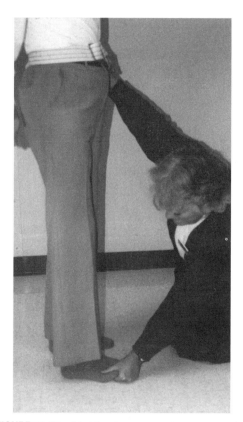

FIGURE 11-22. Facilitating a stepping strategy by manually shifting the patient's center of mass laterally and manually moving the patient's foot into a step.

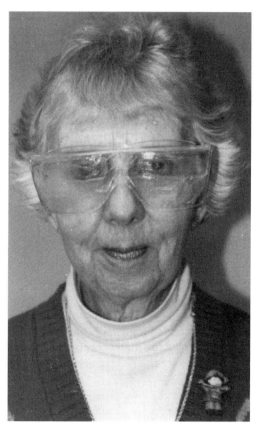

FIGURE 11-23. Training sensory adaptation for postural control. Petroleum jelly-covered glasses used to obscure but not completely remove visual cues for postural control.

postural control. Treatment strategies generally require the patient to maintain balance during progressively more difficult static and dynamic movement tasks while the clinician systematically varies the availability and accuracy of one or more senses for orientation (Shumway-Cook and Horak, 1989, 1990; Herdman, 1999).

Patients who show increased reliance on vision for orientation are asked to perform a variety of balance tasks when visual cues are absent (eyes closed or blindfolded) or reduced (blinders or diminished lighting). Alternatively, visual cues can be made inaccurate for orientation through the use of glasses smeared with petroleum jelly (Fig. 11-23) or Frenzel glasses. Decreasing a patient's sensitivity to visual motion cues can be done by asking the patient to maintain balance during exposure to optokinetic stimuli, such

as moving curtains with stripes, moving large cardboard posters with vertical lines, or even moving rooms.

Patients who show increased reliance on the surface for orientation are asked to perform tasks while sitting or standing on surfaces providing decreased somatosensory cues for orientation, such as carpet or compliant foam surfaces, or on moving surfaces, such as a tilt board. This is shown in Figure 11-24. Finally, to enhance the patient's ability to use remaining vestibular information for postural stability, the patient is asked to balance while both visual and somatosensory inputs for orientation are reduced, such as standing on compliant foam, thick carpet, or an inclined surface with eyes closed. In Figure 11-25 the patient is asked to reach for a glass while standing on foam and wearing petroleum jelly-covered glasses.

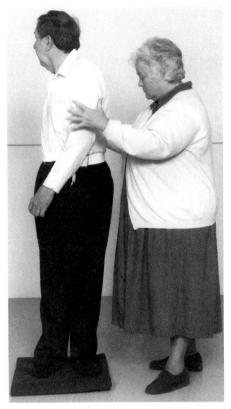

FIGURE 11-24. During balance retraining, facilitating an arm reach in sitting prevents a fall by changing the base of support.

Perceived Limits of Stability

Rehabilitation strategies involving use of postural sway biofeedback have also been used with patients who limit movement of the COM during voluntary sway, suggesting a reduction in perceived stability limits. This can be seen in Figure 11-26, which shows the area of COP displacement in patients following stroke, and neurologically intact adults when they were asked to sway voluntarily in four directions (forward, backward, left, right). The area of perceived stability is also considerably reduced in these patients (Dettman et al., 1987).

Treatment for patients with reduced limits of stability focuses on learning to move the center of mass to various targets within defined limits of stability and then progressively increasing the required distance to reach the targets. Contingent verbal rein-

forcement is given as patients succeed in moving the COM in larger and larger areas. One purpose of this activity is to change perceptions regarding the ability to move the body safely in space.

There is limited evidence that training can influence voluntary excursion of the center of mass. Hamman et al. (1995) examined the effect of a computerized force plate retraining system in improving ability to move the center of mass in two groups of healthy (not balance impaired) adults, aged 20 to 30 years and 60 to 75 years. Subjects were asked to move the center of gravity (COG) cursor to highlighted targets on the computer monitor. Results from this study showed that healthy older adults improved the time taken to move the COG to the highlighted target. Whether this information can be generalized to patients with impaired ability to move the COG is unknown.

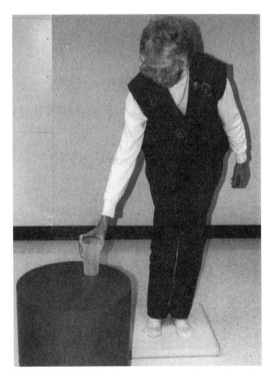

FIGURE 11-25. Training sensory adaptation for postural control. The patient turns to look over her shoulder while standing on foam wearing petroleum jelly-covered glasses to decrease somatosensory and visual inputs and increase reliance on vestibular inputs.

Areas of Stability

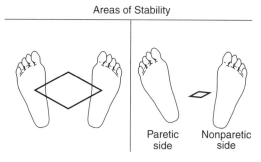

Paretic side   Nonparetic side

A Normal men   B Hemiplegic men

FIGURE 11-26. Poststroke hemiplegic men limit the excursion of the COP during voluntary sway (**B**) more than do normal men (**A**). Participants were asked to sway in each of four directions, forward, backward, left, right. (Adapted with permission from Dettman MA, Linder MT, Sepic SB. Relationships among walking performance, postural stability, and functional assessments of the hemiplegic patient. Am J Phys Med 1987;66:83.)

Intervention at the Functional Task Level

The ability to perform functional movements in a natural (home or community) environment requires the ability to adapt sensory and motor strategies for postural control to changing task and environmental demands. Patients who have a neurological disorder may have difficulty in perceiving relevant factors within a specific task or environment that serve to regulate postural control. Hence they may have difficulty in adapting sensory and movement strategies appropriately. Thus, optimal recovery requires practicing the maintenance of postural control in a wide variety of tasks and environments, which requires adaptation of sensory and motor strategies to changing conditions.

By understanding how various tasks and environments regulate postural control, the clinician can develop a taxonomy of tasks that can be used to guide retraining. When should variability in both task and environmental demands be introduced? As we discussed in Chapter 2, the schema theory of motor learning suggests that the strength of the motor response schema is related to the variability of the task. Remember that a mo-

tor response schema represents the rules and relationships that allow the person to generate a movement or posture that is an appropriate match to the environment. In addition, motor learning and action systems theory also suggests that variability in practice improves retention and transfer of motor skills (Reed, 1982; Schmidt, 1988; Gentile, 1987).

Abreu (1995) examined the effect of environmental predictability on postural control after stroke. The study addressed seated postural stability (defined as the stability of the trajectory of the body COP in both the anteroposterior and mediolateral directions) during a reaching task to two targets that were presented in a predictable versus unpredictable order. They found that in the mediolateral plane, instability of the COP was greatest in the **predictable**, not the unpredictable, reaching task, as was hypothesized. The author suggests that possibly the unpredictable condition requires a greater cognitive effort, which in turn facilitates the development of a more effective movement strategy for postural control. Results from this study suggest that performing postural tasks in unpredictable environments may elicit better postural movement strategies than in predictable environments.

Hanlon (1996) examined whether patients who have had a unilateral stroke learned and retained skills better under random or blocked practice conditions. Hanlon randomly assigned patients aged 26 to 70 years with unilateral cerebrovascular accident to practice a reaching task in random versus blocked conditions. Participants practiced a five-step functional oriented movement sequence (open cupboard door, grasp coffee cup by handle, lift cup off shelf, place on counter, release grasp) 10 times per day. The random practice group practiced the experimental task along with three other upper extremity tasks presented in a random order, while the blocked practice group practiced the experimental task in two blocks of five trials. Results found that the random practice group had significantly better performance on the retention tests than did the blocked practice group, suggesting that random practice was significantly better for learning an upper extremity task following stroke.

These studies suggest that many of the principles of motor learning developed from experiments with healthy, neurologically intact subjects may also apply to patients with neurological injury. Thus, the organization of practice sessions focusing on retraining functional skills related to postural control should incorporate motor learning principles (Chapter 2 reviews these principles).

Putting It All Together

In the task-oriented approach to retraining the patient with postural control problems, therapeutic strategies are used (*a*) to optimize the components of postural control, such as with exercises to improve strength and range of motion; (*b*) to develop and refine task specific sensory and motor strategies used for postural control; and (*c*) to learn to preserve postural control during changing task and environmental conditions.

It is important to realize that one does not work on these goals sequentially but in parallel. Therapeutic strategies for achieving these goals are intertwined; this reciprocal interweaving of exercises, tasks, and activities supports the goals of recovery of postural control, enabling the reestablishment of functional independence.

In addition, rehabilitation of the patient with postural control problems should be organized around learning theory. This will help to ensure that improvements in performance gained through therapy are converted to permanent changes in behavior and retained in varied and novel environments. Patients need to practice the desired behavior (in the case of balance, effective control of the COM) with sufficient duration and intensity to induce plasticity within the central nervous system.

How much practice is enough to induce neural change? Views on this issue are changing. Traditionally practice was restricted to the hours a patient spent in ther-

 LAB ACTIVITY 11-3

OBJECTIVE: Apply the task-oriented approach to retraining posture and balance of a patient with poststroke hemiparesis.

PROCEDURE: Reread the case study in Table 11-5 and your assignment from Lab Activity 11-2. Review the list of functional problems, strategies, and impairments you outlined. Review the sections in this chapter, which summarizes the task-oriented approach to retraining postural control.

ASSIGNMENT: Make a list of short- and long-term goals related to recovery of postural control for Phoebe J. Create a plan of care (including the frequency and duration of your planned treatment) and outline the therapeutic strategies to be used when treating her. Using your plan of care, outline a 60-minute treatment session that details the specific exercises, tasks, and activities to be used in achieving your goals. Finally, recognizing the importance of sustained practice, outline a home program that will enable Phoebe J. to extend her practice time beyond specific therapy sessions.

apy sessions. With increasing awareness that more practice was needed to induce permanent change, patients were given homework, that is, exercises, tasks, and activities to be practiced for varying amounts of time (usually 30 to 60 minutes) daily.

Emerging new views suggest that even this amount of practice may be insufficient to induce permanent change in functional movement behavior in patients following a neurological injury. Edward Taub, a psychologist at the University of Alabama, developed constraint-induced (CI) movement therapy, a new approach to retraining upper limb function based on the concept of learned nonuse (Taub, 1980, 1993). In conjunction with colleagues, he found that significant changes in both the frequency and quality of functional movement of the paretic arm occurred following 10 days of intensive therapy consisting of 6 hours of forced use of the paretic limb; the uninvolved limb was constrained in a sling (Taub et al., 1993; Liepert et al., 1998; Miltner et al., 1999). These authors go on to suggest that the same improvement in function can be found with conventional therapy delivered over the same period and that the critical variable in recovery may not be the nature of the therapy but rather the frequency and intensity with which it is delivered (Liepert et al., 1998).

Motor learning theory also tells us that to optimize motor schemas, practice must occur under varied conditions. Retraining under varied conditions helps a patient learn the principles of postural control rather than a single way to control the center of mass. This ensures that the individual will be able to maintain stability in the face of new and changing task and environmental conditions. The application of this concept can be found in Lab Activity 11-3.

@ EVIDENCE TO SUPPORT THE EFFECT OF BALANCE RETRAINING

Because it is relatively new, we have little evidence examining the effectiveness of a task-oriented approach to the recovery of postural control following a neurological insult. In fact there is limited research examining the effectiveness of training balance (regardless of the approach used) on functional performance and level of disability. Many of the studies examining the effectiveness of balance retraining on improving function and preventing falls have been done with older adults and were reviewed in Chapter 9.

Studies have shown the effectiveness of a physical rehabilitation program in the recovery of function following neurological insult. Because balance retraining is often only one component of a comprehensive physical rehabilitation program, it is difficult to determine its contribution to overall recovery of function. Two studies examining the effectiveness of balance rehabilitation in conjunction with other forms of therapy will be reviewed. The first uses case studies to examine the effect of balance retraining in two

cerebellar patients; the second study uses a randomized control trial to examine the effect of exercise, including balance retraining, following stroke.

Gill-Body et al. (1997) examined the effect of a 6-week staged home-based intervention approach that provided progressive challenges to body stability in standing and walking in two patients with cerebellar dysfunction, a 36-year-old woman with a 7-month history of unsteadiness and dizziness following a surgical resection of a recurrent astrocytoma in the cerebellar vermis and a 48-year-old man with a 10-year history of progressive balance problems due to cerebrotendinous xanthomatosis and diffuse cerebellar atrophy. Patients were seen weekly for outpatient therapy, and they exercised daily at home. The focus of the exercises was on performing activities that challenged postural stability in standing and in walking. Particular emphasis was placed on activities that facilitated the integration of sensory information and control of motor strategies to enhance postural stability. Table 11-6 shows the rehabilitation treatment program and its rationale used with the woman who had a resected cerebellar tumor.

Both clinical (self-report and performance based) and laboratory tests and measures were used to evaluate stance balance and gait before and after treatment. Tests included the Dizziness Handicap Inventory, computed posturography, kinematic analysis of standing balance, and locomotor performance.

Both patients reported improved steadiness during stance and gait (significant improvements on the Dizziness Handicap Index). There was a concomitant improvement on both clinical and laboratory tests of balance. Kinematic analysis showed a decrease in sway in the standing position. Posturography tests showed that the ability to stand under altered sensory conditions improved, as did the ability to respond to external perturbations to balance. The patients could more quickly take a step as needed and were better able to scale the magnitude of postural responses to perturbations of dif-

TABLE 11-6.   Rehabilitation Treatment Program for a Patient With Imbalance and Dizziness Secondary to a Resected Cerebellar Tumor

Rationale	Treatment Activity
Phase 1	
Promote use of VOR and COR for gaze stability	Visual fixation, EO, stationary target, slow head movements
Promote use of saccadic eye movements for gaze stability	Active eye and head movements between two stationary targets
Promote VOR cancellation	EO, moving target with head movement, self-selected speed
Improve ability to use somatosensory and vestibular inputs for postural control	Static stance, EO and EC, feet together, arms close to body, head movements
Improve ability to use vestibular and visual inputs for postural control	Static stance on foam surface, EC intermittently, feet 2.54–5.08 cm (1–2 in) apart
Improve postural contral using all sensory inputs	Gait with narrowed base of support, EO, wide turns to right and left
Improve postural control using visual and vestibular inputs	March in place, EO, on firm and foam surfaces, prolonged pauses in unilateral stance
Phase 2	
Promote use of VOR and COR for gaze stability	Visual fixation, EO, stationary and moving targets, slow and fast speeds, simple static background; imaginary visual fixation, EC
Promote use of saccadic eye movements for gaze stability	Active eye and head movements between two targets, slow and fast speeds
Promote VOR cancellation	EO, moving target with head movement, fast and slow speeds
Improve ability to use somatosensory and vestibular inputs for postural control	Semitandem stance, EO and EC, arms crossed
Improve ability to use vestibular inputs for postural control	Stance on foam, EC intermittently, feet 2.54–5.08 cm apart
Improve postural control using visual and vestibular inputs	Gait with EO with sharp 180° turns to the right and left, firm and padded surfaces
Improve postural control using vestibular and somatosensory inputs	March in place, EC, prolonged pauses in unilateral stance
Improve postural control using all sensory inputs	Walking sideways and backward; standing EO and EC, heel touches forward, toe touches backward
Improve postural control with head moving using all sensory inputs	Gait with EO, normal base of support, slow head movements
Phase 3	
Promote use of VOR and COR for gaze stability	Visual fixation, EO, stationary and moving targets, various speeds, complex static and dynamic backgrounds; imaginary visual fixation, EC
Promote use of saccadic eye movements for gaze stability	Active eye and head movements between two targets, various speeds
Promote VOR cancellation	EO, moving target with head movement, various speeds, complex static and dynamic backgrounds
Improve ability to use somatosensory and vestibular inputs for postural control	Semitandem stance with EC continuously, and with EO on firm and padded surfaces
Improve postural control using vestibular and somatosensory inputs	Gait with EC with base of support progressively narrowed, firm and padded surfaces; march in place slowly, EO and EC on firm and foam surfaces
Improve postural control using visual and vestibular inputs	Gait with EO, rapid sharp turns to right and left, firm and padded surfaces
Improve postural control when head is moving using all sensory inputs	Gait with normal base of support, EO, fast head movements
Improve postural control using all sensory inputs	Braiding; active practice of ankle sway movements; bending and reaching activities

EO, eyes open: EC, eyes closed; VOR, vestibulo-ocular reflex; COR, cervico-ocular reflex.
Reprinted with permission from Gill-Body KM, Popat RA, Parker SW, Krebs DE. Rehabilitation of balance in two patients with cerebellar dysfunction. Phys Ther 1997;77:534–552.

fering sizes. The authors concluded that patients with cerebellar lesions, whether acute or chronic, can significantly improve postural stability by following a structured exercise program (Gill-Body et al., 1997).

Duncan et al. (1998) examined the effect of a structured home-based exercise program that incorporated balance retraining on functional performance in 20 patients who were 30 to 90 days post stroke and who had mild to moderate impairments. Patients were randomly assigned to the experimental home-based exercise program or the usual-care group. The experimental exercise program consisted of 12 weeks of exercise sessions supervised three times a week for 8 weeks and independent for 4 weeks. Exercise sessions lasted 1.5 hours, divided as follows: 10 minutes of warm-up exercises followed by 15 minutes of resistive strength training using proprioceptive neuromuscular facilitation, Theraband (elastic bands), or body weight resistance exercises of major muscle groups; 15 minutes of balance exercises; 15 minutes of functional training of UE, including bimanual tasks; and an aerobic component of progressive walking or progressive bicycle ergometer. The usual-care group received physical therapy and occupational therapy services, either outpatient or home care, that varied in intensity, frequency, and duration. Exercises focused on balance, gait, and functional retraining but included no aerobic conditioning.

Findings were that the experimental home-based group showed significant improvements over the usual-care group on the Fugl Meyer Test (lower extremity function portion) and in gait velocity. The two groups showed equivalent improvements on other measures, including the Berg Balance Test, 6 Minute Walk, Barthel (activities of daily living), Lawton IADL (instrumental activities of daily living), MOS-36 (Medical Outcomes Study Short Form-36), and the Jebson Taylor Hand Function. The authors note that it was difficult to improve aerobic capacity using a home-based program involving walking. There was limited space in the home, and subjects were not safe enough to walk in the community. They stress the importance of showing that home-based postacute rehabilitation is effective in postacute recovery of function following stroke in light of the fact that length of stay in rehabilitation has significantly decreased in the past 5 to 10 years.

The results of these and other studies presented in this chapter are encouraging. They suggest that therapeutic exercises and activities designed for systematic improvement of various aspects of postural control are associated with improved stability. In addition, improvements in balance can have a positive effect on functional skills. More research is needed to examine the effectiveness of balance rehabilitation in general and the task-oriented approach specifically to the recovery of function.

⊘ SUMMARY

1. A task-oriented approach to examining postural control uses a variety of tests, measurements, and observations (*a*) to document functional abilities related to posture and balance control, (*b*) to examine underlying sensory and motor strategies, and (*c*) to determine the underlying sensory, motor, and cognitive systems contributing to postural control.

2. Following completion of the examination, the clinician must interpret results, identifying functional limitations and underlying impairments, and establish the goals and plan of care.

3. The plan of care for retraining postural control in the patient with a neurological deficit varies widely with the constellation of underlying impairments and the degree to which the patient has developed compensatory strategies that are successful in achieving postural demands in functional tasks.

4. The goals of a task-oriented approach to retraining postural control include (*a*) resolution or prevention of impairments, (*b*) development of effective task-specific strategies, and (*c*) adoption of task-specific strategies so that functional tasks can be performed in changing environmental contexts.

5. The goals of interventions aimed at the impairment level are to correct impairments that can be changed and prevent secondary impairments.

6. The goal of intervention at the strategy level is to help patients recover or develop sensory and motor strategies that are effective in meeting the postural demands of functional tasks. This requires that the clinician understand the inherent requirements of the task being performed so those patients can be guided in developing effective strategies for meeting task demands.

7. The goal of intervention at the functional level focuses on having patients practice successfully the performance of a wide variety of functional tasks in many contexts. Since the ability to perform postural tasks in a natural environment requires the ability to modify strategies to changing task and environmental demands, developing adaptive capacities in the patient is a critical part of retraining at the task level.

8. The development of clinical methods based on a systems theory of motor control is just beginning. As systems-based research provides us with an increased understanding of normal and abnormal postural control, new methods for assessing and treating postural disorders will emerge.

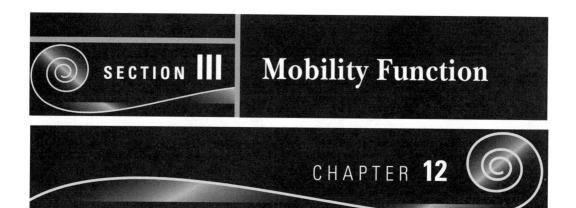

SECTION III — Mobility Function

CHAPTER 12

Control of Normal Mobility

@ INTRODUCTION

A key feature of our independence as human beings is mobility. We define mobility as the ability to independently and safely move oneself from one place to another. Mobility incorporates many types of tasks, including the ability to stand up from a bed or chair, to walk or run, and to navigate through complex environments. During rehabilitation a primary goal of treatment is to help patients regain as much independent mobility as possible. Often, regaining mobility is the primary goal of a patient. This is reflected in the constantly asked question, "Will I walk again?"

In this chapter we discuss many aspects of mobility, including gait, transfers, bed mobility, and stair walking, examining the contributions of the individual, task, and environment to each of these tasks. We begin with a discussion of locomotion, defining the requirements for successful locomotion and discussing the contributions of the different

305

neural and musculoskeletal systems to loco-motor control. In addition, we discuss mechanisms essential for the adaptation of gait to a wide variety of task and environmental conditions. Finally, we consider transitions in mobility, including the initiation of gait and transfers.

Gait is an extraordinarily complex behavior. It involves the entire body and therefore requires the coordination of many muscles and joints. Navigating through complex and cluttered environments requires the use of sensory inputs to assist in the control and adaptation of gait. Finally, locomotor behavior includes the ability to initiate and terminate locomotion, adapt gait to avoid obstacles, and change speed and directions as needed (Patla, 1991). Because of these complexities, understanding both the control of normal gait and the mobility problems of patients with neurological impairments can seem like an overwhelming task.

To simplify the process of understanding the control of gait, we describe a framework for examining gait that we have found useful. The framework is built on understanding the essential requirements of locomotion and how these requirements are translated into goals accomplished during the phases of gait. It is important when examining both normal and abnormal gait to keep in mind both the essential requirements of gait and the conditions that must be met during stance and swing phases of gait to accomplish these requirements.

⊘ ESSENTIAL REQUIREMENTS FOR SUCCESSFUL LOCOMOTION

Locomotion is characterized by three essential requirements: progression, stability, and adaptation (Patla, 1991; Das and McCollum, 1988). **Progression** is ensured through a basic locomotor pattern that produces and coordinates rhythmic patterns of muscle activation in the legs and trunk to move the body in the desired direction. Progression also requires the ability to initiate and termi-nate locomotion and to guide locomotion toward end points that are not necessarily visible (Patla, 1997).

The requirement for **stability** reflects the need to establish and maintain an appropriate posture for locomotion and the demand for dynamic stability of the moving body. Dynamic stability entails counteracting not only the force of gravity but other expected and unexpected forces as well (Patla, 1997).

The third essential requirement of locomotion is the ability to **adapt** gait to meet the goals of the individual and the demands of the environment. Successful locomotion in challenging environments requires that gait patterns be adapted to avoid obstacles, negotiate uneven terrain, and change speed and direction as needed.

Finally, these requirements must be accomplished with strategies that are both energy efficient and effective in minimizing stress to the locomotor apparatus, thus ensuring the long-term structural integrity of the system over the life span of the person (Patla, 1997).

Human gait can be subdivided into a stance (or support) and swing phase. Certain goals must be met during each of these phases of gait to achieve the three task invariants of successful locomotion (progression, stability, and adaptability). During the support phase of gait, we generate both horizontal forces against the support surface to move the body in the desired direction (progression) and vertical forces to support the body mass against gravity (stability). In addition, strategies used to accomplish progression and stability must be flexible to accommodate changes in speed and direction or alterations in the support surface (adaptation).

The goals to be achieved during the swing phase of gait include advancement of the swing leg (progression) and repositioning the limb in preparation for weight acceptance (stability). Both progression and stability require sufficient foot clearance so the toe does not drag on the supporting surface during swing. In addition, strategies used during the swing phase of gait must be sufficiently flexible to allow the swing foot

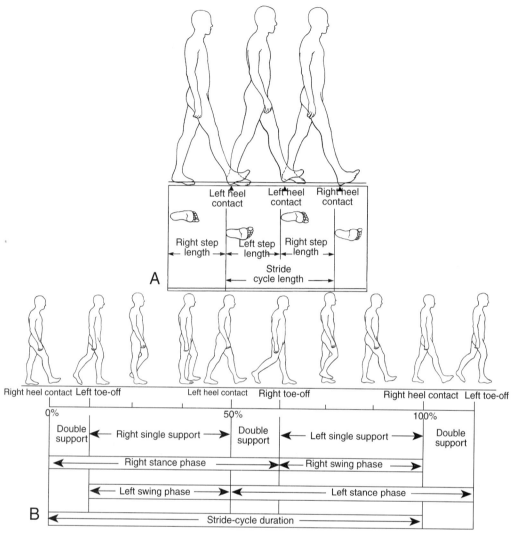

FIGURE 12-1. Temporal and distance dimensions of the gait cycle. (Adapted with permission from Inman VT, Ralston H, Todd F. Human walking. Baltimore: Williams and Wilkins, 1981.)

to avoid any obstacles in its path (adaptation).

The movement strategies used by normal subjects to meet the task requirements of locomotion have been well defined. Kinematic studies describing body motions suggest a similarity in movement strategies across subjects. This is consistent with intuitive observations that we all walk somewhat similarly. In contrast, studies describing the muscles and forces associated with gait suggest that there is a tremendous variation in the way these gait movements are achieved. Thus, there appears to be a wide range of muscle activation patterns used by normal subjects to accomplish the task requirements of gait.

ℰ DESCRIPTION OF THE HUMAN GAIT CYCLE

Think about the human body and the control of gait for a moment. We have discussed the essential requirements for normal gait, that is, progression, stability, and adaptability. The normal human perception–action system has developed elegant control strategies for solving these task requirements.

Although other gait patterns are possible (that is, we can skip, hop, or gallop), humans normally use a symmetrical alternating gait pattern, probably because it provides the greatest dynamic stability for bipedal gait with minimal control demands (Raibert, 1986). Thus, normal locomotion is a bipedal gait in which the limbs move in a symmetrical alternating pattern that can be described by a phase lag of 0.5 (Grillner, 1981).

A phase lag of 0.5 means that one limb initiates its step cycle as the opposite limb reaches the midpoint of its own cycle, as you see in Figure 12-1. Thus, if one complete stride cycle is defined as the time between two ipsilateral foot strikes, such as right heel contact to right heel contact (Fig. 12-1), the contralateral limb begins its cycle midway through the ipsilateral stride cycle.

Traditionally, all descriptions of gait, whether kinematic, electromyographic (EMG), or kinetic, are described with reference to different aspects of the gait cycle. Thus, an understanding of the various phases of gait is necessary for understanding descriptions of normal locomotion.

Phases of the Step Cycle

As we mentioned earlier, the single limb cycle consists of two main phases: stance, which starts when the foot strikes the ground, and swing, which begins when the foot leaves the ground (Fig. 12-1). At freely chosen walking speeds, adults typically spend approximately 60% of the cycle duration in stance and 40% in swing. As you see in Figure 12-1, approximately the first and the last 10% of the stance phase are spent in double support, that is, the period when both feet are in contact with the ground. Single-support phase is the period when only one foot is in contact with the ground, and in walking, this consists of the time when the opposite limb is in swing phase (Murray et al., 1984; Rosenrot et al., 1980).

The stance phase is often further divided into five subphases: (*a*) initial contact, (*b*) the loading response (together taking up

about 10% of the step cycle during double-support phase), (*c*) midstance, (*d*) terminal stance (about 40% of stance phase, which is in single support), and (*e*) preswing (the last 10% of stance, in double support). The swing phase is often divided into three subphases: initial swing, midswing, and terminal swing, all of which are in single support phase and in total make up 40% of the step cycle (DeLuca et al., 1992).

Typically, researchers and clinicians use EMG, kinematic, and kinetic analysis to study gait. For a review of the technology used to analyze gait from these various perspectives, refer to the technology boxes in Chapter 7.

Temporal and Distance Factors

Gait is often described with respect to temporal and distance parameters such as velocity, step length, step frequency (cadence), and stride length (Fig. 12-1). Velocity of gait is defined as the average horizontal speed of the body measured over one or more strides. In the research literature, it is usually reported in the metric system, such as in meters per second (DeLuca et al., 1992). In contrast, in the clinic, gait is usually described in nonmetric terms (feet) and either distance or time. For example, one might report that the patient is able to walk 50 feet or the patient is able to walk continuously for 5 minutes. Because of this difference in convention between the clinic and the lab, we offer information in both metric and nonmetric terms.

Cadence is the number of steps per unit of time, usually reported as steps per minute. Step length is the distance from one foot strike to the foot strike of the other foot. For example, the right step length is the distance from the left heel to the right heel when both feet are in contact with the ground and the right foot is in front. Stride length is the distance covered in two steps, for example from one heel strike to the next heel strike by the same foot. Thus, right stride length is defined by the distance between one right heel strike and the next right heel strike.

Normal and abnormal gait are often described with reference to these variables. When performing clinical assessment, there is an advantage to measuring step length rather than stride length. This is because you won't be able to note any asymmetry in step length if you evaluate only stride length.

How fast do people normally walk? Normal young adults tend to walk about 1.46 m/second (3.26 miles per hour), have a mean cadence (step rate) of 1.9 steps/second (112.5 steps/minute) and a mean step length of 76.3 cm (30.05 inches) (Craik, 1989). The application of this concept can be found in Lab Activity 12-1.

As you probably found, walking velocity is a function of step length and step frequency, or cadence. When people increase walking speed, they typically lengthen their step and increase their pace. Thus, there is a linear relationship between step length and step frequency over a wide range of walking speeds (Grieve, 1968; Inman et al., 1981). However, once an upper limit to step length is reached, continued increases in speed come from step rate.

Although normal adults have a wide range of walking speeds, self-selected speeds tend to stay within a small range of step rates, with averages of about 110 steps/minute for men and about 115 steps/minute for women (Finley and Cody, 1970; Murray et al., 1984). Preferred step rates appear to be related to minimizing energy requirements (Ralston, 1976; Zarrugh et al., 1974). In fact, it has been found that in locomotion we exploit the pendular properties of the leg and elastic properties of the muscles. Thus, swing phase requires little energy expenditure. A person's comfortable or preferred walking speed is at his or her point of minimal energy expenditure per unit distance. At slower or higher speeds, passive pendular models of gait break down, and much more energy expenditure is required (Mochon and McMahon, 1980).

As we increase walking speed, the proportion of time spent in swing and stance changes, with stance phase becoming shorter in relation to swing (Herman et al., 1976; Murray, 1967). Finally, the stance-to-swing proportions shift from the 60:40 dis-

 LAB ACTIVITY 12-1

OBJECTIVE: To learn to calculate temporal and distance parameters of gait.

PROCEDURE: Materials needed for this lab: roll of white paper 0.5 m (18 to 20 inches) wide, moleskin cut into 1-inch triangles and squares, one bottle each of red and blue water-soluble ink, masking tape, cotton swabs, and a stopwatch. Tape a strip of paper 6 m (20 feet) long to the floor at the beginning of each trial. Seat the subject on a chair at one end of the paper. Place one triangle and one square of moleskin on the approximate midline of the sole of each shoe, on the toe and heel respectively. Use red ink to saturate the moleskin on the right shoe and blue ink to saturate the moleskin on the left shoe. Have your subject walk down the paper pathway at a comfortable pace. Use the stopwatch to record the time to walk the entire length of the paper. Repeat these procedures, asking subjects to walk at their fastest pace. You may wish to repeat the lab, asking subjects to walk with a variety of assistive devices, such as a cane or walker.

ASSIGNMENT: From the ink prints on the paper, calculate the following for each leg:

1. Step length: vertical distance between heel marker of one foot and the next heel marker of the opposite foot
2. Stride length: vertical distance between heel marker of one foot and heel marker of the **same** foot on the next step
3. Step width: horizontal distance between heel markers of one foot and the next foot
4. Cadence: number of steps taken per unit of time (the amount of time taken to walk across the paper divided by the total number of steps)

Establish norms (means and standard deviations) for each of these parameters for your subjects. Compare your norms to those presented in this chapter. How do spatial and temporal factors change as a function of gait speed? How do they change if an assistive device is used for gait? (This lab activity is adapted from Boenig, 1977).

tribution of walking to 40:60 distribution as running velocities are reached. Double support time also disappears during running.

As walking speed slows, stance time increases, while swing times remain relatively constant. The double support phase of stance increases most. For example, double support takes up 25% of the cycle time with step durations of about 1.1 seconds and 50% of the cycle time when cycle duration increases to about 2.5 seconds (Herman et al., 1976). In addition, variability increases at lower speeds, probably because of decreased postural stability during the single support period, which also lengthens with slower speeds.

Within an individual, joint angle patterns and EMG patterns of lower extremity muscles are quite stable across a range of speeds, but the amplitude of muscle responses increases with faster speeds (Murray et al., 1966; Winter, 1983; Zarrugh et al., 1974). In contrast, joint torque patterns appear more variable, though they also show gain increases as walking velocity increases.

Kinematic Description of Gait

Another way of describing normal versus abnormal gait is through the kinematics of the gait cycle, that is, the movement of the joints and segments of the body through space. Figure 12-2 shows the normal movements of the pelvis, hip, knee, and ankle in the sagittal, frontal, and transverse planes (DeLuca et al., 1992).

The elegant coordination of motion at all of the joints ensures the first requirement of gait: the smooth forward progression of the center of body mass. While motion at each individual joint is quite large, the coordinated action of motion across all of the joints results in the smooth forward progression of the body.

In the 1950s Saunders and colleagues wrote a paper that has significantly affected our ideas regarding the determinants of normal and pathological gait (Saunders et al., 1953). In that paper they identified "determinants" of normal walking that they proposed were responsible for saving the body energy by minimizing the displacement of the body's center of gravity during gait. This theory is based on simple kinematic arguments. For example, it was noted that if one measured sagittal-plane hip motion during gait, one would see a large amount of flexion and extension (Fig. 12-2). It was proposed that if gait were accomplished solely through these hip movements, the center of mass (COM) would follow these large motions of the hip, and you would see large vertical displacements of the COM. This so-called compass gait is seen in people who walk with a stiff knee (Perry, 1992).

According to the theory, the addition of pelvic rotation about the vertical axis to motion at the hip would change the gait pattern, allowing stride length to increase and the amplitude of the sinusoidal oscillations of the COM to decrease. It was suggested that this should result in a smoother path of the COM and a less abrupt transition from step to step.

It was also proposed that the addition of pelvic tilt (rotation of the pelvis about an anteroposterior axis) would flatten the path of the COM even further. Pelvic tilt occurs during swing, when the swing hip lowers in preparation for toe-off. In normal gait, a lateral shift in the pelvis occurs as stance is changed from one limb to another. The width of the step contributes to the magnitude of the lateral shift of the COM.

It was next proposed that the addition of knee flexion would significantly improve the coordinated efficiency of gait, with knee flexion during stance further flattening the vertical movements of the COM and knee flexion during swing shortening the vertical length of the swing limb and allowing the foot to clear the ground.

Furthermore, it was proposed that ankle motion also makes an important contribution to smooth gait (Fig. 12-2). In particular, plantar flexion of the stance ankle would allow a smooth transition from step to step and contribute to the initial velocity of the swing limb (Perry, 1992).

It was also proposed that motion at the three major articulations within the foot is also important in the control of progression and stability during gait. For example, the subtalar joint, the junction between the talus and calcaneus, allows the foot to tilt medially (inversion) and laterally (eversion). Eversion of the foot begins as part of the loading

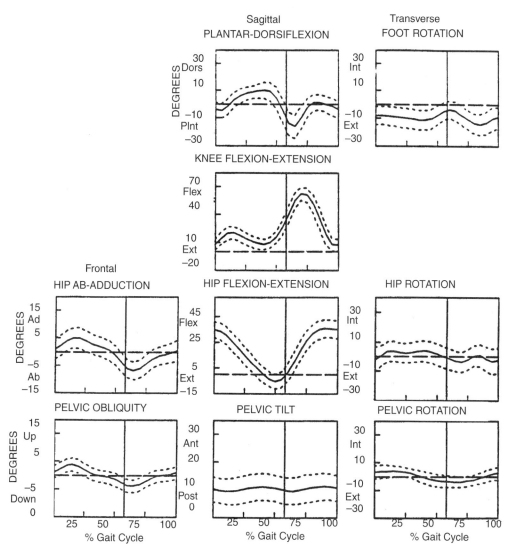

FIGURE 12-2.   Normal movements of the pelvis, hip, knee, and ankle in sagittal, frontal, and transverse planes during the gait cycle. (Adapted with permission from DeLuca PA, Perry JP, Ounpuu S. The fundamentals of normal walking and pathological gait. AACP and DM Inst. Course 2. 1992.)

response, immediately after heel strike, and reaches its peak by early midstance. Following this, the motion slowly reverses, reaching the peak of inversion at the onset of preswing. During swing, the foot drifts back to neutral and then into inversion just before heel strike. Subtalar motion is an essential component of shock absorption during limb loading. In addition, rigidity in this area contributes to foot stability as weight is transferred to the forefoot in terminal stance.

The midtarsal joint is the junction of the hindfoot and forefoot. During loading, the arch flattens quickly; this should allow forefoot contact and thus contribute to shock absorption. Finally, motion at the metatarsophalangeal joints would allow the foot to roll over the metatarsal heads rather than the tips of the toes during terminal stance (Perry, 1992).

Researchers have noted that this theory of the determinants of gait has a logical appeal, but for many years little research tested the theory rigorously (Vaughan and Sussman, 1993). However, recent work has begun to investigate whether the gait determinants reduce the vertical movement of the body during walking, thus decreasing the energy cost. Gard and Childress (1997, 1999) investigated one of the determinants of gait, pelvic obliquity, to determine its effect on the trunk's vertical displacement during walking. Contrary to the predictions of Saunders et al. (1953), they found that pelvic obliquity did not significantly decrease the peak-to-peak vertical movement of the trunk but simply reduced the mean elevation of the trunk by 2 to 4 mm and shifted the phase of the vertical displacement of the trunk by about 10 to 15 degrees (Gard and Childress, 1997).

They also examined a second determinant of gait, stance phase knee flexion, and found that it did not significantly decrease the amplitude of the trunk's vertical displacement. Their data and previous work by others support the concept that stance phase knee flexion serves a different function, shock absorption (Gard and Childress, 1999; Lafortune et al., 1996).

Walking is energy efficient, but what is responsible for this efficiency? Saunders et al. (1953) suggested that minimization of vertical COM motion is responsible for energy-efficient gait. However, Farley and Ferris (1998) suggest that it is not minimizing vertical COM motion that reduces the metabolic cost of walking but the smooth mechanical transfer of kinetic and gravitational energies. In fact, the COM must fluctuate in a sinusoidal fashion to achieve efficient transfer of mechanical energy. Research has shown that during walking the body vaults over a relatively stiff stance limb and the COM reaches its highest point at the middle of the stance phase. Thus, the gravitational potential energy of the COM is at its highest during midstance phase. In contrast, the kinetic energy of the COM reaches its minimum value at midstance, since the horizontal ground reaction force decelerates the body during the first half of the stance phase and accelerates it during the second half of the stance phase (Farley and Ferris, 1998).

In summary, the step cycle is made up of a complex series of joint rotations, which when coordinated into a whole, provide for a smooth forward progression of the COM. Though Saunders et al. (1953) originally predicted that this reduced the energy cost of walking, it is now clear that it is other factors, such as the transfer of mechanical energy, which require sinusoidal fluctuation of the COM, that reduce the metabolic cost of walking.

The application of this concept can be found in Lab Activity 12-2.

Muscle Activation Patterns

Next, we examine the muscle responses during locomotion in terms of their function at each point in the step cycle (Basmajian and De Luca, 1985; DeLuca et al., 1992). Despite the variability between subjects and conditions in the EMG patterns that underlie a typical step cycle, certain basic characteristics have been identified.

In general, muscles in the stance limb act to support the body (stability) and propel it forward (progression). Muscle activity in the swing limb is largely confined to the beginning and end of the swing phase, since the leg swings much like a jointed pendulum under the influence of gravity (McMahon, 1984). Typical EMG patterns during the different phases of the step cycle are shown in Figure 12-3.

Remember, there are two goals to be accomplished during the stance phase: (*a*) securing the stance limb against the impact force of foot strike and supporting the body against the force of gravity (stability), and (*b*) subsequent generation of force, to propel the body forward into the next step (progression).

To accomplish the first goal, that is, absorb impact for postural stability, knee flexion occurs at the initiation of stance, and there is a distribution of the impact of foot strike from heel contact to the foot-flat stance. At the initiation of stance, eccentric activation of the knee extensors (quadriceps) controls the small knee flexion wave that is used to absorb the impact of foot strike. Eccentric activation of the ankle dor-

LAB ACTIVITY 12-2

OBJECTIVE: To begin to learn to observe the kinematics of gait.

PROCEDURE: You need a large room where your partner can walk for 20 to 30 feet and you can observe him or her from the side (sagittal plane). Your partner should wear shorts. Have your partner walk back and forth. Choose a reference leg, and observe the following from the sagittal plane:

1. Observe stance versus swing phase of gait.
2. Within the stance phase, identify heel strike, midstance, and push-off.
3. Within the swing phase, identify early swing and late swing.
4. Observe the hip at these five points in the gait cycle and determine whether the hip is flexed, extended, or in a neutral position (thigh segment vertical).
5. Observe the knee at these five points in the gait cycle and determine whether the knee is flexed or extended.
6. Observe the ankle at these five points in the gait cycle and determine whether the ankle is dorsiflexed, plantarflexed, or neutral (90 degrees).

ASSIGNMENT: Create a graph that plots angular change at each of the three joints as a function of the events observed in the gait cycle. Create a graph for each joint similar to the ones shown in Figure 12-2. On the x-axis mark the five events you were observing across the step cycle. On the y-axis is the angular displacement of the joint. Represent neutral by a line. Flexion of the joint is above the line, and extension is below the line. Roughly graph the motions you observed at each of the three joints on the graphs. Now compare your results with those found in Figure 12-2. How closely do your graphs approximate those shown in Figure 12-2? If your graphs differ significantly from those shown in 12-2, observe your partner walking again and determine why there is a discrepancy between the two. Is your partner walking with an atypical gait? Alternatively, were there errors in your observations?

siflexors (anterior tibialis) decelerates the foot upon touchdown, opposing and slowing the plantar flexion that results from heel strike. Thus, both muscle groups initially act to oppose the direction of motion. In addi-

tion, postural stability during the stance phase involves activating extensor muscles at the hip, knee, and ankle, which keeps the body from collapsing under the force of gravity. Activation of the hip extensor muscles controls forward motion of the head, arm, and trunk as well. By midstance, the quadriceps is predominantly inactive, as are the pretibial muscles.

The second goal in the stance phase is generating a propulsive force to keep the body in motion. The most common strategy used to generate propulsive forces for progression involves the concentric contraction of the plantarflexors (gastrocnemius and soleus) at the end of stance phase of gait. The ability of the body to move freely over the foot in conjunction with the concentric contraction of the gastrocnemius means the COM of the body will be anterior to the supporting foot by the end of stance, creating a forward fall critical to progression. The hip and knee extensors (hamstrings and quadriceps, respectively) may exhibit a burst of activity late in stance as a contribution to propulsion. This activity, however, typically is less important than the activity observed during the impact absorption phase.

The primary goal to be accomplished in the swing phase of gait is to reposition the limb for continued forward progression. This requires both accelerating the limb forward and making sure the toe clears the ground.

Forward acceleration of the thigh in the early swing phase is associated with a concentric contraction of the quadriceps (Fig. 12-3*B*, part 1). By midswing, however, the quadriceps is virtually inactive as the leg swings through, much like a pendulum driven by an impulse force at the beginning of swing phase. However, the iliopsoas contracts to aid in this forward motion, as shown in Figure 12-3*B*, parts 2 and 3. The hamstrings become active at the end of swing to slow the forward rotation of the thigh in preparation for foot strike (Fig. 12-3*B*, part 4). Knee extension at the end of swing in preparation for loading the limb for stance phase occurs not as the result of muscle ac-

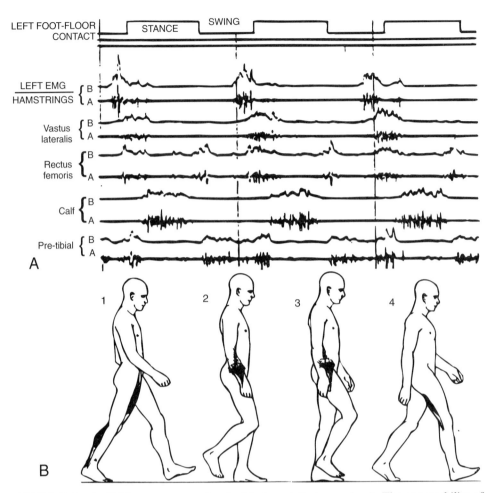

FIGURE 12-3. **A.** EMG patterns associated with the adult step cycle. **A.** The repeatability of muscle activity across three gait cycles. *A,* Raw EMG. *B,* Rectified and integrated EMG. All muscles are recorded from the left leg. The vertical lines are left foot-to-floor contact. **B.** Muscle activity from toe-off until heel strike: *1.* Plantarflexors rotate the foot around the ankle and quadriceps straighten the knee, generating a ground reaction force that propels the body forward. *2, 3.* Contraction of the iliopsoas tugs the right leg forward while the knee flexes passively. *4.* Hamstrings contract near the end of swing to brake the movement and the heel strikes. (**A** adapted with permission from Murray MP, Mollinger LA, Gardner GM, Sepic SB. Kinematic and EMG patterns during slow, free, and fast walking. J Orthop Res 1984;2: 272–280. B adapted with permission from Lovejoy Co. Evolution of human walking. Scientific American 1988;5:121.)

tivity but as the result of passive nonmuscular forces (Winter, 1984).

Foot clearance is accomplished through flexion at the hip, knee, and ankle, which results in an overall shortening of the swing limb compared to the stance limb. Again, flexion of the hip is accomplished through activation of the quadriceps muscle. Flexion at the knee is accomplished passively, since rapid acceleration of the thigh will also produce flexion at the knee. Activation of the pretibial muscles produces ankle dorsiflexion late in swing to ensure toe clearance and to prepare for the next footfall.

Joint Kinetics

Thus far, we have examined the kinematics or movements of the body during the step cycle and looked at the patterns of muscle activity in each of the phases of gait. What are the typical forces that these movements and muscle responses create during locomotion? The dominant forces at a joint do not necessarily mirror the movements of the joint, as you will see in the discussion that follows.

Determination of the forces generated during the step cycle is considered a kinetic analysis. The kinetic or force parameters associated with the normal gait pattern are less stereotyped than the kinematic or movement parameters. The active and passive muscle forces (called joint moments) that generate locomotion are themselves quite variable.

Stance Phase

Remember, the goals during stance phase include stabilizing the limb for weight acceptance and shock absorption and generating propulsive forces for continued motion. Fig. 12-4 shows the averaged joint angle and joint moment changes observed during one stride cycle. Note that the support moment (top trace of joint moment graph) during the stance phase of the step cycle (0 to 60% of stride) is the algebraic sum of the joint moments at the hip, knee, and ankle (lower traces) (Winter, 1980). This net extensor moment keeps the limb from collapsing while bearing weight, allowing stabilization of the body and thus accomplishing the stability requirements of locomotion.

However, researchers have shown that people use a wide variety of force-generating strategies to accomplish this net extensor moment. For example, one strategy for achieving a net extensor moment involves use of a dominant hip extensor moment to counter a knee flexor moment. Alternatively, a knee and ankle extensor moment can be combined to counterbalance a hip flexor moment and still maintain the net extensor support moment (Winter, 1980, 1984, 1990; Winter et al., 1990).

Why is it important to have this flexibility in the individual contributions of joint torques to the net extensor moment? Apparently this flexibility in the way torques are generated is important to controlling balance during gait.

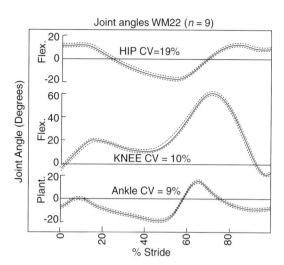

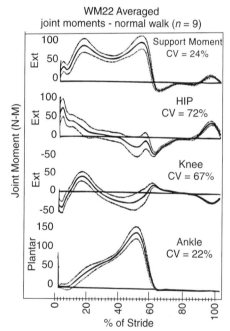

FIGURE 12-4. *Top.* Joint angle changes in the hip, knee, and ankle associated with the adult step cycle. *Bottom.* Individual joint moments (ankle, knee, hip) and the net support moment associated with the adult step cycle. Stance phase is approximately the first 60% of the cycle. CV, coefficient of variation. (Adapted with permission from Winter DA. Kinematic and kinetic patterns of human gait: variability and compensating effects. Human Movement Science 1984;3:51–76.)

Winter and his colleagues have researched gait extensively and suggest that balance during unperturbed gait is very different from balance during stance (Winter et al., 1991). In walking, the center of gravity does not stay within the support base of the feet and thus the body is in a continuous state of imbalance. The only way to prevent falling is to place the swinging foot ahead of and lateral to the center of gravity as it moves forward.

In addition, the mass of the head, arms, and trunk, called the HAT segment, must be regulated with respect to the hips, since the HAT segment represents a large inertial load to keep upright. Winter and colleagues propose that the dynamic balance of the HAT is the responsibility of the hip muscles, with almost no involvement of the ankle muscles. They suggest that this is because the hip has a much smaller inertial load to control, that of the HAT segment, as compared to the ankles, which have to control the entire body. Thus, they propose that balance during ongoing gait is different from stance balance control, which relies primarily on ankle muscles (Winter et al., 1991).

They note that the hip muscles are also involved in a separate task, contributing to the extensor support moment necessary during stance, and view the muscles controlling the HAT segment and those controlling the extensor support moment as two separate synergies. We mentioned earlier that the net extensor moment of the ankle, knee, and hip joints during stance was always the same, but the individual moments were highly variable from stride to stride and individual to individual. One reason for this variability is so that the balance control system can continuously alter the anterior and posterior motor patterns on a step-to-step basis. However, the hip balance adjustments must be compensated for by appropriate knee moments to preserve the net extensor moment essential for the stance phase of gait (Winter, 1990; Winter et al., 1991).

Swing Phase

The major goal during swing is to reposition the limb, making sure the toe clears the ground. Researchers have found that the joint moment patterns during the swing phase are less variable than during stance phase, indicating that adults use fairly simi-

lar force-generating patterns to accomplish this task. This is illustrated by the large standard deviations around the mean joint torques during stance (0 to 60% of stride) as compared to the small standard deviations in swing (60% to 100% of stride), shown in Figure 12-4, bottom graph.

At normal walking speeds, early in swing, a flexor moment at the hip contributes to flexion of the thigh. Early hip flexion is assisted by gravity, reducing the need for a large flexor hip joint moment.

Once swing phase has been initiated, it is often sustained by momentum. Then, as swing phase ends, an extensor joint moment may be required to slow the thigh rotation and prepare for heel strike (Woollacott and Jensen, 1996). Thus, even though the thigh is still flexing, there is an extensor moment on the thigh at this point.

What controls knee motions during swing? Interestingly, during swing, joint torque at the knee is used to constrain rather than generate knee motion. In early swing, an extensor moment slows knee joint flexion and contributes to reversal of the knee joint from flexion to extension. Later in swing, a flexor knee joint moment slows knee extension to prepare for foot placement (Winter, 1980, 1983; Cavanagh and Gregor, 1975).

At the end of swing phase and during the initial part of stance phase, a small dorsiflexing ankle moment helps control plantarflexion at heel strike. So even though the ankle motion is plantarflexion, the ankle joint force is a dorsiflexion moment.

Moving through the stance phase, ankle plantarflexion moment increases to a maximum point just after knee flexion, when the ankle begins to plantarflex. The ankle joint torque is the largest of all of the moments of the lower limb and is the main contributor to the acceleration of the limb into swing phase.

Therefore, many of these examples show that the joint torque is opposite that of the limb movement itself. In other words, the joint torque shows us that the combined forces may be acting to brake the movement or control footfall, rather than simply accelerate the limb.

@ CONTROL MECHANISMS FOR GAIT

How is locomotor coordination achieved? What control mechanisms ensure that the task requirements are met for successful locomotion? Much of the research examining the neural and nonneural control mechanisms essential for locomotion has been done with animals. It is through this research on locomotion in animals that scientists have learned about pattern formation in locomotion, the integration of postural control to the locomotor pattern, the contribution of peripheral and central mechanisms to adaptation and modulation of gait, and the role of the various senses in controlling locomotion.

The following section reviews some of the research on locomotor control in animals, relating it to experiments examining the neural control of locomotion in humans.

Pattern Generators for Gait

Research in the past 25 years has greatly increased our understanding of the nervous system's control of the basic rhythmic movements underlying locomotion. Results of these studies indicate that central pattern generators within the spinal cord play an important role in the production of these movements (Grillner, 1973; Smith, 1980; Wallen, 1995). A rich history of research has enhanced our understanding of the neural basis of locomotion.

In the late 1800s, Sherrington and Mott (Sherrington, 1898; Mott and Sherrington, 1895) performed some of the first experiments to determine the neural control of locomotion. They severed the spinal cord of animals to eliminate the influence of higher brain centers and found that the hindlimbs continued to exhibit alternating movements.

In a second set of experiments, in monkeys, they cut the sensory nerve roots on one side of the spinal cord, eliminating sensory inputs to stepping on one side of the body. They found that the monkeys did not use the deafferented limbs during walking. This led them to the conclusion that locomotion required sensory input. They created a model of locomotor control that attributed the control of locomotion to a set of reflex chains, with the output from one phase of the step cycle acting as a reflexive sensory stimulus to activate the next phase.

Graham Brown (1911) performed an experiment only a few years later showing the opposite result. He found that by making bilateral dorsal (sensory) root lesions in spinalized animals, he could see rhythmic walking movements. Why did the two labs get different results? It appears that it is because Sherrington cut sensory roots on only one side of the spinal cord, not both.

In more recent experiments, Taub and Berman (1968) found that animals did not use a limb when the dorsal roots were cut on one side of the body but would begin to use the limb again when dorsal roots on the remaining side were sectioned. Why? Since the animal has appropriate input coming in from one limb and no sensation from the other, the animal prefers not to use it. Interestingly, researchers have found that they can make animals use a single deafferented limb by restraining the intact limb. These results are the rationale behind a therapy approach called the constraint-induced (or forced use) paradigm. In this approach, hemiplegic patients are forced to use their hemiplegic arm, since the intact side is restrained (Wolf et al., 1989; Taub et al., 1993).

Recent studies have confirmed and extended the results of Graham Brown. These studies have found that muscle activity in spinalized cats is similar to that seen in normal cats walking on a treadmill (Forssberg et al., 1977), with the extensor muscles of the knee and ankle activated prior to paw contact in stance phase. This demonstrates that extension is not simply a reflex response to contact but is part of a central program. In addition, the spinalized cat is capable of fully recruiting motor units within the spinal cord when increasing gait from a walk to a gallop (Smith et al., 1979).

Can a spinalized cat adapt the step cycle to clear obstacles? Yes. If a glass rod touches the top of the cat's paw during swing phase, it activates a flexion response in the stimulated leg, with simultaneous extension of the contralateral leg. This lifts the swing leg up and over the obstacle and gives postural support in the opposite leg. Interestingly, the exact same stimulation of the dorsal surface of the paw during stance causes increased extension, probably to get the paw quickly out of the way of the obstacle. Thus, the identical stimulus to the skin activates functionally separate sets of muscles during different phases of the step cycle, to compensate appropriately for different obstacles perturbing the movement of the paw (Forssberg et al., 1977).

Research using the lamprey to study the pattern-generating circuits in the spinal cord has shown that different network units are precisely coordinated to achieve a proper timing of the different muscle groups. The spinal circuitry has been characterized in great detail in this simple vertebrate. Studies have shown that different modulatory systems act upon the networks to change the rate of burst activity. For example, brainstem systems activate two types of glutamate receptors (NMDA [*N*-methyl D-aspartate] and non-NMDA) within the spinal network to activate locomotion. The relative amount of activation of these two types of receptors determines the rate of burst activity. In addition, serotonin systems reduce the burst rate (Wallen, 1995).

As you can see from this research, although the spinal pattern generators are able to produce stereotyped locomotor patterns and perform certain adaptive functions, descending pathways from higher centers and sensory feedback from the periphery allow the rich variation in locomotor patterns and adaptability to task and environmental conditions.

Descending Influences

Descending influences from higher brain centers are also important in the control of locomotor activity. Much research has focused on identifying the roles of higher centers in controlling locomotion, through transecting the brain of animals along the neuraxis and observing the subsequent locomotor behavior (Patla, 1991). The three preparations that are most often studied are the spinal, the decerebrate, and the decorticate preparations, as in Figure 12-5.

In the spinal preparation (which can be made at a level to allow the observation of only the hind limbs or of all four limbs as part of the preparation), one needs an external stimulus to produce locomotor behavior. This can be either electrical or pharmacological.

The decerebrate preparation leaves the spinal cord, brainstem, and cerebellum intact. An area in the brainstem called the mesencephalic locomotor region appears to be important in the descending control of locomotion. Decerebrate cats do not normally walk on a treadmill, but they begin to walk normally when tonic electrical stimulation is applied to the mesencephalic locomotor region (Shik et al., 1966). Weight support and active propulsion are locomotor characteristics seen in this preparation.

When spinal pattern–generating circuits are stimulated by tonic activation, they produce, at best, a bad caricature of walking because of the lack of important modulating influences from the brainstem and cerebellum. This is because normally, within each step cycle, the cerebellum sends modulating signals to the brainstem that are relayed to the spinal cord via the vestibulospinal, rubrospinal, and reticulospinal pathways, which act directly on motor neurons, to fine-tune the movements according to the needs of the task (Grillner and Zangger, 1979).

The cerebellum also may have an important role in modulation of the step cycle. Experiments suggest that two tracts are involved in this modulation. First, the dorsal spinocerebellar tract is hypothesized to send information from muscle afferents to the cerebellum and is phasically active during locomotion. Second, the ventral spinocerebellar tract is hypothesized to receive information from spinal neurons concerning the central pattern generator output and to send this information to the cerebellum (Arshavsky et al., 1972a, b).

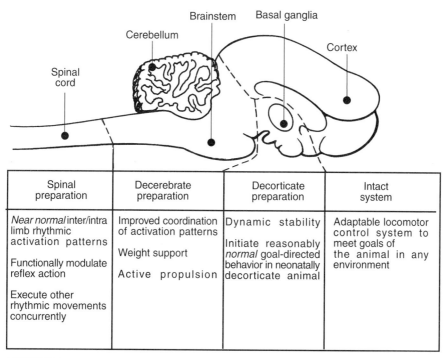

FIGURE 12-5.   Diagram of the brain and spinal cord showing the sites of lesions used in the study of the contributions of various neural subsystems to gait. (Adapted with permission from Patla AE. Understanding the control of human locomotion: a prologue. In: Patla AE, ed. Adaptability of human gait. Amsterdam: North-Holland, 1991:7.)

It is possible that the cerebellum has an additional role in the modulation of the step cycle. It has been hypothesized that the cerebellum may also modulate activity, not to correct error but to alter stepping patterns. For example, as an animal crosses uneven terrain, the legs must be lifted higher or not so high depending on visual cues about the obstacles encountered. The muscle response patterns may be modulated through the following steps. First, the locomotor rhythm is conveyed to the cerebellum. The cerebellum extrapolates to specify when the next flexion or extension is to occur. The cerebellum facilitates descending commands that originate from visual inputs to alter the flexion or extension phase at precisely the correct time (Keele and Ivry, 1990).

The decorticate preparation also leaves the basal ganglia intact, with only the cerebral cortex removed. In this preparation, an external stimulus is not required to produce locomotor behavior, and the behavior is reasonably normal goal-directed behavior. However, the cortex is important in skills such as walking over uneven terrain.

In this preparation vision may have a major role in modulating locomotor outputs. As reviewed in Chapter 3, the two major pathways involved in visual processing from the primary visual cortex go to the posterior parietal cortex and inferotemporal cortex, often called the "where and what" pathways, or more recently, the "perception and action" pathways (Milner and Goodale, 1993). These pathways help us visually recognize objects and events from different viewpoints and process this information from an egocentric perspective so that we can move efficiently in space. In addition, visual input to the superior colliculus is involved in orienting to novel stimuli in the visual field.

It has been hypothesized that the hippocampus is the site that codes topological information, while the parietal cortex (receiving visual and somatosensory information) provides a metric representation of three-dimensional space. The frontal cortex, along with the basal ganglia, would transform this information into appropriate spatially directed locomotor movements in an egocentric frame (Paillard, 1987; Patla, 1997).

Sensory Feedback and Adaptation of Gait

One of the requirements of normal locomotion is the ability to adapt gait to a wide-ranging set of environments. Sensory information from all of the senses is critical to our ability to modify how we walk. In animals, when all sensory information is taken away, stepping patterns tend to be very slow and stereotyped. The animal can neither maintain balance nor modify its stepping patterns to make gait truly functional. Gait ataxia is a common consequence among patients with sensory loss, particularly loss of proprioceptive information from the lower extremities (Sudarsky and Ronthal, 1992).

There are two ways that equilibrium is controlled during locomotion: reactively and proactively. One uses the reactive mode when, for example, there is an unexpected disturbance, such as a slip or a trip. One uses the proactive mode to anticipate potential disruptions to gait and modify movement to minimize the disruption. As in stance, the somatosensory, visual, and vestibular systems all play a role in reactive and proactive postural control of locomotion. The next section describes how sensory information is used to modify ongoing gait.

Reactive Strategies for Modifying Gait

All three sensory systems—somatosensory, visual, and vestibular—contribute to reactive

or feedback control of gait. Research on animals and humans has contributed to our understanding of the somatosensory contributions to gait.

Somatosensory Systems

Researchers have shown that animals that have been both spinalized and deafferented can continuously generate rhythmic alternating contractions in muscles of all of the joints of the leg, with a pattern similar to that seen in the normal step cycle (Grillner and Zangger, 1979). Does this mean that sensory information plays no role in the control of locomotion? No. Though these experiments have shown that animals can still walk in the absence of sensory feedback from the limbs, the movements show characteristic differences from those in the normal animal. These differences help us understand the role that sensory input plays in the control of locomotion (Smith, 1980).

First, sensory information from the limbs contributes to appropriate stepping frequency. For example, the duration of the step cycle is significantly longer in deafferented cats than in a chronic spinal cat without deafferentation.

Second, joint receptors and muscle spindle afferents from the stretched hip flexors appear to play a critical role in normal locomotion, with the position of the ipsilateral hip joint contributing to the onset of swing phase (Smith, 1980; Grillner and Rossignol, 1978; Pearson, 1995). Studies on decerebrate cats have shown that input from muscle spindles can reset the locomotor rhythm. Activation of both ankle extensor Ia afferents and group II flexor afferents both reset the rhythm to extension in fictive locomotion. In addition, small movements about the hip joint produce entrainment of the locomotor rhythm. This continues after anesthesia of the joint capsule and gradually reduces in strength when more hip muscles are denervated. This suggests that afferents from muscles around the hip influence the rhythm-generating neurons (Pearson, 1995).

The Golgi tendon organ (GTO) afferents (the Ib afferents) from the leg extensor muscles also can strongly influence the timing of the locomotor rhythm by inhibiting flexor burst activity and promoting extensor activity. A decline in their activity at the end of the stance phase may be involved in regulating the transition from stance to swing. In addition, they may provide a mechanism for automatically compensating for changes in loads carried by extensor muscles. For example, when one walks up an incline, the load increase on the extensor muscles increases the feedback from the GTOs and automatically increases the activity in the extensor motor neurons. Note that this activity of the GTOs is exactly the opposite of their activity when they are activated passively, when the animal is at rest. At rest, the GTOs inhibit their own muscle and excite the antagonist muscles, while during locomotion they excite their own muscle and inhibit antagonists (Pearson et al., 1992; Pearson, 1995).

Third, cutaneous information from the paw of the chronic spinal cat has a powerful influence on the spinal pattern generator in helping the animal navigate over obstacles, as mentioned earlier (Forssberg et al., 1977).

Human research, similar to animal research, has shown that reflexes are highly modulated in locomotion during each phase of the step cycle to adapt them functionally to the requirements of each phase (Stein, 1991). Stretch reflexes in the ankle extensor muscles are small in the early part of the stance phase of locomotion, since this is the time that the body is rotating over the foot and stretching the ankle extensors. A large reflex at this phase of the step cycle would slow or even reverse forward momentum.

On the other hand, the stretch reflex is large when the COM is in front of the foot during the last part of stance phase, since this is the time when the reflex can help in propelling the body forward. This phase-appropriate modulation of the stretch reflex is well suited to the requirements of the task of locomotion as compared to stance. Stretch reflex gains are further reduced in running, probably because a high gain reflex response would destabilize the gait in running. Stretch reflex gain changes alter quickly (within 150 msec) as a person moves from

stance to walking to running (Stein, 1991).

As was shown in research on cats, cutaneous reflexes actually showed a complete reversal from excitation to inhibition during the different phases of the step cycle. For example, in the first part of swing phase, when the tibialis anterior is active, the foot is in the air and little cutaneous input would be expected unless the foot strikes an object. If this happens, a rapid flexion is necessary to lift the foot over the object to prevent tripping. This is when the reflex is excitatory to the tibialis anterior. However, in the second tibialis anterior burst, the foot is about to contact the ground, a time when a lot of cutaneous input occurs. Limb flexion would not be appropriate at this time, since the limb is needed to support the body. In addition, at this time the reflex shows inhibition of the tibialis anterior (Stein, 1991).

These studies have shown that spinal reflexes can be appropriately integrated into different phases of the step cycle to remain functionally adaptive. The same outcome occurs in the integration of compensatory automatic postural adjustments into the step cycle. Studies were performed in which subjects walked across a platform that could be perturbed at various points in the step cycle. Results showed that automatic postural responses were incorporated appropriately into the different step cycle phases (Nashner, 1980). For example, postural muscle responses were activated at about 100 msec latencies in gastrocnemius when this muscle was stretched faster than normal in response to backward surface displacements pitching the body forward. This helped slow the body's rate of forward progression to realign the COM with the backward-displaced support foot. Similar responses occurred in tibialis anterior when this muscle was shortened more slowly than normal by forward surface displacements that displaced the body backward. This helped increase the rate of forward progress to realign the body with the forward-displaced foot.

Previous research on the control of **steady-state** walking has shown that one of the main control issues is keeping the HAT segment well balanced and that the trunk and hip muscles play an active role in this control (Winter et al., 1990). The work discussed earlier on **reactive control** of balance during gait has shown that the distal perturbed leg muscles are important in this type of control (Nashner, 1980; Dietz et al., 1984; Berger et al., 1984b). However, when a slip occurs, there is not only stretch of the ankle musculature but a challenge to upper body balance as well. Thus it is possible that proximal hip and trunk muscle activity may be a primary contributor to both steady-state gait and to the recovery of balance during slips.

Recent studies recording from bilateral leg, thigh, hip, and trunk muscles have shown that proximal muscles are **not** the primary muscles contributing to recovery from balance threats during slips in healthy young adults. Though proximal muscle activity was often present during the first slip trial in young adults, it tended to adapt away during subsequent trials. However, activity in anterior bilateral leg muscles as well as anterior and posterior thigh muscles showed early (90 to 140 msec), high magnitude (4 to 9 times the activity in normal walking) and relatively long-duration bursts (Tang et al., 1998). As shown previously for recovery of balance during quiet stance, patterns of muscle response to balance threats during walking were activated in a distal-to-proximal sequence. As you see in Figure 12-6, for a forward slip at heel strike, first the tibialis anterior on the ipsilateral side was activated (TAi), followed by the rectus femoris (Rfi) and biceps femoris (Bfi) and then the gluteus medius (GMEi) and abdominal muscles (Abi) (in initial trials).

Many falls in older adults begin with trips. How is balance recovery accomplished during trips? Research analyzing responses to a tripping perturbation have found that the type of strategy used to maintain stability depends on when in the swing phase the trip occurs. As you see in Figure 12-7, if the trip occurs early in the swing phase of walking, the most common movement outcome was an elevating strategy of the swing limb, with muscle responses occurring at 60 to 140 msec. Figure 12-7 shows the increased flexion at the hip, knee, and ankle (broken lines) after contact with the obstacle (*arrow*)

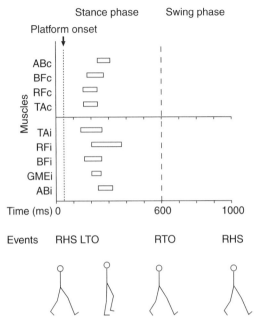

FIGURE 12-6. Organization of the postural responses of the anterior muscles and the biceps femoris (BF) in response to a forward slip at heel strike. The horizontal bars indicate the duration of postural activity in these muscles. The stick figures indicate the events during normal walking. RHS, right heel strike; LTO, left toe-off; RTO, right toe-off; TA, tibialis anterior; RF, rectus femoris; AB, rectus abdominis; GME, gluteus medius; i, ipsilateral to the perturbed side; c, contralateral side (Adapted with permission from Tang PF, Woollacott MH, Chong RKY. Control of reactive balance adjustments in perturbed human walking: roles of proximal and distal postural muscle activity. Exp Brain Res 1998;119:141–152.)

in the trial in which the subject tripped compared to the control trial (solid lines). The elevating strategy consisted of a flexor torque component of the swing limb, with the temporal sequencing of the swing limb's biceps femoris occurring prior to the swing limb's rectus femoris to remove the limb from the obstacle before accelerating the limb over it. An extensor torque component in the stance limb generated an early heel off to increase the height of the body.

Use of the elevating strategy would be dangerous if a trip occurred late in the swing phase, since flexion of the swing limb as it is approaching the ground would increase, not decrease, instability; thus, a lowering strategy was used by subjects, as you see in Figure 12-8. Note the early plantarflexion of the ankle.

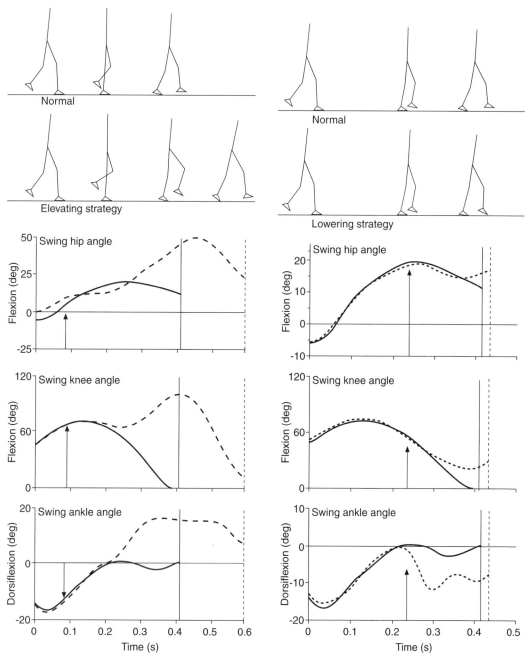

FIGURE 12-7. Hip, knee, and ankle trajectories of the swing limb in response to a trip during early swing phase of walking, showing the elevation strategy. Normal trial, solid line; perturbed trial, broken line. Time 0, toe-off; arrow, contact of foot with obstacle; vertical solid line, normal heel contact; vertical broken line, perturbed heel contact. (Adapted with permission from Eng JJ, Winter DA, Patla AE. Strategies for recovery from a trip in early and late swing during human walking. Exp Brain Res 1994;102:344.)

FIGURE 12-8. Hip, knee, and ankle trajectories of the swing limb in response to a trip during late swing phase of walking, showing the lowering strategy. Normal trial, solid line; perturbed trial, broken line. Time 0, toe-off; arrow, contact of foot with obstacle; vertical solid line, normal heel contact; vertical broken line, perturbed heel contact. (Adapted with permission from Eng JJ, Winter DA, Patla AE. Strategies for recovery from a trip in early and late swing during human walking. Exp Brain Res 1994;102:345).

The lowering strategy was accomplished by inhibitory responses in the swing limb vastus lateralis and an excitatory response of the swing limb biceps femoris, resulting in a shortened step (Eng et al., 1994).

More recent work has shown that the nervous system also takes advantage of passive dynamics to control the recovery from a trip during swing phase of gait. Kinematic data were analyzed using inverse dynamics techniques (Technology Box 12-1) to determine the joint moment and mechanical power (kinetic) profiles and to partition the joint moments into active and passive components. Results showed that the nervous system used the passive dynamics of the musculoskeletal system to aid in balance recovery. Active control of one joint, the knee joint, passively contributed to the flexion at the hip and ankle joints following a trip in early swing (Eng et al., 1997). Thus, to understand the interactions between passive and active components of the control systems it is important to consider both the passive and active joint moments produced during balance recovery in addition to the muscle response patterns of involved muscles.

How do humans modify gait when walking or running on surfaces with varying compliance or compressibility? If humans used the same muscle stiffness for all surfaces, the dynamics of walking and running would be strongly affected by surface stiffness or compliance. Although no studies have examined *walking* on compliant surfaces, recent work on *running* (Ferris et al., 1998) has shown that humans adjust muscle stiffness according to the surface they are running across. They found that the central nervous system modulates joint displacements and joint moments according to surface stiffness, probably to keep COM movement and ground contact time the same. Research on animals has shown that this is done within one step of moving onto the new surface. The previously mentioned research on human stretch reflex and GTO contributions to the step cycle suggests that proprioceptive feedback may be a factor in this stiffness modulation (Pearson et al., 1992; Stein, 1991). However, research has also shown that when lower limb

TECHNOLOGY BOX 12-1

KINETIC ANALYSIS-INVERSE DYNAMICS
INVERSE DYNAMICS is a process that allows researchers to calculate the joint moments of force (torque) responsible for movement—in this case, locomotion. Researchers begin by developing a reliable model of the body using anthropometric measures such as segment masses, COM, joint centers, and moments of inertia. Because these variables are difficult to measure directly, they are usually obtained from statistical tables based on the person's height, weight, and sex (Winter, 1990).

Using extremely accurate kinematic information on the limb trajectory during the step cycle in combination with a reliable model, researchers can calculate the torque acting on each segment of the body. They can then partition the net torque into components that are due to gravity, the mechanical interaction among segments (motion-dependent torques), and a generalized muscle torque. This type of analysis allows researchers to assess the roles of muscular and nonmuscular forces in the generation of the movement (Winter et al., 1990).

reflexes are temporarily blocked by ischemia, adults run with a normal ground contact time, suggesting that leg stiffness is unchanged (Dietz et al., 1979). Thus, there may be multiple contributions to stiffness regulation.

Vision
Work with humans suggests that vision modulates locomotion in a feedback manner in a variety of ways. First, visual flow cues help us determine our speed of locomotion (Lackner and DeZio, 1988). Studies have shown that if one doubles the rate of optic flow past persons as they walk, 100% perceive that their stride length has increased. In addition, about half of the subjects perceive that the force exerted during each step is less than normal. However, other subjects perceive that they have nearly doubled their stepping frequency (Lackner and DeZio, 1992).

Visual flow cues also influence the alignment of the body with reference to gravity and the environment during walking. For example, when researchers tilted the room surrounding a treadmill on which a person was running, it caused the person to incline the trunk in the direction of the tilted room to compensate for the visual illusion of body tilt in the opposite direction (Lee and Young, 1986).

Vestibular System

An important part of controlling locomotion is stabilizing the head, since it contains two of the most important sensors for controlling motion: the vestibular and visual systems (Berthoz and Pozzo, 1988, 1994). The otolith organs, the saccule and the utricle, detect the angle of the head with respect to gravity, and the visual system also provides us with the so-called visual vertical.

Adults appear to stabilize the head, and thus gaze, by covarying both pitch (forward) rotation and vertical displacement of the head to give stability to the head in the sagittal plane (Pozzo et al., 1990, 1992). The head is stabilized with precision (within a few degrees) that is compatible with the efficiency of the vestibulo-ocular reflex, an important mechanism for stabilizing gaze during head movement.

It has been hypothesized that during complex movements, such as walking, postural control is not organized from the support surface upward in what is called a bottom-up mode but is organized in relation to the control of gaze in what is called a top-down mode. In this mode, head movements are independent from the movements of the trunk. It has been shown that the process for stabilizing the head is disrupted in patients with bilateral labyrinthine lesions (Berthoz and Pozzo, 1994).

Proactive Strategies

Proactive strategies for adapting gait focus on the use of sensory inputs to modify gait patterns. Proactive strategies are used to modify and adapt gait in two ways. First, vision is used to identify potential obstacles in the environment and to navigate around them. Second, prediction is used to estimate the potential destabilizing effects of simultaneously performing tasks like carrying an object while walking, and anticipatory modifications to the step cycle are made accordingly.

Proactive visual control of locomotion has been classified into avoidance and accommodation. Avoidance strategies include (*a*) changing the placement of the foot, (*b*) increasing ground clearance to avoid an obstacle, (*c*) changing the direction of gait when it is perceived that objects cannot be cleared, and (*d*) stopping. Accommodation strategies involve longer-term modifications, such as reducing step length when walking on an icy surface and shifting the propulsive power from ankle to hip and knee muscles when climbing stairs (Patla, 1997).

Most avoidance strategies can be successfully carried out within a step cycle. An exception occurs during change of direction, which requires planning one step cycle in advance. It has been suggested that there are various rules associated with changing the placement of the foot. For example, when possible, step length is increased rather than shortened, and the foot is placed inside rather than outside of an obstacle as long as the foot need not cross the midline of the body. Adapting strategies for foot placement does not involve simply changing the amplitude of the normal locomotor patterns but is complex and task specific (Patla, 1997).

The decision to step over an obstacle or to move around it is related to the object size compared to body size. For example, when the ratio of the size of the obstacle to the length of the leg is 1:1, subjects prefer to go around it (Warren, 1995). It is probable that this choice relates to stability issues, since the risk of tripping increases with the height of the object to be stepped over.

Experience with an object also determines avoidance strategy. For example, perceived fragility of an obstacle influences the amount of toe clearance, with clearance being larger for the more fragile objects (Patla, 1997).

How do we sample the environment for proactive visual control? Visual processing time is shared with other tasks, so the terrain is typically sampled for less than 10% of travel time during walking over even surfaces. However, when uneven surfaces are simulated by requiring subjects to step on specific locations, visual monitoring goes up to about 30% (Patla, 1997).

How do we navigate in a large scale spatial environment? Humans use a piloting strategy, which requires a mental representation of the spatial environment. These cognitive maps include both topological information (relationships of landmarks in the environment) and metric information (specific distances and directions). Topological information is needed when obstacles constrain our path. The fact that most animals can also accurately take shortcuts to reach a goal supports the concept that metric information is also used in navigation (Patla, 1997).

Nonneural Contributions to Locomotion

So far, we have looked at neural contributions to the control of locomotion, but there are also important musculoskeletal and environmental contributions. Biomechanical analyses of locomotion in the cat have determined the contributions of both muscular and nonmuscular forces to the generation of gait dynamics (Hoy and Zernicke, 1985, 1986; Hoy et al., 1985; Smith and Zernicke, 1987). This involves a type of kinetic analysis called inverse dynamics. To understand more about inverse dynamics, refer to Technology Box 12-1.

As we have said in earlier chapters, nonmuscular forces, such as gravity, play a role in the construction of all movement. When an inverse dynamics analysis of limb dynamics is used, it is possible to determine the relative importance of the muscular and nonmuscular contributions. For example, during locomotion, each segment of the cat hindlimb is subjected to a complex set of muscular and nonmuscular forces. Changes in speed lead to changes in the interactive patterns among the torque components (Hoy and Zernicke, 1985; Wisleder et al., 1990).

Very often in cat locomotion, high passive extensor torques at a joint must be counteracted by active flexor torques generated by the muscles when the animal is moving at one speed or in one part of the step cycle. When the speed is increased or the animal moves to a different part of the cycle, the passive torques that must be counteracted completely change. How does the dialogue between the passive properties of the system and the neural pattern generating circuits occur? This is still unclear, although the discharge from somatosensory receptors plays a role (Hoy et al., 1985; Smith and Zernicke, 1987; Wisleder et al., 1990). What is revealed in the dynamic analysis of limb movements is the intricacies of the interaction among active and passive forces.

The results from these studies suggest that in normal locomotion there is a continuous interaction between the central pattern generators and descending signals. Higher centers contribute to locomotion through feed-forward modulation of patterns in response to the goals of the individual and to environmental demands. As noted briefly earlier, sensory inputs are also critical for feedback and feed-forward modulation of locomotor activity to adapt it to changing environmental conditions.

℮ INITIATING GAIT AND CHANGING SPEEDS

How do we initiate walking? Before we describe the initiation of gait, let's do Lab Activity 12-3.

Research studies confirm what you no doubt noticed from your own experiment: the initiation of gait from quiet stance begins with the relaxation of specific postural muscles, the gastrocnemius and the soleus (Carlsoo, 1966; Herman et al., 1973). In fact, the initiation of gait has the appearance of a simple forward fall and regaining of one's balance by taking a step. This reduction in the activation of the gastrocnemius and soleus is followed by activation of the tibialis anterior, which assists dorsiflexion and moves the COM forward in preparation for toe-off. But as you noticed and as recent research on gait confirms, the initiation of gait is more than a simple fall.

LAB ACTIVITY 12-3

OBJECTIVE: To clarify the movements essential to the initiation of gait.

PROCEDURES: Get up and stand next to a wall with your shoulder touching the wall. First try to start walking with the foot that is next to the wall. Now try to start walking with the foot that is away from the wall.

ASSIGNMENT: In each condition, such as gait initiation with the leg nearest versus away from the wall, note the following: What muscles contract and relax? Which way does the body move in the process of preparing to take a step? Under which condition is it easiest to initiate gait? When you tried to initiate gait with the leg farther from the wall, did you notice that you had more problems? Why? Could it be because you couldn't easily shift your weight in preparation for stepping (Larsson, 1985)?

In tracing the center of pressure during the initiation of gait in normal adults, the following sequence of events is evident. Prior to movement onset, the center of pressure is positioned just posterior to the ankle and midway between both feet, as you see in Figure 12-9. As the person begins to move, the center of pressure first moves posteriorly and laterally toward the swing limb and then shifts toward the stance limb and forward.

Movement of the center of pressure toward the stance limb occurs simultaneously with hip and knee flexion and ankle dorsiflexion as the swing limb prepares for toe-off. Then the center of pressure moves quickly toward the stance limb. Toe-off of the swing limb occurs with the center of pressure shifting from lateral to forward movement over the stance foot (Mann et al., 1979).

What neural patterns are correlated with these shifts in center of pressure? As the center of pressure moves posteriorly and toward the swing limb, both limbs are stabilized against backward sway by activation of anterior leg and thigh muscles, the tibialis anterior and the quadriceps. Subsequent activation of the tibialis anterior causes

dorsiflexion in the stance ankle, pulling the lower leg over the foot as the body moves forward in preparation for toe-off. Anterior thigh muscles are activated to keep the knee from flexing so that the leg rotates forward as a unit. Activation of hip abductors counters lateral tilt of the pelvis toward the swing limb side as this limb is unloaded. Also, activation of the peroneals stabilizes the stance ankle. After toe-off, the gastrocnemius and hamstring muscles in the stance leg are used for propelling the body forward (Herman et al., 1973; Mann et al., 1979). How long after initiation does it take to reach a steady velocity in gait? Steady state is reached within one to three steps, depending on the magnitude of the velocity one is trying to achieve (Breniere and Do, 1986; Cook and Cozzens, 1976).

The Walk–Run Transition

As we increase our speed during walking or decrease our speed during running, there comes a point at which a gait transition oc-

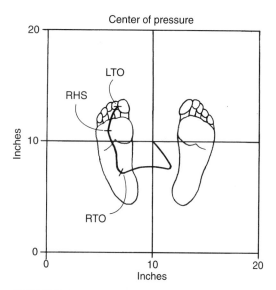

FIGURE 12-9. Trajectory of the center of pressure during the initiation of gait from a balanced, symmetrical stance. Prior to movement, the center of pressure is midway between the feet. LTO, left toe-off; RTO, right toe-off; RHS, right heel strike. (Adapted with permission from Mann RA, Hagy JL, White V, Liddell D. The initiation of gait. J Bone Joint Surg 1979;61-A:232–239.)

curs. The selection of this transition point occurs over a relatively narrow range of speeds across adults. Since humans are capable of walking and running at both higher and lower speeds than the transition speed, a number of researchers have tried to determine the factors that influence this transition (Hreljac 1993a, 1995a,b; Kram et al., 1997).

It has traditionally been assumed by many researchers that both humans and other animals change gait at a speed that minimizes their metabolic energy consumption, since many animals select a transition speed within a particular gait that minimizes metabolic energy cost (Hoyt and Taylor, 1981; Grillner et al., 1979; Cavagna and Franzetti, 1986; Alexander, 1989). If this were the case, the preferred transition speed for humans between a walk and a run would be about 2.24 to 2.36 m/second (Margaria, 1976). However, it has been noted that the preferred transition speed is more typically 1.88 to 2.07 m/second (Thorstensson and Roberthson, 1987; Hreljac, 1993a). Thus, recent research has attempted to determine the primary factors contributing to this transition.

A recent set of studies showed that subjects changing from a walk to a run at these lower speeds perceived that their sense of exertion decreased by 26%, even though the energetic cost increased by 16% (Hreljac, 1993a). Thus it is unlikely that the energetic cost of locomotion is the primary factor contributing to the speed of gait transition. In horses it has been shown that the transition from trot to gallop occurs when the ground reaction forces reach a critical level, with peak forces decreasing by about 14% when the horses shifted from a trot to a gallop (Farley and Taylor, 1991). Since ground reaction forces are related to musculoskeletal forces, this may be a way to prevent injuries due to high musculoskeletal forces. However, it has been shown that in humans there is an increase in ground reaction forces during the transition from a walk to a run, so this doesn't appear to be a critical factor for the transition from walk to run (Hreljac, 1993b).

Instead, it has been proposed that peak ankle angular velocity and acceleration are critical components in triggering this transition (Hreljac, 1995a). Why would this be the case? It has been hypothesized that high levels of activity in ankle dorsiflexors close to the time of toe-off at the walk–run transition point are necessary to rotate the foot quickly to prevent toe drag and to position the heel for the next stance phase. At this time there is also cocontraction of the ankle plantarflexors, requiring increased output from the dorsiflexors to rotate the foot. Thus one outcome of the gait transition would be a reduction in muscular stress or fatigue in the dorsiflexors (Hreljac, 1995a). Shifting to a run would remove the stress from the dorsiflexors and transfer it to the larger muscles of the upper leg.

It has also been shown that body size is moderately correlated (r = .54 to .60) with the preferred transition speed. This follows from the assumption that people of different heights would reach the same ankle angular accelerations at different walking speeds (Hreljac, 1995b).

⊘ STAIR WALKING

Understanding the sensory and motor requirements associated with stair walking is critical to retraining this skill. Stairs are a significant hazard even among the nondisabled population. Stair walking accounts for the largest percentage of falls in public places, with four out of five falls occurring during stair descent. Stair walking is similar to level walking in that it involves stereotyped reciprocal alternating movements of the lower limbs (Simoneau et al., 1991; Craik et al., 1982).

As with locomotion, successful negotiation of stairs has three requirements: (*a*) the generation of primarily concentric forces to propel the body upstairs or eccentric forces to control the body's descent downstairs (progression) while (*b*) controlling the COM within a constantly changing base of support (stability) and (*c*) the capacity to adapt strategies used for progression and stability to accommodate changes in stair environment, such as height, width, and the presence or absence of railings (adaptation) (McFadyen and Winter, 1988).

Sensory information is important for controlling the body's position in space (stability) and to identify critical aspects of the stair environment so that appropriate movement strategies can be programmed (adaptation). Researchers have shown that normal subjects change movement strategies used for negotiating stairs when sensory cues about stair characteristics are altered (Simoneau et al., 1991; Craik et al., 1982).

Similar to gait, stair climbing has been divided into two phases, a stance phase lasting approximately 64% of the full cycle and a swing phase lasting 36% of the cycle. In addition, each phase of stair walking has been further subdivided to reflect the objectives to be achieved during each phase.

Ascent

During ascent, the stance phase is subdivided into weight acceptance, pull-up, and forward continuance, while swing is divided into foot clearance and foot placement. During stance, weight acceptance is initiated with the middle to front portion of the foot. Pull-up occurs because of extensor activity at the knee and ankle, primarily concentric contractions of the vastus lateralis and soleus muscles. Stair ascent differs from level walking in two ways: (*a*) forces needed to accomplish ascent are twice as great as those needed to control level gait, and (*b*) the knee extensors generate most of the energy to move the body forward during stair ascent. Finally, during the forward continuance phase of stance, the ankle generates forward and lift forces; however, ankle force is not the main source of power behind forward progression in stair walking. In controlling balance during stair ascent, the greatest instability comes with contralateral toe-off, when the ipsilateral leg takes the total body weight and the hip, knee, and ankle joints are flexed (McFadyen and Winter, 1988).

The objectives of the swing phase of stair climbing are similar to level gait and include foot clearance and placing the foot appro-

priately so weight can be accepted for the next stance phase. Foot clearance is achieved through activation of the tibialis anterior, dorsiflexing the foot, and activation of the hamstrings, which flex the knee. The rectus femoris contracts eccentrically to reverse this motion by midswing. The swing leg is brought up and forward through activation of the hip flexors of the swing leg and motion of the contralateral stance leg. Final foot placement is controlled by the hip extensors and ankle foot dorsiflexors (McFadyen and Winter, 1988).

Descent

Walking upstairs is accomplished through concentric contractions of the rectus femoris, vastus lateralis, soleus, and medial gastrocnemius. In contrast, walking downstairs is achieved through eccentric contractions of these same muscles, which work to control the body with respect to the force of gravity. The stance phase of stair descent is subdivided into weight acceptance, forward continuance, and controlled lowering, while swing has two phases: leg pull-through and preparation for foot placement (Craik et al., 1982; McFadyen and Winter, 1988).

Weight acceptance phase is characterized by absorption of energy at the ankle and knee through the eccentric contraction of the triceps surae, rectus femoris, and vastus lateralis. Energy absorption during this phase is critical, since ground reaction forces as much as two times body weight have been recorded when the swing limb first contacts the stair. Activation of gastrocnemius prior to stair contact is responsible for cushioning the landing (Craik et al., 1982).

The forward continuance phase reflects the forward motion of the body and precedes the controlled lowering phase of stance. Lowering of the body is controlled primarily by the eccentric contraction of the quadriceps muscles and to a lesser degree by the eccentric contraction of the soleus muscle.

During swing, the leg is pulled through by activation of the hip flexor muscles. However, by midswing, flexion of the hip and knee is reversed, and all three joints extend in preparation for foot placement. Contact is made with the lateral border of the foot and is associated with tibialis anterior and gastrocnemius activity prior to foot contact.

Adapting Stair-Walking Patterns to Changes in Sensory Cues

Researchers have shown that neurologically intact people adapt the movement strategies they use for going up and down stairs in response to changes in sensory information about the task. For example, when normal subjects wear large collars obstructing their view of the stairs, anticipatory activation of the gastrocnemius prior to foot contact is reduced. This anticipatory activity is further reduced when the subject is blindfolded. In this study, subjects still managed a soft landing by changing the control strategy used to descend stairs. Subjects moved more slowly, protracting swing time and using the stance limb to control the landing (Craik et al., 1982).

Foot clearance and placement are critical aspects of movement strategies used to descend stairs. Good visual information about stair height is critical. When normal subjects wear blurred lenses and cannot clearly define the edge of the step, they slow down and modify movement strategies so that foot clearance is increased and the foot is placed farther back on the step to ensure a larger margin of safety (Simoneau et al., 1991). Thus, information from the visual system about the step height appears to be necessary for optimal programming of movement strategies used to negotiate stairs.

◉ MOBILITY OTHER THAN GAIT

Although mobility is often thought of solely in relation to gait or locomotion, many other aspects of mobility are essential to independence in daily life activities. The ability to change positions, whether moving from sit to stand, rolling, rising from a bed, or moving from one chair to another, is a fundamental part of mobility. These various types of mobility activities are often grouped together as transfer tasks.

Retraining motor function in the patient with a neurological impairment includes the recovery of these diverse mobility skills. This requires an understanding of (*a*) the essential characteristics of the task, (*b*) the sensory motor strategies that normal individuals typically use to accomplish the task, and (*c*) the adaptations required for changing environmental characteristics.

All mobility tasks share three essential task requirements: motion in a desired direction (progression), postural control (stability), and the ability to adapt to changing task and environmental conditions (adaptation). The following sections briefly review some of the research on these other aspects of mobility function. As you will see, compared to the tremendous number of studies on normal gait, there have been relatively few studies examining these other aspects of mobility function.

Transfers

Transfers are an important aspect of mobility function. One cannot walk if one cannot get out of a chair or rise from a bed. Inability to change positions safely and independently is a great hindrance to the recovery of normal mobility.

Several researchers have studied transfer skills from a biomechanical perspective. As a result, we know quite a bit about typical movement strategies used by neurologically intact adults when performing these tasks. However, use of a biomechanical approach has provided us with little information about the perceptual strategies associated with these various tasks. In addition, because most often research subjects are constrained to carry out the task in a unified way, we have little insight into ways in which sensory and movement strategies are modified in response to changing task and environmental demands.

Sit to Stand

Sit-to-stand (STS) behaviors emerge from interaction among characteristics of the task, the individual, and constraints imposed by the environment. While the biomechanics of STS have been described, many important questions have not yet been studied by motor control researchers. For example, how do the movements involved in STS vary as a function of the speed of the task; the characteristics of the support, including height of the chair; the compliance of the seat; and the presence or absence of hand rests? In addition, do the requirements of the task vary with the nature of the task immediately following? That is, do we stand up differently if we are intending to walk instead of stand still? What perceptual information is essential to establishing efficient movement strategies when performing STS?

The essential characteristics of the STS task include (*a*) generating sufficient joint torque needed to rise (progression), (*b*) ensuring stability by moving the COM from one base of support (the chair) to a base of support defined solely by the feet (stability), and (*c*) modifying movement strategies used to achieve these goals according to the environmental constraints, such as chair height,

the presence of arm rests, and the softness of the chair (adaptation).

The STS task has been divided into two, three or four phases, depending on the researcher. Each phase has its own unique movement and stability requirements. A four-phase model of STS is shown in Figure 12-10 (Schenkman et al., 1990; Millington et al., 1992). This figure also shows the movements of the joints and the muscle activity used by a normal subject when completing this task.

The first phase, called the weight shift or flexion momentum stage, begins with the generation of forward momentum of the upper body through flexion of the trunk. The body is quite stable during this phase, since the COM, though moving forward, is still within the base of support of the chair seat and the feet. Muscle activity includes activation of the erector spinae, which contract eccentrically to control forward motion of the trunk (Schenkman et al., 1990; Millington et al., 1992).

Phase 2 begins as the buttocks leave the seat and entails the transfer of momentum

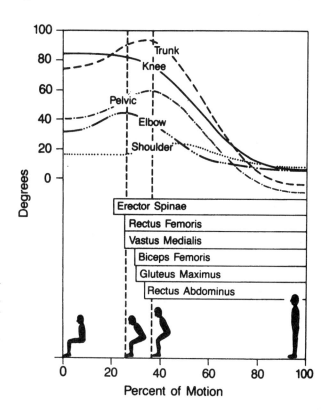

FIGURE 12-10. Diagram of the four phases of the sit-to-stand movement showing the kinematic and EMG patterns associated with each phase. (Adapted with permission from Millington PJ, Myklebust BM, Shambes GM. Biomechanical analysis of the sit-to-stand motion in elderly persons. Arch Phys Med Rehabil 1992;73:609–617.)

from the upper body to the total body, allowing lift of the body. Phase 2 involves both horizontal and vertical motion of the body and is considered a critical transition phase. Stability requirements are precise, since it is during this phase that the COM of the body moves from the base of support of the chair to that of the feet. The body is inherently unstable during this phase because the COM is far from the center of force. Because the body has developed momentum prior to liftoff, vertical rise of the body can be achieved with little lower extremity muscle force. Muscle activity in this phase is characterized by coactivation of hip and knee extensors, as you see in Figure 12-10 (Schenkman et al., 1990).

Phase 3 of the STS task is referred to as the lift or extension phase and is characterized by extension at the hips and knees. The goal in this phase is primarily to move the body vertically; stability requirements are less than in phase 2, since the COM is well within the base of support of the feet. The final phase of STS is the stabilization phase, the period following complete extension when task-dependent motion is complete and body stability in the vertical position is achieved (Schenkman et al., 1990).

STS requires the generation of propulsive forces in both the horizontal and vertical directions. However, the horizontal propulsive force responsible for moving the COM anterior over the base of support of the foot must change to a braking impulse to bring the body to a stop. Braking the horizontal impulse begins even before liftoff from the seat. Thus, there appears to be a programmed relationship between the generation and braking of forces for the STS task. Without this coordination between propulsive and braking forces, the person could easily fall forward upon achieving the vertical position.

Horizontal displacement of the COM appears to be constant despite changes in the speed of STS. The horizontal trajectory of the COM is probably the invariant feature controlled in STS to ensure that stability is maintained during rise of the body (Millington et al., 1992).

This strategy could be referred to as a momentum transfer strategy, and its use requires (*a*) adequate strength and coordination to generate upper body movement prior to liftoff, (*b*) the ability to contract trunk and hip muscles eccentrically to apply braking forces to slow the horizontal trajectory of the COM, and (*c*) concentric contraction of hip and knee muscles to generate vertical propulsive forces that lift the body (Schenkman et al., 1990).

Accomplishing STS using a momentum transfer strategy requires a trade-off between stability and force requirements. The generation and transfer of momentum between the upper body and total body reduce the requirement for lower extremity force because the body is already in motion as it begins to lift. On the other hand, the body is in a precarious state of balance during the transition stage when momentum is transferred.

An alternative strategy that ensures greater stability but requires greater amounts of force to achieve liftoff includes flexing the trunk sufficiently to bring the COM well within the base of support of the feet prior to liftoff. However, the body has zero momentum at liftoff. This strategy has been referred to as a zero-momentum strategy and requires the generation of larger lower extremity forces to lift the body to vertical (Schenkman et al., 1990).

Another common strategy used by many older adults and people with neurological impairments is the use of armrests to assist in STS. Use of the arms assists in both the stability and force generation requirements of the STS task.

Understanding the different strategies that can be used to accomplish STS, including the trade-offs between force and stability, will help the therapist when retraining STS in the patient with a neurological deficit. For example, the zero-momentum strategy may be more appropriate for a patient with cerebellar pathology who has no difficulty with force generation but who has a major problem with controlling stability. On the other hand, the patient with hemiparesis, who is very weak, may need to rely more on a momentum strategy to stand up. The frail elderly person who is both weak and unstable may need to rely on armrests to accomplish STS.

Supine to Stand

The ability to assume a standing position from supine is an important milestone in mobility skills. This skill is taught to a wide range of patients with neurological impairments, from young children with developmental disabilities first learning to stand and walk to frail older people prone to fall. The movement strategies used by normal individuals moving from supine to stand have been studied by a number of researchers. An important theoretical question addressed by these researchers is whether rising to stand from supine follows a developmental progression and whether by the age of 4 or 5 years the mature, or adultlike, form emerges and remains throughout life (VanSant, 1988a). The application of this concept can be found in Lab Activity 12-4.

Researchers have studied supine-to-stand movement strategies in children aged 4 to 7 years and young adults aged 20 to 35 years (VanSant, 1988b). These researchers found that while there was a slight tendency toward age-specific strategies for moving from supine to stance, there was also great variation among subjects of the same age. Their findings do not appear to support the traditional assumption of a single mature supine-to-stance pattern that emerges after the age of 5 years.

The three most common movement strategies for moving from supine to stand are shown in Figure 12-11. For analysis of strategies used for moving from supine to stand, the body is divided into three components, the upper extremities, lower extremities, and axial region, which includes trunk and head. Movement strategies are described in relation to the various combinations of movement patterns within each of these segments. The research on young adults suggests that the most common pattern uses symmetrical movement patterns of the trunk and extremities and the use of a symmetrical squat to achieve the vertical po-

LAB ACTIVITY 12-4

OBJECTIVE: To observe the strategies used to move from supine to stand in healthy adults.

PROCEDURES: For this lab you will need a stopwatch, four or five partners, and room to observe each person moving from supine (flat on the floor) to standing. Time each person as he or she moves from supine to a full standing position. Observe the movement patterns used by each individual. Pay specific attention to use of arms, symmetry of foot placement, and trunk rotation.

ASSIGNMENT: Were all subjects able to arise without physical assistance of another? How did times vary across subjects? How many strategies did you observe among the five subjects? Did any two subjects move in the same way? How do your results compare with VanSant's (1988) results shown in Figure 12-11? What are the primary muscles in each of the strategies? How would weakness or loss of joint range of motion affect each of these strategies?

sition (Fig. 12-11A). However, only one-fourth of the subjects studied used this strategy.

The second most common movement pattern involved asymmetrical squat on arising (12-11B), while the third most common strategy involved asymmetrical use of the upper extremities, a partial rotation of the trunk, and assumption of stance using a half-kneel position (12-11C).

Additional studies have characterized movement patterns used to rise from supine in adults aged 30 to 39 years and found some differences in movement strategies compared to younger adults (Green and Williams, 1992). In addition, this study looked at the effect of physical activity levels on strategies used to stand up. The study findings were that strategies used to stand up are influenced by lifestyle factors, including level of physical activity.

Many factors probably contribute to determining the type of movement strategy used to move from supine to stance. Traditionally, nervous system maturation, specifi-

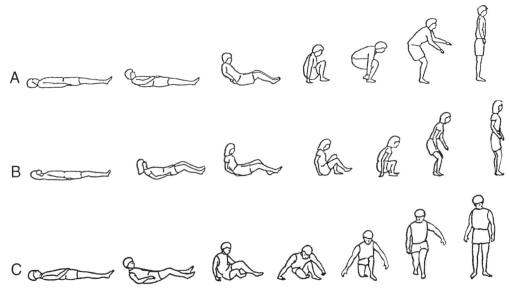

FIGURE 12-11. Three most common movement strategies identified among young adults for moving from supine to stand. **A.** Symmetrical trunk and symmetrical squat. **B.** Symmetrical trunk and asymmetrical squat. **C.** Asymmetrical trunk movement. (Adapted with permission from VanSant AF. Rising from a supine position to erect stance: description of adult movement and a developmental hypothesis. Phys Ther 1988;68:185–192.)

cally the maturation of the neck-on-body righting reactions and body-on-body righting reactions, were considered the most significant factors affecting the emergence of a developmentally mature supine-to-stance strategy. However, a switch from an asymmetrical rotation to symmetrical sit-up strategy may be constrained by the ability to generate sufficient abdominal and hip flexor strength.

Developmental changes in moving from supine to stance are considered further in the chapter on age-related aspects of mobility.

Rising From Bed

Clinicians are often called upon to help patients relearn the task of getting out of bed. In therapeutic texts on retraining motor control in the patient with neurological impairments, therapists are instructed to teach patients to move from supine to side lying, then to push up to a sitting position and from there to stand up. These instructions are based on the assumption that this pattern is the one typically used to rise from a bed (Carr and Shepherd, 1983; Bobath, 1978).

To test these assumptions, researchers examined movement patterns used by young adults to rise from a bed (McCoy and VanSant, 1993). These studies report that movement patterns used by nondisabled people to rise from a bed are extremely variable. The researchers found 89 patterns among 60 subjects! In fact, no subject used the same strategy consistently in 10 trials of getting out of bed.

Figure 12-12 shows one of the most common strategies used by young adults to rise from a bed. Essential components of the strategy include pushing with the arms or grasping the side of the bed and then pushing with the arms, flexing the head and trunk, pushing into a partial sit position, and rolling up into stance. Another common strategy was a push-off pattern with the arms, rolling to the side and coming to a symmetrical sitting position prior to standing up.

While the authors of this study have not specifically stated the essential features of this task, its similarity to the STS task suggests they share the same invariant characteristics. These include (*a*) the need to generate momentum to move the body to vertical, (*b*) stability requirements for controlling the COM

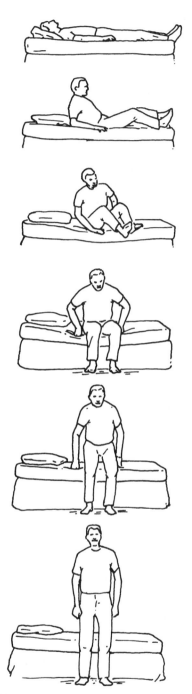

FIGURE 12-12. Most common movement strategy used by young adults for getting out of bed. (Adapted with permission from Ford-Smith CD, VanSant AF. Age differences in movement patterns used to rise from a bed in subjects in the third through fifth decades of age. Phys Ther 1992;73:305.)

as it changes from within the support base defined by the horizontal body to that defined by the buttocks and feet, and finally to a base of support defined solely by the feet; and (*c*) the ability to adapt how one moves to the characteristics of the environment.

In preparation for understanding why patients move as they do, it may be helpful to reexamine descriptions of movement strategies used to rise from a bed in light of these essential task characteristics. This may make it possible to determine common features across diverse strategies that are successful in accomplishing invariant requirements of the task. It would also become possible to examine some trade-offs between movement and stability requirements in the different strategies. For example, in the roll-off strategy, is motion achieved with greater efficiency at the expense of stability? Alternatively, the come-to-sit pattern may require more force to keep the body in motion, but stability may be inherently greater.

This research demonstrates the tremendous variability of movement strategies used by neurologically intact subjects when getting out of bed. It suggests the importance of helping patients with neurological impairments to learn a variety of ways to get out of bed.

Rolling

Rolling is an important part of bed mobility skills and an essential part of many other tasks, such as rising from bed. Movement strategies used by unimpaired adults to roll from supine to prone are very variable. Figure 12-13 shows one of the most common movement patterns used by adults to roll from supine to prone (Richter et al., 1989). Essential features of this strategy include a lift-and-reach arms pattern, with the shoulder girdle initiating motion of the head and trunk, and a unilateral lift of the leg.

A common assumption in the therapeutic literature is that rotation between the shoulders and pelvis is an invariant characteristic in rolling patterns used by normal adults (Bobath, 1978); however, in this study many of the adults did not show this pattern. Simi-

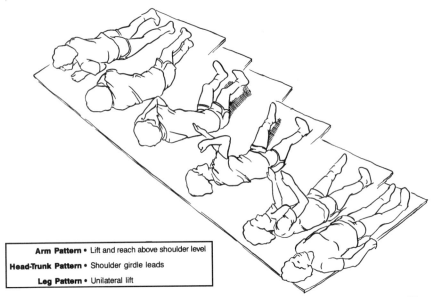

| **Arm Pattern** • Lift and reach above shoulder level |
| **Head-Trunk Pattern** • Shoulder girdle leads |
| **Leg Pattern** • Unilateral lift |

FIGURE 12-13. Most common movement strategy used by young adults when rolling from supine to prone. (Adapted with permission from Richter RR, VanSant AF, Newton RA. Description of adult rolling movements and hypothesis of developmental sequences. Phys Ther 1989;69:63–71.)

lar to the findings from studies on rising from a bed, the great variability used by normal subjects to move from supine to prone suggests that therapists may use greater freedom in retraining movement strategies for patients with neurological impairments. Clearly, there is no one correct way to accomplish this movement.

ⓔ SUMMARY

1. The three major requirements for successful locomotion are (*a*) progression, defined as the ability to generate a basic locomotor pattern that can move the body in the desired direction; (*b*) stability, defined as the ability to support and control the body against gravity; and (*c*) adaptability, defined as the ability to adapt gait to meet the individual's goals and the demands of the environment.

2. Normal locomotion is a bipedal gait in which the limbs move in a symmetrical alternating pattern. Gait is divided into a stance and swing phase, each of which has its own intrinsic requirements.

3. During the support phase of gait, hori-

zontal forces are generated against the support surface to move the body in the desired direction (progression), while vertical forces support the body mass against gravity (stability). In addition, strategies used to accomplish both progression and stability must be flexible to accommodate changes in speed and direction or alterations in the support surface (adaptation).

4. The goals to be achieved during the swing phase of gait include advancement of the swing leg (progression) and repositioning of the limb in preparation for weight acceptance (stability). Both the progression and stability goals require sufficient foot clearance that the toe does not drag on the supporting surface during swing. In addition, strategies used during the swing phase of gait must be sufficiently flexible to allow the swing foot to avoid any obstacles in its path (adaptation).

5. Gait is often described with respect to temporal distance parameters such as velocity, step length, step frequency (called cadence), and stride length. In addition, gait is described with refer-

ence to changes in joint angles (kinematics), muscle activation patterns (EMG), and the forces used to control gait (kinetics).

6. Many neural and nonneural elements work together in the control of gait. Though spinal pattern generators are able to produce stereotyped locomotor patterns and perform certain adaptive functions, descending pathways from higher centers and sensory feedback from the periphery allow rich variation in locomotor patterns and adaptability to task and environmental conditions.

7. One of the requirements of normal locomotion is the ability to adapt gait to a wide-ranging set of environments, and this requires use of sensory information from all of the senses, both reactively and proactively.

8. An important part of controlling locomotion is stabilizing the head, since it contains two of the most important motion control sensors, the vestibular and visual systems. In neurologically intact adults, the head is stabilized with great precision, allowing gaze to be stabilized through the vestibulo-ocular reflex.

9. Stair walking is similar to level walking in that it involves stereotyped reciprocal alternating movements of the lower limbs and has three requirements: (*a*) the generation of primarily concentric forces to propel the body upstairs or eccentric forces to control the body's descent downstairs (progression), while (*b*) controlling the COM within a constantly changing base of support (stability) and (*c*) the capacity to adapt strategies used for progression and stability to accommodate changes in stair environment, such as height, width, and the presence or absence of railings (adaptation).

10. Although mobility is often thought of in relation to gait, many other aspects of mobility are essential to independence. These include the ability to move from sit to stand, rolling, rising from a bed, or moving from one chair to another. These skills are referred to as transfer tasks.

11. Transfer tasks are similar to locomotion in that they share common task requirements: motion in a desired direction (progression), postural control (stability), and the ability to adapt to changing task and environmental conditions (adaptation). Researchers have found great variability in the types of movement strategies used by neurologically intact young adults when performing transfer tasks.

12. Understanding the stability and strength requirements for different types of strategies used to accomplish transfer tasks has important implications for retraining these skills in neurologically impaired patients with various types of motor constraints.

CHAPTER 13

A Life Span Perspective of Mobility

ⓔ INTRODUCTION

It is wonderful to see children develop their first mobility skills as they begin to crawl, creep, walk, and run—finally navigating expertly through complex environments. How do these skills develop? When do they begin to emerge? What key features of normal locomotor development should we incorporate into our measurement tools so that we can better understand the delayed or disordered development of the child with central nervous system (CNS) pathology?

Falls and the injuries that often accompany them are a serious problem in the older adult. Many of these falls occur during walking. Problems with balance and gait are considered major contributors to falls in the older adult. Nevertheless, not all older adults have difficulties with mobility skills. As with balance control, it is important to distin-

guish between age-related changes in mobility affecting all older adults and pathology-related changes, which affect only a few.

This chapter discusses mobility skills from a life span perspective. We first review the development of mobility skills in neurologically intact children and summarize research from theoretical perspectives that explore the factors contributing to the emergence of this complex ability. In the latter half of the chapter, we discuss how mobility skills change in the older adult.

ⓔ DEVELOPMENT OF LOCOMOTION

Independent locomotion may at first seem to be a fairly simple and automatic skill, but it is an intricate motor task. A child learning to walk must activate a complex pattern of muscle contractions in many body segments to produce a coordinated stepping movement, resulting in progression. The child must be strong enough to support body weight and stable enough to compensate for shifts in balance while walking to accomplish the goal of stability. Finally, the child must develop the ability to adapt gait to changing environmental circumstances, allowing navigation around and over obstacles and across uneven surfaces (Thelen and Ulrich, 1991).

In the following section, we summarize research evidence suggesting that in the development of locomotion, these three requirements emerge sequentially during the first years of life. How does this complex behavior develop? What are the origins of this behavior during prenatal development?

Prenatal Development

Researchers have traced the origins of locomotor rhythms to embryonic movements that begin in the first stages of development. Ultrasound techniques have been used to document the movements of human infants prenatally. This research has shown that all movements except those observed in the earliest stages of embryonic development (7 to 8 weeks) are also seen in neonates and young infants. Isolated leg and arm movements develop in the embryo by 9 weeks of age, while alternating leg movements, similar to walking movements seen after birth, develop in the infant by about 16 weeks of embryonic age (De Vries et al., 1982; Prechtl, 1984).

Animal research has also explored the prenatal development of locomotor circuitry. Detectable limb movements appear to emerge in a cephalocaudal sequence, with movements in the forelimbs preceding those in the hindlimbs (Bradley and Smith, 1988). Intralimb coordination develops prior to interlimb coordination, with the first detectable movements occurring at proximal joints and movement progressing distally with development. Finally, interlimb coordination develops, first with alternating patterns, then with synchronous patterns (Stehouwer and Farel, 1984).

Many newborn animals, such as the rat, do not normally show coordinated locomotor movements until about 1 week after birth (Bradley and Bekoff, 1989). If, however, rats are placed in water at birth, they swim, demonstrating the maturity of their locomotor system. In addition, adult forms of locomotion can be elicited in 3-day-old kittens by placing them on a treadmill (Bradley and Smith, 1988). However, gait in kittens is uncoordinated because of their poor postural abilities.

These findings suggest that a primary constraint on emerging locomotor behavior is the immaturity of the postural system and thus the inability to achieve upright stability. In addition, these findings remind us to be careful about assuming that because a behavior is not evident, there is no neural circuitry for it.

Early Stepping Behavior

Because locomotor patterns develop for some months before birth, it is not surprising to find that stepping behavior can be elicited in newborns under the right conditions (Prechtl, 1984; Forssberg, 1985; Thelen et al., 1989). For example, when newborn infants are held upright under the arms, tilted slightly forward with the soles of the feet touching a surface, they often perform coordinated movements that look much like erect locomotion. Surprisingly, stepping becomes progressively more difficult to elicit during the first month of life and disappears in most infants by about 2 months of age, reappearing many months later with the onset of self-generated locomotion.

This pattern of appearance and disappearance of newborn stepping was found in a study that examined 156 children longitudinally (Forssberg, 1985). It was found that 94 infants stepped at 1 month, 18 stepped at 3 months, but only 2 stepped at 4 and 5 months. Then, at 10 months, after a 4- to 8-month period of no stepping, all 156 infants stepped with support, and 18 stepped without support. Thus, the stepping pattern appeared to be temporarily lost in 98% to 99% of the infants.

What causes these changes? Different theoretical approaches explain changes in infant behavior in different ways. From a reflex hierarchy perspective, newborn stepping is thought to result from a stepping reflex. Its disappearance is assumed to be mainly the result of inhibition by maturing higher neural centers. Figure 13-1 illustrates seven phases in the development of infant locomotion, beginning with the observation of this reflex (phase 1) and its disappearance (phase 2), continuing with its reappearance (phase 3), the emergence of assisted locomotion (phase 4), and concluding with three phases of erect independent walking. In the last three phases the hands gradually move from a high guard position (phase 5) to the side (phase 6), and the trunk and head become more erect (phase 7) (McGraw, 1945).

In contrast to a reflex-hierarchical model, researchers using a systems approach have examined the emergence of stepping in relation to the contributions of multiple neural and nonneural systems. In particular, these studies have explored the conditions leading to the emergence of newborn stepping and the changes that cause its disappearance.

Esther Thelen, a psychologist, and her colleagues have applied a dynamical systems approach to the study of locomotor development (Thelen et al., 1989). This approach views locomotion as an emergent property of many interacting complex processes, including sensory, motor, perceptual, integrative, respiratory, cardiac, and anatomical systems. According to a dynamical systems approach, moving and developing systems have certain self-organizing properties, that is, they can spontaneously form patterns that arise simply from the interaction of the different parts of the system.

A dynamical systems model stresses that actions always occur within specific contexts. As a result, a given neural code will produce different behavioral outcomes according to the contributions of the other elements of the system, as in the position of the child with relation to gravity. Thus, dynamical systems researchers suggest that the specific leg trajectory seen in newborn stepping is not coded precisely anywhere in the nervous system. Instead, the pattern emerges through the contributions of many elements. These include the neural substrate, anatomical linkages, body composition, activation or arousal level, and the gravitational conditions in which the infant is kicking (Thelen et al., 1989).

From a dynamical systems perspective, the disappearance of the neonatal stepping pattern at about 2 months of age results from changes in a number of components of the system that reduce the likelihood of seeing this behavior. For example, body build changes greatly in the first 18 months of life. Infants add a lot of body fat in the first 2 months of life and then slim down toward the end of the first year. It has been suggested that the stepping pattern goes away at 2 months because infants have insufficient strength to lift the leg, which is now heavier, during the step cycle (Thelen et al., 1989).

When 4-week-old infants are submerged up to their trunk in water, making them more buoyant and counteracting gravity, stepping increases in frequency (Thelen et al., 1984). This suggests that their weight is a factor that affects the step cycle. Further support for the weight hypothesis related to the disappearance of newborn stepping comes from research examining newborn kicking patterns. Supine kicking has the same spatial and temporal pattern as newborn stepping. For example, the swing phase of locomotion is similar to the flexion and extension phases of the kick, while the stance phase is similar to the pause between kicks. As stepping speeds up, the stance phase is reduced, and as kicking speeds up, the pause phase is reduced (Thelen et al., 1989).

This suggests that the same pattern generator may be responsible for both supine kicking and newborn stepping. Yet supine kicking continues as newborn stepping disappears. One explanation for the persistence of supine kicking is that it requires less strength than stepping, since the infants are not working against gravity (Thelen et al., 1984).

Hans Forssberg, a Swedish physiologist and pediatrician, examined the nervous sys-

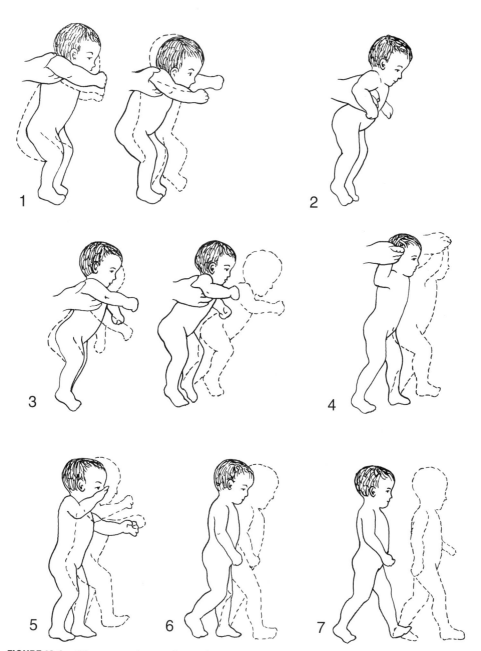

FIGURE 13-1. The seven phases of erect locomotion according to McGraw. *1.* Stepping reflex. *2.* Its disappearance. *3.* Its reappearance. *4.* Assisted locomotion. *5–7.* Three phases of erect independent walking, in which the hands gradually move from a high guard position (*5*) to the side (*6*), and the trunk and head become more erect (*7*). (Adapted with permission from McGraw MB. The neuromuscular maturation of the human infant. NY: Hafner Press, 1945.)

tem contribution to the emergence of loco-motion in more detail. He postulated that human locomotion is characterized by the interaction of many systems with certain hi-erarchical components (Forssberg, 1985). His research suggests that an innate pattern generator creates the basic rhythm of the step cycle, which can be seen in newborn stepping. In the first year, the gradual devel-opment of descending systems from higher neural centers gives the child the ability to control this locomotor activity. Adaptive systems for equilibrium control, organized at a higher level than those controlling the pattern generator, develop over a longer period.

According to this research, the emergence of walking with support is not the result of critical changes in the stepping pattern per se but appears to be due to maturation of the equilibrium system. In addition, the gradual emergence of mature gait over the next year is hypothesized to result from a new, higher-level control system influencing the original lower-level network and modifying it (Forssberg, 1985).

Forssberg's research, using electromyography (EMG) and motion analysis, has examined how the locomotor pattern changes over the first 2 years of development. Studies using motion analysis techniques have shown a gradual transformation of the locomotor movement from a synchronous pattern of joint movements in newborn stepping to a more adultlike dissociated pattern of joint motion by the end of the first year of development. The transformation to adultlike gait patterns happens during the latter part of the second year. At this point, heel strike begins to occur in front of the body. Figure 13-2 shows the kinematics of neonatal versus adult stepping movements. Note that the infant shows high levels of hip flexion compared to the adult.

The EMG analysis supported the findings of the motion analysis. For example, in the neonate, the motor pattern was characterized by a high degree of synchronized activity. In other words, the extensor muscles of different joints were active simultaneously, and there was much coactivation of agonist and antagonist muscles at each joint. As with the movement patterns, the EMG patterns began to look more mature during the latter part of the second year, with asynchronous patterns emerging at the joints (Forssberg, 1985).

Neonatal locomotion may be similar to that of quadrupeds who walk on the their toes, such as cats, dogs, and horses. For example, newborns show high knee and hip flexion and do not have heel strike. Since extensor muscle activity occurs prior to foot

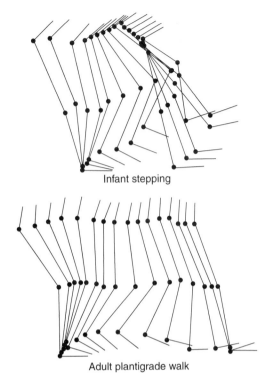

Infant stepping

Adult plantigrade walk

FIGURE 13-2.   Stick figures taken from motion analysis of one step cycle of walking in an infant versus an adult. Note the high amounts of hip flexion in the infant. (Reprinted with permission from Forssberg H. Ontogeny of human locomotor control: 1. Infant stepping, supported locomotion and transition to independent locomotion. Exp Brain Res 1985;67:481.)

touchdown, it appears to be driven by an innate locomotor pattern generator, as has been found in quadrupeds, rather than being reflexively activated by the foot in contact with the ground. It has also been suggested that the neural network for stepping must be organized at or below the brainstem level, since anencephalic infants (infants born without a cerebral cortex) can perform a similar pattern of stepping (Peiper, 1961).

Interestingly, some researchers believe the abnormal gait patterns found in many patients with neurological pathology are actually immature locomotor patterns. Thus, children with cerebral palsy, mentally retarded children, and children who habitually toe-walk may persist in using an immature locomotor pattern, while adults with acquired neurological disease may revert to immature locomotion because of the loss of higher center modulation over the locomotor pattern generator (Forssberg, 1985).

So what are the elements that contribute to the emergence of locomotion in the infant? Remember that in development, some elements of the nervous and musculoskeletal system may be functionally ready before others, but the system must wait for the maturation of the slowest component before the target behavior can appear. A small increase or change in the development of the slowest component can act as the control parameter, becoming the impetus that drives the system to a new behavioral form.

The research we just discussed shows that many of the components that contribute to independent locomotion are functional before the child takes any independent steps. Function of the locomotor pattern generator is present in a limited capacity at birth and is improved during the second half of the first year as the tight intralimb synergies become dissociated and capable of more complex modulation and control. As we noted in Chapter 8, infants are able to use optic flow information at birth to modulate head movements and by 5 to 6 months of age for modulation of stance. Motivation to navigate toward a distant object is clearly present by the onset of creeping and crawling, and voluntary control over the limbs is certainly present by this time for many behaviors (Thelen et al., 1989).

So what is the constraint that keeps upright bipedal locomotion from emerging before 9 to 12 months of age? Most researchers believe that it is primarily limitations in balance control and possibly also limitations in strength (Forssberg, 1985; Thelen et al., 1989; Woollacott et al., 1989).

For example, when an infant is creeping, one foot can be picked up at a time, so there is always a tripod stance available; hence balance is much less demanding. Normal infants who are about to take their first steps have developed motor coordination within the locomotor pattern generator, and they have functional visual, vestibular, and somatosensory systems and the motivation to move forward. Infants may also have sufficient muscle strength at least to balance, if

not for use in propelling the body forward. But they cannot use these processes in effective locomotion until the postural control system can effectively control the shift of weight from leg to leg to avoid a fall. When these processes hit a particular threshold for effective function, the dynamic behavior of independent bipedal locomotion can emerge.

There are three requirements for successful locomotion: a rhythmic stepping pattern (progression), the control of balance (stability), and the ability to modify gait (adaptation). Clearly, a rhythmic stepping pattern develops first. It is present in limited form at birth and is refined during the first year of life. Stance stability develops second, toward the end of the first year and the beginning of the second year of life. As we discuss in the next section, it appears that adaptability is refined in the first years after the onset of independent walking.

Maturation of Independent Locomotion

Bril and Breniere, two French researchers, studied the emergence of locomotion and hypothesized that learning to walk is a two-stage process (Bril and Breniere, 1993; Breniere and Bril, 1998). In the initial phase (3 to 6 months after onset of walking), infants learn to control balance, and in the second phase, which lasts through 5 years of independent walking, the locomotor pattern is progressively refined.

They studied children longitudinally during the first 6 years of life to see how gait patterns change as independent locomotion develops. Significant changes in emerging gait patterns are summarized in Figure 13-3. Figure 13-3A shows the decrease in the duration of the double-support phase of gait that shows a dramatic drop in the first 4 months of walking, then continues to drop until about 35 months of independent walking. Figure 13-3B shows the dramatic increase in step length that occurs in the first 4 months of walking, along with a decrease in step width that continues through about 10 months of walking. They noted that in newly

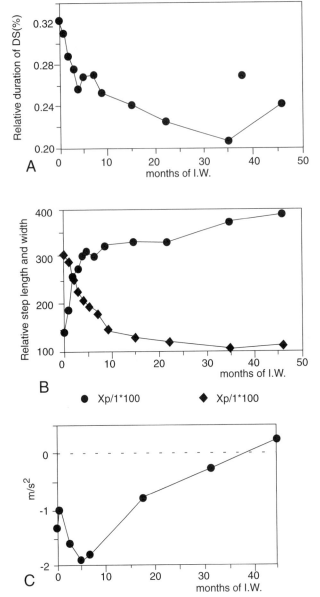

A

B

● Xp/1*100   ◆ Xp/1*100

C

FIGURE 13-3. Changes in walking parameters during the first 4 years of walking. **A.** The relative duration of the double-support phase. **B.** Changes in relative step length and width. **C.** Changes in vertical acceleration of the center of gravity. DS, double support; I.W., independent walking. (Reprinted with permission from Bril B, Breniere Y. Posture and independent locomotion in childhood: learning to walk or learning dynamic postural control? In: Savelsbergh GJP, ed. The development of coordination in infancy. Amsterdam: North Holland, 1993, 337–358.)

walking children, velocity was very low, with the swing phase very short and double-support phase long, probably because the children needed a long double-support phase to regain balance.

The authors asked what factors might constrain the development of these postural abilities during walking (Breniere and Bril, 1998). They proposed that high levels of strength are required to control gravitational forces tending to destabilize the upper body. In fact, it has been predicted that re-

quirements of musculotendinous forces at the hip may reach 6 to 8 times body weight at certain points in the stance phase of gait (McKinnon and Winter, 1993). Thus, Breniere and Bril hypothesized that newly walking children may lack muscular strength to control balance. In order to test this hypothesis the authors measured vertical center of gravity acceleration under the assumption that vertical ground reaction forces reflect the ability of the musculoskeletal system to compensate for body weight.

In adults, the vertical acceleration of the center of mass at heel strike is positive, indicating that they have both the muscular capacity and the control to counter destabilizing forces associated with initial contact. In contrast, Breniere and Bril (1998) found, as you see in Figure 13-3*C*, that at the onset of independent walking, the vertical acceleration of the center of mass at heel strike was always negative, indicating an initial deficit in muscular capacity. In the first 5 months of independent walking the infants increased walking velocity substantially, in large part by increasing the step length. This increases the vertical instability, and interestingly, the vertical acceleration of the center of mass becomes even more negative. Thus, during this period, muscle strength appears to remain low compared to balance requirements. As you see in Figure 13-3*C*, by about 6 months of independent walking the vertical acceleration of the center of mass at heel strike finally showed a change in direction toward positive values, indicating a change in postural control. Now the infants stopped walking by falling and began to control this forward falling during walking. The vertical acceleration of the center of mass at heel strike finally reached 0 value at about 3 to 4 years of walking experience (4 to 5 years of age), showing that they could control the inertial and gravity forces induced by walking (Fig. 13-3*C*). By 5 years of walking experience, 3 of the 5 children showed positive values similar to those of adults (Breniere and Bril, 1998). Since the changes in step width, step length, and double-support phase relate to the mastery of balance control, their findings support the idea that it is during the first phase of walking that a child learns to integrate posture into locomotor movements.

Studies of changes in EMG characteristics and kinematics from the onset of walking through the mastery of mature forms of gait have been performed by other laboratories (Okamoto and Kumamoto, 1972; Sutherland et al., 1980).

In the first days of independent walking, stepping patterns are immature. Push-off motion in the stance phase is absent, the step is very wide, and the arms are held high. The infant appears to generate force to propel the body forward by leaning forward at the trunk. The swing phase is short because the infant is unable to balance on one leg. By 10 to 15 days of independent walking, the infant begins to reduce cocontraction, and at 50 to 85 days after walking onset, the muscle patterns begin to show a reciprocal relationship. Interestingly, if infants are supported during walking, the reciprocal relationship between muscles emerges, but with the additional requirement of stabilizing the body while walking independently, the coactivation returns (Okamoto and Kumamoto, 1972).

Other common gait characteristics in the first year of walking include a high step frequency, absence of the reciprocal swinging movements between the upper and lower limbs, a flexed knee during stance phase, and increased hip flexion, pelvic tilt, and hip abduction during swing phase. There is also ankle plantarflexion at foot strike and decreased ankle flexion during swing, giving a relative foot drop (Sutherland et al., 1980).

By 2 years of age, the pelvic tilt and abduction and the external rotation of the hip are diminished. At foot strike, a knee flexion wave appears, and reciprocal swing in the upper limb is present in about 75% of the children. The relative foot drop disappears as the ankle dorsiflexes during swing. By the end of age 2, the infant begins to show a push-off in stance. During the years from 1 to 7, the muscle amplitudes and durations gradually reduce toward adult levels. By age 7, most muscle and movement patterns during walking look very similar to that of the adult (Sutherland et al., 1980).

Sutherland et al. (1980) list five important characteristics that determine mature gait, including (*a*) duration of single-limb stance, (*b*) walking velocity, (*c*) cadence, (*d*) step length, and (*e*) the ratio of pelvic span to step width.

Duration of single-limb stance increases steadily from 32% in 1-year-olds to 38% in 7-year-olds (39% is a typical adult value). Walking velocity and cadence decrease steadily, while step length increases. Step length, which is short in the newly walking child because of lack of stability of the supporting limb, lengthens with increasing balance abilities. Finally, the ratio of pelvic span, which is defined as body width at the level of the pelvis, to step width increases until age 2.5, after which it stabilizes. By 3 years of age, the gait pattern is essentially mature, though small improvements continue through age 7 (Sutherland et al., 1980).

Table 13-1 summarizes some of the characteristic changes in the step cycle from the initiation of independent walking through the development of mature patterns at about age 3 (Gallahue, 1989). These changes can be seen more graphically in Figure 13-4.

Run, Skip, Hop, and Gallop

Running is often described as an exaggerated form of walking. It differs from the walk because it has a brief flight phase in each step. The flight phase that distinguishes a run from a walk is seen at about the second year of age. Until this time, the infant's run is more like a fast walk, with one foot always in contact with the ground. By 4 years of age, most children can hop (33%) and gallop (43%). The development of the gallop precedes the hop slightly. In one study, by 6.5 years, the children were skillful at hopping and galloping. However, only 14% of 4-year-olds could skip (step-hop) (Clark and Whitall, 1989).

If central pattern generators (CPGs) control walking, are there separate CPGs for hopping, galloping, and skipping? Probably not. Then why do they emerge in a fixed order of appearance? It is possible to explain their emergence from the dynamical systems perspective. Remember that walking and running are patterns of interlimb coordination in which the limbs are 50% out of phase with one another. This is the easiest stepping pattern to produce and thus appears earliest. Running appears later than walking, probably because of its increased strength and balance requirements. Galloping requires that the child produce an asymmetrical gait with unusual timing and a differentiation in force production in each limb, and it may produce additional balance requirements. Hopping

TABLE 13-1. Developmental Sequence for Walking

I. Walking
   A. Initial stage
      1. Difficulty maintaining upright posture
      2. Unpredictable loss of balance
      3. Rigid, halting leg action
      4. Short steps
      5. Flat-footed contact
      6. Toes turn outward
      7. Wide base of support
      8. Flexed knee at contact followed by quick leg extension
   B. Elementary stage
      1. Gradual smoothing out of pattern
      2. Step length increased
      3. Heel–toe contact
      4. Arms down to sides with limited swing
      5. Base of support within the lateral dimensions of trunk
      6. Out-toeing reduced or eliminated
      7. Increased pelvic tilt
      8. Apparent vertical lift
   C. Mature stage
      1. Reflexive arm swing
      2. Narrow base of support
      3. Relaxed, elongated gait
      4. Minimal vertical lift
      5. Definite heel–toe contact
II. Common Problems
   A. Inhibited or exaggerated arm swing
   B. Arms crossing midline of body
   C. Improper foot placement
   D. Exaggerated forward trunk lean
   E. Arms flopping at sides or held out for balance
   F. Twisting of trunk
   G. Poor rhythmical action
   H. Landing flatfooted
   I. Flipping foot or lower leg in or out

Reprinted with permission from Gallahue DL. Understanding motor development: infants, children, adolescents. Indianapolis: Benchmark Press, 1989:236.

emerges next, possibly because it requires the ability to balance the body's weight on one limb and requires additional force to lift the body off the ground after landing. Skipping (a step-hop) emerges last, possibly because one locomotor coordination pattern is imbedded in another pattern, and thus it requires additional coordination abilities (Clark and Whitall, 1989).

It has been proposed that developmental milestones such as walk, run, gallop, hop,

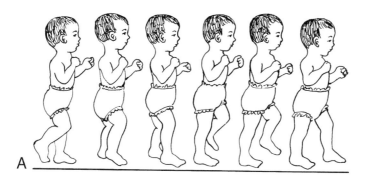

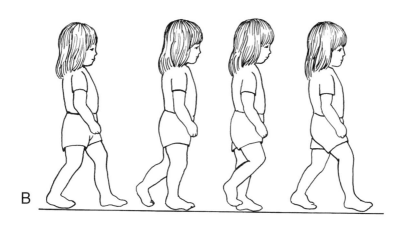

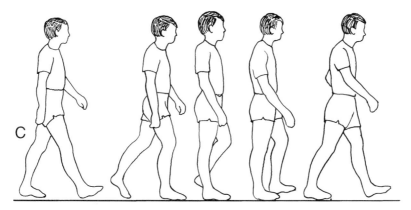

FIGURE 13-4.   Body motions associated with developing gait. **A.** Initial forms of gait. **B.** Elementary forms of gait. **C.** Mature forms of gait. (Adapted from Gallahue DL. Understanding motor development: Infants, children, adolescents. Indianapolis: Benchmark, 1989:237.)

and skip are better indicators of balance development than chronological age. For example, in a study that compared EMG (timing and amplitude) and kinetic (center of pressure [COP] and torque production) characteristics of reactive postural responses in children, the highest level of significance between groups across development was found when children were grouped by these developmental milestones rather than chronological age (Sundermier et al., in press).

Development of Adaptation

How do children learn to adapt their walking patterns so they can navigate over and around obstacles? As we mentioned in Chapter 12, both reactive and proactive strategies are used to modify gait to changes in the environment. There has been very little research examining the development of adaptation in normal children. As a result, we know little about how children learn to compensate for disturbances to their gait nor how they develop proactive strategies to modify gait in advance of obstacles.

Reactive Strategies

Reactive strategies for adapting gait relate to the integration of compensatory postural responses into the gait cycle. Researchers have looked at compensatory postural muscle responses to perturbations during locomotion and compared them to those during perturbed quiet stance.

In response to fast-velocity stance perturbations, children respond with both an automatic postural response and a monosynaptic reflex response. As children mature, the stretch reflex response gets smaller in amplitude as the postural response gets faster. In very young children there is considerable coactivation of antagonist muscles (Berger et al., 1985).

Perturbations during gait produce a monosynaptic reflex response in children aged 1 to 2.5 years but not in older children, as you see in Figure 13-5. This figure shows

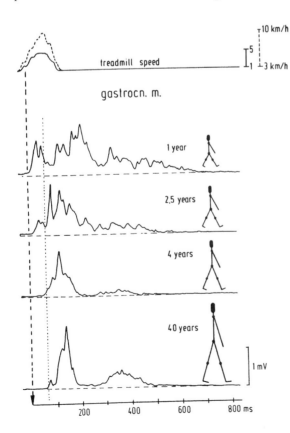

FIGURE 13-5. Examples of the gastrocnemius EMG responses of individual children of 1, 2.5, and 4 years of age and of an adult whose balance is perturbed during walking on a treadmill by a brief increase in treadmill speed. *Left vertical line,* onset of the treadmill acceleration. *Dotted line,* onset of the EMG response. Note the large monosynaptic reflex in the youngest children before the automatic postural response. This disappears by 4 years of age. (Reprinted with permission from Berger W, Quintern J, Dietz V. Stance and gait perturbations in children: developmental aspects of compensatory mechanisms. Electroencephal Clin Neurophysiol 1985;61:385–388.)

the 1-year-old having large monosynaptic reflexes before the automatic postural response, but the reflex is reduced in the 2.5- year-old and has disappeared in the 4-year-old and adult. Similar to stance perturbations, automatic postural responses to gait perturbations become faster with age, with mature responses occurring by about 4 years. Coactivation of antagonist muscles also is reduced with age.

Changes in the characteristics of compensatory postural activity are associated with increased stability during gait and increased ability to compensate for perturbations to gait (Berger et al., 1985). This study suggests that children as young as a year old who are capable of independent locomotion can integrate compensatory postural activity into slow walking when gait is disturbed, though their responses are immature.

Compensatory Stepping Skills During Balance Recovery

The ability to step independently is a fundamental skill required both for locomotion and for balance recovery when threats to balance are large, requiring a step. Interestingly, it appears that the ability to take independent steps in walking does not automatically translate into the ability to use a step for balance recovery. In a study examining the emergence of the ability to step in response to increasing velocities of balance threats, standers (children who could stand but not walk), new walkers (children capable of three steps but with less than 2 weeks' walking experience), intermediate walkers (children with 1 to 3 months' walking experience) and advanced walkers (children with 3 to 6 months' walking experience) were given backward support surface translations. Results showed that the ability to adapt balance responses to increasing balance threats is not present in new standers and new walkers, since almost no children in these two categories were able to take a step to recover balance. Stepping to recover balance begins to develop in infants with 1 to 3 months of walking experience and is relatively refined by 6 months of walking experience (Roncesvalles et al., 2000).

Proactive Strategies

Proactive strategies for adapting gait use sensory information to modify gait patterns in advance of obstacles to gait. When do children begin integrating these strategies into the step cycle? It has been suggested that children first learning to walk acquire feedback control of balance before feed-forward control (Hass and Diener, 1988). The results of experiments by Bril and Breniere (1993) support this idea, since children seem to spend the first 4 to 5 months of walking learning to integrate balance into the step cycle. However, there is little research on the development of proactive strategies to help clinicians understand the emergence of this important aspect of mobility.

Head and Trunk Stabilization During Gait

An important part of controlling locomotion is learning to stabilize the head. Adults stabilize the head with great precision, allowing a steady gaze. Thus, control of the head, arm, and trunk (HAT) segment is a critical part of controlling mobility. How do children control the HAT during locomotion, ensuring stabilization of the head and gaze?

Assaiante and Amblard (1993, 1995) performed experiments in children ranging from early walkers through 10 years of age to explore changes in control of these body segments. They suggest that balance and locomotion can be organized according to one of two stable reference frames, either the support surface on which the subject stands and moves or the gravitational reference of vertical.

They noted that when using the support surface as reference, the subject organized balance responses from the feet up toward the head, using mainly proprioceptive and cutaneous cues. In contrast, when the subject stabilized the head using vision and vestibular information, balance was organized from the head down toward the feet. These researchers explored the changing use of these two strategies in balance control during locomotor development in children.

They also noted that the head can be stabilized on the trunk in one of two modes, in an en bloc mode, in which it moves with the trunk, or in an articulated mode, in which it moves freely, minimizing movements away from vertical. This study explored locomotor strategies through kinematic analysis of walking in infants and children up to 8 years of age.

The authors found that from the acquisition of stance until about 6 years of age, children organize locomotion from the bottom up, using the support surface as a reference and controlling head movements in an en bloc mode, which serves to reduce the degrees of freedom to be controlled. During this period the children gradually learn to stabilize the hips, then the shoulders, and finally the head. At about 7 years of age, with mastery of control of the head, the head control changes to an articulated mode, and top-down organization of balance during locomotion becomes dominant. The authors hypothesized that at 7 to 8 years of age, information specifying head position in relation to gravity becomes more available to the equilibrium control centers and thus allows the child to use an articulated mode of head control. They suggest that there may be a transient dominance of vestibular processing in locomotor balance at this age (Assaiante and Amblard, 1995).

Other research has shown that during the first 10 to 15 weeks of independent walking there is a substantial increase in head and trunk stabilization, after which these parameters do not change for about a year. Hip stabilization in space is present at the onset of walking, while head and trunk stabilization improves considerably during the following 3 to 4 months (Ledebt et al., 1995).

Studies of the development of canal and otolith vestibulo-ocular reflexes (VORs) have shown that their developmental time course is different. Canal VOR is relatively stable in young walkers. However, the onset of walking is a transition point in otolith VOR development, with clear changes in the slow-phase velocity of the VOR. It has therefore been proposed that otolith VOR development may play a critical role in the development of postural control during the first months of walking. The authors noted that though the canal VOR does not change during this period, it is very different from that of older children, which suggests that it is still immature. They propose that this may be related to the fact that new walkers adopt a stiff neck posture during walking, also used by adults with bilateral vestibular deficits. This strategy reduces the amplitude of head rotations in the pitch and roll planes to limit instability in the movement of the visual field due to problems with gaze stabilization (Wiener-Vacher et al., 1996).

Initiation of Gait

Chapter 12, on locomotion in adults, showed that gait initiation involves anticipatory shifts in the center of pressure backward and toward the stepping foot, which cause a forward and lateral shift of the center of gravity toward the stance leg. Recent research has shown that an anticipatory backward shift in the center of pressure is present in children as young as 2.5 years of age and becomes habitual by 6 years of age (Ledebt et al., 1998).

In adults, the anticipatory changes in the center of pressure are accompanied by inhibition of the soleus muscle and activation of the tibialis muscles prior to heel-off (Herman et al., 1973; Breniere et al., 1981). In a recent study using motion analysis and muscle response patterns to characterize step initiation in both prewalkers and in children with 1 month to 4 years of walking experience (Assaiante et al., in press), anticipatory postural adjustments before step initiation were not found in prewalkers but were present in children with as little as 1 to 4 months of walking experience. These adjustments included a clear anticipatory lateral tilt of the pelvis and of the stance leg to unload the opposite leg shortly before its swing phase. In addition, there was an anticipatory activation of the hip abductor muscle of the leg in stance phase prior to heel off, suggesting control of pelvis stabilization. These anticipatory postural adjustments did not occur consistently until 4 to 5 years of age. Between 1 and 4 years of age there was a shift from the use of both upper and lower parts of the body (an en bloc strategy) in the lateral shift of the body toward the stance leg to the inclusion of only the pelvis and leg (articulated operation) in the older children, similar to findings from adults. Accompanying these kinematic changes were lower use of hip and knee muscles and greater use of ankle muscles in the older children during the gait initiation process (Assaiante et al., in press). The application of this concept can be found in Lab Activity 13-1.

Development of Other Mobility Skills

The first part of this chapter describes the emergence of independent locomotion. We now turn briefly to a review of some of the information on the emergence of other mobility behaviors during development, including rolling, prone progression, and movement from lying in a supine position to stance.

There are two approaches to describing motor development in infants and children. One approach relies on normative studies that describe the age at which various motor behaviors emerge. Normative studies have given rise to norm-referenced scales that compare an infant's motor behavior with the performance of a group of infants of the same age. Normative studies can provide clinicians with rough guidelines about the relative ages associated with specific motor milestones. However, they have universally reported that there is huge variability in the time at which normal children achieve motor milestones (Palisano, 1993).

Another approach to describing motor development is with reference to the stages associated with the emergence of a single behavior, such as rolling or coming to stand. Clinicians often use stages in the emergence of a skill as the basis for a treatment progression, with the assumption that a mature and stable adultlike pattern is the last stage in the progression. However, recent research has raised doubts about the concept that there is a consistent stable sequential pattern during the emergence of a particular motor behavior (Fishkind and Haley, 1986; Horowitz and Sharby, 1988).

 LAB ACTIVITY 13-1

OBJECTIVE: To examine the kinematics of developing gait.

PROCEDURE: Observe gait patterns in one or two infants of the following ages: 8 to 10 months (prewalkers), 12 to 18 months (new walkers), and 18 to 24 months (experienced walkers). Repeat Lab Activity 12.1 to document age-related changes in spatial and temporal aspects of gait across these age groups. To gather information on age-related kinematic changes, repeat Lab Activity 12.2 with these age groups.

Also observe and describe the following gait characteristics in each child: (*a*) ability to maintain an upright posture, (*b*) ability to control stability (how often the child falls within a fixed period), (*c*) initial contact at foot strike, and (*d*) position of arms.

ASSIGNMENT: Compare your descriptions across the children. How do each of the parameters change with age and experience in walking? Compare your descriptions of the development of gait to those described in Table 13-1. When do gait parameters begin to approximate those of adults?

Given these cautions about timing, variability, and the sequential nature of the emergence of motor skills, we review some of the studies that have examined the stages in the emergence of rolling, prone progression, and the assumption of the vertical position from supine. As we mentioned in Chapter 7, much of the information we have on the emergence of motor behavior in children is largely the result of efforts in the 1920s and 1930s by two developmental researchers, Arnold Gesell and Myrtle McGraw, who observed and recorded the stages of development in normal children (McGraw, 1945).

Development of Rolling

Rolling is an important part of mobility because rotation or partial rotation is a part of movements used to achieve supine-to-sit or supine-to-stand behavior. Babies first roll from the side-lying position to the supine position at 1 to 2 months of age and from supine to side lying at 4 to 5 months. Infants roll from prone to supine at 4 months of age and from supine to prone at 6 to 8 months. Infants change their rolling pattern as they mature, from a log-rolling pattern, in which the entire body rolls as a unit, to a segmental pattern. By 9 months of age, most infants use a segmental rotation of the body on the pelvis (McGraw, 1945; Touwen, 1976).

Development of Prone Progression

According to McGraw (1945), the prone progression includes nine phases that take the infant from the prone position to creeping and crawling and span the months from birth to 10 to 13 months. Figure 13-6 illustrates the nine phases reported by McGraw and the relative time in which the behavior was seen. Graphed is the age at which the behavior was seen and the percent of children in which the behavior was observed. The first phase is characterized by lower extremity flexion and extension in a primarily flexed posture. In phase 2, spinal extension begins, as does the development of head control. In the third phase, spinal extension continues cephalocaudally, reaching the thoracic area. The arms can extend and support the chest off the surface. Propulsion movements begin in the arms and legs during phases 4 and 5. In phase 6, the creeping position is assumed. Phase 7 is characterized by fairly disorganized attempts at progression; however, by phases 8 and 9, organized propulsion in the creeping position has emerged.

Keep in mind that McGraw placed great emphasis on the neural antecedents of maturing motor behavior. Her emphasis was on describing stages of motor development that could be related to the structural growth and maturation of the central nervous system. Current research has shown that many factors contribute to the emergence of motor skill during development, including but not limited to maturation of the CNS (Thelen and Ulrich, 1991).

Development of Supine to Stand

Just as the pattern used to roll changes as infants develop, so does the movement pattern used to achieve stance from a supine posi-

tion. The pattern initially seen in infants moving from supine to stand includes rolling to prone, then moving onto all fours and using a pull-to-stand method to achieve the erect position. With development, the child learns to move from the all-fours position to a plantigrade position and from there to erect stance. By age 2 to 3 years, the supine-to-prone portion is modified to a partial roll and sit-up pattern, and by ages 4 to 5, a symmetrical sit-up pattern emerges (Fig. 13-7). This is considered a mature or adult-like movement pattern used for this task (McGraw, 1945). But as you remember from Chapter 12, researchers have found tremendous variability in how adults move from supine to stand. Just as was true for adults, most likely strength in the abdominals and hip flexors plays a major roll in the type of pattern used by infants when moving from supine to stand (VanSant, 1988a).

✆ LOCOMOTION IN THE OLDER ADULT

Falls and the injuries that often accompany them are a serious problem in the older adult. In fact, falls are the seventh leading cause of death in people over 75 years of age (Ochs et al., 1985). Of adults over 75 years who have had an injurious fall, 45% acquire a fear of falling, and 26% of these people begin avoiding situations that require refined balance skills, which leads to further declines in walking and balance skills.

Many of the falls among the elderly occur during walking. It is therefore important to understand the changes in the systems contributing to normal gait in the elderly to understand the cause of increased falls in this population. As we stated in the first section of this chapter, many researchers now believe that balance control is a primary contributor to stable walking. In addition, decreased balance control is a major factor affecting loss of independent mobility in many elderly. The following sections describe locomotor changes commonly seen in the older adult and the systems contributing to these changes.

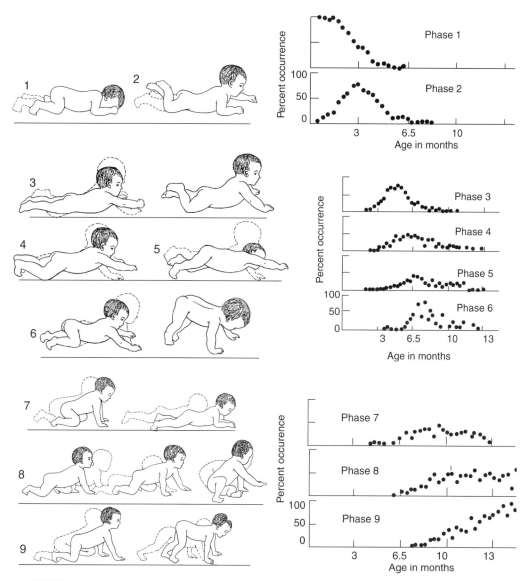

FIGURE 13-6.   *Left.* The nine phases of prone progression as reported by McGraw. *Right.* Graphs for each phase showing the ages at which the behavior was seen (x-axis) and the percent of children in whom the behavior was observed (y-axis). (Adapted with permission from McGraw MG. The neuromuscular maturation of the human infant. NY: Hafner, 1945.)

Dysmobility: Aging or Pathology?

Again, age-related changes in locomotion may be due to primary or secondary aging phenomena. Primary factors affecting aging include changes in gene expression that result in changes in hormonal function, aging, and death. Also, individuals may have a genetic predisposition to specific diseases, which results in an inevitable decline of neu-

ronal function within a particular system. Secondary, or experiential, factors include nutrition, exercise, stress level, and acquired pathologies, among others. The extent to which gait disorders in the elderly are due to primary or secondary factors is an important point to consider as we begin to look at the literature on changes in gait characteristics in the older adult.

The older clinical literature referred to

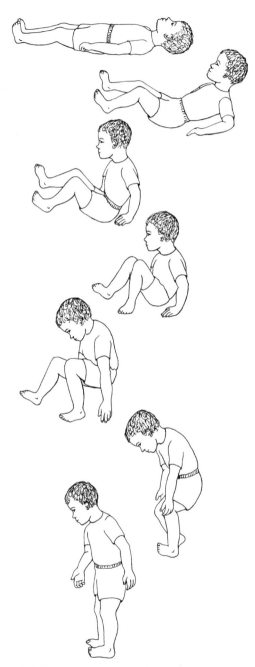

FIGURE 13-7. Common pattern used to move from supine to stand in children aged 4 to 5. The child uses a symmetrical pattern. (Adapted with permission from VanSant AF. Age differences in movement patterns used by children to rise from a supine position to erect stance. Phys Ther 1988;68:1130–1138.)

many walking patterns as age-related gait disorders. These diverse gait disorders included gait apraxia (slow, halting, short-stepped, shuffling, or sliding gait), hypokinetic-hypertonic syndrome (slow, deliberate gait but without shuffling or sliding), and marche à petit pas (small, quick shuffling steps, followed by a slow cautious, unsteady gait), vestibular dysfunction gait (difficulties in turning), and proprioceptive dysfunction gait (cautious, with a tendency to watch the feet and make missteps) (Craik, 1989).

As with the postural control literature, care must be taken when reviewing studies discussing age-related changes in gait. When interpreting the results of a study, one should examine carefully the population studied, and ask questions such as these: What criteria were used in selecting older subjects? Did researchers exclude anyone with pathology under the assumption that pathology is not a part of primary aging? Results vary tremendously depending on the composition of older adults under study. For example, one study noted that in an unselected group of subjects 60 to 99 years old, walking velocities were much slower than those for young adults and also slower than reported in other published studies on older adults (Imms and Edholm, 1981). It is quite possible that the subjects in the study were less fit and that many complained of symptoms likely to impair gait. In contrast, a study that screened 1184 older adults and chose 32 who had no pathology found no changes in the gait parameters tested (Gabell and Nayak, 1984).

Thus, more recent research has begun to indicate that many gait disorders considered to be age-related, such as gait apraxia, hypokinetic-hypertonic syndrome, and marche à petit pas, are manifestations of pathology rather than characteristics of a generalized aging process. However, as we note in the following sections, distinctive changes in gait occur in many healthy older adults.

Temporal and Distance Factors

Studies examining changes in walking patterns with age have used a number of experimental approaches. In one approach, which we might call a naturalistic approach, adults were observed walking spontaneously in a natural setting. This paradigm was used to minimize the constraints on walking style that are often necessary when quantifying gait parameters in a laboratory setting.

In these studies, researchers observed people of different ages walking along the streets of New York City (Drillis, 1961) and Amsterdam (Molen, 1973). In the first study, of 752 pedestrians in New York City, as age increased from 20 to 70 years, there was a decrease in walking velocity, step length, and step rate (no statistical analysis was reported). In the second study, on 533 pedestrians in Amsterdam, similar results were found. Gender differences were also found; both younger and older women walked more slowly and with shorter step length and higher cadence than men.

While there are advantages in allowing subjects to walk in a natural environment, the disadvantages include being unable to control for such variables as goals, such as taking a stroll versus hurrying to work, and relative health of the subjects (Craik, 1989).

Laboratory studies have also repeatedly demonstrated that walking speed decreases with age. One of the earlier studies outlines three stages of age-related changes in walking (Spielberg, 1940). Stage 1 changes were found in adults between 60 and 72 years of age and included decreases in walking speed, shorter step length, lower cadence, and less vertical movement of the center of gravity. Subjects between 72 and 86 years of age showed stage 2 gait changes, including the disappearance of normal arm–leg synergies, along with overproduction of unnecessary movements. In stage 3, including subjects ages 86 to 104 years, there was a disintegration of the gait pattern, arrhythmia in the stepping rate, and an absence of arm swing movement. It was later pointed out that these changes are not typical in healthy older adults, and the study probably included adults with symptoms of Parkinson's disease and other motor pathology (Murray et al., 1969).

Kinematic Analysis

Later studies of age-related changes in gait focused on a kinematic analysis of stepping patterns in older adults. In one study, subjects were healthy men with normal strength and range of motion ranging in age from 20 to 87 years of age. Those over 65 years of age were given a neurological exam to exclude the possibility of neurological deficits contributing to the observed changes. Participants were photographed in the laboratory using interrupted-light photography at 20 Hz while walking at their preferred and fast speeds (Murray et al., 1969).

Men over 67 years of age showed significantly ($p < .01$) slower walking speeds (118 to 123 cm/second) than the young adults (150 cm/second). Stride length was also significantly shorter, especially during fast walking. Vertical movement of the head during the gait cycle was smaller, while lateral movement was larger. The stride tended to be wider for men over 74. Toeing out was also greater for men over 80. Beyond 65, stance phase was longer, with a commensurate shortening of time in swing phase.

Finally hip, knee, and ankle flexion were less than in young adults, and the whole shoulder rotation pattern was shifted to a more extended position, with less elbow rotation as well. Figure 13-8 is adapted from their study, showing the differences in the limb positions of a younger versus an older man at heel strike.

Interestingly, the researchers concluded that the men studied did not have a pathological gait pattern. Instead, they said, walking was guarded, possibly with the aim to increase stability. Gait patterns were similar to those used by someone walking on a slippery surface or in darkness. Doesn't this sound like a postural control problem? From reading this description, one might hypothesize that gait changes in the elderly person relate more to the loss of balance control than to changes in the step cycle itself (Murray et al., 1969).

In a second study, age-related changes in gait patterns were investigated in women, and similar changes were noted, including

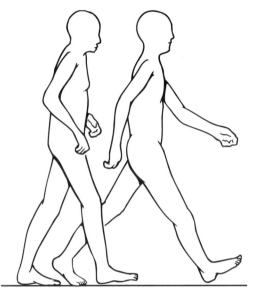

FIGURE 13-8.   The walking pattern of a young adult versus a healthy older man. (Adapted with permission from Murray MP, Kory RC, Clarkson BH. Walking patterns in healthy older men. J Gerontol 1969:24:169–178.)

reduced walking speeds and shorter steps. These changes occurred in the 60- to 70-year-old group (Murray et al., 1970).

How do these slower walking speeds affect function in daily life? Many of the previous studies report that older adults are unable to walk faster than 1.4 m/second. This is the minimal speed required to cross a street safely. Lundgren-Lindquist et al. (1983) have shown that none of the 205 subjects studied who were 79 years old could cross a street before the traffic light changed when walking at their preferred speed. Thus, many of the older adults studied would not be considered functional walkers on city streets with heavy traffic.

Muscle Activation Patterns

The previous studies show clear changes in certain kinematic characteristics of the gait cycle in the average older adult. How do these changes relate to changes in muscle response patterns? In a study comparing patterns of muscle activity in younger (19 to 38 years) and older (64 to 86 years) women, average EMG activity levels in gastrocnemius, tibialis anterior, biceps femoris, rectus

femoris, and peroneus longus were higher in the older group than in the younger group (Finley et al., 1969).

In addition, there were changes in the activity of individual muscles at specific points in the step cycle. For example, at heel strike, peroneus longus and gastrocnemius were moderately to highly active in the older women but showed little or no activity in the younger group. The authors suggested that this increased activity resulted from an effort to improve stability during the stance phase of gait. For example, increased coactivation of agonist and antagonist muscles at a joint may be used to improve balance control by increasing joint stiffness. This is a strategy often seen in subjects who are unskilled in a task or who are performing in a situation that requires increased control (Woollacott, 1989). The application of this concept can be found in Lab Activity 13-2.

Kinetic Analysis

We just noted several studies indicating that older adults show higher levels of muscle re-

---

 LAB ACTIVITY 13-2

OBJECTIVE: To examine age-related changes in the spatial, temporal, and kinematic parameters of gait.

PROCEDURES: Find two older adults from your community, one who is very active and well balanced and one who has complaints of gait and balance problems. Repeat Lab Activity 12.1 to document age-related changes in spatial and temporal aspects of gait with both older adults. To gather information on age-related kinematic changes, repeat Lab Activity 12.2 with both older adults.

ASSIGNMENT: Compare the data you have gathered from healthy young adults to that gathered on your two older subjects. What parameters of gait are similar between the young and the elderly? What parameters differ? How similar or dissimilar are gait parameters between the two older adults? How do your data compare with those described in Table 13-2?

TABLE 13-2.	Summary of Gait Changes in the Older Adult

Temporal and distance factors
   Decreased velocity
   Decreased step length
   Decreased step rate
   Decreased stride length
   Increased stride width
   Increased stance phase
   Increased time in double support
   Decreased swing phase
Kinematic changes
   Decreased vertical movement of the center of gravity
   Decreased arm swing
   Decreased hip, knee, ankle flexion
   Flatter foot on heel strike
   Decreased ability to covary hip/knee movements
   Decreased dynamic stability during stance
Muscle activation patterns
   Increased coactivation (increased stiffness)
Kinetic changes
   Decreased power generation at push-off
   Decreased power absorption at heel strike

sponses and different activation sequences among leg muscles than young adults during walking. But how do these changes in muscle activation patterns change the dynamics of gait?

Using the method of inverse dynamics, moments of force and the mechanical power generated and absorbed at each joint can be calculated. This process allows the amount of power generated by muscles to be estimated. Remember from Chapter 12 that an increase in muscle energy is needed to initiate swing, while a decrease in energy is needed to prepare for heel strike.

Using inverse dynamics techniques, Winter and colleagues compared the gait patterns of 15 healthy adults aged 62 to 78 years to 12 adults aged 21 to 28 years. They found that older adults had significantly shorter stride and longer double-support time than young adults. In addition, in elderly subjects, plantar flexors generated significantly less power at push-off, while the quadriceps muscle absorbed significantly less energy during late stance and early swing (Winter et al., 1990).

These researchers concluded that the re-

duction of plantar flexor power during push-off could explain the shorter step length, flat-footed heel strike, and increased double-support duration. Two alternative explanations were proposed for a weaker push-off in the older adult. One explanation suggested that a reduction in muscle strength in the ankle plantar flexors in the older adults could be responsible for the weaker push-off. An alternative explanation argued that reduced push-off could be an adaptive change used to ensure a safer gait, since high push-off power thrusts upward and forward and is thus destabilizing (Winter et al., 1990).

In this study, an index of dynamic balance was computed to determine the ability to coordinate the anteroposterior balance of the HAT segment while maintaining an appropriate extensor moment in the ankle, knee, and hip during stance phase. It was found that the older adults showed a reduced ability to covary movements at the hip and knee. This means that older adults had trouble controlling the HAT segment while maintaining an extensor moment in the lower stance limb. In evaluating the older group individually, it was noted that two-thirds were within the normal young adult range, while one-third had very low covariances of moments at the hip and knee. It was concluded that some older adults may have had problems with dynamic balance during locomotion, indicative of balance impairments not detected in their medical history or simple clinical tests (Winter et al., 1990).

Numerous research studies have described changes in gait patterns found among many older adults. These changes are summarized in Table 13-2.

Changes in Adaptive Control

Many falls by older adults occur while walking and may be due to slipping and tripping. Several research groups have examined proactive adaptive strategies during gait in the elderly. In addition, studies on age-related changes in reactive balance control have recently been published (Tang and Woollacott, 1998, 1999).

Proactive Adaptation

Proactive adaptation depends in large part on the ability to use visual information to alter gait patterns in anticipation of upcoming obstacles (Patla, 1993). One group of researchers asked whether a possible cause of poor locomotor abilities in older adults might be a reduced ability to sample the visual environment during walking (Patla et al., 1992). They wanted to know whether visual sampling of the environment changed with age.

In their experiment, subjects wore opaque liquid crystal eyeglasses and pressed a switch to make them transparent whenever they wanted to look at the environment. Subjects walked across a floor that either was unmarked or had footprints marked at regular intervals, on which the subjects were supposed to walk. When subjects were constrained to land on the footprints, the young subjects sampled frequently, though for shorter intervals than older subjects, who tended to sample less often but for longer periods. Thus, older adults seem to monitor the terrain much more than the young adults (Patla, 1993).

What is the minimum time required to implement an avoidance strategy in the younger versus older adult? In a second study, healthy young and older adults were asked to walk along a walkway, and when cued by a light at specific points along the walkway, either to lengthen or shorten their stride to match the position of the light (Patla et al., 1992).

Compared with young adults, older adults had more difficulty in modulating their step length when the cue was given only one step duration ahead. Young adults succeeded 80% of the time, while older adults succeeded 60% of the time when lengthening the step and only 38% of the time when shortening the step. The two groups were equally successful when the cue was given two step durations in advance (Patla et al., 1992).

The authors suggest that older adults have more difficulty in shortening a step because of balance constraints. Shortening the step requires regulating the forward pitch of

the HAT segment, which if not controlled, could result in a fall. Remember that in the review of Winter's study presented earlier, older adults had more trouble than young adults controlling dynamic balance during gait.

These results suggest that the older adult may need to begin making modifications to gait patterns in the step prior to a step requiring obstacle avoidance. This may be one cause of increased visual monitoring.

What strategies do older adults use to avoid obstacles during walking? To answer this question, researchers analyzed the gait of 24 young and 24 older (mean age 71 years) healthy adults while they stepped over obstacles of varying heights. Obstacles were made the height of a 1- or 2-inch door threshold or a 6-inch curb, and performance was compared to a 0-mm condition (tape marked on the walkway). No age-related changes in foot clearance over the obstacles were found, but older adults used a significantly more conservative strategy when crossing obstacles. Older adults used a somewhat slower approach speed, a significantly slower crossing speed, and a shorter step length. Also, four of the 24 older adults inadvertently stepped on an obstacle, while none of the young adults did (Chen et al., 1991).

Reactive Adaptation

Trips

Research on falls (Overstall et al., 1977; Gabell et al., 1985) has indicated that 35% to 47% of falls in older adults result from tripping over an object. In order to study the determinants of balance recovery from a trip, Chen (1993) used a biomechanical model simulation. He showed that the critical muscles for recovery from a trip are the hip flexors of the swing leg and the ankle plantarflexors of the stance leg. In addition, he found that rate of torque development rather than available strength was critical to balance recovery. Thus the critical factor to recovery of balance following a trip appears to be how quickly restorative forces can be generated. Figure 13-9 shows the effects of different joint torques and torque development rates on balance recovery after tripping. Figure 13-9*A* shows a stick figure of the response to tripping if one had maximum joint torques and torque development rates, while Figure 13-9*B–C* shows a response if a subject had 75% and 50% of reference torques and rates available. For subject C, the swing foot recontacts the ground, tripping again, with his upper body center of mass in front of his base of support, causing an additional perturbation to balance (Schultz, 1995).

Studies on ability to develop ankle torques in young versus older adults have shown that older adults have slower torque development rates than the young, suggesting that this may be a contributor to falls following trips (Thelen et al., 1996).

Slips

Slips also account for a high percentage (27% to 32%) of falls and subsequent injuries in community-dwelling older adults (Gabell et al., 1985). This phenomenon suggests that although active and healthy older adults preserve a mobility level comparable to that of young adults, these older adults may have difficulty generating efficient reactive postural responses when they slip. A study by Tang and Woollacott (1998) tested the hypothesis that active and healthy older adults use a less effective reactive balance strategy than young adults during an unexpected forward slip at heel strike while walking. They predicted that less effective balance strategies would be manifested by slower and smaller postural responses, altered temporal and spatial organization of the postural responses, and greater upper trunk instability after the slip in older adults.

In the study, young adults (n = 33; age, 25 ± 4 years) and community-dwelling older adults (n = 32; age, 74 ± 14 years) walked down a ramp and across a force plate that moved forward at heel strike, creating a forward slip. Both muscle response characteristics and body segment movements used in the recovery of balance were analyzed.

The researchers noted that older adults were less stable after the slips than young adults. For example, when recovering from a

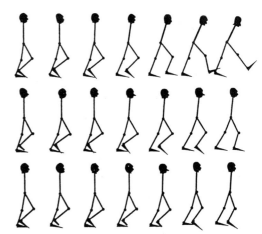

FIGURE 13-9.   A. Stick figure of the response to tripping if a subject had maximum joint torques and torque development rates. **B, C.** Response that would be seen if a subject had 75% and 50% of reference torques and rates available. For the hypothetical subject in **C**, the swing foot recontacts the ground, tripping again, with his upper body center of mass in front of his base of support, causing an additional perturbation to balance (Reprinted with permission from Schultz AB: Muscle function and mobility biomechanics in the elderly: an overview of some recent research. J Gerontol 1995;50A [special issue]:60-63.)

slip, older adults tended to trip more, as the advancing swing limb caught on the surface. Trips occurred 66% of the time in older adults, compared to 15% in the younger adults. Older adults also showed greater trunk hyperextension and higher arm elevation in response to the slip than the young adults, as you see in Figure 13-10*A*. The figure shows a stick figure taken from the motion analysis of the movements of a young and an older adult responding to a forward slip at heel strike. Note the backward extension of the trunk and the raising of the arm in the older adult at the onset of the slip. In addition, older adults had an earlier contralateral foot strike and shortened stride length, suggesting a more conservative balance strategy and an attempt to quickly reestablish the base of support after the slip.

What changes in neuromuscular response characteristics could be the cause of these difficulties in regaining balance in the older adults? A summary of the analysis is shown in Figure 13-10*B*. Older adults (dark bars) showed longer onset latencies and smaller

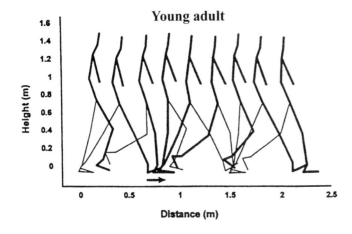

Young adult

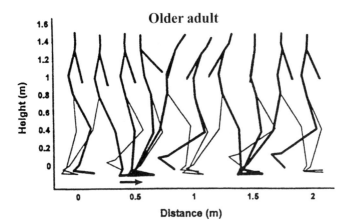

Older adult

FIGURE 13-10. A. Stick figures taken from the motion analysis of the movements of a young and an older adult responding to a forward slip at heel strike. Note the backward extension of the trunk and the raising of the arm in the older adult at the onset of the slip (*arrow*). **B.** Means and standard deviations of onset latencies, burst durations, and burst magnitudes of postural responses in young (bars with light shading) and older (bars with darker shading) adults for the anterior muscles of the perturbed leg. TAi, ipsilateral tibialis anterior; RFi, ipsilateral rectus femoris; GMEi, ipsilateral gluteus medius; ABi, ipsilateral gluteus medius. (Reprinted with permission from Tang PF, Woollacott MH. Inefficient postural responses to unexpected slips during walking in older adults. J Gerontol 1998;53:M471–M480.)

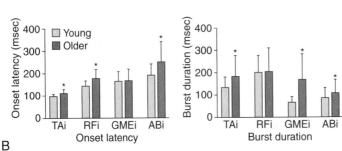
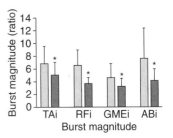

B

magnitudes in the postural muscles activated in balance recovery (for example, tibialis anterior, rectus femoris, and abdominal muscles of the perturbed leg) compared to the younger adults (light bars). These delayed and weaker muscle responses thus contributed to the trunk hyperextension and trips seen in the older adults during recovery. In order to compensate for these deficiencies in responses, the older adults showed longer muscle response burst dura-

tion (Fig. 13-10*B*) and the use of the arms to aid in recovery. They also showed a longer coactivation time for the agonist–antagonist muscle pairs at the ankle, knee, and trunk of the perturbed leg, possibly to stiffen the joints as an additional aid in balance control (Tang and Woollacott, 1998).

How do older adults adapt their responses to balance threats at different phases in the gait cycle? When young adults undergo a balance threat at midstance rather than at heel strike, the threat to stability is less, and they reduce the amplitude of responses appropriately. However, when older adults experience a midstance slip, their responses are actually the same size as at heel strike, showing little to no adaptation. Why is this the case? It is possible that their reduced response capacity (smaller burst magnitudes) at heel strike (Fig. 13-10*B*) is the key constraint. They may be showing a normal response at midstance but simply do not have the response capacity to increase the response to appropriate levels for the increased balance threat at heel strike (Tang and Woollacott, 1999).

Gait Changes in Fallers Versus Nonfallers

How do the walking characteristics of older adults who fall compare to those with no history of falls? While the previous studies have shown that the gait characteristics of healthy older adults show few differences from those of younger adults, older individuals with a history of falls show significant differences in walking patterns (Heitmann et al., 1989; Wolfson et al., 1995). Wolfson et al. (1995) have shown that both stride length (nonfallers, 0.82 ± 0.22 m; fallers, 0.53 ± 0.21 m) and walking speed (nonfallers, 0.64 ± 0.21 m/second; fallers, 0.37 ± 0.17 m/second) are significantly reduced in older adults who fall.

Heitmann et al. (1989) have found that older female subjects with poor balance performance have increased step width during gait. Other studies reported that step width at the heel was significantly larger in older persons with a history of falls walking at a fast speed of 6 km/hour than the step width of subjects without a history of falls. It was also noted that older fallers had balance problems unrelated to gait because they were unable to stand as long as nonfallers with feet in tandem position and eyes open. Of course, it is likely that older adults with a history of falls have an undiagnosed pathological condition. Therefore, it is important to examine these subjects carefully to determine underlying pathology that may contribute to gait

disturbances (Heitmann et al., 1989; Gehlsen and Whaley, 1990).

Role of Pathology in Gait Changes in the Elderly

What is the role of secondary aging factors, particularly the role of pathology, in gait abnormalities observed in older adults? In many studies examining apparently healthy older adults, participants are considered pathology free if they have no known neurological, cardiovascular, or musculoskeletal disorder. Yet, when this population is examined carefully, many show subtle pathologies. For example, a study on idiopathic gait disorders among older adults found that on closer medical evaluation, this type of gait pattern could actually be attributed to a number of specific disease processes (Sudarsky and Ronthal, 1983). This suggests that in many instances pathological conditions may be an underlying contributing factor in gait pattern changes seen in older adults. Pathology within a number of systems has the potential to affect locomotor skills in the older adult.

Cognitive Factors

The ability to divide attention between two or more tasks is an important aspect of locomotion during many activities of daily life. For example, an older adult may be required to walk across a street while talking to a friend and/or while looking both ways to avoid oncoming traffic. In the past 10 years a number of studies have addressed the ability of older adults simultaneously to perform locomotor and other cognitively demanding tasks to determine whether attentional problems are a factor contributing to falls.

In order to study attention it is helpful to define it. Attention is defined here as the information-processing capacity of an individual. An assumption regarding this information-processing capacity is that it is limited for any individual and that performing any task requires a given portion of capacity. Thus, if two tasks are performed together and they require more than the total capacity, the performance in either or both deteriorates.

Traditionally locomotion as been considered to be automatic, but it is possible that it still requires attention. In fact, a study by La-Joie et al. (1993) showed that when young adults were asked to perform an auditory reaction time task while sitting, standing, and walking, the reaction time increased from sitting through walking, and it was higher in the single-support phase than in the double-support phase of the step cycle. They concluded that gait is not completely automatic and requires attention.

It has been suggested that as the functional capacity of older adults is stressed while walking and performing a secondary motor or cognitive task, problems in gait or in the performance of a secondary task will be revealed because of either (*a*) a limited capacity to perform either task, requiring more attentional resources or (*b*) limitations in the information-processing capacity of the older adults causing problems in allocating attention efficiently between the two tasks.

In order to determine if older adults show problems with attention when performing a secondary task while walking, Eichhorn et al. (1998) asked older (mean age 73 years) and young (mean age 24 years) adults to respond vocally to a tone cue (say "soft" to a low and "loud" to a high tone) as quickly as possible while walking. They found that the reaction time of the older adults on the auditory task was significantly slower when walking, while that of the younger adults was not. Thus older adults showed problems performing both tasks efficiently when they were performed simultaneously.

In a slightly more complex walking task, Chen et al. (1996) asked healthy older (mean age 72 years) and young (mean age 24 years) adults to walk down a walkway and step over a virtual object (a band of light) while responding vocally when a red light was turned on at the end of the walkway. Figure 13-11 shows the experimental setup. They found that both young and older adults showed increased obstacle contact when performing the secondary task, but it was greater in the older adults. Thus, decre-

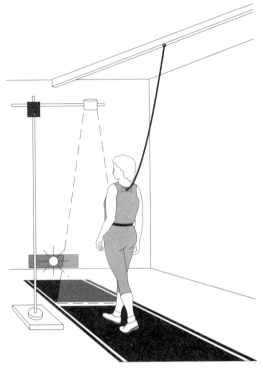

FIGURE 13-11. Experimental setup for study of attentional demands associated with performing a secondary task while avoiding an obstacle. Young and older adults walked down a walkway and stepped over a virtual object (a band of light) while responding vocally when a red light was turned on at the end of the walkway. (Adapted with permission from Chen HC, Schultz AB, Ashton-Miller JA, et al. Stepping over obstacles: Dividing attention impairs performance of old more than young adults. J Gerontol 1996;51A:M116–122.)

ments in obstacle avoidance occur in both younger and older adults when performing a secondary cognitive task, but older adults show higher decrements. This decreased ability to avoid obstacles when performing a secondary cognitive task may contribute to many falls in older adults.

Studies have shown that after repeated falls, older persons develop a fear of falling, and this fear may contribute to changes in gait characteristics as well. For example, it has been shown that preferred walking pace, anxiety level, and depression are good predictors of the extent of fear of falling in community-dwelling older adults (Tinetti et al., 1990). Older adults who avoid activities because of a fear of falling tend to walk with a slower pace and have higher levels of anxiety and depression than adults with little fear of falling. This has led several investigators to propose that slowed gait velocity among older adults is a conscious strategy used to ensure safe gait rather than the consequence of specific constraints on walking speed (Craik, 1989; Murray et al., 1969; Winter et al., 1990).

In other studies examining balance control in older adults with a fear of falling, researchers were not sure whether these adults had real problems with balance control or the fear of falling itself was affecting stability in an artifactual way (Maki et al., 1991). Thus, it is possible that cognitive factors, such as fear of falling, may contribute to changes in gait patterns in older adults.

Sensory Impairments

As noted in Chapter 9, pathologies within visual, proprioceptive, and vestibular systems are common among many older adults, reducing the availability of information from these senses for posture and gait. If reduction in sensory function is part of normal aging, it is important to determine ways to optimize environmental factors and use training to improve stability during walking in older adults.

Muscle Weakness

Decreased muscle strength has been indicated as a contributor to locomotor changes in the older adult. In the section on kinetics of the gait cycle, we noted that Winter et al. (1990) reported a significant decrease in push-off power during gait in healthy older adults, which was possibly related to decreased muscle strength. Chapter 9 discusses in detail issues related to age-related reductions in muscle strength.

Effects of Exercise Programs on Gait Function

A number of studies have examined the effect of various exercise programs on gait function in older adults. Meier (1992) gave intensive daily physical therapy to six nurs-

ing home residents over a 5-week period and found a high degree of improvement in gait in this group compared to six controls. Sauvage et al. (1992) used a 12-week moderate to high-intensity strengthening and aerobic exercise program on a nursing home resident population and found significant improvements in clinical mobility scores, strength, muscular endurance, and some gait parameters, including velocity. High-intensity resistance training has also been shown to increase knee extensor muscle strength and muscle size and to enhance functional mobility in frail adults in their 90s. Mean tandem gait speed was increased in this group by 48% after an 8-week training program. In addition, two of the frail older subjects no longer used canes as an aid in walking at the end of the training period (Fiatarone et al., 1990).

Another study (Lord et al., 1996b) used a 22-week randomized controlled trial of exercise to determine if a program of regular exercise could improve gait patterns in older women (mean age 71 years) and whether improvements were mediated by increased lower limb strength. They found improvements in muscle strength; increased walking speed, cadence, and stride length; and shorter stride times due to reduced swing and stance durations. No changes were found in an age-matched control group. They noted that increased cadence was associated with improved ankle dorsiflexion strength, and increased stride length was associated with increased hip extension strength.

As might be expected, subjects with slower initial walking speeds showed the greatest improvements, and those with higher velocities showed little change. Older women with gait speeds of less than about 1 m/second, who have difficulties with functional activities such as crossing roads in urban environments, benefited most from the intervention (Lord et al., 1996b; Lloyd, 1990). These studies suggest that both exercise and strength training programs have positive effects on gait parameters in older adults, especially those with slow gait velocities prior to training.

Gait Initiation

Gait initiation requires dynamic balance control, since it is a transitional phase between static standing balance and dynamic balance requirements associated with walking. One way of examining the ability to control gait initiation is to measure both center of gravity (COG) changes reflecting body position and COP changes reflecting weight shifts and muscular control during dynamic postural changes. Gait initiation requires the separation of the COG and COP. This separation between the COG and COP, known biomechanically as the COG–COP moment arm, helps predict an individual's ability to tolerate dynamic unsteadiness. A small moment arm indicates that the COP and COG are being kept closely aligned during gait initiation, minimizing dynamic unsteadiness. It has been shown (Chang and Krebs, 1999) that length of COG–COP moment arm during gait initiation clearly differentiates healthy older adults, who show a COG–COP moment arm of 21 ± 8 cm, from disabled older adults, who show a moment arm of 15 ± 3 cm. This shortened moment arm may be either the result of muscle weakness (a primary impairment) or a compensatory strategy used to minimize dynamic unsteadiness.

Stair Walking

Research has documented that walking on stairs is associated with the highest proportion of falls in public places and that most of these falls occur as subjects walk down the stairs. To determine the physical requirements of stair walking in older adults, characteristics of stair descent were studied in a group of 36 healthy women aged 55 to 70 (Simoneau et al., 1991). Participants were asked to walk down a set of stairs under conditions of poor or distorted visual inputs. For example, (*a*) stairs were painted black, (*b*) vision of the stair was blurred (stairs were painted black and the subject wore a headband with a light-scattering plastic shield), or (*c*) stairs were painted black with a white stripe at the edge of each tread. A striped corridor surrounded the stairs.

High-speed film analysis showed significantly slower cadence, larger foot clearance, and more posterior foot placement while subjects walked under the blurred condition as compared to the other two stair color conditions. The authors further observed that foot clearance was larger than that obtained during previous pilot work from their laboratory on young adults. They concluded that older subjects walked with larger foot clearance during stair descent than did young adults and that gait patterns during stair descent were affected by visual conditions.

Age-Related Changes in Other Mobility Skills

Sit to Stand

The task of rising from a seated position is often associated with falling in older adults (Tinetti et al., 1986). Research indicates that 8% of community dwelling older adults over 65 years of age show some problems in rising from a chair or bed. As a result, several studies have examined the sit-to-stand (STS) task in older adults (Alexander et al., 1991; Millington et al., 1992; Pai et al., 1994).

One study compared movement strategies, forces used, and the time taken to rise from sitting among young adults, older adults able to rise without armrests (old able), and older adults unable to rise without armrests (old unable). Average times to rise from a chair were similar in the young and old able groups (1.56 versus 1.83 seconds) but significantly longer in the old unable group (3.16 seconds). In addition, the hand forces used by the old able group were significantly less than those used by the old unable group.

The old able were mainly different from the young in the amount of time they spent in the initial phase of rising from the chair, which included the time from start to liftoff from the seat. They flexed their legs and trunks more during trials in which they used no hands to help themselves rise. A second study (Pai et al., 1994) showed that the peak vertical momentum of the center of mass of elderly adults was significantly smaller than for young adults, probably because of lower levels of muscle strength in the older adults.

While none of the elderly subjects reported significant musculoskeletal or neurological impairment, a significantly larger proportion of the old unable group had a history of vertebral fractures, decreased vision, dizziness, poor balance, and falls. Every old unable subject also had muscle weakness in the lower extremities, decreased proprioception in the hands and feet, and spinal and lower extremity deformities, such as kyphosis and osteoarthritis (Alexander et al., 1991; Millington et al., 1992).

Rising From a Bed

Are there age-related differences in movement patterns used in rising from a bed? To answer this question, adults ranging in age from 30 to 59 years of age were videotaped while rising from a bed (Ford-Smith and VanSant, 1993). As reported for young adults, there was considerable variability in patterns for rising from a bed among the slightly older group, aged 50 to 59. As mentioned in Chapter 12, the most common patterns of bed rising in the 30- to 39-year-old group involved a grasp and push pattern with the upper extremities, a roll-off or come-to-sit pattern, and a synchronous lifting of the lower limbs off the bed with one limb extending to the floor in front of the other. The slightly older group, consisting of 50- to 59-year-olds, tended to use a more synchronous lifting pattern, with both legs moved to the floor simultaneously, as is seen in Figure 13-12. No studies on patterns used by the elderly when rising from the bed have been published to date. Since many elderly people report falls at night associated with getting out of bed, such a study is essential.

Supine to Stand

Moving from a supine to a standing position is an important task, even in older adults. The ability to stand up after a fall is a key element for functional independence. A number of studies have examined patterns of supine-to-stand movements across the life span and have shown that there is a progression across childhood to adulthood from

asymmetrical to symmetrical movement patterns, with older adults more likely to show asymmetrical patterns like those seen in children (VanSant, 1990). A recent study investigated the relationship of age, activity level, lower extremity strength and range of motion to the movement patterns and time required to rise to a standing position from the floor (Thomas et al., 1998). They confirmed previous results regarding movement patterns and found that symmetrical movement patterns were associated with younger age, greater plantarflexion and hip extension strength, and greater dorsiflexion range of motion. This suggests that symmetrical patterns like those seen in young adults require higher levels of extensor muscle strength; however, alternative asymmetrical standing strategies are available to older adults with extensor weakness.

℮ COMPARING GAIT CHARACTERISTICS OF INFANTS AND ELDERLY: TESTING THE REGRESSION HYPOTHESIS

It has been suggested that changes in the gait pattern among the elderly are related to the reemergence of immature walking patterns seen in young infants. Thus, it is hypothesized that as aging occurs, there is a regression to immature reflex patterns that characterized movement in young infants. This regression is thought to result from loss of higher-center control over the primitive reflexes that reemerge in the very old (Shaltenbrand, 1928). What are the similarities and differences between the gait characteristics of the very young and the very old?

Both groups show a shorter duration of single-limb stance and a greater relative duration of double support. This has been interpreted in both groups as an indication of decreased balance abilities (Murray et al., 1969; Sutherland et al., 1980; Gabell and Nayak, 1984; Bril and Breniere, 1993).

The gait of young walkers has also been described as having a wide base of support

Sequence

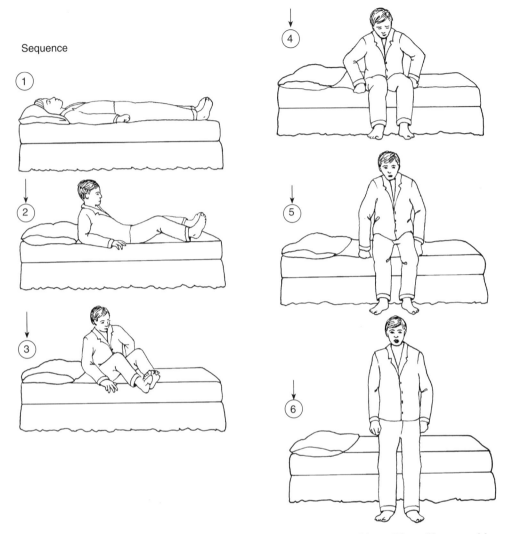

FIGURE 13-12. Frequent pattern of rising from a bed seen in subjects 50 to 59 years old. (Adapted with permission from Ford-Smith CD, VanSant AF. Age differences in movement patterns used to rise from a bed in subjects in the third through fifth decades of age. Phys Ther 1993;73:305.)

along with toeing-out, a characteristic observed in the elderly as well (Murray et al., 1969; Bril and Breniere, 1993). It has been suggested in both groups that an increased base of support is used to ensure better balance control.

Finally, both young children (Forssberg, 1985) and older adults (Finley et al., 1969) show coactivation of agonist and antagonist muscles during gait. This again has been described as a way of increasing joint stiffness, which helps in balance control (Woollacott, 1986).

Clearly, there are many similarities in the gait characteristics of the young child and the older adult. These similarities appear to relate to difficulties with balance control common to both groups. Thus, it is not necessarily true that similarities between the very old and very young are due to a reappearance of primitive reflexes. In this case, the reason is a functional one: the two groups, often for different reasons, have difficulties with the balance system but use similar strategies to compensate for those difficulties.

SUMMARY

1. There are three requirements for successful locomotion: (*a*) the ability to generate a rhythmic stepping pattern to move the body forward (progression), (*b*) postural control (stability), and (*c*) the ability to adapt gait to changing task and environmental requirements (adaptation). In the development of locomotion, these three factors emerge sequentially, with the stepping pattern appearing first, equilibrium control next, finally followed by adaptive capabilities.

2. The emergence of independent gait is characterized by the development of many interacting systems with certain hierarchical components. An innate pattern generator creates the basic rhythm of the step cycle, which can be seen in newborn stepping. In the first year, the gradual development of descending systems from higher neural centers gives the child increasing control over this locomotor behavior. The control of equilibrium, organized at a higher level than that of the pattern generator, develops over a longer period, as do adaptive systems essential to the integration of reactive and proactive strategies into gait.

3. The development of locomotion behavior begins before birth and continues until the emergence of mature gait at about 7 years of age. Stepping behavior is present at birth and can be elicited in most infants if they are supported and inclined slightly forward. This early behavior resembles quadrupedal stepping, with flexion of the hip and knee, synchronous joint motion, and considerable coactivation of agonist and antagonist muscles.

4. In many infants, early stepping disappears at about 2 months of age, possibly because of biomechanical changes in the infant's system, such as an increase in relative body weight. Early stepping gradually transforms into a more mature pattern over the first 2 years of life.

5. Researchers seem to agree that the ability to integrate postural control into the locomotor pattern is the most important rate-limiting factor on the emergence of independent walking.

6. The most significant modifications to the gait pattern occur during the first 4 to 5 months of independent walking. Most of these changes reflect the child's growing ability to integrate balance control with locomotion.

7. Studies characterizing gait patterns in older adults have consistently shown that healthy older adults have reduced walking speed, shorter strides, and shorter steps than young adults.

8. Proactive locomotor abilities also change with age, with older adults taking more time to monitor the visual environment and to alter an upcoming step to avoid an obstacle and using strategies such as slowing of approach and cross-over time when stepping over obstacles.

9. Changes in the characteristics of gait in older adults are influenced by balance ability, leg muscle strength, and changes in the availability of sensory information. Cognitive factors, such as fear of falling and attentional problems, may also be important contributors.

10. When evaluating gait patterns of older people, consideration must be given to the underlying mechanisms contributing to these changes. In this way, one can differentiate between contributions related to pathology and aging per se. Only after the systems contributing to walking pattern dysfunction are identified can a clinician design effective and appropriate interventions to improve gait and thus help older adults achieve a safe and independent lifestyle.

Abnormal Mobility

ℰ INTRODUCTION

Impaired mobility function, specifically disorders of gait, is one of the earliest and most characteristic symptoms of a wide variety of neurological disorders. Mobility is a critical part of maintaining independence and an essential attribute of quality of life (Patla and Shumway-Cook, 1999). Impaired mobility is a critical determinant of independence and a major contributor to physical disability (Guralnik et al., 1995). When impairments in mobility restrict the ability of the individual to move about the residence or the community to perform necessary activities of daily life, disability results. This chapter describes impaired mobility function, including abnormalities of gait, stair walking, and transfers, in the patient with neurological pathology.

ℰ ABNORMAL GAIT

While abnormal gait is characteristic of many neurological disorders, the constellation of underlying problems that produces disordered gait varies from patient to patient, even among patients with the same pathology. The type of gait abnormality observed depends on the type and extent of central nervous system (CNS) pathology, the constellation of resulting impairments, and the extent to which the patient is able to compensate for those impairments. Understanding the contribution of these elements to gait abnormalities can be difficult. As a result, technology such as electromyography (EMG), kinematic, and kinetic analysis is often necessary to distinguish impairment from compensation. Technology is thus used extensively in studies examining gait problems in the patient with a neurological disorder.

Classification Systems

While a number of classification schemes have been proposed, there is little consensus on the best framework for classifying gait disorders. The most common framework for understanding and classifying disorders of gait is based on the neurological diagnosis itself, such as parkinsonian gait, cerebellar ataxic gait, or spastic cerebral palsy gait.

Another approach has classified gait disorders into three groups according to the suspected level of CNS involvement (Nutt et al., 1993; Nutt and Horak, 1997). This classification is based on Hughlings Jackson's concept of the CNS as a hierarchy with low, middle, and high levels of sensorimotor processing. Examples of the types of gait disorders found at each level are summarized in Table 14-1. Gait disorders at the lowest level of the CNS hierarchy reflect problems arising from peripheral sensory (such as sensory ataxic gait) or motor systems (such as amputee gait). Gait disorders arising from disturbances in peripheral function are often well compensated if the CNS is intact.

Middle-level sensorimotor deficits, such as those resulting from stroke or Parkinson's disease, are thought to result from the faulty execution of posture and locomotor patterns. CNS problems at middle levels affect the organization and execution of movement patterns related to posture and gait. Gait disorders found at the highest level of the sensorimotor hierarchy (for example, cautious gait, frontal gait apraxia) are the least understood. Highest-level dysfunction results in improper selection of postural and locomotor patterns appropriate to task and conditions (Nutt et al., 1993; Nutt and Horak, 1997).

Alternatively, researchers have classified gait according to the primary pathophysiological mechanism producing disordered gait. Crenna and Inverno (1994) have suggested a conceptual framework based on four main impairments contributing to disordered gait in patients with supraspinal le-

TABLE 14-1. A Proposed Classification System for Gait Abnormalities Based on a Hierarchical Organization of Pathologies Affecting the CNS

I. Lowest-level gait disorders
   A. Peripheral skeletomuscle problems
      Arthritic gait
      Myopathic gait
      Peripheral neuropathic gait
   B. Peripheral sensory problems
      Sensory ataxic gait
      Vestibular ataxic gait
      Visual ataxic gait
II. Middle-level gait disorders
   Hemiplegic gait
   Paraplegic gait
   Cerebellar ataxic gait
   Parkinsonian gait
   Choreic gait
   Dystonic gait
III. Highest-level gait disorders
   Cautious gait
   Subcortical disequilibrium
   Frontal disequilibrium
   Isolated gait ignition failure
   Frontal gait disorder

Reprinted with permission from Nutt JG, Marsden CD, Thompson PD. Human walking and higher-level gait disorders, particularly in the elderly. Neurology 1993;43:271.

sions: (*a*) defective muscle activation (paretic component); (*b*) abnormal velocity-dependent recruitment of muscle during lengthening (spastic component), (*c*) loss of selectivity in motor output (cocontraction component), and (*d*) changes in mechanical properties of muscle tendon system (nonneural component). This conceptual framework has found support from Knutsson and colleagues' work, which has identified similar components in the gait of adult stroke patients (Knutsson and Richards, 1979). A limitation of this approach is that to date, the classification system is based solely on problems within the motor systems and does not include gait disorders due to sensory or perceptual problems.

In this chapter we use both a pathophysiological and diagnostic framework to discuss disorders of gait. We begin with a patho-physiological framework to examine how impairments in motor, sensory, perceptual, and cognitive systems contribute to disorders of gait and consider some common compensatory strategies used to maintain function in light of these impairments. Finally, we use our case studies to summarize gait problems from a diagnostic perspective. Regardless of the type of classification system used, understanding the effects of sensory, motor, and cognitive impairments on mobility function, as well as the types of patients likely to have these problems, is essential knowledge for examining and treating the patient with mobility problems.

Impairments in Motor Systems

Motor problems affecting gait include disruptions to both neuromuscular and musculoskeletal systems. In patients with neurological pathology, musculoskeletal problems are secondary to primary neuromuscular problems that limit movement.

Neuromuscular Impairments

The neuromuscular control of gait includes the generation of the basic locomotor patterns for progression and the control of posture for maintaining orientation and stability. The nervous system must be able to generate the basic locomotor patterns and maintain an appropriate posture for locomotion. In addition, since the mass of the head, arms, and trunk is large and a significant amount of time is spent in single-leg support, balance is inherently unstable and the control of dynamic equilibrium is essential (Patla, 1995).

Spasticity

Because spasticity is a frequent accompaniment of neurological disorders, many researchers have looked at its effect on gait. Spasticity can impact gait in two ways. First, spasticity results in the inappropriate activation of a muscle at points during the gait cycle when it is being rapidly lengthened. In addition, spasticity alters the mechanical properties of a muscle, producing increased stiffness, a musculoskeletal problem (Dietz et al., 1981). Increased stiffness affects the freedom of body segments to move rapidly with regard to one another; this limits the transfer of momentum during gait, affecting the progression requirements of locomotion.

In order to determine the contribution of spasticity to disordered gait, a number of researchers have examined activation levels of muscles in response to stretch during perturbed and nonperturbed gait. Some studies have examined activation of spastic muscles during lengthening contractions in unperturbed gait (Knutsson and Richards, 1979; Sinkjaer et al., 1996; Crenna, 1998). Others have used perturbations to gait either by rapid stretching of the calf muscles using mechanical devices fixed to the subject's leg (Andersen and Sinkjaer, 1996; Llewellyn et al., 1986) or abruptly changing belt speed during treadmill walking (Berger et al., 1984c).

Regardless of the methods used, a key to understanding the contribution of spasticity to disordered gait requires knowing when muscles undergo lengthening during the gait cycle. This allows the researcher to examine the activity of spastic muscles during critical lengthening periods. For example, Figure 14-1A summarizes data from 10 healthy children showing the lengthening phases in representative lower limb muscles including the quadriceps, medial hamstring, soleus, and tibialis anterior. As can be seen in this graph, the quadriceps is lengthened twice over the gait cycle, in early stance phase during knee yielding associated with loading, and when the knee flexes during toe-off. One would expect therefore that the effect of a spastic quadriceps muscle would be greatest during these two points in the gait cycle. In contrast, the hamstrings have one lengthening period in late swing, associated with knee extension in preparation for initial contact. Therefore, one would expect the effect of spasticity in the hamstrings to be heightened activation of this muscle during late swing.

In patients for whom spasticity is the primary impairment contributing to disordered

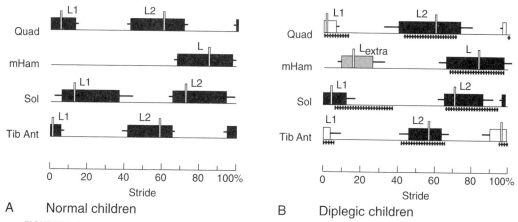

FIGURE 14-1.   Lengthening phases in representative lower limb muscles including the quadriceps (Quad), medial hamstring (mHam), soleus (Sol) and tibialis anterior (Tib Ant) in normal healthy children **(A)** and children with spastic cerebral palsy **(B)**. (Adapted with permission from Crenna P. Spasticity and "spastic" gait in children with cerebral palsy. Neurosci Biobehav Rev 1998;22:573.)

gait, one in fact does see heightened activity in spastic muscles undergoing lengthening. However, often spasticity is not the sole contributor to disordered gait. This is best illustrated in Figure 14-1*B*, which shows the activation of four representative muscles in a child with spastic diplegia. In this figure the filled boxes represent muscle activity that is comparable to normal. However, the clear boxes represent an absence of muscle activity that is normally seen (see, for example, Quad L1), while the hatched boxes represent muscle activity that is found in children with cerebral palsy but never in the normal control children. Thus one can see from looking at this figure that spasticity is not the only component contributing to disordered gait (Crenna, 1998).

The following section briefly reviews the effects of spasticity in certain key muscles.

Plantarflexor Spasticity.   Spasticity in the ankle plantarflexors (triceps surae) is a common problem following neurological injury and has been reported in patients with stroke, cerebral palsy, and following traumatic brain injury (Perry, 1992; Knutsson and Richards, 1979; Crenna and Inverno, 1994).

Knutsson and Richards (1979) studied 26 adult patients with spastic hemiplegia sec-ondary to stroke and found that 9 of 26 patients (about one-third) showed a "spastic" pattern of gait, characterized primarily by abnormal activation of the triceps surae muscles during the early part of the stance phase of walking. Figure 14-2*A* compares averaged EMG activity (normalized to 239 mV) of the triceps surae during the gait cycle in 10 normal control subjects and 9 patients with spastic hemiparesis. Compared to normal controls, in the patients with spastic hemiparesis, the triceps surae activation began early in the stance phase and had relatively lower peak amplitude. Following initial contact, stretch of the triceps surae resulted in the early activation of the muscles. The resultant shortening of the muscle before the body passed ahead of the foot pulled the lower leg backward and produced knee hyperextension. This is seen in the graph of knee angle during the gait cycle. Figure 14-2*B* is a stick figure of lower limb motion in a normal subject versus one who is hemiparetic. It illustrates the effect of premature contraction of the triceps surae in the hemiparetic limb. The force produced by the triceps surae creates a backward thrust of the knee, leaving the muscle unable to build tension for push-off.

Crenna and Inverno (1994) identified

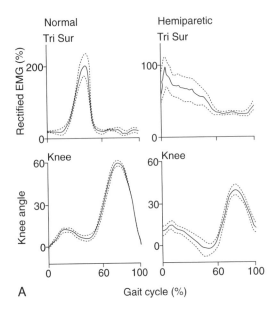

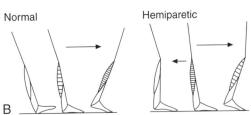

FIGURE 14-2. The effect of spastic triceps surae (Tri Sur) on gait in patients with hemiplegia. **A.** Comparison of averaged EMG activity (normalized to 239 mV) of the triceps surae during the gait cycle in 10 normal control subjects and 9 patients with spastic hemiparesis, along with the corresponding knee angular changes. Note the high activation of triceps surae during the entire stance phase in the patients with hemiparesis. **B.** Effect of early triceps surae activation on knee position in normal and hemiparetic gait. (Adapted with permission from Knutsson E. Can gait analysis improve gait training in stroke patients? Scand J Rehab Med 1994(Suppl);30:78)

spasticity as one of four contributing factors to disordered gait in children with spastic forms of cerebral palsy (diplegia and hemiplegia). The effect of a spastic muscle on gait parameters in stance versus swing is shown in Figure 14-3. It compares activity of the soleus muscle when it is being lengthened in early stance (Fig. 14-3A) and in swing (Fig. 14-3B) in a normal control child and a child with spastic diplegia. The child with diplegia shows excessive activation of the soleus (in-

creased EMG amplitude) in the early stance-lengthening phase. Interestingly, there was no excessive activation of the soleus muscle in the child with spastic diplegia when the soleus muscle underwent a second lengthening during swing phase of gait (Fig. 14-3B).

Sinkjaer et al. (1996) found that impaired gait in patients with multiple sclerosis was in part due to impaired stretch reflex modulation of the soleus muscle and concomitant increased ankle joint stiffness. During normal walking the soleus stretch reflex is modulated in a phase-dependent way (shown in Figure 14-4A), with stance phase showing a large-magnitude stretch response, the transition from stance to swing phase showing a minimal response, and the swing phase showing a response that is 50% of the stance phase magnitude. In 5 of the 7 multiple sclerosis patients studied, the soleus muscle's response to stretch during walking was faster (shorter onset latency) and increased in amplitude by 241%, and there was virtually no phase-dependent modulation of the stretch reflex during the different phases of gait (Fig. 14-4B). Interestingly, the two patients who showed some stretch reflex modulation were also those who walked fastest; therefore, the authors suggest that locomotor impairments are strongly linked to stretch reflex modulation in this population of patients.

Thus, spasticity in the plantarflexors can contribute to pathological gait patterns in both stance and swing phase of gait. Research has shown that in stance phase, plantarflexor spasticity affects foot position at initial contact, impacting the stability component of gait. Spastic plantarflexors limit dorsiflexion, preventing heel strike at initial contact. When initial contact is made with a flat foot, the ground reaction force vector is anterior to the knee, producing knee extension. This is shown in Figure 14-5. Major compensations for excessive plantar flexion include hyperextension of the knee and/or forward trunk lean. Patients also compensate by shortening the step length of the other limb. Which compensatory strategy is used depends on a number of factors. Knee mobility is critical to the hyperexten-

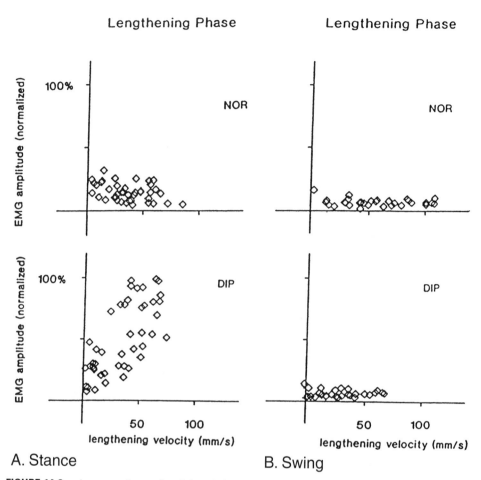

FIGURE 14-3. A comparison of activity of the soleus muscle when it is being lengthened in early stance (**A**) and in swing (**B**) in a normal control child (NOR) and a child with spastic diplegia (DIP). (Adapted with permission from Crenna P, Inverno M. Objective detection of pathophysiological factors contributing to gait disturbance in supraspinal lesions. In: Fedrizzi E, Avanzini G, Crenna P. Motor development in children. New York: Libbey, 1994:110.)

sion strategy. In contrast, good hip and trunk extensors are necessary for the trunk flexion strategy (Perry, 1992).

In the swing phase of gait, spasticity in the plantarflexors results in inadequate toe-off due to an extended knee position at terminal stance. Inability to flex the knee adequately makes toe-off more difficult and requires the hip and knee flexors to work harder to lift the limb and clear the foot during swing. Spastic plantarflexors affect forward foot clearance during swing; the consequence is toe drag (Fig. 14-6). In terminal swing, spastic plantarflexors resist extension at the knee and dorsiflexion of the foot, critical to positioning the leg for heel strike at initial contact. Compensatory strategies include a shortened stride and reduced gait velocity.

Spasticity in the plantarflexors in conjunction with other ankle joint muscles produces coronal plane problems at the foot. A combination of excessive activity of the triceps surae and posterior tibialis muscles produces inversion and an equinovarus foot position. An equinovarus foot position in the sagittal plane is shown in Figure 14-7*A* and in the frontal plane in 14-7*B*. This is seen clinically as the elevation of the first metatarsal head from the floor with the subsequent foot contact made on the lateral border of the foot only.

In contrast, in equinovalgus gait, foot contact is made with the medial border of the

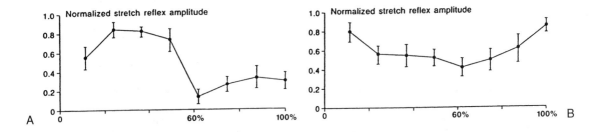

FIGURE 14-4. Normal modulation of the soleus stretch reflex during the different phases of gait (**A**) in comparison to minimal modulation in patients with multiple sclerosis (**B**), who have a spastic soleus muscle. Normal subjects (**A**) show a large stretch response in stance phase and minimal response to stretch in the transition from stance to swing (60% of gait cycle); in the swing phase the stretch reflex is 50% of that in stance phase. In contrast, patients with multiple sclerosis (**B**) show very little modulation of stretch reflex amplitude throughout the gait cycle. (Adapted with permission from Sinkjaer T, Andersen JB, Nielsen JF. Impaired stretch reflex and joint torque modulation during spastic gait in multiple sclerosis patients. J Neurol 1996;243:570.)

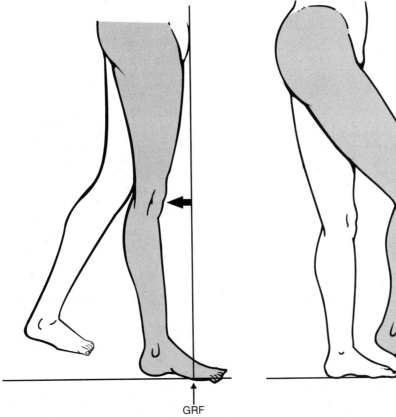

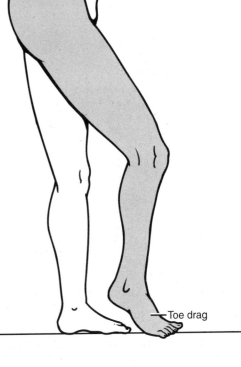

FIGURE 14-5. When initial contact is made with a flat foot, the ground reaction force (GRF) vector is anterior to the knee, producing knee extension.

FIGURE 14-6. Spastic plantarflexors affect forward foot clearance during swing; the consequence is toe drag.

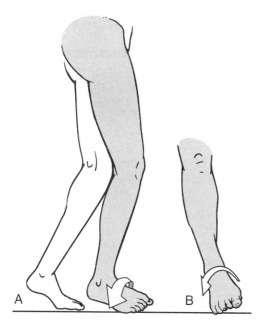

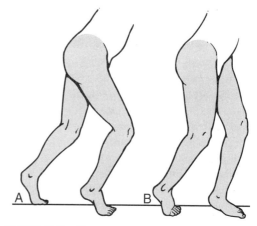

FIGURE 14-8. Hamstring spasticity producing excessive knee flexion in both swing (**A**) and stance (**B**) phase of gait is a frequent problem in certain types of cerebral palsy and manifests as a crouched gait pattern.

FIGURE 14-7. A combination of excessive activity of the triceps surae and posterior tibialis muscle produces inversion and an equinovarus foot position, illustrated from both the sagittal (**A**) and frontal (**B**) planes.

foot. Equinovalgus gait can result from excessive activation of the triceps surae in conjunction with the peroneus brevis muscle. An alternative cause of valgus gait is weakness or inaction by the ankle invertors, for example a weak or inactive soleus. Thus, flaccid paralysis can also lead to a valgus foot posture.

Quadriceps Spasticity.   Like plantar-flexor spasticity, quadriceps spasticity can also result in excessive knee extension in the stance phase of gait. Remember that during weight acceptance, a brief flexion of the knee assists in absorbing the shock of loading. Quadriceps spasticity results in an excessive response to knee flexion and subsequent lengthening of the quadriceps, triggering a stretch reflex response that can limit flexion and result in hyperextension of the knee (Perry, 1992; Montgomery, 1987).

Hamstring Spasticity.   Hamstring spasticity producing excessive knee flexion is a frequent problem in certain types of cerebral palsy and manifests as a crouched gait pattern, shown in Figure 14-8. In the terminal

swing phase of gait, excessive activation of the hamstring muscle prevents the knee from fully extending, resulting in knee flexion at initial contact (14-8*A*). Excessive knee flexion persists throughout the stance phase of gait (14-8*B*), increasing the demand on the quadriceps muscle to prevent collapse of the limb into flexion. A shortened step results.

Hip Adductor Spasticity.   Hip adductor spasticity produces a contralateral drop in the pelvis during stance, as the femur is drawn in medially. Adductor spasticity can result in scissors gait, which is characterized by excessive adduction. During the swing phase of gait, as the hip flexes, excessive adduction produces a severe medial displacement of the entire limb. This results in a reduced base of support, affecting stability. In severe cases, the adducted swing leg catches on the stance limb and impedes progression (Perry, 1992; Montgomery, 1987).

In summary, spasticity contributes to disordered gait through the inappropriate activation of a muscle during the portions of the gait cycle when it is lengthened and through changes in stiffness resulting from alterations in the mechanical properties of the muscle itself.

Weakness and Paresis
Analysis of abnormal gait in various neurological pathologies has shown that spastic-

ity is not the only component of disordered gait. Other factors, including deficient recruitment of motor units, the so-called paretic component, can produce gait abnormalities. Paresis is a primary neuromuscular impairment affecting the number, type, and discharge frequency of motor neurons essential for force production during gait (Perry, 1992; Duncan and Badke, 1987).

Like spasticity, paresis affects both the neural and nonneural components of force production. Its neural component results from insufficient supraspinal recruitment of motor neurons in specific leg muscles either during certain parts of the gait cycle or throughout the gait cycle. Nonneural contributions to paresis reflect secondary changes in the muscle fibers themselves that affect the patient's ability to generate tension.

Muscles in gait act both concentrically to generate motion and eccentrically to control motion. Thus, weakness can result in both the inability to generate forces to move the body forward, such as the effect of weak plantarflexors in terminal stance, and unrestrained motions resulting from lack of control, such as foot slap following heel strike because of loss of eccentric control by the tibialis anterior and uncontrolled plantarflexion.

How much does weakness affect the ability to walk independently? This depends on what muscles are weak, the extent of the weakness, and the capacity of other muscles to substitute for weak muscles in achieving the requirements of gait. Walking normally does not tax the various lower extremity muscle groups to their full capacity (Patla, 1995; Buchner and DeLateur, 1991). The only muscles that come close to their maximum output during gait are the ankle plantarflexors, which normally provide a major source of propulsive power. In the presence of plantarflexor weakness, alternative power sources are used, resulting in a change in locomotor characteristics such as stride length and velocity. While trunk strength is needed to keep the head, arms, and trunk upright, researchers have shown that no significant trunk deviations occur in gait unless weakness in the trunk muscles is significant, that

is, less than a grade 3 on a manual muscle test (Perry, 1992).

What is the effect of lower extremity weakness on gait speed? Several researchers have shown a positive association between lower extremity muscle strength and walking speed. The association appears to be curved and includes both a threshold of strength for walking to occur and a ceiling at which strength can further increase without changing walking velocity (Rantanen, et al., 1999). In other words, a person needs at least a minimum level of strength to walk at a given speed. When strength increases above the minimum required level, a reserve capacity of strength related to walking speed occurs. The association between strength and walking speed is strongest below the reserve capacity threshold, but at levels of strength above threshold an increase in strength no longer affects functional performance. Rantanen et al. (1999) found a strong relationship between knee extension strength and severity of walking disability among older women (see Fig. 15.4).

The following section briefly reviews the effect of weakness in select groups of lower extremity muscles on gait.

Plantarflexor Weakness.   In Knutsson and Richard's study of gait in hemiparetic subjects, 9 of 26 (about one-third) showed a "paretic" pattern of gait rather than a spastic pattern (Knutsson and Richards, 1979). The paretic component resulted from a lack of muscle activation in gait. As shown in Figure 14-9A, EMG activity indicated a complete lack of phasic activation of the paretic calf muscles in stroke patients (broken line) compared to the normal controls (solid line). As shown in Figure 14-9B, there was relatively low activity of the tibialis anterior in the subjects with hemiparesis (broken line) compared to normal controls (solid line). Strong hyperextension of the knee in the stance phase and lack of knee flexion characterized this gait pattern in the swing phase. This can be seen in Figure 14-9C, an angle diagram showing changes in knee motion in normal subjects (solid line) and in patients (broken line). Interestingly, for sev-

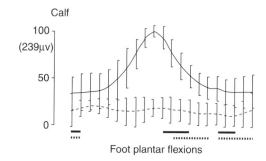

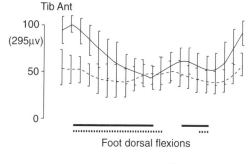

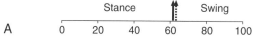

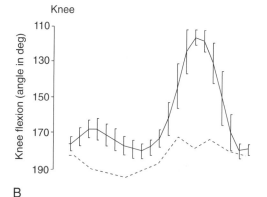

FIGURE 14-9. The effects of paresis on gait. **A.** Rectified, integrated EMG activity from ankle plantarflexors and dorsiflexors across the gait cycle in normal healthy controls (*solid lines*) and a group of hemiparetic subjects (*broken line*). EMG in the patients' group shows lack of phasic activation of the calf muscles and relatively low activity of the tibialis anterior (Tib Ant). **B.** Angle diagram showing changes in knee motion in normal subjects (*solid line*) and in patients (*broken line*). (Adapted with permission from Knutsson E, Richards C. Different types of disturbed motor control in gait of hemiparetic patients. Brain 1979;102:420.)

eral of the patients examined, poor muscle recruitment in gait was associated with preserved recruitment when the muscle was activated voluntarily, suggesting that the injury disturbs the central generation of programmed gait activation but leaves the capacity to activate muscle voluntarily relatively intact.

During the stance phase of gait, weak or inactive plantarflexors cannot restrain forward motion of the tibia through an eccentric contraction. This results in excessive ankle dorsiflexion and an increased knee flexion from 15 to 30 degrees. Persisting knee flexion during the stance phase of gait increases the demands on the quadriceps muscle, which eccentrically contracts to stabilize the knee. This increases the energy required for walking (Perry, 1992).

In addition, weak plantarflexors also result in loss of heel rise at terminal stance and a loss of terminal stance knee extension. This can also result in pelvic retraction, defined as excessive backward rotation of the pelvis, during terminal stance. Dynamic backward rotation occurs in terminal stance and is usually associated with persistent heel contact due to calf muscle weakness (Perry, 1992).

Quadriceps Weakness. A weak quadriceps (grades 3+ to 4) will lead to difficulty controlling knee flexion during loading. A very weak quadriceps (grades 0 to 3) will lead to trouble stabilizing the knee during midstance. The primary compensation for this is hyperextension of the knee during midstance, since the forward movement of the body weight will serve as the knee extensor force. When hyperextension is continued into preswing, it prevents the knee from freely moving during the swing phase. This can slow progression and result in toe drag.

Compensation for weak quadriceps involves a forward trunk lean, which brings the body vector anterior to the knee, resulting in knee hyperextension. While this is an effective compensatory strategy for stabilizing the knee, there are disadvantages to the use of a knee hyperextension strategy as a compensation for weak quadriceps. First, it limits knee flexion during loading and increases the impact of body weight on the structures of the stance limb. It traumatizes the internal structure of the knee and can damage these structures in the long term. The advantage of the knee hyperextension strategy is that it allows a more stable posture and therefore may be a reasonable and appropriate strategy for patients with a very weak quadriceps (Perry, 1992).

Hip Flexor Weakness.   Normal gait requires only a grade 2+ (poor plus) muscle strength in the hip flexors (Perry, 1992). Hip flexor weakness, producing inadequate hip flexion, primarily affects the swing phase of gait. Knee flexion is lost in swing when there is inadequate hip flexion, so the patient is unable to develop sufficient momentum at the hip to indirectly flex the knee. As a result, toe clearance is reduced or lost. A shortened step is also associated with inadequate hip flexion and can affect the position of the foot at heel strike. When the hip cannot be flexed at the initiation of swing, limb advancement and thus progression are hampered. At the same time, placement of the foot in preparation for weight acceptance is affected, challenging stability.

Patients use several compensatory strategies to achieve foot clearance during swing despite inadequate hip flexion, and these are shown in Figure 14-10. The first uses a posterior tilt of the pelvis and activation of the abdominal muscles to advance the swing limb (Fig. 14-10*A*). The second uses circumduction, defined as hip hike; forward rotation of the pelvis; and abduction of the hip to advance the limb (Fig. 14-10*B*). The other strategies used to advance the limb despite hip flexor weakness include contralateral vaulting (Fig. 14-10*C*), involving coming up onto the forefoot of the stance limb, or leaning the trunk toward the opposite limb (Fig. 14-10*D*).

Hip Extensor Weakness.   Hip extensor weakness can also produce a forward trunk lean that threatens stability. Backward lean in stance compensates for hip extensor weakness by bringing the center of mass behind the hips; it is used for stability. However, tibialis anterior activity is needed to prevent falls in the backward direction (Perry, 1992).

Hip Abductor Weakness.   Weak hip abductors (gluteus medius) can result in drop of the pelvis on the side contralateral to the weakness, called a Trendelenburg gait. A common compensation for hip abductor weakness is a lateral shift of the center of mass over the stance leg in conjunction with lateral lean of the trunk toward the stance leg. This shift of the upper body over the stance side moves the ground reaction force (GRF) in the same direction. When the GRF passes directly through the center of the femoral head, the internal moment generated by the hip abductors, which normally produces a stabilizing force, is no longer needed (Perry, 1992; Gage, 1991). When the problem is a painful hip, this same compensatory mechanism is used to reduce the proportion of force passing through the hip joint (Gage, 1991).

In summary, paresis, like spasticity, is a major factor contributing to disordered gait in the patient with neurological pathology. Unlike spasticity, which affects gait only during lengthening contractions, paresis affects both control of movement through loss of eccentric contractions and generation of movement through loss of concentric contractions.

Coordination Problems

Coordination problems, or difficulties coordinating multijoint movements, are a hallmark of neurological pathology. However, multijoint coordination problems are not immediately observable by looking at one

FIGURE 14-10.   Compensatory strategies used to advance the swing leg despite inadequate hip flexion. **A.** Activation of the abdominal muscles in conjunction with a posterior tip of the pelvis. **B.** Circumduction. **C.** Contralateral vaulting. **D.** Leaning the trunk toward the opposite limb.

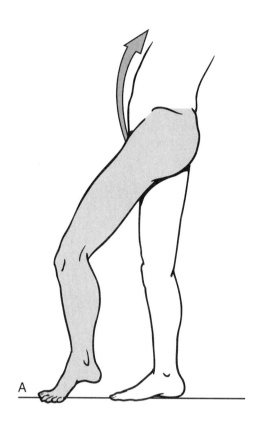

A

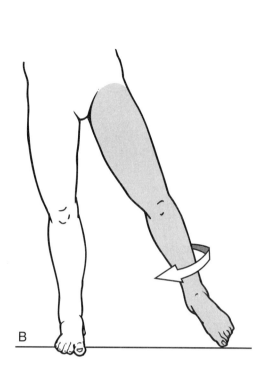

B

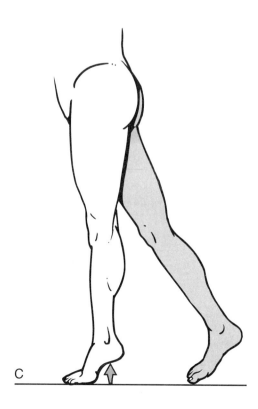

C

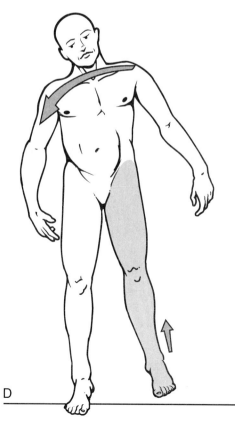

D

joint at a time; but require examining movement across multiple joints. As will be seen in the following discussion, multijoint coordination problems can manifest in many ways.

Abnormal Synergies. Abnormal synergies are defined as the simultaneous recruitment of muscles at multiple joints and body segments resulting in stereotyped and relatively fixed patterns of movement. The presence of abnormal synergies reflects loss of fractionation of movement (muscle recruitment) and is due to corticospinal lesions.

Abnormal synergies manifest in gait as either total extension (Fig. 14-11A) or total flexion (Fig. 14-11B). This can been seen in the EMG traces as simultaneous activation of either extensors (Fig. 14-11A) during the stance phase of gait or flexors (Fig. 14-11B) during swing. Thus persistent flexion of the knee throughout the swing cycle is often associated with the use of a flexor synergy, or total flexor pattern at all three joints. Use of the flexor synergy results in inability to extend the knee while flexing the hip during terminal swing. Knutsson and Richards (1979) reported that mass patterns of flexion and extension were one of four characteristic gait patterns found in hemiparetic stroke patients.

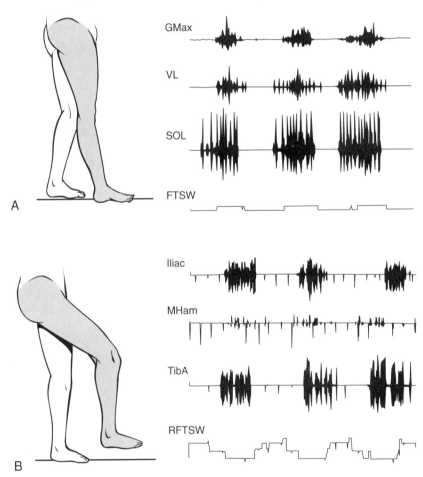

FIGURE 14-11. Synergies manifest in gait as either total extension or total flexion. *Right.* EMG traces of extensor muscles **(A)** and flexor muscles **(B)** *Left.* Excessive extension in stance **(A)** and flexion in swing **(B)**. GMax, gluteus maximus; VL, vastus lateralis; SOL, soleus; FTSW, foot switch; Iliac, iliacus; MHam, medial hamstrings; Tib A, tibialis anterior; RFTSW, right foot switch. (Adapted with permission from Perry J. Gait analysis: normal and pathological function. Thorofare, NJ: Slack, 1992:313.)

Disordered Patterns of Activation: Control Problems.   Central lesions of the CNS result in impaired programming affecting leg muscle activation. Impaired programming can manifest in gait as (*a*) inability to recruit a muscle appropriately, (*b*) increased activation of a muscle that is unrelated to spasticity mediated stretch, or (*c*) inability to modulate a muscle's activity throughout the gait cycle (Patla, 1995).

Loss of the ability to selectively recruit the tibialis anterior muscle during gait following stroke is a common example of impaired programming. Inability to activate the tibialis anterior results in a flat foot at foot strike; alternatively, the heel may strike but the foot drops quickly (foot slap) because eccentric contraction of the anterior tibialis is inadequate. The presence of a rapid foot drop following heel strike suggests that the underlying impairment is an inactive tibialis anterior rather than a spastic or contracted gastrocnemius or soleus (Perry, 1992; Montgomery, 1989; Knutsson and Richards, 1979).

Overactivity of the hamstring muscle unrelated to stretch has been reported both in adult patients following stroke (Knutsson and Richards, 1979) and in children with cerebral palsy (Crenna, 1998; Perry, 1992). Hamstring hyperactivity can manifest as either premature or prolonged activation of the hamstrings (Crenna, 1998; Perry, 1992). It was originally thought that hamstring overactivity was the result of spasticity, such as velocity-dependent hyperactivity of the stretch reflex. However, researchers have found that performing a dorsal rhizotomy, which involves selectively cutting the sensory nerve roots, does not decrease hamstring hyperactivity in children with cerebral palsy. This suggests that the basis for hamstring hyperactivity is abnormal coordination, not a simple hyperactive stretch reflex (Crenna, 1998; Perry, 1992).

Coactivation of Agonist and Antagonist Muscles.   Normal gait is characterized by a remarkable degree of selectivity of muscle activity. There is a reciprocal recruitment pattern during gait such that coactivation of agonist and antagonist is minimized. Cocon-

traction is defined as the loss of selective recruitment of physiologically antagonistic muscles. Coactivity among antagonist muscles during gait has been reported in many patients with supraspinal lesions, including stroke and cerebral palsy. Researchers have hypothesized several possible reasons for the presence of coactivation, including (*a*) pathologically disorganized central programs, (*b*) additional postural support activity, (*c*) immature gait programs, and (*d*) compensatory programming, that is, the use of coactivation to increase stiffness (Knutsson, 1994; Crenna, 1998).

A coactivation pattern of activity was found in 4 of 26 stroke patients (Knutsson and Richards, 1979). Increased coactivation in the leg muscle groups began at the end of the swing phase and continued throughout the stance phase of gait. Knutsson suggests that while this pattern is not commonly seen in adult-onset spastic hemiparesis, it is a common finding in cerebral palsy (Knutsson, 1994). Crenna and colleagues reported that coactivation of lower extremity muscles was a common finding among children with spastic-type cerebral palsy (Crenna, 1998). Figure 14-12 shows a comparison of coactivation between hamstrings and quadriceps in a normal control child versus a child with spastic diplegia. Note that the filled areas (activity in both muscles greater than 20% of maximum locomotor output) cover a much greater part of the step cycle in the child with spastic diplegia than in the normal child.

Musculoskeletal Impairments

Problems in the musculoskeletal system include weakness, loss of range of motion, contractures, and changes in alignment. Passive properties of the muscle–tendon system contribute to development of torques during walking. Thus abnormal joint stiffness and limited range of motion not only reduce joint motion but affect the ability of muscles to generate power at various speeds (Patla, 1995).

In both children with cerebral palsy and adults with hemiplegia, changes in the passive properties of the musculoskeletal system

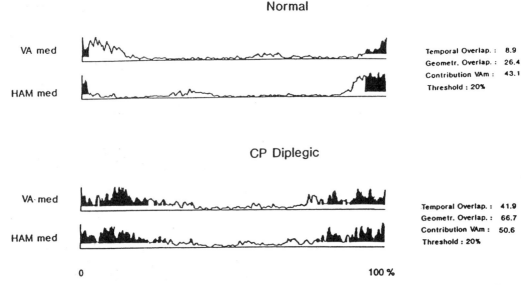

FIGURE 14-12. Quantitative assessment of cocontraction between quadriceps (VA med) and hamstrings (HAM med) in a normal and an age-matched child with spastic diplegia, walking at comparable speed. Filled areas represent coactivation of agonist and antagonist muscles. (Reprinted with permission from Crenna P, Inverno M. Objective detection of pathophysiological factors contributing to gait disturbance in supraspinal lesions. In: Fedrizzi E, Avanzini G, Crenna P. Motor Development in Children. New York: Libbey, 1994:112.)

have been found to be relevant factors in disordered locomotion. Among these patient populations, both soft tissue contractures and bony constrictions limit joint range of motion, constrain movement, and increase the workload on the muscles, affecting a patient's ability to meet the requirements of gait. In general, decreased joint mobility during stance restricts forward motion of the body over the supporting foot, affecting progression. In swing, decreased joint mobility reduces foot clearance, affecting progression, and appropriate foot placement for weight acceptance, affecting stability. Limited range of motion also limits a patient's ability to modify movement strategies, affecting adaptation. For example, a patient with limited ankle and knee flexion cannot increase limb flexion during the swing phase of gait to step over an obstacle.

As we mentioned in Chapter 10, musculoskeletal limitations in the patient with neurological dysfunction most often are secondary to a CNS lesion. Musculoskeletal impairments that particularly affect gait include ankle extensor contractures, knee and hip flexor contractures, and reduced pelvic and spinal mobility.

A wide range of musculoskeletal problems occurring at the ankle, knee, and hip joints can reduce a patient's ability to use a heel strike strategy during the initiation of stance and result in low heel contact, foot-flat contact, forefoot contact, contact made with the medial or lateral border of the foot, and/or foot slap during loading. During stance, a smooth progression over the supporting foot requires a minimum of 5 degrees of ankle dorsiflexion; thus, ankle plantarflexor contractures can impair a patient's ability to move the limb over the foot. The effect of a plantarflexion contracture on foot strike varies with its severity. A 15-degree plantarflexion contracture is common in adults with acquired disability and usually results in a low heel contact and early flat-foot during loading. A 30-degree contracture is fairly common in children with spastic cerebral palsy and produces a forefoot contact at foot strike (Perry, 1992).

Plantarflexor contractures limit tibial advancement over the stationary foot during stance. If the contracture is elastic, that is, able to lengthen in response to body weight, the only result may be an inappropriate foot position at foot contact, since body weight will lengthen the plantarflexors, allowing the tibia to advance (Perry, 1992). However, if the contracture is not elastic, recurvatum results. Recurvatum occurs when the knee has sufficient mobility to move posteriorly past neutral. Knee hyperextension can occur quickly or slowly and usually begins in mid-stance or terminal stance and continues into preswing. Excessive knee extension means the tibia cannot advance over the stationary foot in the stance phase (Perry, 1992). Plantarflexor contractures also affect foot clearance during swing by preventing sufficient ankle flexion to allow toe clearance.

Hip flexion contractures result in inadequate hip extension, which can affect both stability and progression. During midstance, if the hip cannot extend to neutral, the trunk will flex forward, bringing the center of mass anterior to the hip joint. Gravity will pull the trunk forward into more flexion, and this places an additional demand on the hip extensors to prevent collapse of the forward trunk and loss of stability (Perry, 1992). Hip flexion contractures that limit hip extension have a great effect on terminal stance, since it is during this phase that the hip is normally hyperextended. Lack of hip extension produces an anterior pelvic tilt and an inability to move the thigh posterior to the hip. This results in a shortened step length and reduces forward progression of the body.

One way to compensate for a hip flexion contracture is to flex the knees. This allows the pelvis to be normally aligned despite the hip flexion contracture. Flexion of the hips and knees is called a crouched gait and is often seen in spastic cerebral palsy as a compensatory gait pattern for inadequate hip extension (Perry, 1992; Montgomery, 1987). However, this compensatory strategy has its own limitations, since it increases the demands on the quadriceps muscle to control the knee. Increased knee flexion also requires either excessive ankle dorsiflexion or heel rise onto the forefoot during stance and thus constrains progression (Perry, 1992; Montgomery, 1987).

Knee flexion contractures can result in inadequate knee extension that will keep the knee from fully extending in terminal swing. This will affect placement of the foot in preparation for stance. Knee flexion contractures prevent the knee from fully extending at the end of swing. This affects the patient's ability to place the foot appropriately for weight transfer, reducing stability and increasing the need for muscular action to control the knee (Perry, 1992; Montgomery, 1987).

In summary, a wide variety of motor impairments contribute to disorders of gait in patients with neurological dysfunction. These impairments can occur alone or in combination, which can make sorting out their relative contributions difficult. We now turn our attention to sensory impairments that also contribute to disordered gait.

Sensory Impairments

The control of gait is based on the integration of both peripheral sensory inputs and descending supraspinal inputs. Sensation is a critical determinant for maintaining gait in natural environments where we must constantly modify how we move in response to changes in our surroundings. Sensory inputs play several important roles in the control of locomotion. Sensory inputs serve as a trigger for the initiation of swing. Thus, loss of proprioceptive cues that normally signal hyperextension in the hip and the termination of stance can result in delayed initiation of swing phase (Smith, 1980). In addition, sensory inputs are necessary for adapting locomotor patterns to changes in environmental demands. This includes signaling unanticipated disruptions to gait, as well as the ability to predict and anticipate upcoming obstacles. Thus the effects of sensory impairments on gait are varied, depending on which sense is affected and the age at which the sensory loss occurs.

Somatosensory Deficits

Abnormal somatosensory inputs result in gait ataxia. Gait problems in patients with sensory ataxia can be due to interruption of either peripheral or central proprioceptive pathways. When this occurs, the patient is usually no longer aware of the position of the legs in space or even of the position of the body itself. With a mild dysfunction, walking may not appear to be obviously abnormal if the patient can see well. However, ataxia is worse when visual cues are reduced or inappropriate. Staggering and unsteadiness increase, and some patients lose the ability to walk (Katoka et al., 1986).

Normally, proprioceptively mediated stretch reflexes are modulated throughout the gait cycle. They are facilitated in gastrocnemius and soleus at the end of stance phase, allowing for compensation of ground irregularities and assisting push-off, but inhibited during swing phase to prevent stretch reflex–mediated plantarflexion during ankle dorsiflexion (Sinkjaer et al., 1996). Loss of proprioceptive inputs results in reduced modulation throughout the gait cycle.

Visual Deficits

Vision is critical to feed-forward control of equilibrium during gait. Visual inputs are used to regulate gait on a local level (step by step) and on a more global level (route finding) (Patla, 1995). Loss of vision affects stability and adaptation aspects of gait. Visually impaired and blind patients tend to walk slowly. In addition, they appear able to use auditory cues to assist in locating obstacles in space (Ashmead et al., 1989).

Vision is critical for obstacle avoidance during gait, since visual inputs regarding upcoming obstacles are used to alter gait patterns in an anticipatory manner. For example, loss of the visual field on one side (hemianopsia) can affect a patient's ability to perceive threats to stability on the impaired side. This is shown in Figure 14-13, which illustrates a bus coming from the right that may not be perceived by a patient with hemianopsia (Tobis and Lowenthal, 1960). Thus, loss of visual inputs affect both route finding and obstacle avoidance.

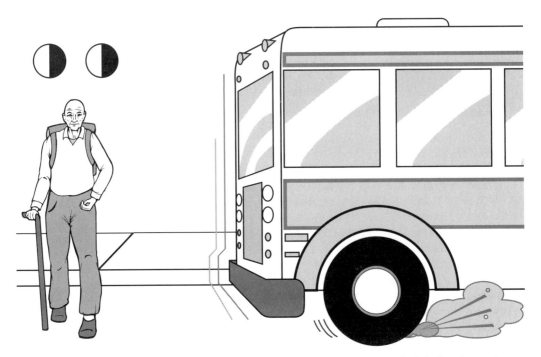

FIGURE 14-13. Functional effects of visual hemianopsia. The patient with right hemianopsia does not perceive the bus coming from the right. (Adapted with permission from Tobis JS, Lowenthal M. Evaluation and management of the brain damaged patient. Springfield IL: Charles C Thomas, 1960:78.)

Vestibular Deficits

The functional consequence of loss of vestibular inputs appears to depend on the age of the individual at the time of the sensory loss. For example, individuals who lost vestibular function as infants had nearly normal posture and gait control (Horak et al., 1988). However, loss of vestibular function in adulthood can produce gait ataxia and difficulty in stabilizing the head in space.

Adult patients with vestibular deficits may walk more slowly than unimpaired individuals. Other changes include a prolonged double-support phase, and a 6.5% longer cycle time than normal subjects (Takahashi et al., 1988). Interestingly, when vestibular patients were asked to walk at a normal velocity, using a metronome to establish the pace, their double-support phase duration came closer to normal. It is not clear why vestibular patients seem to prefer a slower gait and whether practicing at faster speeds would improve the kinematics of their gait cycle.

It has been reported that patients with vestibular deficits may also show impairments in head stabilization during gait, especially in the dark (Takahashi et al., 1988; Pozzo et al., 1991). Gaze is equally stable for vestibular deficit patients and normal subjects during sitting and standing. However, when walking, the ability to stabilize gaze is impaired, and thus patients have complaints of impaired vision and oscillopsia. In addition, eye movements compensate for head movements more effectively during active head rotations than during similar movements made while walking. It has been suggested that this may be due to the predictable nature of active voluntary head movements versus the passive head movements made during locomotion (Grossman and Leigh, 1990).

When normal subjects walk or run in the dark, the amplitude and velocity of head rotation are less than during normal walking. However, these parameters increase for subjects with bilateral vestibular deficits when they walk in the dark (Pozzo et al., 1991).

Perceptual and Cognitive Impairments

As mentioned in Chapter 6, perceptual and cognitive problems can have a devastating effect on functional movement capability, including mobility function.

Body Image and Scheme Disorders

Body image deficits can result in a number of gait deviations, including trunk lean toward the stance leg, resulting in loss of stability. Impaired body image can also result in inappropriate foot placement and difficulty in controlling the center of body mass relative to the changing base of support of the feet (Perry, 1992). Patients with unilateral spatial neglect, defined as the inability to perceive and integrate stimuli on one side of the body, affecting the left side tend to veer to the right when walking, or bump into objects on the left side when walking or propelling a wheelchair (Warburg, 1994).

Suzuki et al. (1997) used a dual task methodology to examine the relationship between unilateral spatial neglect and gait in 31 stroke patients, 15 with left hemiplegia (right hemisphere damage) and 19 with right hemiplegia (left hemisphere damage). They created a video face test using a video monitor placed in front of the patient, which showed a video of scenery associated with walking along a corridor. Faces appeared on the video periodically, positioned to the right or left of midline. The ability to perceive faces presented on the right versus left side was examined while patients were sitting, standing, or stepping continuously. Results from this interesting study are summarized in Table 14-2. Their study found that many of the patients with unilateral spatial neglect (see for example patients 1, 5 and 6) were able to observe all 15 faces presented on the side contralateral to the lesion when sitting or standing; however, they were unable to perceive faces (score of 0) while stepping. In contrast, patients 8 and 12 in Table 14-2 show unilateral spatial neglect (as indicated by 0 scores) in sitting, standing, and stepping. These findings indicate that in

TABLE 14-2   Scores on the Video Face Test in Patients With Unilateral Spatial Neglect: Number of Correct Identifications of Faces Presented on the Right or Left Side in Sitting, Standing, and Walking

Subject No.	Hemisphere Lesion Side	Sitting		Standing		Stepping	
		RT	LT	RT	LT	RT	LT
1	Right	15	15	15	15	14	0
2	Right	15	15	15	15	15	7
3	Right	14	15	15	15	13	7
4	Right	14	13	15	15	15	0
5	Right	15	15	15	15	15	0
6	Right	15	15	15	15	15	0
7	Right	15	15	15	15	15	9
8	Right	15	0	15	0	15	0
9	Right	15	15	15	15	15	15
10	Right	14	15	15	15	15	15
11	Left	14	15	15	15	10	15
12	Left	0	15	0	15	0	15

RT, right; LT, Left.
Total possible, 15.
Reprinted with permission from Suzuki E, Chen W, Kondo T. Measuring unilateral spatial neglect during stepping. Arch Phys Med Rehabil 1997;78:176.

some patients unilateral spatial neglect is context specific.

Interestingly, two of the patients (9 and 10) with unilateral spatial neglect who performed normally on the video face test in stepping (score of 15) required more assistance to step during the test, suggesting that they allocated attention to the video task rather than to the stepping task. Other subjects were able to keep stepping with minimal or no assistance (Suzuki et al., 1997).

Spatial Relation Disorders

Purposeful locomotion toward a goal that is not visible from the start requires navigational strategies that depend on stored spatial knowledge (Patla, 1995). The impact of deficits in spatial cognition on mobility is considerable and particularly affects the ability to navigate safely through the environment, avoiding collisions with obstacles that are not readily perceived. Inability to remember the relationship of one place to another, called topographical disorientation,

can significantly affect route-finding aspects of locomotion (Patla, 1995).

Pain

Pain can cause patients to alter movement patterns used for gait. An antalgic gait is defined as a gait pattern that results from pain. Compensatory strategies used in the presence of pain are movements that (a) reduce weight bearing time on the painful limb, such as shortening stance phase of gait; (b) avoid impact loads; (c) reduce joint excursion, for example by limiting knee flexion during the stance phase of gait; and (d) decreasing joint compressive forces by minimizing activity in muscles that cross the joint, for example side-bending over a painful hip to bring the center of mass closer to the joint's center of rotation, reducing the need for hip abductor activity and concomitant joint compressive forces (Eyring and Murray, 1965). Antalgic gaits are often characterized by decreased gait velocity, shortened stance phase on the painful limb, a tendency to stiffen the limb to minimize joint motion, and a reduction in forceful foot contact or push-off.

Cognitive Impairments

Cognitive impairments also impact mobility function, specifically the ability to initiate gait, to adapt gait patterns to changing environmental demands, and to navigate to both familiar and unfamiliar locations. Cognitive impairments, as discussed in Chapter 6, include deficits affecting memory, attention, and executive functions. A more complete discussion of higher-order gait disorders resulting from impaired cognitive function can be found elsewhere (Nutt et al., 1993; Nutt and Horak, 1997).

Many studies have found that dementia is a major risk factor for falls (Alexander et al., 1995; Tinetti et al., 1988). Alexander et al. (1995) studied 17 subjects with Alzheimer's disease. They found that the patients with Alzheimer's disease walk at half the speed of healthy older adults, have a higher obstacle contact rate, and tend to land closer to the obstacle. These factors may contribute to falls, particularly trips. In addition, falls during gait may be the result of impaired insight resulting in patients attempting tasks that are beyond their physical capabilities (Nutt and Horak, 1997).

Researchers have shown that posture, balance, and gait, though considered "automatic," require attentional resources (Teasdale et al., 1993; LaJoie et al., 1993). Thus, impairments in attention have the potential to impact the ability to safely carry out activities such as gait, particularly when distracters are present (Kerns and Mateer, 1996).

⊘ A CASE STUDY APPROACH TO UNDERSTANDING GAIT DISORDERS

We now turn to summarizing gait disorders by diagnosis, using our case studies as examples. Again, as in Chapter 10, it is important to remember that there is great heterogeneity among patients even with the same diagnosis. Thus not all patients who have had a stroke will have a gait disorder similar to that of Phoebe J.

Phoebe J.: Gait Problems Following Cerebral Vascular Accident

Stroke is considered to be a leading cause of disability throughout the world (Dombovy et al., 1987). The ability to walk is often a primary factor in determining residential status and level of productivity following a stroke. As a result, retraining the ability to walk is a critical part of the rehabilitation process following a stroke.

It is likely that Phoebe J., our patient with left hemiparesis, will walk only half as fast as healthy adults, since the average gait velocity among patients who have had a stroke is 37 m/minute, compared with 82 m/minute for healthy adults. However, the speed of walking depends greatly on the degree of recovery. Researchers have shown a relationship between walking speed and Brunnstrom's stages of recovery following stroke (Brandstater et al., 1983). These data are summarized in Table 14-3. Patients in stage 6, defined by Brunnstrom as having the ability to perform isolated joint movements freely in a well-coordinated manner, walk considerably faster (0.65 m/second, or 39 m/minute) than do patients in stage 3, defined as having the ability to voluntarily initiate movements only within a full-limb synergy and with marked spasticity (0.16 m/second, or 9.6 m/minute). Patients who were at stage 1 or 2 were unable to walk (Brandstater et al., 1983).

Researchers have also shown that patients with the slowest gait (0.08 to 0.24 m/second, or 4.8 to 14.4 m/minute) have significant muscle weakness and a primitive mass synergy pattern (DeQuervain et al., 1996). Patients with intermediate gait velocity (0.4 to .7 m/second, or 24 to 42 m/minute) had mild weakness and were able to isolate joint movements. The one patient who walked at a nearly normal gait velocity (1.04 m/second, or 62.4 m/minute) had no weakness but showed marked hemianopsia and apraxia.

TABLE 14-3.   Characteristics of Hemiplegic Gait According to Stage of Motor Recovery

Variable	Stage of motor recovery				Total patients n = 23	Normal n = 5
	3	4	5	6		
Walking speed (m/sec)	0.16 ± 0.07	0.17 ± 0.08	0.40 ± 0.15	0.65 ± 0.11	0.31 ± 0.21	1.14 ± 0.10
Stride period (sec)	2.8 ± 0.7	2.8 ± 0.7	2.0 ± 0.4	1.4 ± 0.1	2.3 ± 0.8	1.2 ± 0.1
Cadence (steps/min)	45 ± 9	45 ± 9	63 ± 11	85 ± 9	57 ± 18	104 ± 9
Stride length (m)	0.41 ± 0.12	0.44 ± 0.16	0.73 ± 0.20	0.91 ± 0.09	0.60 ± 0.25	1.32 ± 0.12
Stance period (sec)						
Aff. side	1.9 ± 0.7	1.9 ± 0.8	1.2 ± 0.3	0.89 ± 0.11	1.6 ± 0.7	0.68 ± 0.07
Unaff. side	2.5 ± 0.7	2.3 ± 0.8	1.5 ± 0.3	0.95 ± 0.13	1.9 ± 0.8	0.68 ± 0.08
Swing period (sec)						
Aff. side	0.89 ± 0.21	0.88 ± 0.33	0.74 ± 0.12	0.53 ± 0.07	0.78 ± 0.25	0.48 ± 0.03
Unaff. side	0.34 ± 0.11	0.44 ± 0.11	0.52 ± 0.12	0.47 ± 0.06	0.44 ± 0.12	0.48 ± 0.03
Stance/swing ratio						
Aff. side	2.4 ± 1.3	2.6 ± 1.7	1.7 ± 0.5	1.7 ± 0.3	2.1 ± 1.2	1.4 ± 0.1
Unaff. side	8.1 ± 3.2	6.0 ± 3.1	2.9 ± 0.7	2.1 ± 0.4	5.0 ± 3.2	1.4 ± 0.1
Double support (percent of stride)	54 ± 14	50 ± 15	34 ± 9	29 ± 5	43 ± 15	17 ± 2
Stance symmetry (aff/unaff)	0.77 ± 0.11	0.82 ± 0.14	0.83 ± 0.09	0.94 ± 0.17	0.83 ± 0.12	1.00 ± 0.03
Swing symmetry (unaff/aff)	0.41 ± 0.16	0.55 ± 0.21	0.70 ± 0.13	0.91 ± 0.19	0.62 ± 0.23	0.99 ± 0.02
Stance/swing ratio symmetry (aff/unaff)	0.33 ± 0.18	0.47 ± 0.22	0.59 ± 0.19	0.88 ± 0.30	0.53 ± 0.27	1.01 ± 0.06

Reprinted with permission from Brandstater M, deBruin H, Gowland C, et al. Hemiplegic gait: analysis of temporal variables. Arch Phys Med Rehabil 1983;64:585.

Phoebe J. is also likely to show disruption of other spatial temporal parameters associated with her hemiparetic gait, including increased double-support time, decreased stance time by the involved leg, and a shortened step by the noninvolved leg. This will result in significant step asymmetry (Olney and Richards, 1996). We are likely to find an invariant relationship between stride length and walking rate. We will want to examine muscle strength in the affected and unaffected leg, as well as her ability to shift weight laterally, since researchers have shown that the biomechanical determinants of maximum walking speed following cerebrovascular accident are muscle strength of the affected and unaffected side during knee extension and postural control, specifically right-left weight shift (Suzuki et al., 1999).

If we perform a kinematic analysis of Phoebe J.'s gait, we may identify characteristic patterns in both the stance and swing phase of gait that occur in many patients with hemiparesis. In the stance phase of hemiplegic gait we may observe (*a*) equinovarus foot position, leading to a forefoot or flat-foot strike during loading; (*b*) knee hyperextension in midstance with a forward lean of the trunk; and (*c*) limited hip extension during stance phase, resulting in an inability to place the hemiparetic leg in a trailing position during terminal stance. The pelvis may be retracted on the stance leg and drop on the swing side because of abductor weakness. In the swing phase of gait we may observe (*a*) toe drag, impeding progression because of inadequate flexion at the hip, knee, and ankle; (*b*) delayed hip flexion until after toe-off; (*c*) reduced knee flexion during preswing and swing; and (*d*) inappropriate foot placement because of incomplete knee extension and ankle dorsiflexion at the end of swing (Montgomery, 1987; Olney and Richards, 1996).

If we have the available technology, we may do an EMG analysis of Phoebe J.'s gait to determine the muscle patterns used for walking and possibly the underlying cause of abnormal gait patterns. By analyzing the activation of muscles during gait, we may be able to place Phoebe J. into one or more of the following categories of gait disorders: (*a*) "spastic pattern" characterized by exaggerated stretch response, (*b*) "paretic pattern" characterized by decreased or absent centrally generated patterned muscle activation, or (*c*) "coactivation pattern" produced by abnormal coactivation of multiple muscle groups (Knutsson and Richards, 1979; Knutsson, 1981, 1994). These patterns were described in more detail in early sections of this chapter.

If we analyze her energy expenditure while walking, we may be surprised to find the oxygen cost for walking is quite low despite the abnormal appearance of her gait. The inefficiency associated with abnormal gait patterns appears to be offset by slow speed. This suggests that walking is not physiologically stressful for the typical stroke patient unless there are cardiovascular problems as well (Waters, 1992; Waters et al., 1988). But this study examined energy costs in stroke patients based on time walked. When distance walked is considered, energy expenditure associated with hemiparetic gait is twice that of normal gait, because it takes stroke patients, who walk at half the velocity of normal adults, twice as long to cover that same distance (Montgomery, 1987).

Finally, Phoebe J. is likely to show asymmetry in gait initiation (Hesse et al., 1997). Hemiparetic patients demonstrate significant differences in timing, step length, mediolateral displacement of the center of pressure (COP), and pattern of velocity of center of mass movements when starting with the affected versus unaffected leg. Figure 14-14*A* shows the movement of the COP during gait initiation for a control subject with an anticipatory shift of the COP over the stance leg prior to initiating stepping. Figure 14-14*B* shows the movement of the COP of a hemiparetic subject initiating gait with the affected side, while Figure 14-14*C* shows gait initiation with the unaffected side. This figure illustrates that when patients initiate gait

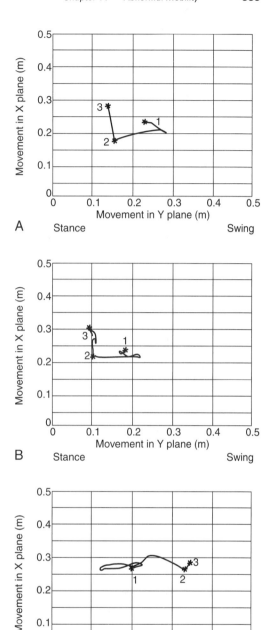

FIGURE 14-14. Movement of the COP during gait initiation for a control subject (**A**) and a hemiparetic subject initiating gait with the affected (**B**) and unaffected (**C**) sides. Note the similarities in gait initiation between the upper and middle traces. (Adapted with permission from Hesse S, Reiter F, Jahnke M, et al. Asymmetry of gait initiation in hemiparetic stroke subjects. Arch Phys Med Rehabil 1997;78:722.)

with the affected limb, there is nearly normal anticipatory movement of the COP over the unimpaired leg in preparation for step initiation. In contrast, when stepping is initiated with the unimpaired leg, there is a reduction in movement of the COP over the affected leg associated with minimizing the amount of time in which the body is supported by the paretic limb alone.

Differences in causes of gait abnormalities among patients who have had a stroke suggest that therapy and training should be adapted to individual patients. Thus for patients with paretic patterns of activity, exercises for strength involving eccentric, concentric, and isometric contractions are indicated in addition to the use of orthoses or other supports for weight bearing. In contrast, spasticity components of disordered gait require therapeutic interventions that reduce the response of the muscle to stretch (Knutsson, 1998).

Laurence W.: Gait Problems in Parkinson's Disease

Laurence W. is likely to have significant gait problems, since both gait and balance are major clinical problems in Parkinson's disease (Brown and Steiger, 1996). The degree of his gait abnormality will depend on the progression of his disease. Blin et al. (1990, 1991) studied 21 patients at various stages in the clinical progression of the disease (Hoehn and Yahr stage I through IV). Compared to normal elderly controls, patients with Parkinson's disease showed a slower walking velocity, a shorter and more variable stride length, and longer stride duration. In addition, patients with Parkinson's disease showed an increased duration of stance and double-support phase and a concomitant decrease in the swing phase. Table 14-4 compares selected gait characteristics in Parkinson's disease patients with those of healthy age-matched controls.

Researchers have found a significant relationship between walking velocity in patients with Parkinson's disease and the stages of disability as described by the Schwab Classification of Progression (Schwab, 1960) or the

Hoehn and Yahr Classification (Hoehn and Yahr, 1967).

Kinematic analysis of Laurence W.'s gait may indicate a reduction in the speed and amplitude of leg movements (resulting in characteristic short shuffling steps) and arm movements (resulting in diminution of arm swing). Specific alterations in the stance phase of gait may include (*a*) lack of heel strike; instead, patients make contact with the foot flat or with the forefoot; (*b*) incomplete knee extension during midstance; (*c*) inability to extend the knee and plantarflex the ankle in terminal stance, resulting in decreased forward thrust of the body; (*d*) forward trunk lean; (*e*) diminished trunk motion; and (*f*) reduced or absent arm swing. Decreased motion of the joints is apparent in swing phase as well. While dorsiflexion may be exaggerated during the swing phase, decreased hip and knee flexion leads to diminished toe clearance. In addition, reduced speed and amplitude of motion of the swing leg also affect forward thrust of the body (Knutsson, 1972; Stern et al., 1983).

An EMG study of Laurence W.'s gait may allow us to describe him as having one of three types of muscle activation patterns: (*a*) continuous EMG activity instead of cyclical activity, (*b*) reduced amplitude of muscle activation, or (*c*) abnormal coactivation of muscles (Knutsson, 1972).

Laurence W. will likely demonstrate problems with freezing while walking, particularly when he is turning or moving through doorways. Gait in patients with Parkinson's disease has been characterized by an inability to control momentum. If a patient is unable to generate sufficient momentum, forward progression is arrested. This is often referred to as freezing, or gait ignition failure. Freezing episodes are transient, lasting seconds to minutes. Freezing most often affects gait initiation (start hesitation) during turns, in narrow spaces, and when approaching obstacles (Fahn, 1995; Giladi et al., 1997). We may be able to help Laurence W. reduce his freezing episodes using trick maneuvers such as counting or stepping over real or imagined lines (Stern et al., 1980).

In addition to freezing, Laurence W.'s gait

TABLE 14-4.   Comparison of Selected Gait Characteristics in Patients With Parkinson's Disease Compared to Healthy Age-Matched Controls

	PD patients (n = 21)		Controls (n = 58)		PD patients versus controls	
	Mean	SD	Mean	SD	z	P
Velocity (m/sec)	0.44	0.20	0.83	0.23	5.25	<0.01
Stride length (m)	0.57	0.26	0.97	0.22	4.95	<0.01
Stride duration (sec)	1.29	0.16	1.19	0.15	2.17	<0.05
Swing duration (sec)	0.40	0.08	0.46	0.05	2.88	<0.01
Stance duration (sec)	0.88	0.16	0.74	0.12	3.50	<0.01
Swing velocity (m/sec)	1.36	0.44	2.12	0.46	5.03	<0.01
Peak velocity	2.00	0.66	3.28	0.72	5.31	<0.01
Double support duration (sec)	0.23	0.08	0.13	0.05	5.21	<0.01
Relative double support duration (sec)	35.8	9.80	21.8	6.80	5.24	<0.01
Stride duration variability	5.51	5.10	4.75	2.30	0.12	NS
Stride length variability	6.68	4.27	5.17	3.80	1.92	<0.05

Reprinted with permission from Blin O, Ferrandez AM, Serratrice G. Quantitative analysis of gait in Parkinson patients: increased variability of stride length. J Neurosci 1990;98:95.

will also be characterized by unrestrained momentum that leads to uncontrolled progression, called a propulsive gait pattern. Propulsive gait disorders may be due to an exaggerated forward inclination of the body, resulting in an anterior displacement of the center of mass beyond the supporting foot. In some instances, however, propulsive gait is seen in patients who have normal vertical posture but seem unable to oppose forward momentum (Knutsson, 1972).

Laurence W., like many patients with Parkinson's disease, is likely to have problems with gait initiation leading to akinesia (defined as loss of willed movement). Gait initiation was kinematically studied in 31 patients with Parkinson's disease (Rosin et al., 1997). Gait initiation was divided into two phases, movement preparation time and movement execution. Patients with Parkinson's disease had significantly longer movement preparation time but not execution time. In addition, while initiation of ankle, knee, hip, arm, and trunk movements was delayed, the sequencing and timing of submovements was comparable between groups. The authors suggest that gait initia-

tion problems in Parkinson's disease were not the result of dyscoordinated movements but rather were due to a deficit within the basal ganglia's internal cueing for movement sequences (Rosin et al., 1997).

Laurence W. is taking medication to help control the symptoms of Parkinson's disease. You may notice that he shows considerable fluctuations in his motor performance, both throughout the course of the day and from one day to the next. Contributions to motor fluctuations include variation in levels of anti–Parkinson's disease medications, time of day, fatigue, stress, diet, and change in responsiveness to the medication (Marsden and Fahn, 1994; Nutt et al., 1984). A number of studies have examined the effect of medication (levodopa) on various gait parameters (Morris et al., 1996b; MacKay-Lyons, 1998; Blin et al., 1991; Pedersen et al., 1991). Gait parameters particularly sensitive to changes in drug levels are walking velocity and stride length (MacKay-Lyons 1998; Blin et al., 1991; Morris et al., 1996a). In contrast, other variables such as cadence, stride time, and swing duration did not vary as a function of medication cycle (Blin et al., 1991; Pedersen et al., 1991). Morris et al. (1996a) concluded that characteristics of gait in patients with mild Parkinson's disease are reproducible during the "on" phase of medication (both across 30 minutes of peak dosage and over 24-hour intervals) but are more variable during the "off" phase. In contrast, MacKay-Lyons (1998) found extensive variability throughout the entire levodopa cycle in patients with moderately severe Parkinson's disease. Not all fluctuations in motor performance are predictable, however. Poewe (1994) found that approximately 15% of patients with Parkinson's disease develop random fluctuations in motor performance that were not related to levodopa doses. This led Poewe to categorize fluctuations in motor performance in patients with Parkinson's disease as either predictable or random.

Laurence W. may rely heavily on visual cues during walking. Prokop and Berger (1996) found that when an optical flow pattern was imposed during stepping on a treadmill, patients with Parkinson's disease continuously modulated their speed in response to changing visual flow patterns, while healthy controls did not (Prokop and Berger, 1996). It has been hypothesized that increased reliance on visual cues to regulate gait is the result of impaired proprioceptive reflexes (Bronstein et al., 1990). In contrast to patients with spasticity, patients with Parkinson's disease show a reduced reflex sensitivity (Berardelli et al., 1983; Tatton et al., 1984).

Zach C.: Gait Problems Following Traumatic Cerebellar Injury

Zach C., our 18-year-old with cerebellar damage following a motor vehicle accident, is likely to have significant gait problems, since a hallmark of cerebellar disorders is ataxic gait. His gait is probably characterized by a wide base of support and irregularity of stepping in distance and direction, leading to veering and lurching in different directions (Palliyath et al., 1998). He is likely to walk more slowly than his age-matched peers and probably has a reduced step and stride length. Palliyath et al. (1998) quantified gait in 10 patients with cerebellar ataxia, 6 with

hereditary cerebellar cortical atrophy and 4 with olivopontocerebellar atrophy. Mean quantitative differences in gait characteristics between patients and normal controls are shown in Table 14-5. Patients were on average slower than normal controls and showed more variability across all measures. Patients showed reduced step and stride length and motion at the ankle, knee, and hip. Interestingly, despite current clinical assumptions that cerebellar ataxic gait is characterized by increased step width and high steppage, in this study there was no significant difference in step width or toe clearance between the two groups. This may be due to a high variability in gait characteristics and the low number of subjects in this study.

In discussing the pathophysiology of gait disorders in cerebellar disorders, the authors suggest that while the stepping generator in the spinal cord, responsible for the gross pattern of rhythmic movements in locomotion, is intact in these patients, modulation of the spinal generator is diminished by loss of supraspinal cerebellar signals.

Sara L.: Gait Problems in Spastic Diplegia Forms of Cerebral Palsy

Sara L., our 3-year-old with a spastic diplegia form of cerebral palsy, will likely begin walking much later than her age-matched peers. She will probably walk much more slowly, averaging 40 m/minute (Crenna et al., 1991). She is likely to have reduced stride length and step width. When she needs to change her walking speed, she will probably modulate cadence rather than stride length, possibly because of static or dynamic contractures that limit motion (Abel and Damiano, 1996).

Sara L. will probably walk with a characteristic crouched gait pattern (Perry, 1992; Gage, 1991). Crouched gait (Fig. 14-8) results from excessive hip and knee flexion in conjunction with excessive ankle plantarflexion and anterior pelvic tilt during stance and swing phases of gait. Foot strike is abnormal, with an equinovarus foot posture and most often forefoot contact. This foot position is continued through the stance phase of gait. Excessive plantarflexion and knee and hip

TABLE 14-5. Comparison of Selected Gait Characteristics in Patients With Cerebellar Ataxia Compared to Healthy Age-Matched Controls

Descriptor	Control (mean ± SD)	Patient (mean ± SD)	p from t test
Cadence (steps/min)	111.00 ± 7.60	102.20 ± 15.90	0.14
Step length (% height)	0.48 ± 0.20	0.29 ± 0.07	0.02*
Stride length (% height)	0.96 ± 0.40	0.59 ± 0.14	0.02*
Step width (% height)	0.16 ± 0.08	0.14 ± 0.03	0.68
Step length symmetry	1.00 ± 0.06	0.97 ± 0.17	0.64
Stride length symmetry	1.02 ± 0.02	1.00 ± 0.04	0.35
Step width symmetry	0.98 ± 0.06	1.02 ± 0.12	0.31
Stance time (sec)	0.66 ± 0.12	0.79 ± 0.17	0.07
Swing time (sec)	0.39 ± 0.05	0.43 ± 0.06	0.18
Step time (sec)	0.54 ± 0.04	0.61 ± 0.11	0.13
Stride time or gait cycle (sec)	1.08 ± 0.08	1.21 ± 0.22	0.11
Gait velocity (mm/sec)	0.90 ± 0.39	0.47 ± 0.17	0.01*
Ankle angle range of motion	31.50 ± 6.20	23.20 ± 5.10	0.004*
Ankle angle at heel strike	102.50 ± 5.90	103.00 ± 8.50	0.90
Heel-off time (% gait cycle)	44.00 ± 4.00	50.00 ± 8.00	0.04*
Toe-off time (% gait cycle)	66.00 ± 1.00	68.00 ± 3.00	0.04*
Knee angle range of motion	58.50 ± 2.10	53.90 ± 7.70	0.10
Knee angle range of motion during stance	11.50 ± 4.90	7.50 ± 3.80	0.07
Time of peak flexion of knee during swing (% gait cycle)	2.70 ± 1.90	75.50 ± 3.20	0.02*
Hip angle range of motion	34.30 ± 5.90	31.30 ± 4.70	0.23
Foot height (cm)	11.90 ± 1.20	11.50 ± 1.90	0.62

Reprinted with permission from Palliyath S, Hallett M, Thomas SL, Lebiedowska MK. Gait in patients with cerebellar ataxia. Move Disord 1998;13:962.

flexion are seen during loading and continue through the stance phase of gait. Excessive flexion persists into terminal stance, and the preswing phase is minimal or absent because of inability to extend the hip and knee. The swing phase of gait also shows excessive knee and hip flexion (Fig. 14-8B). Often, foot-to-floor clearance is greater than normal because of excessive flexion of the swing limb (Gage, 1991; Crenna et al., 1991).

If Sara L. had spastic hemiplegia cerebral palsy instead of spastic diplegia, she would likely present with a genu recurvatum gait pattern instead of a crouched gait pattern. This gait pattern is characterized by knee hyperextension during stance and excessive ankle plantarflexion. Hip flexion and forward lean of the trunk may occur as the patient leans forward to balance over a plantarflexed foot. This is shown in Figure 14-15. Loading is onto the forefoot because of inadequate knee extension and excessive plan-

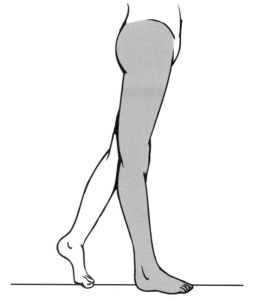

FIGURE 14-15. Genu recurvatum in stance due to excessive activity of the triceps surae in a child with spastic hemiplegia cerebral palsy.

tarflexion during swing. During swing, toe drag constrains progression, requiring contralateral trunk lean to free the foot and advance the thigh. The genu recurvatum gait pattern is more common in unilateral motor impairments, such as spastic hemiplegia (Gage, 1991; Crenna et al., 1991).

An EMG analysis of Sara L.'s gait may allow us to separate her problems into one of four categories: (*a*) defective recruitment of motor units, referred to as a paresis or weakness pattern; (*b*) abnormal velocity-dependent recruitment during muscle stretch, the so-called spasticity pattern; (*c*) nonselective activation of antagonist muscles with a loss of a normal reciprocal inhibitory pattern, called the cocontraction pattern, or (*d*) problems associated with musculoskeletal restraint due to changes in mechanical properties of muscles, the nonneural problem pattern (Crenna et al., 1991).

Interestingly, in children with spastic hemiplegic cerebral palsy, a cocontraction pattern of muscle activity was found in both the hemiplegic leg and the uninvolved leg. Thus, researchers are now considering the possibility that cocontraction is a compensatory strategy aimed at stiffening a joint to compensate for postural instability or paresis (Crenna et al., 1991; Berger et al., 1982; Leonard et al., 1991). The particular gait profile seen in an individual will reflect a combination of the factors just listed. Thus, each individual with cerebral palsy will present a slightly different gait pattern.

When walking, Sara L.'s heart rate and oxygen rates are higher than those of her age-matched peers. Researchers believe that this is because the flexed posture, which is typical of the crouch gait pattern, requires additional muscle activity for stability. Interestingly, the physiological costs of walking decrease in normal children as they get older. In contrast, the physiological costs of walking increase as children with cerebral palsy get older. Why does this happen? Increased physiological costs of walking are not due to an increase in motor abnormalities in cerebral palsy, since it is a nonprogressive disease. Instead, researchers believe that oxygen rates associated with walking in-

crease as children with cerebral palsy get older because changes in body morphology, including increased body weight and size, interact with impaired motor control. This results in an increase in the physiological cost of gait in older children. As a result, the older child with cerebral palsy may walk less and increasingly rely on a wheelchair (Waters, 1992).

℮ DISORDERS OF MOBILITY OTHER THAN GAIT

Stair Walking

Like level walking, stair walking involves reciprocal movements of the legs through alternating stance and swing phases. Climbing up stairs requires the generation of concentric forces at the knee and ankle (mostly the knee) for forward and vertical progression. Stability demands are greatest during the single-limb stance phase, when the swing leg is advancing to the next step (McFadyen and Winter, 1988).

In contrast to stair ascent, descent is achieved largely through eccentric contractions of the hip, knee, and ankle extensors, which control body position in response to the accelerating force of gravity. Energy absorption and a controlled landing are ensured through anticipatory activation of the gastrocnemius prior to foot contact with the step (McFadyen and Winter, 1988).

This means that in the patient with a neurological deficit, decreased concentric control will primarily affect stair ascent, while decreased eccentric control will primarily affect stair descent. Patients with a CNS lesion tend to stair-walk slowly, to require the use of rails for support and progression, and in severe cases of dyscontrol, to be unable to use a reciprocal pattern for stair walking. Instead, they bring both feet to the same step prior to progressing to the next step.

Impaired visual sensation affects anticipatory aspects of this task. For example, gastrocnemius activity, which precedes foot contact, is less when visual cues are reduced (Simoneau et al., 1991).

Transfers and Bed Mobility

During the performance of transfer activities, such as sit to stand (STS), rolling, and rising from a bed, healthy young adults tend to use momentum to move the body smoothly and efficiently from one position to another. An alternative strategy for transfer tasks is the zero-momentum, or force control, strategy (see Chapter 12).

There are many reasons patients with neurological impairments may use a force control strategy during transfers. Postural control problems limiting stability, cardiovascular problems such as orthostatic hypotension, and dizziness may require a patient to move slowly and make interim stops during the task. For example, when rising from a bed, a patient with orthostatic hypotension must sit for a moment on the side of the bed before standing up or risk a sudden drop in blood pressure and loss of balance. The overreliance on a force control strategy and upper extremity control during transfer tasks, however, can limit these patients' adaptability in response to changing environmental conditions. For example, they may find it difficult to stand up independently from a chair without arms (Schenkman et al., 1990; Carr and Shepherd, 1998).

Many studies have examined pathological gait in neurologically dysfunctional patients. In contrast, few studies have systematically explored problems constraining other mobility skills in these patients. Much of the information available comes from anecdotal descriptions of characteristic patterns used by stroke patients to achieve these skills (Davies, 1985; Charness, 1986).

Sit to Stand

Many impairments can constrain the ability to move from sit to stand (STS) effectively and efficiently. Impaired force control affects the STS task in two ways. The inability to activate trunk, hip, and knee muscles concentrically limits the generation of propulsive forces to move and lift the body. Loss of eccentric control limits the patient's ability to control horizontal motions of the center of mass and thus impairs stability (Schenkman et al., 1990; Carr and Shepherd, 1998).

Decreased spinal mobility and diminished motion in the hips, knees, and ankles restrict a patient's ability to move freely. This affects momentum and force control strategies but primarily the momentum control strategy. This is because the ability to transfer momentum from one body segment to another requires freedom of motion in the joints (Schenkman et al., 1990; Carr and Shepherd, 1998).

Decreased postural control impairs the ability to control movements of the center of mass and constitutes a major constraint on the STS task. One of the most frequently seen problems in patients with impaired stability is falling backward when trying to stand up. This results when the patient generates propulsive forces to lift the body before the center of mass is adequately positioned within the base of support of the feet.

Sensory impairments affect a patient's ability to determine the position of the body in space, particularly placement of the center of mass with respect to the supporting surface. Force control problems limit the patient's ability to control horizontal movements of the center of mass from over the buttocks to the new base of support, the feet.

Perceptual impairments, including impaired body image, inappropriate internal representations of stability limits, and abnormal motion perception (dizziness) also affect a patient's ability to accomplish STS safely.

Finally, cognitive impairments can significantly limit a patient's ability to perform a task safely. For example, a patient may try to sit down before he or she is appropriately positioned with respect to a chair.

Bed Mobility Skills

Bed mobility skills include changing position while in bed (rolling supine to side-lying or prone), and getting out of bed, either to a chair or standing up. Researchers have found that normal young adults use a variety of momentum-related strategies when performing bed mobility skills. There is enormous variety in how people move; in fact, none of the young adults tested used exactly the same strategy twice.

In contrast, neurologically impaired patients frequently use force control movement strategies, which are characterized by frequent starts and stops. As mentioned previously, there are many reasons a force-control strategy may be more appropriate in the neurologically impaired patient than a momentum strategy (Richter et al., 1989).

The most common approach to rolling shown by normal young adults involves reaching and lifting with the upper extremity, flexing the head and upper trunk, and lifting the leg to roll onto the side, then over to prone. Most healthy young adults did not show rotation between the shoulders and pelvis, assumed by many clinicians to be an invariant feature of rolling (Richter et al., 1989). Because bed mobility skills are primarily initiated by movement of the head, upper trunk, and shoulders, impairments that affect these structures, such as weakness and/or range of motion limitations, limit performance of these skills.

☺ SUMMARY

1. While abnormal gait is a common characteristic of many neurological pathologies, the constellation of underlying problems that produce disordered gait vary from patient to patient depending on (*a*) primary impairments such as inadequate activation of a muscle; (*b*) secondary impairments, such as contractures; and (*c*) compensatory strategies developed to meet the requirements of mobility in the face of persisting impairments.

2. Musculoskeletal impairments constrain movement and increase the workload on the muscles, affecting a patient's ability to meet the requirements of gait. Decreased joint mobility during stance restricts forward motion of the body over the supporting foot, affecting progression. In swing, decreased joint mobility reduces foot clearance, affecting progression, and appropriate foot placement for weight acceptance, affecting stability.

3. Neuromuscular impairments affecting gait include weakness, abnormalities of muscle tone, and task-specific control problems. Task-specific control problems consist of (*a*) the inability to recruit a muscle during an automatic task such as posture or gait; (*b*) inappropriate activation of a muscle during gait, which is not related to stretch of the muscle; (*c*) coactivation of agonist and antagonist muscles around a joint, which increases stiffness and decreases motion; and (*d*) problems related to scaling the amplitude of muscle activity during gait.

4. Sensory disorders can lead to problems in the following areas of locomotor control: (*a*) signaling terminal stance and thus triggering the initiation of swing, (*b*) signaling unanticipated disruptions to gait, and (*c*) detecting upcoming obstacles important for modifying gait to changes in task and environmental conditions.

5. Impairments can manifest as problems affecting the patient's abilities to meet the progression, stability, and adaptation goals inherent in both the stance and the swing phase of gait. A careful analysis of movement patterns can lead the clinician to generate multiple hypotheses about the possible underlying causes of gait problems.

6. During the performance of transfer activities such as STS, rolling, and rising from a bed, healthy young adults tend to use a momentum strategy, which requires the generation of concentric and eccentric contractions to control motion and ensures stability. In contrast, a force control strategy, characterized by frequent starts and stops, is frequently used by neurologically dysfunctional patients. This is related to impairments affecting both stability and progression aspects of the movement. This is also the strategy most commonly taught by clinicians when retraining transfer tasks.

CHAPTER 15

Clinical Management of the Patient With a Mobility Disorder

℮ INTRODUCTION

Management of mobility problems is often a key to return of functional independence in the patient with neurological pathology. Consider Phoebe J., the 67-year-old woman with left hemiparesis. Prior to her stroke, she was living independently with her spouse in her own home. In the hospital, she is dependent in all mobility functions, requiring assistance in moving about her bed, transferring to her wheelchair or commode, and standing up. At this point she is unable to walk, even with the assistance of another.

Since mobility is essential to many basic activities of daily living (BADLs), such as toileting, transfers, and dressing, as well as many instrumental activities of daily living (IADLs), such as shopping, cleaning, and cooking, regaining mobility function will be a critical determinant of Phoebe J.'s ability to recover functional independence and return to living in her own home. Given the importance of mobility to recovery of functional independence, a critical issue for Phoebe J.'s therapist will be to determine the most effective way to examine and retrain mobility skills.

This chapter presents a task-oriented approach to examining and treating the patient with mobility dysfunction, with a main focus on examination and treatment of gait. We begin with examination, reviewing some of the tests and measurements that can be used to document functional abilities related to mobility. As part of examination, we explore the process of observational gait analysis, an approach to describing strategies used to accomplish the main tasks of gait. The second half of the chapter addresses issues related to retraining mobility skills in the patient with neurological impairments.

☺ EXAMINATION

In a task-oriented approach, examination of mobility function analyzes performance at three levels: (*a*) the functional task level, (*b*) the essential strategies used to accomplish the requirements of mobility tasks, and (*c*) the underlying sensory, motor, and cognitive impairments that constrain mobility.

Examination at the Functional Level

Temporal and Distance Factors

Examination of functional mobility often focuses on determining the distance a patient can walk, the time it takes to traverse this distance, and the level of assistance needed (Katz et al., 1970; Lawton, 1971; Keith et al., 1987). The patient can be asked to walk a specified distance, such as 150 feet, and the time taken to walk that distance recorded.

Alternatively, the patient can be asked to walk for a specified time, and the distance walked recorded.

Temporal Factors: Gait Velocity

A number of researchers have suggested that velocity alone can be used as a measure of functional gait, since it is simple, quick, and appears to be a composite measure of temporal and distance variables (Richards et al., 1995; Brandstater et al., 1983; Murray et al., 1970). Converting the patient's self-selected gait velocity to a percentage of normal can be an effective way to communicate locomotor abilities to patients, their families, and insurers (Montgomery, 1987; Bohannon, 1997). In order to find the patient's percentage of normal gait velocity reference, it is necessary to know the normal values. In some cases a standard reference value of 80 m/minute is used. Bohannon (1997) published normative values for comfortable and maximum gait speed based on data from 230 healthy individuals. Reference values are both gender and age (by decades) specific and include both actual gait speed (cm/second) and gait speed normalized to height (actual gait speed [cm/second] divided by height [cm]). Norms from this study (converted to m/minute) are shown in Table 15-1.

TABLE 15-1.	Reference Values for Gait Speed: Comfortable Versus Maximum Velocity by Decade of Age and Gender

Gender, Decade	Comfortable (m/min)		Maximum (m/min)	
	Men	Women	Men	Women
20s	83.6	84.4	151.9	148.0
30s	87.5	84.9	147.4	140.5
40s	88.1	83.5	147.7	127.4
50s	83.6	83.7	124.1	120.6
60s	81.5	77.8	115.9	106.4
70s	79.8	76.3	124.7	104.9

Adapted with permission from Bohannon RW. Comfortable and maximum walking speed of adults aged 20 to 79 years: reference values and determinants. Age Ageing 1997;26:15–19.

What is the best distance to use when calculating gait velocity? One common method calculates gait speed measured over 10 meters (33 feet) indoors (Collen et al., 1990). Alternatively, patients have been asked to walk 5 meters, turn, and walk back (so-called 2 × 5 m test) (Collen et al., 1990). Guralnik et al. (1994) calculated gait speed over two distances, 2.44 m (8 feet) and 4 m (13.2 feet) in their study of disability rates among older women. This study found that the 4-m walk was the distance of choice because it was demonstrated to be feasible in the home as well as the clinical setting and the longer distance improved measurement accuracy (Guralnik et al., 1994). The application of this concept can be found in Lab Activity 15-1.

What is the effect of surface type on gait velocity? While walking speed is one of the most widely used outcome measures related to gait during rehabilitation, most studies have measured walking speed in environmental conditions that do not necessarily mimic those found in either a home or community setting. For example, one study found that at least 68% of surfaces encountered in a home setting are carpeted (Kay D., unpublished thesis, LaTrobe University, Melbourne, Australia). Other differences between clinic and home environments include presence of furniture and other obstacles, distractions (phone ringing, dog barking), carrying an external load, and lighting.

Stephens and Goldie (1999) examined gait velocity in stroke patients walking 10 meters across two surfaces, parquet and carpet, to determine the effect of surface on walking speed. Patients were significantly slower on the carpeted surface (44.76 m/minute) than on the parquetry (47.61 m/minute), suggesting that carpet is a more challenging surface for patients with stroke. These authors suggest that during gait retraining, patients should practice on the types of surfaces they expect to walk on once discharged.

Being able to calculate a patient's self-selected gait velocity, regardless of surface type, is important, since it represents a cumulative quality score of a patient's ability and confidence in walking (Richards et al.,

LAB ACTIVITY 15-1

OBJECTIVE: To determine gait velocity under self-paced and fast-paced conditions.

PROCEDURE: Measure a 10-m (33 feet) walking course. You will be calculating a steady-state gait velocity, so you want to be walking at a constant speed, not speeding up or slowing down. Starting about 2 feet before the first mark, begin walking at a comfortable pace, and keep walking for at least 2 feet after the second mark. Using a stopwatch, calculate the time it takes to walk the marked 10 meters. Repeat this three times, recording the time for each trial. Now, repeat the test walking the 10 meters as fast as you can and record the time. You may also wish to try this test using various types of assistive devices, such as a single-point cane, a pick-up walker, or a front-wheeled walker.

ASSIGNMENT: Average the three trials for each condition and calculate gait velocity (divide the total walking distance of 10 meters by the elapsed time in seconds, and multiply by 60 to get meters per minute) for both the self-paced and fast-paced conditions. Convert self-selected gait velocity to a percentage of normal (you may use either the norm 82 m/minute or refer to Table 15-1 for age- and gender-specific norms). Compare self-selected gait velocity to fast-paced velocity and calculate the percentage increase in gait speed. How does using an assistive device change your gait velocity?

1995; Brandstater et al., 1983). It can also be used to infer level of disability related to mobility, since patients who walk at less than 30% of normal do not usually become community ambulators (Montgomery, 1987).

Distance Factors: 3-, 6-, or 12-Minute Walk

Independent mobility in the community requires not just sufficient speed but endurance as well (Hesse et al., 1994). Thus, measuring the distance a patient can walk is an important outcome when retraining gait. Activity of daily living (ADL) scales, such as the Functional Independence Measure (FIM), measure independence in walking based on distance measures (Keith et al., 1987).

The 12-minute walking test was designed to examine exercise tolerance in patients with chronic respiratory disease (McGavin et al., 1976). However, because the 12-minute test is time-consuming and fatiguing to the patient, several researchers examined the validity of a shorter version of the test, comparing the performance of patients at 2, 6, and 12 minutes (Butland et al., 1982). These researchers concluded that while the 12-minute test has excellent test–retest reliability, both the 2- and 6-minute tests are equally reliable, though slightly less sensitive in discriminating a patient's level of exercise tolerance. They concluded that the shorter durations could be used when assessing exercise tolerance (Butland et al., 1982).

This research was applied to the development of a 3-minute walk test, assessing walking endurance in the patient with neurological dysfunction (Shumway-Cook, unpublished data). In the Three-Minute Walk Test patients are asked to walk at a comfortable speed, and the distance walked in 3 minutes is measured. A premeasured established path is laid out for this test. Standardized instructions are given to patients to walk at a comfortable pace, using whatever assistive device they would use when walking outside their homes and stopping to rest whenever they need to. Patients are allowed to rest as needed, though the clock is not stopped during the rest period. Thus, an increased number of rest periods is reflected in a shorter distance traveled.

Findings recorded during the Three-Minute Walk Test include distance covered, average gait velocity, number of rests required, number of deviations from a 15-inch path, and heart rate before and after the walk. As part of a study examining the effects of exercise on balance mobility and the likelihood of falls in older adults with a history of recurrent falls, scores on the Three-Minute Walk Test were compared between healthy adults aged 65 to 90 with no neurological impairments and adults in the same age range with a history of imbalance and falls. Findings from this study were that neurologically intact older adults were able to walk 727 ± 148 feet in 3 minutes (73 m/minute) with no loss of balance, compared with 323 ± 166

feet (32 m/minute) in the group of fallers. In addition, the older adults with a history of imbalance lost balance an average of four times during the 3-minute test (Shumway-Cook et al., 1997b).

Other Temporal and Distance Factors

A number of authors have advocated the inclusion of other temporal and distance factors, such as cadence, step, and stride length, including right-left asymmetry in step and stride length in the examination of gait (Holden et al., 1984; Robinson and Smidt, 1981). These factors are usually documented over a short distance, such as 20 to 30 feet. Characteristics of constant velocity gait are determined, and thus the first and last 5 feet are not used in the calculations. Patients are usually given one practice trial, followed by two data collection trials, separated by rest periods.

A number of methods for quantifying temporal and distance factors in the clinic, including a footprint analysis using either inked feet and white butcher paper (Holden et al., 1984) or floor grids (Robinson and Smidt, 1981) have been suggested.

Technological Devices for the Clinic

The use of laboratory methods, such as motion analysis, electromyography (EMG), and force plates, for analyzing gait is expensive and time consuming and requires special expertise; as a result it is not realistic in clinical settings. However, a growing number of simple devices to quantify spatial and temporal aspects of gait in the clinic are being developed. These devices vary in their complexity and cost but can improve the therapist's ability to measure specific gait parameters in the clinical setting. Examples include portable stride analyzers (insoles that contain four compression-closing switches connected to a light-weight mobile data collection box worn on a belt) and various types of instrumented walkways.

Energy Efficiency

An important aim of gait retraining is to reduce the energy cost of walking (Kerrigan et al., 1998). Bernardi et al. (1999) examined the physiological cost (energy, cardiac, and ventilatory cost per meter walked) of walking in 96 subjects (14 normal controls and 82 disabled patients). This study confirmed that walking speed was the best single measure of walking impairment. The study also found a negative linear correlation between preferred speed and physiological cost (energy, cardiac, and/or ventilatory), indicating that the energy cost of walking is speed dependent. Patients requiring cane, crutches, or a walker had a walking energy cost twice as high as that of subjects who did not use assistive devices when walking.

This study also examined whether heart rate could be used as a measure of walking energy cost. Overall walking cardiac cost (WCC) was calculated as the number of heartbeats per unit distance (WCC = HR_w/S, where HR_w is heart rate walking [beats per minute] and S is the speed in m/minute). Results suggested that heart rate was a good measure of walking energy cost (WEC) in young adults. However, in older adults and in some patients it was less reliable because of other factors that can influence heart rate, such as anxiety, irregular rhythm, drugs, and cardiovascular adaptation to physical exercise.

Thus, researchers have shown that a healthy individual's comfortable walking speed is associated with the minimum metabolic cost; walking more slowly or faster than this speed increases the metabolic cost of gait. The slower gait velocities used by most patients are associated with a much higher metabolic cost than those of healthy controls. Thus, if during gait retraining patients can increase their comfortable walking speed, they can decrease their metabolic cost of walking (Bernardi et al., 1999).

Scales for Examining Mobility

Measurement of spatial and temporal aspects of gait, while important, is limited to examining gait under static conditions (walking at a comfortable speed over level ground in ideal ambient conditions). A number of mobility scales have been developed to examine a broader range of walking skills that are more characteristic of mobility

in community environments. These include starts and stops, changes in direction and speed, stepping over and around obstacles, and the integration of multiple tasks such as talking, turning to look at something, and carrying objects during gait. Thus, these tests include not only the examination of unimpeded gait, defined as a closed skill task, but also the ability to modify and adapt gait to both expected and unexpected disturbances to locomotion. When selecting a test, clinicians should keep in mind the severity of mobility impairment in the patient being tested and choose an appropriate scale to avoid a ceiling (a test that is too easy) or floor (a test that is too difficult) effect.

Duke Mobility Skills Profile

The Duke Mobility Skills Profile (Duncan, 1993) was developed to quantify performance in ambulatory older adults. The test examines multiple mobility tasks, including unimpeded gait, transfers, and stairs. Skills are scored 0, 1, or 2 based on the criteria shown in Table 15-2. This test has good test–retest and interrater reliability.

Dynamic Gait Index

Shumway-Cook developed the Dynamic Gait Index to evaluate and document a patient's ability to modify gait in response to changing task demands in ambulatory patients with balance impairments. The test is shown in Table 15-3. Preliminary research has shown that the test has good interrater and test–retest reliability and can be used as a predictor of falls among the elderly (Shumway-Cook et al., 1997a). For example, a population of 15 healthy older adults with no neurological impairments or history of imbalance received a mean score of 21 ± 3 on the Dynamic Gait Index. In contrast, an equal number of older adults with a history of falls and imbalance but no neurological diagnosis such as stroke or Parkinson's disease received a mean score of 11 ± 4.

Physical Performance and Mobility Examination

The Physical Performance and Mobility Examination (PPME) was developed to measure physical function and mobility in hospitalized and frail older adults (Winograd et

TABLE 15-2.   Duke Mobility Skills Profile

1. Can this person walk?
   Yes—go to question three   yes=1 _____
   No—go to question two   no=0 _____
2. Can this person sit upright without human assistance for 60 seconds?   yes=1 _____
                                                                                       no=0 _____

3. Does gait meet criteria?   yes=1 _____
   (no device, symmetrical, step length twice foot length)   no=0 _____
4. Can this person descend stairs step-over-step without holding railing?   yes=1 _____
                                                                                       no=0 _____

                                                                                       Total _____

Soc. Sec. #: _____
day: _____

Mobility Skills Protocol
(modified 10/26/89)

Equipment – Straight-back hard-seated chair, tape measure, 12-inch ruler, shoebox, stopwatch, pencil, white tape

1. *Sitting balance*
   Will you sit forward in the chair, arms folded across chest, for 1 minute? (patient sits in
      standardized chair (straight-back kitchen-type chair), without leaning back for 1 minute.
   2 = can sit upright, unsupported for 60 seconds.
   1 = can sit upright independently *with support* for 60 seconds holding onto arm of chair or leaning
      against back of chair
   0 = cannot sit upright independently for 60 seconds   _____

2. *Sitting reach*
   Will you reach forward and get this ruler out of my hand? (45 degrees plane forward—put ruler 12
      inches beyond dominant hand reach).
   2 = reaches forward and successfully grasps item
   1 = cannot grasp or requires arm support
   0 = does not attempt reach
   C = contraindicated
   R = refused   _____

3. *Transfer*
   Will you show me how to get from your chair to the bed (or to another chair)?
   2 = performs independently (without help from a person), appears steady and safe
   1 = performs independently (without help from a person) but appears unsteady
   0 = cannot do or requires help from a person to complete the task
   C = contraindicated
   R = refused

4. *Rising from a chair*
   a. Will you get up from the chair without using your arms to push up? (patient seated in straight-
      back kitchen chair, arms folded across chest or out in front)
      1 = done on 1st try
      0 = not done on 1st try
      C = contraindicated
      R = refused   _____
   b. Will you get up from the chair using your arms to push up? (subject can put hands on arms of
      chair or on chair seat for assistance; subject can hold onto assistive device if desired while
      standing up)
      ***** NOTE – (score = 1 if scored 1 on 4a)
      1 = can do independently
      0 = can't do independently
      C = contraindicated
      R = refused   _____

5. *Standing balance*
    a. Will you stand the way you usually stand for 1 minute?
       2 = steady, without holding onto walking aid or other object for support for 60 seconds
       1 = steady, but uses walking aid or other object for support for 60 seconds
       0 = cannot stand upright for 60 seconds
       C = contraindicated
       R = refused
                                                                            _____

6. *Picking up object off the floor*
    (drop pencil 1 foot in front of subject (out of base of support). Will you pick this pencil up from
       the floor?
    2 = performs independently (without help from object/person)
    1 = performs with some help (holds onto a table, chair, assistive device, person, etc.) or is unsteady
       (staggers or sways, has to catch self to to keep from falling, etc.)
    0 = unable to pick up object and return to standing
    C = contraindicated
    R = refused
                                                                            _____

7. *Walking*
    (measure 10-foot pathway)
    Will you walk in your usual way (with or without assistive device) from here to here (indicate
       distance to patient—allow 3 to 5 feet for warm-up).
    2 = meets all standards for gait characteristics
    1 = fails any standard or uses assistive device
    0 = unstable, can't do (requires intervention to keep from falling or staggers, trips)
    C = contraindicated
    R = refused
    standards for gait (tested only in subject's preferred manner)
    1. symmetrical step length
    2. walks along straight path
    3. distance between stance toe and heel of swing foot at least 1 ft length
                                                                            _____

8. *Turning*
    Will you walk along the path, then turn and come back?
    2 = no more than three continuous steps, no assistive device
    1 = fails criteria for a score of 2 but completes task without intervention
    0 = unable to turn; requires intervention to prevent falling
    C = contraindicated
    R = refused
                                                                            _____

9. *Abrupt stop*
    Will you walk as fast as you can and stop when I say stop? (walk with subject and announce "stop"
       after 6 to 8 steps)
    2 = stops within one step without stumbling or grabbing
    1 = cannot stop within one step or stumbles, uses assistive device
    0 = requires intervention to avoid fall
    C = contraindicated
    R = refused
                                                                            _____

10. *Obstacle*
    (place shoebox in walking path)
    Will you walk at your normal pace and step over the shoebox that is in the way?
    2 = steps over without interrupting stride
    1 = catches foot, interrupts stride, uses assistive device
    0 = cannot step over box
    C = contraindicated
    R = refused
                                                                            _____

11. *Standing Reach*
    (45 degree plane forward—put ruler 12 inches beyond dominant hand reach)
    Will you reach forward and get this ruler from me?
    2 = reaches forward and successfully grasps ruler without stepping or holding on
    1 = reaches forward but cannot grasp ruler without stepping or holding onto device
    0 = does not attempt to shift weight
    C = contraindicated
    R = refused   _____

12. *Stairs* (must have at least 2 steps)
    Try to go up and down these stairs without holding on to the railing.
    Ascending
    2 = steps over step, does not hold on to railing or device
    1 = one step at a time or must hold on to railing or device
    0 = unsteady, can't do
    C = contraindicated
    R = refused   _____
    Descending
    2 = steps over step, does not hold on to railing or device
    1 = one step at a time or must hold onto railing or device
    0 = unsteady, can't do
    C = contraindicated
    R = refused   _____
13. Preferred assistive device:
    _____ wheelchair (= 1)
    _____ walker (= 2)
    _____ quad cane (= 3)
    _____ straight cane (= 4)
    _____ other _____ (= 5)
    _____ none (= 0)

_____

Reprinted with permission from Duncan P. Duke Mobility Skills Profile. Center for Human Aging, Duke University, 1989.

---

al., 1994). The PPME was designed to assess function without overtaxing frail or acutely ill subjects. Six mobility tasks integral to everyday life were chosen for the test, which does not examine constituent abilities, such as strength and range of motion. This test includes both high-level tasks, such as standing up five times from a chair, and lower-level tasks, such as bed mobility and transfer skills. The test is summarized in Table 15-4. Shown are the list of tasks, a description of how the task is to be performed, and the response dimensions.

Mobility Scale for Acute Stroke Patients

The Mobility Scale was developed by Simondson and colleagues to assess mobility function in stroke patients in an acute hospital setting (Simondson et al., 1996). Patients are asked to perform five tasks, which incor-porate functional movements from bed mobility to walking. Performance relative to level of assistance needed to complete each task is graded on a 6-point ordinal scale (1, unable, to 6, unassisted and safe). This test is shown in Table 15-5. Interrater and test–retest reliability are excellent (Simondson et al., 1996).

Rivermead Mobility Index

The Rivermead Mobility Index (RMI) (Collen et al., 1991), shown in Table 15-6, quantifies mobility function using 15 activities; 14 of these activities are scored via the patient's self-report (1, yes; 0, no). Item 5, standing unsupported for 10 seconds, is directly observed. The RMI is simple and quick and can be used in a variety of environments. It has been shown to be both a reliable and valid test of mobility function (Forlander and Bohannon, 1999).

TABLE 15-3. Dynamic Gait Index

1. Gait level surface_____

   Instructions: Walk at your normal speed from here to the next mark (20 feet)

   Grading: Mark the lowest category that applies.

   (3) Normal: Walks 20 feet, no assitive devices, good speed, no evidence of imbalance, normal gait pattern.

   (2) Mild impairment: Walks 20 feet, uses assistive devices, slower speed, mild gait deviations.

   (1) Moderate impairment: Walks 20 feet, slow speed, abnormal gait pattern, evidence of imbalance.

   (0) Severe impairment: Cannot walk 20 feet without assistance, severe gait deviations, or imbalance.

2. Change in gait speed_____

   Instructions: Begin walking at your normal pace (for 5 feet), when I tell you to "go", walk as fast as you can (for 5 feet). When I tell you "slow," walk as slowly as you can (for 5 feet).

   Grading: Mark the lowest category that applies.

   (3) Normal: Able to smoothly change walking speed without loss of balance or gait deviation. Shows a significant difference in walking speeds between normal, fast, and slow speeds.

   (2) Mild impairment: Is able to change speed but demonstrates mild gait deviations, or no gait deviations but unable to achieve a significant change in velocity, or uses an assistive device.

   (1) Moderate impairment: Makes only minor adjustments to walking speed, or accomplishes a change in speed with significant gait deviations, or changes speed but loses significant gait deviations, or changes speed but loses balance but is able to recover and continue walking.

   (0) Severe impairment: Cannot change speeds, or loses balance and has to reach for wall or be caught.

3. Gait with horizontal head turns_____

   Instructions: Begin walking at your normal pace. When I tell you look right, keep walking straight but turn your head to the right. Keep looking to the right until I tell you, "look left," then keep walking straight and turn your head to the left. Keep your head to the left until I tell you, "look straight," then keep walking straight but return your head to the center.

   Grading: Mark the lowest category that applies.

   (3) Normal: Performs head turns smoothly with no change in gait

   (2) Mild impairment: Performs head turns smoothly with slight change in gait velocity, i.e., minor disruption to smooth gait path or uses walking aid.

   (1) Moderate impairment: Performs head turns with moderate change in gait velocity, slows down, staggers but recovers, can continue to walk.

   (0) Severe impairment: Performs task with severe disruption of gait, i.e., staggers outside 15-inch path, loses balance, stops, reaches for wall.

4. Gait with vertical head turns_____

   Instructions: Begin walking at your normal pace. When I tell you, "look up," keep walking straight, but tip your head and look up. Keep looking up until I tell you, "look down." Then keep walking straight and turn your head down. Keep looking down until I tell you, "look straight," then keep walking straight, but return your head to the center.

   Grading: Mark the lowest category that applies.

   (3) Normal: Performs head turns with no change in gait.

   (2) Mild impairment: Performs task with slight change in gait velocity, i.e., minor disruption to smooth gait path or uses walking aid.

   (1) Moderate impairment: Performs task with moderate change in gait velocity, slows down, staggers but recovers, can continue to walk.

   (0) Severe impairment: Performs task with severe disruption of gait, i.e., staggers outside 15-inch path, loses balance, stops, reaches for wall.

5. Gait and pivot turn_____

   Instructions: Begin walking at your normal pace. When I tell you, "turn and stop," turn as quickly as you can to face the opposite direction and stop.

   Grading: Mark the lowest category that applies.

   (3) Normal: Pivot-turns safely within 3 seconds and stops quickly with no loss of balance.

   (2) Mild impairment: Pivot-turns safely in more than 3 seconds and stops with no loss of balance.

   (1) Moderate impairment: Turns slowly, requires verbal cueing, requires several small steps to catch balance following turn and stop.

   (0) Severe impairment: Cannot turn safely; requires assistance to turn and stop.

6. Step over obstacle_____

   Instructions: Begin walking at your normal speed. When you come to the shoebox, step over it, not around it, and keep walking.

   Grading: Mark the lowest category that applies.

   (3) Normal: Is able to step over box without changing gait speed; no evidence of imbalance.

   (2) Mild impairment: Is able to step over box but must slow down and adjust steps to clear box safely.

   (1) Moderate impairment: Is able to step over box but must stop, then step over. May require verbal cueing.

   (0) Severe impairment: Cannot perform without assistance.

7. Step around obstacles_____

   Instructions: Begin walking at your normal speed. When you come to the first cone (about 6 feet away), walk around the right side of it. When you come to the second cone (6 feet past first cone), walk around it to the left.

   Grading: Mark the lowest category that applies.

   (3) Normal: Is able to walk around cones safely without changing gait speed; no evidence of imbalance.

   (2) Mild impairment: Is able to step around both cones but must slow down and adjust steps to clear cones.

   (1) Moderate impairment: Is able to clear cones but must significantly slow speed to accomplish task or requires verbal cueing.

   (0) Severe impairment: Unable to clear cones, walks into one or both cones, or requires physical assistance.

8. Steps_____

   Instructions: Walk up these stairs as you would at home (i.e., using the rail if necessary). At the top, turn around and walk down.

   Grading: Mark the lowest category that applies.

   (3) Normal: Alternating feet, no rail.

   (2) Mild impairment: Alternating feet, must use rail.

   (1) Moderate impairment: Two feet to a stair; must use rail.

   (0) Severe impairment: Cannot do safely.

TABLE 15-4. Physical Performance and Mobility Examination

Tasks	Description	Response dimension
1. Bed mobility	Sit up in bed from lying down	Need for assistance, time to complete
2. Transfers	Stand up from bed (from sitting) move to chair, sit down, stand up from chair once	Need for assistance, use of arms
3. Multiple chair stands	Stand up from chair 5 times	Need for assistance, use of arms, time to complete
4. Standing balance	Ability to hold 4 positions for 10 seconds, feet apart, feet together, semitandem, tandem	Need for assistance, time
5. Step up	Step up one step with handrail	Need for assistance, use of handrail
6. Ambulation	Walk 5 meters, 2 trials	Time at usual pace, number of steps

Reprinted with permission from Winograd CH, Lemsky CM, Nevitt MC, et al. Development of a physical performance and mobility examination. J Am Geriatr Soc 1994;42:743–749.

TABLE 15-5. Mobility Scale for Acute Stroke Patients

Activities
1. Bridging from supine, buttocks clear of bed, return to supine
2. Sitting from supine, legs over bed, return to supine (let patient choose side)
3. Balance sitting on a standardized stool for 3 minutes, feet on the floor
4. Sit to vertical stand from a standardized chair with no arm rests
5. Gait, assessed indoors on a level surface along a measured walkway of 10m, with or without a gait aid

For activities 1, 2, and 4 ask the patient to perform the activity three times and record the best of three attempts. Ask patient to perform activities 3 and 5 once; record the overall assistance provided for the duration of the activity.

Rating scale
1. Unable to do activity; patient makes no contribution or is unable to complete activity.
2. Maximum assistance of one to two people; patient makes minimal contribution to activity.
3. Moderate assistance of one individual, hands-on for most of activity. Patient is able to perform some part of the activity independently.
4. Minimum assistance, hands-on for part of the activity.
5. Supervised (verbal input, no hands on).
6. Unassisted and safe, no verbal input.

Reprinted with permission from Simondson J, Goldie P, Brock K, Nosworthy J. The Mobility Scale for acute stroke patients: intrarater and interrater reliability. Clin Rehab 1996;10:295–300.

Determining Level of Disability Related to Mobility

An important part of rehabilitation of persons with gait disorders is predicting their level of disability. However, there are few guidelines to assist the clinician in the prediction process. The relationship between impairments, functional limitations, and level of disability is not clear. Gait velocity, a functional measure, has been shown to relate to strength, an impairment measure, but neither measure has been shown to correlate well with home versus community independence, a disability measure (Perry et al., 1995).

Hoffer et al. (1973) suggested a classification of walking disability including unable (a person who cannot meet the requirements of walking within the home or community), physiological walker (an individual who walks for therapeutic but not functional purposes); household (an individual who can safely perform the tasks that define mobility at home) and community walker (no limitations to the individual's ability to meet the demands of moving within the community). However, beyond defining the levels, Hoffer did not provide specific criteria that would discriminate among the four levels.

Hoffer's classification was expanded and modified by Perry et al. (1995). This classification system is summarized in Table 15-7. Perry and colleagues studied 147 stroke patients to identify the best combination of measures that predicted mobility status (Perry et al., 1995). Measures used to predict level of ambulation included a self-report questionnaire regarding walking abilities, calculation of stride characteristics using a foot switch stride analyzer, a test of proprioception, and the Upright Motor Control Test. This test is shown and explained in Figure 15-1.

The study determined that velocity was the only single measure that predicted walking classification. A velocity of 25 m/minute predicted community ambulation. The mean walking velocity of the highest category of community walkers among the stroke subjects was 48 m/minute, compared to the normal population value of 80 m/minute. Interestingly, while patients who walked this speed were considered community ambulators, this speed was not fast enough to cross a street safely.

In addition to gait velocity, four ambulation tasks were found to be critical to determining level of mobility disability. These in-

---

TABLE 15-6. Rivermead Mobility Index

Ask the patient each question. Score 1 for yes, 0 for no. Observe for question 5.

Topic and Question	Date
1. Turning over in bed: Do you turn over from your back to your side without help?	
2. Lying to sitting: From lying in bed, do you get up to sit on the edge of the bed on your own?	
3. Sitting balance: Do you sit on the edge of the bed without holding on for 10 seconds?	
4. Sitting to standing: Do you stand up from any chair in less than 15 seconds and stand there for 15 seconds using hands and/or an aid if necessary?	
5. Standing unsupported: Ask to stand. Observe standing for 10 seconds without any aid.	
6. Transfer: Do you manage to move from bed to chair and back without any help?	
7. Walking indoors with an aid if necessary: Do you walk 10 meters, with an aid if necessary, but with no standby help?	
8. Stairs: Do you manage a flight of stairs without help?	
9. Walking outside on even ground: Do you walk around outside on pavements without help?	
10. Walking inside with no aid: Do you walk 10 meters inside with no AFO, brace, splint, or other aid (including furniture or walls) without help?	
11. Picking up off floor: Do you manage to walk 5 meters, pick something up from the floor, and then walk back without help?	
12. Walking outside on uneven ground: Do you walk over uneven ground, such as grass, gravel, snow, ice, without help?	
13. Bathing: Do you get into and out of a bath or shower by yourself unsupervised and without help?	
14. Up and down four steps: Do you manage to go up and down four steps with no rails but using an aid if necessary?	
15. Running: Do you run 10 meters without limping in 4 seconds (fast walk, not limping, is acceptable)?	

AFO, ankle–foot orthosis.
Reprinted with permission from Collen FM, Wade DT, Robb GF, Bradshaw CM. The Rivermead Mobility Index: a further development of the Rivermead Motor Assessment. Int Disabil Studies 1991;13:50–54.

---

cluded the ability to manage (*a*) changes in surface levels and terrain irregularity, (*b*) obstacle avoidance, (*c*) distance, and (*d*) manual handling of loads. Interestingly, while the ability to manage a change in level, such as curbs, was found to be critical to leaving home, the ability to manage stairs was not.

Perry's findings were consistent with a study by Lerner-Frankiel et al. (1990),who examined the mobility requirements associated with a range of IADLs in the Los Angeles area. These researchers wanted to determine whether the criteria used by clinicians to judge independence in the community were consistent with the actual distances and velocities needed to function independently. This study determined that to be a community ambulator, patients need to be able to walk at more than 33% of a normal adult's velocity, or about 1 mph. Community ambulators needed to be able to walk a minimum of 300 m, or about 1000 feet. Patients who walked at less than 30% of normal speed did not usually become community ambulators because it took too long to cover the required distances involved in IADL activities.

TABLE 15-7.   Perry's Proposed Scheme for Classifying Mobility Function

Discriminant Functions	Functional Walking Category					
	Physiological	Limited Household	Unlimited Household	Most-Limited Community	Least-Limited Community	Community
Bathroom	4.32[a]	11.78[a]	16.93[c]	16.96[c]	16.60[c]	17.89
Bedroom	3.39[a]	8.35[a]	12.68[c]	11.83[c]	11.25[c]	10.83
Enter/exit	1.80[b]	3.67[b]	5.47[a]	7.83[c]	7.24[c]	7.05
Curb	−0.14[b]	1.94[b]	4.77[a]	7.04[c]	7.94[c]	8.40
Grocery	−0.06[c]	−0.37[c]	−0.01[c]	−0.03[a]	1.61[c]	1.58
Shopping center, uncrowded	0.21[c]	0.74[c]	1.54[c]	1.34[a]	3.79[c]	2.98
Shopping center, crowded	0.30[c]	0.02[c]	0.05[c]	−0.22[c]	−2.10[a]	1.19
Constant	−6.70	−33.51	−76.24	−88.13	−92.45	−101.47

[a] Questionnaire item had a strong influence on placement between the two adjacent walking groups.
[b] Questionnaire item had moderate influence on placement between the two adjacent walking groups.
[c] Questionnaire item had minimal or no influence on placement between the two adjacent walking groups.

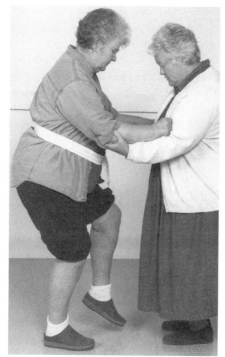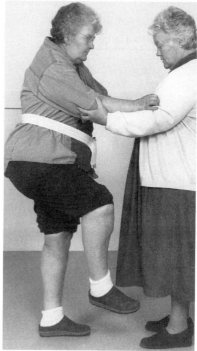

A   B

FIGURE 15-1.   Upright motor control test. **A.** Knee extension: This test involves extension in control of the body weight during single-limb stance. The patient bends both knees to approximately 30 degrees and then lifts the unaffected leg off the ground. Knee extension grades: strong, straightens the flexed knee to full extension; moderate, supports body weight on the flexed knee; weak, unable to support body weight on the flexed knee. **B.** Knee flexion: This test involves knee flexion of the unloaded leg during single-limb stance. The patient stands as straight as possible and brings the knee and foot on the affected side up toward chest as high and as fast as possible, repeated three times. Knee flexor grades: strong, joint flexes more than 60 degrees; weak, joint flexes less than 60 degrees or cannot complete three efforts in 10 seconds. (Adapted with permission from Perry J, Garrett M, Gronley JK, Mulroy, SJ. Classification of walking handicap in the stroke population. Stroke 1995;26:982.)

In addition, they were unable to cross intersections safely, a factor that severely limits mobility within the community.

In addition to distance and temporal parameters, they found two more requirements associated with community ambulation: (*a*) the ability to achieve 80 m/minute velocity for approximately 13 to 27 m to cross a street safely in the normal time allotted by stoplights and (*b*) the ability to negotiate 7- to 8-inch curbs independently (with assistive devices as needed).

The study also found that clinicians generally underestimated the distance and speed needed to function independently within a community environment (Lerner-Frankiel et al., 1990). This may be because tests of normal ADL skills, for example the FIM, often define complete independence in locomotor skills as being able to walk 150 feet safely (Keith et al., 1987). However, this standard may underestimate the requirements for being truly independent within the community.

Patla and Shumway-Cook (1999) suggest that classifying levels of mobility disability first requires an understanding of the external factors that determine the complexity and difficulty of mobility in various environments. They define eight external factors, which they call dimensions, that operationally define the demands of community mobility. These include distance and time parameters, ambient conditions (defined by light levels and weather), terrain characteristics (including both geometric properties, such as curbs and stairs, and physical properties, such as compliance and friction), external physical loads, attentional demands, postural transitions (stop, start, head turns, changes in direction), and traffic level (avoiding collisions with stationary or moving people and objects).

Patla and Shumway-Cook argue that current approaches classifying mobility disability based solely on distance and temporal parameters are insufficient, since they do not consider performance with respect to other dimensions critical to determining the complexity and risk associated with mobility. For example, going to the drugstore when it is sunny and dry involves a different level of risk than going to the drugstore when it is snowy and dark. Risk is defined as the threat to successfully completing performance of the task. In the case of going to the drugstore when it is snowy and dark, the loss of ambient light increases the risks in successfully completing the task by increasing the difficulty in route finding, avoiding obstacles, and maintaining balance. Snow increases risk because slick surfaces and heavy attire may hinder the individual's capacity for maintaining stability while walking.

Thus, functional mobility within a community environment requires not only the ability to walk safely in fairly simple and predictable environments but also the ability to modify and adapt gait to both expected and unexpected disturbances and challenges to locomotion. Mobility disability is defined not by the number of tasks a person can or cannot perform but rather by the range of environmental contexts under which tasks can be carried out. The more disabled one is, the more restrictive the dimensions under which one can safely move about. For example, the patient can walk only a limited distance or at a certain speed; the patient cannot carry any physical load because an assistive device is required; or the patient can walk (steady state) but cannot safely perform postural transitions, such as start, stop, or turn. These concepts are being tested in a study designed to measure the impact of specific environmental factors on mobility in older adults to determine the role of environment in the emergence of mobility disability in community-dwelling older adults.

Limitations of Functional Gait Measures

All functional measures, whether of mobility, balance, or general motor control, are indicators of end product only and do not provide information about the way performance is achieved. Thus, these measures do not provide insight into underlying impairments that require treatment. However, functional measures are good indicators of overall function and therefore are important indices of change.

Examination at the Strategy Level

Quantitative measures such as gait speed provide an objective measure of function but do not describe the quality of performance (the ways in which gait patterns deviate from normal). Therefore, examination of gait must include a systematic description of the strategies used by patients to meet the requirements inherent in locomotion.

Visual Gait Analysis

Visual gait analysis is the most common method for examining gait in clinical practice (Krebs et al., 1985). Visual gait analysis is the observation of kinematic patterns of movement used for gait. Observation of atypical kinematic patterns of movement is used to identify major gait deficits; however, nonobservable deficits, such as weakness, coordination, and spasticity, can only be inferred from observation and require confirmation with appropriate testing. Visual gait analysis is used as both an evaluative tool, such as to monitor change over time, and as a diagnostic tool, such as to determine the causal factors producing atypical gait (Winter, 1993; Lord et al., 1998). In visual gait analysis the observer describes characteristics of gait without the aid of any electronic devices.

Many standardized forms are available to help clinicians structure their approach to visual gait analysis. Some forms of visual gait analysis that are helpful in guiding a clinical examination of gait patterns in the patient with neurological impairments follow.

Rancho Los Amigos Gait Analysis Form

The Gait Analysis Form, shown in Table 15-8, from the physical therapy department of Rancho Los Amigos Hospital in Downey, California, is a comprehensive approach to movement analysis during gait. The form is based on the framework for analyzing gait suggested by Perry (1992) and shown in Figure 15-2. Gait is broken down into component parts. The observer focuses on one period of gait at a time, such as stance versus swing, considers the functional tasks to be performed in those periods, such as weight acceptance, single-limb support and limb advancement, and observes motion at each of the major joints, such as ankle, knee, hip, pelvis, and trunk, in each of the phases of gait, such as initial contact, loading response, and midstance.

Gait Assessment Rating Scale

The Gait Assessment Rating Scale (GARS), developed by Wolfson and colleagues, is shown in Table 15-9 (Wolfson et al., 1990). The GARS also allows the quantification and documentation of three categories of gait abnormalities: a general category, a lower extremity category, and a trunk, head and arms (HAT) category. The GARS has been used to document gait problems in healthy elderly adults as well as in older adults with a history of falls. The GARS has been shown to have high interrater reliability and is a sensitive indicator of changes in gait function among older adults.

Rivermead Visual Gait Assessment

The Rivermead Visual Gait Assessment (RVGA) shown in Table 15-10 has also been proposed as a method to structure visual gait assessment. A total of 20 observations are made, and a four-point scale is used to quantify degree of abnormality with 0 indicating normal ability; 1, mild; 2, moderate; and 3, severe abnormality. The RVGA is divided into three parts: observations of the upper limb position, observations made during stance phase, and those made during the swing phase of gait. Visual gait analysis includes observation of one side of the body at a time. A global score can be calculated by summing total numbers of deviation scores ranging from 0 (normal) to 59 (severely abnormal gait). This test has been shown to have good reliability and validity (Lord et al., 1998).

Essential Components of Gait From Carr and Shepherd

Carr and Shepherd (1998) have described a simpler approach to clinical gait analysis based on observation of a limited group of what they describe as the essential components of walking. They suggest that

TABLE 15-8. Rancho Los Amigos Gait Analysis Form

GAIT ANALYSIS: FULL BODY

RANCHO LOS AMIGOS MEDICAL CENTER
PHYSICAL THERAPY DEPARTMENT

Reference Limb:
L ☐ R ☐

| | Major Deviation |
| | Minor Deviation |

	Weight Accept		Single Limb Support		Swing Limb Advancement			
	IC	LR	MSt	TSt	PSw	ISw	MSw	TSw
Trunk Lean: B/F								
Lateral Lean: R/L								
Rotates: B/F								
Pelvis Hikes								
Tilt: P/A								
Lacks Forward Rotation								
Lacks Backward Rotation								
Excess Forward Rotation								
Excess Backward Rotation								
Ipsilateral Drop								
Contralateral Drop								
Hip Flexion: Limited								
Excess								
Inadequate Extension								
Past Retract								
Rotation: IR/ER								
Ad/Abduction: Ad/Ab								
Knee Flexion: Limited								
Excess								
Inadequate Extension								
Wobbles								
Hyperextends								
Extension Thrust								
Varus/Valgus: Vr/Vl								
Excess Contralateral Flex								
Ankle Forefoot Contact								
Foot-Flat Contact								
Foot Slap								
Excess Plantar Flexion								
Excess Dorsiflexion								
Inversion/Eversion: Iv/Ev								
Heel Off								
No Heel Off								
Drag								
Contralateral Vaulting								
Toes Up								
Inadequate Extension								
Clawed								

MAJOR PROBLEMS:

Weight Acceptance

Single Limb Support

Swing Limb Advancement

Excessive UE Weight Bearing ☐

Name _____

Diagnosis _____

© 1991 LAREI, Rancho Los Amigos Medical Center, Downey, CA 90242

Reprinted with permission from Rancho Los Amigos Medical Center's Physical Therapy Department and Pathokinesiology Laboratory, Downey, California.

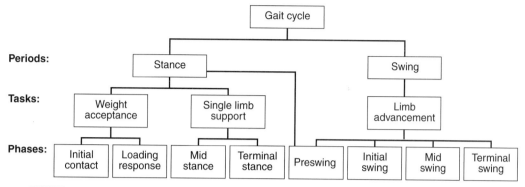

FIGURE 15-2. Conceptual framework for analyzing gait suggested by Perry (1992).

during gait analysis observation should focus on the following key elements:

Stance phase

- Extension at the hip with dorsiflexion at the ankle to move the body forward
- Lateral horizontal shift of the pelvis to the stance side
- Flexion at the knee during loading and again during terminal stance (push-off)
- Plantarflexion at heel contact, followed by dorsiflexion (shank moving over the stance foot) and then plantarflexion at push-off

Swing phase

- Flexion at the hip and knee
- Drop in pelvis at toe-off on swing side
- Rotation of pelvis forward on swing side
- Extension of knee and dorsiflexion of ankle just prior to heel contact

We have taken Carr and Shepherd's framework of essential components and added a simple ordinal scale to it (Table 15-11). We have found it a useful guide to simplify gait analysis in the clinic (Shumway-Cook, unpublished observation).

Clinicians can develop their own simple tools to guide their visual gait analysis. Regardless of the type of form used, the process of gait analysis can be facilitated by videotaping the patient's gait. Though sometimes time consuming, in the long run videotaping provides the clinician more time to observe gait and therefore increases the reliability and validity of the observational gait analysis.

Replaying the tape, particularly with stop-frame and slow-motion features, allows repeated viewing of gait patterns without fatiguing a patient.

Systematically observing and documenting gait abnormalities is the first step toward understanding and hypothesizing possible causes for these deviations. Table 15-12 illustrates a diagnostic chart developed by Winter to serve as a framework for understanding possible causes of abnormalities observed during a visual gait analysis. The chart has three columns: the first is the observed abnormality; the second lists the possible causes of the abnormality; and the third describes the type of biomechanical or neuromuscular evidence that might be gathered to determine which of the possible causes is likely to be producing the observed abnormality. Thus, results of a visual gait analysis are tied to hypotheses regarding possible underlying causes and the types of diagnostic tests needed to confirm the cause. This information can be used by a clinician when determining appropriate interventions for retraining gait. The application of this concept can be found in Lab Activity 15-2.

Limitations to Visual Gait Analysis

Studies have shown that a major limitation of most observational gait analysis is poor reliability even among highly trained and experienced clinicians (Krebs et al., 1985). In addition, a detailed qualitative gait analysis is time consuming and often unrealistic in a busy clinical environment. Finally, there is no strong evidence to indicate that most ob-

TABLE 15-9. Gait Assessment Rating Scale

GENERAL CATEGORIES

1. Variability—a measure of inconsistency and arrhythmicity of stepping and of arm movements.
   0 = fluid and predictably paced limb movements
   1 = occasional interruptions (changes in velocity), approximately <25% of time
   2 = unpredictability of rhythm approximately 25–75% of time
   3 = random timing of limb movements

2. Guardedness—hesitancy, slowness, diminished propulsion and lack of commitment in stepping and arm swing
   0 = good forward momentum and lack of apprehension in propulsion
   1 = center of gravity of HAT projects only slightly in front of push-off, but still good arm–leg coordination
   2 = HAT held over anterior aspect of foot and some moderate loss of smooth reciprocation
   3 = HAT held over rear aspect of stance phase foot and great tentativity in stepping

3. Weaving—an irregular and wavering line of progression
   0 = straight line of progression on frontal viewing
   1 = a single deviation from straight (line of best fit) line of progression
   2 = two to three deviations from line of progression
   3 = four or more deviations from line of progression

4. Waddling—a broad-based gait characterized by excessive truncal crossing of the midline and side bending
   0 = narrow base of support and body held nearly vertically over feet
   1 = slight separation of medial aspects of feet and just perceptible lateral movement of head and trunk
   2 = 3 to 4 inches of separation between feet and obvious bending of trunk to side so that COG of head lies well over ipsilateral stance foot
   3 = extreme pendular deviations of head and trunk (head passes lateral to ipsilateral stance foot) and further widening of base of support

5. Staggering—sudden and unexpected lateral partial losses of balance
   0 = no losses of balance to side
   1 = a single lurch to side
   2 = two lurches to side
   3 = three or more lurches to side

LOWER EXTREMITY CATEGORIES

1. % Time in Swing—a loss in the percentage of the gait cycle constituted by the swing phase
   0 = approximately 3:2 ratio of duration of stance to swing phase
   1 = a 1:1 or slightly less ratio of stance to swing
   2 = markedly prolonged stance phase but with some obvious swing time remaining
   3 = barely perceptible portion of cycle spent in swing

2. Foot Contact—the degree to which heel strikes the ground before the forefoot
   0 = very obvious angle of impact of heel on ground
   1 = barely visible contact of heel before forefoot
   2 = entire foot lands flat on ground
   3 = anterior aspect of foot strikes ground before heel

3. Hip ROM—the degree of loss of hip range of motion seen during a gait cycle
   0 = obvious angulation of thigh backward during double support (10 degrees)
   1 = just barely visible angulation backwards from vertical
   2 = thigh in line with vertical projection from ground
   3 = thigh angled forward from vertical at maximum posterior excursion

4. Knee ROM—the degree of loss of knee range of motion seen during a gait cycle
   0 = knee moves from complete extension at heel strike (and late stance) to almost 90 degrees (70 degrees) during swing phase
   1 = slight bend in knee seen at heel-strike and late-stance and maximal flexion at midswing is closer to 45 degrees than 90 degrees
   2 = knee flexion at late stance more obvious than at heel strike; very little clearance seen for toe during swing
   3 = toe appears to touch ground during swing, knee flexion appears constant during stance, and knee angle during swing appears 45 degrees or less

TRUNK, HEAD, AND UPPER EXTREMITY CATEGORIES

1. Elbow Extension—a measure of the decrease of elbow range of motion
   0 = large peak-to-peak excursion of forearm (approximately 20 degrees), with distinct maximal flexion at end of anterior trajectory
   1 = 25% decrement of extension during maximal posterior excursion of upper extremity
   2 = almost no change in elbow angle
   3 = no apparent change in elbow angle (held in flexion)

2. Shoulder Extension—a measure of the decrease of shoulder range of motion
   0 = clearly seen movement of upper arm anterior (15 degrees) and posterior (20 degrees) to vertical axis of trunk
   1 = shoulder flexes slightly anterior to vertical axis
   2 = shoulder comes only to vertical axis, or slightly posterior to it during flexion
   3 = shoulder stays well behind vertical axis during entire excursion

3. Shoulder Abduction—a measure of pathological increase in shoulder range of motion laterally
   0 = shoulders held almost parallel to trunk
   1 = shoulders held 5–10 degrees to side
   2 = shoulders held 10–20 degrees to side
   3 = shoulders held greater than 20 degrees to side

4. Arm–Heel strike Synchrony—the extent to which the contralateral movements of an arm and leg are out of phase
   0 = good temporal conjunction of arm and contralateral leg at apex of shoulder and hip excursions all of the time
   1 = arm and leg slightly out of phase 25% of the time
   2 = arm and leg moderately out of phase 25–50% of time
   3 = little or no temporal coherence of arm and leg

5. Head Held Forward—a measure of the pathological forward projection of the head relative to the trunk
   0 = earlobe vertically aligned with shoulder tip
   1 = earlobe vertical projection falls 1 inch anterior to shoulder tip
   2 = earlobe vertical projection falls 2 inches anterior to shoulder tip
   3 = earlobe vertical projection falls 3 inches or more anterior to shoulder tip

6. Shoulders Held Elevated—the degree to which the scapular girdle is held higher than normal
   0 = tip of shoulder (acromion) markedly below level of chin 1 to 2 inches
   1 = tip of shoulder slightly below level of chin
   2 = tip of shoulder at level of chin
   3 = tip of shoulder above level of chin

7. Upper Trunk Flexed Forward—a measure of kyphotic involvement of the trunk
   0 = very gentle thoracic convexity, cervical spine flat, or almost flat
   1 = emerging cervical curve, more distant thoracic convexity
   2 = anterior concavity at midchest level apparent
   3 = anterior concavity at midchest level very obvious

HAT, head, arms, truck; COG, center of gravity; ROM, range of motion.
Reprinted with permission from Wolfsan L, Whipple R, Amerman P, Tobin JN. Gait assessment in the elderly: a gait abnormality rating scale and its relation to falls. J Gerontol 1990; 45:M12–M19.

servational gait analysis forms are sensitive to changes in gait patterns in response to therapy.

An alternative to observational gait analysis is the use of technological systems to quantify movement patterns, muscle activation patterns, and forces used in gait. However, this technology is beyond the reach of the average clinician. In addition to being extremely expensive, this equipment re-

quires considerable time and technical expertise to use.

Gait analysis is an integral part of almost every motor control evaluation in the patient with neurological dysfunction. Gait itself is complex, and understanding the complications of gait is even more difficult. Therefore, it is essential that a clinician have a systematic and consistent approach to observing and analyzing gait. Despite its lim-

LAB ACTIVITY 15-2

OBJECTIVE: To perform a visual gait analysis.

PROCEDURE: Get a partner. Choose one or more of the visual gait analysis forms presented in this chapter. Observe your partner walking at his or her comfortable gait speed, first from the sagittal plane, then from the frontal plane. You may wish to videotape several cycles of gait from both the sagittal plane and frontal plane. If you have access to a patient with an atypical gait pattern, you may wish to repeat this assignment with him or her.

ASSIGNMENT: Complete the gait analysis form you have chosen. If you use several forms, consider the ease of using each form. How long did it take you to complete a visual gait analysis? If you have analyzed an atypical gait pattern, refer to Table 15-12 and determine the possible causes of the gait abnormalities you observed. What further tests will you need to complete to determine which of the possible causes are present in your patient?

itations, an observational gait analysis form provides a framework for systematically observing gait and is therefore an essential part of the examination of gait.

Examination at the Impairment Level

A complete examination of mobility includes identifying underlying impairments that may be constraining mobility. The physical examination of underlying systems important to gait is often referred to as a static evaluation, since it evaluates factors such as strength, range of motion, and tone in passive situations, such as while the patient is sitting or lying down. In contrast, a dynamic evaluation examines these systems while the patient is performing functional movements, such as gait. Examination of underlying impairments was discussed in Chapter 6 and will not be repeated in this chapter.

Do Impairments Predict Gait Performance?

Static examination of factors such as strength, range of motion, and spasticity are important; however, they do not always predict gait performance in patients with neurological lesions. Nadeau et al. (1997) studied the relationship between plantarflexor strength and gait speed in subjects with hemiplegia. An instrumented dynamometer was used to evaluate muscular parameters (static torque, dynamic torque, power, and maximal rate of tension development) in ankle plantarflexors in the hemiparetic limb of patients who had had a stroke. Muscular parameters were compared to gait speed, performance on the Up and Go Test and Fugl Myer Assessment, and level of plantarflexor spasticity.

Results showed that subjects with hemiparesis were significantly weaker than controls. Dynamometric assessment showed that in subjects with hemiparesis, ankle plantarflexion torque was on average 50% that of normal controls. In addition, torque values for the subjects with hemiparesis declined more rapidly in the initial stages of movement than they did for controls. There was no relationship between dynamometric data and spasticity at the ankle (as measured passively while the patient was sitting), suggesting that plantarflexor strength was not associated with hyperactivity or spasticity at the ankle joint.

Comfortable gait speed in the hemiplegic subjects was 45 m/minute, or 76% of that of elderly controls. Maximal plantarflexor parameters as measured with a dynamometer were not significantly related to gait performance, suggesting that the strength of the plantarflexors was not the most important determinant of gait velocity in subjects with hemiplegia. Some patients with good plantarflexor strength walked at relatively slow gait speeds; in contrast, some patients with decreased plantarflexor strength could walk at relatively fast velocities (over 60 m/minute). These individuals produced the faster gait using alternative movement strategies, such as increased use of hip flexors for pull-off during swing as a substitute for decreased push-off in terminal stance (Nadeau et al., 1997).

While ankle strength may not predict gait performance, knee strength may. The Up-

TABLE 15-10   The Rivermead Visual Gait Assessment

Patient:_____

Scoring: 0 = normal   **Deviations:** 1 = mild   2 = moderate   3 = severe (please circle)

Upper Limb Position

1   Shoulder Depressed/Retracted/Elevated   0   1   2   3
2   Elbow flexed   ≤45 degrees (=0)   45 to 90 degrees (=1)   >90 degrees (=2)   0   1   2

Stance Phase   *For trunk deviations, 0 = midline*

3   Trunk flexed/extended   3   2   1   0   1   2   3
                                                                  ◄─────────────►
                                              Inclined: backward   forward

4   Trunk side flexed   3   2   1   0   1   2   3
                                                                  ◄─────────────►
                                              Direction: left   right

5   Trunk and pelvis: lateral displacement   3   2   1   0   1   2   3
                                                                  ◄─────────────►
                                              Amount: excessive   reduced

6   Contralateral drop pelvis   0   1   2   3
7   Hip extension decreased   0   1   2   3
8   *with backward rotation*   0   1   2   3
9A   Knee **flexion** excessive: *at initial contact*   0   1   2   3
10A   *throughout range*   0   1   2   3
                                           or
9B   Knee **extension** excessive: *at initial contact*   0   1   2   3
10B   *throughout range*   0   1   2   3
11A   Ankle in excessive **plantar**flexion   0   1   2   3
                                           or
11B   Ankle in excessive **dorsi**flexion   0   1   2   3
12   Inversion excessive   0   1   2   3
13   Plantarflexion decreased at toe-off   0   1   2   3

Swing Phase   *For trunk deviations, 0 = midline*

14   Trunk flexed   3   2   1   0   1   2   3
                                                                  ◄─────────────►
                                              Direction: backward   forward

15   Trunk side flexed   3   2   1   0   1   2   3
                                                                  ◄─────────────►
                                              Direction: left   right

16   Hike pelvis (elevation)   0   1   2   3
17   Backward rotation pelvis   0   1   2   3
18   Decreased hip flexion   0   1   2   3
19   Decreased knee flexion   0   1   2   3
20   Ankle in excess plantarflexion   0   1   2   3

Any other deviations noted..   0   1   2   3
                                 0   1   2   3

        Reference limb_____

            Walking aid_____

                AFO_____

        Total score_____/59   **Date**_____

Reprinted with permission from Lord FM, Wade DT, Robb GF, Bradshaw CM. The
Rivermead Mobility Index: a further development of the Rivermead Motor
Assessment. Int Disabil Studies 1991;13:54.

TABLE 15-11.   A Simple Guide for Visual Gait Analysis Based on The Essential Components of Gait Suggested by Carr and Shepherd (1998)

1 = present; 0 = partially present or absent

Stance Phase

	Behavior to Observe	Score
Pelvis	Lateral horizontal shift of the pelvis to the stance side	
Hip	Extension of the hip	
Knee	Flexion during loading	
	Extension mid stance	
	Flexion at push-off	
Ankle	Dorsiflexion at heel contact followed by plantarflexion	
	Dorsiflexion (shank moving over the stance foot)	
	Plantarflexion at push-off	

Swing Phase

	Behavior to Observe	Score
Pelvis	Drop in pelvis at toe off on swing side	
	Rotation of pelvis forward on swing side	
Hip	Flexion during swing	
Knee	Flexion during swing	
	Extension just prior to heel contact	
Ankle	Dorsiflexion	
	Total Score	

right Motor Control Test, described in Figure 15-1, examines hip, knee, and ankle flexion and extension strength in the standing position. Perry and colleagues found that a combination of gait velocity and knee extension control was highly predictive of mobility function in stroke patients. A combination of a strong grade of knee extension on the Upright Motor Control Test (Figure 15-1: single-limb stance of the affected leg, able to extend the knee from 30 degrees of flexion) and a gait velocity of 16 m/minute predicted community ambulation. A moderate or weak knee extension score would require at least 24 m/minute and 32 m/minute, respectively, to achieve community-level ambulation. In these patients the loss of knee control required the substitution of other mechanisms to achieve the required gait speed.

While strength may not always correlate with gait parameters, sensation appears to. In the study by Nadeau et al. (1997), the patients with the lowest sensory scores tended to be the slowest walkers, supporting the findings of Brandstater et al. (1983) that the quality of gait is poorest in patients with sensory deficit following stroke. This is also consistent with the finding of Perry et al. (1995) that proprioception was a strong predictor of independent mobility function following stroke and that of Lord et al. (1996a), who found that sensory impairments predicted gait performance in older adults.

Thus the relationship between impairment and gait parameters is complex and depends on many factors, including the type and extent of impairment, the functional level of the patient, and the capacity for compensation by other systems.

Measuring Mobility: Do We Really Need All These Tests and Measures?

As you can see, examination of mobility using a task-oriented approach is complex. It uses a range of tests and measures to quan-

TABLE 15-12. Winter's Framework for Understanding Atypical Gait Patterns

Observed Abnormality	Possible Causes	Biomechanical and Neuromuscular Diagnostic Evidence
Foot slap at heel contact	Below-normal dorsiflexor activity at heel contact	Below-normal tibialis anterior EMG or dorisflexor moment at heel contact
Forefoot or flat-foot initial contact	(a) Hyperactive plantarflexor activity in late swing	(a) Above-normal plantarflexor EMG in late swing
	(b) Structural limitation in ankle range	(b) Decreased dorsiflexion range of motion
	(c) Short step-length	(c) See (a), (b), (c) and (d) immediately below
Short step length	(a) Weak push-off prior to swing	(a) Below-normal plantarflexor moment or power generation (A2) or EMG during push-off
	(b) Weak hip flexors at toe-off and early swing	(b) Below-normal hip flexor moment or power (H3) or EMG during late push-off and early swing
	(c) Above-normal knee extensor activity during push-off	(c) Above-normal quadriceps EMG or knee extensor moment or power absorption (K3) in late stance
	(d) Excessive deceleration of leg in late swing	(d) Above-normal hamstring EMG or knee flexor moment or power absorption (K4) late in swing
Stiff-legged weight bearing	(a) Above-normal extensor activity at the ankle, knee, or hip early in stance	(a) Above-normal EMG activity or moments in hip extensors, knee extensors, or plantarflexors early in stance
Stance phase with flexed but rigid knee	(a) Above-normal extensor activity during weight acceptance at the ankle and hip with reduced knee extensor activity	(a) Above-normal EMG activity or moments in hip extensors and plantarflexors in early and middle stance
	(b) Excessive ankle dorsiflexion	(b) Hyperactivity of dorsiflexors or excessive dorsiflexion of ankle orthosis
Weak push-off accompanied by observable pull-off	(a) Weak plantarflexor activity at push-off Normal or above-normal hip flexor activity during late push-off and early swing	(a) Below-normal plantarflexor EMG, moment or power (A2) during push-off Normal or above normal hip flexor EMG or moment or power (H3) during late push-off and early swing
Hip hiking in swing with or without circumduction of lower limb	(a) Weak hip, knee, or ankle flexor activity during swing	(a) Below-normal tibialis anterior EMG or hip or knee flexors during swing
	(b) Overactive extensor synergy during swing	(b) Above-normal hip or knee extensor EMG or moment during swing
Trendelenburg gait	(a) Weak hip abductors	(a) Below-normal EMG in hip abductors: gluteus medius and minimus, tensor fasciae latae
	(b) Overactive hip adductors	(b) Above-normal EMG in hip adductors, adductor longus, magnus and brevis, and gracilis

Reprinted with permission from Winter DA. Knowledge base for diagnostic gait assessments. Med Prog Technol 1993;19:72.

tify functional status and predict level of disability, describe gait strategies, and document underlying impairments. In this time of health care reform, when the amount of time available to examine and treat a patient is shrinking rapidly, do we really need all of these measures? Is it necessary to measure functional mobility, perform a visual gait analysis, and examine underlying impairments? We argue that each provides essential information when establishing a plan of care for the patient.

For example, a static examination of underlying impairments determines the resources and constraints affecting gait and other aspects of mobility function. A dynamic evaluation using visual gait analysis can help a clinician determine the extent to which current strategies meet the requirements of gait in the face of underlying impairments. Functional measures, whether a single measure such as gait velocity or multiple measures available through mobility scales, document level of function and predict disability. These measures are important for justifying the need for therapy and serve as outcome measures, quantifying change over time and in response to intervention. Thus, a clinician can use information from all three levels of assessment to develop a comprehensive plan of care designed to maximize functional mobility status.

✐ TRANSITION TO TREATMENT

Setting Goals

As is true for goal setting related to other physical skills, clinicians need to establish both long- and short-term goals during mobility retraining that are objective, measurable, and meaningful.

Long-Term Goals

Long-term goals are often stated in terms of functional performance. They usually reflect ambulation outcomes with respect to level of independence. Examples of long-term goals: the patient will be able to walk independently a minimum of 1000 feet with the use

of a cane and orthosis; the patient will be able to walk independently with a quad cane, 50 feet while turning the head to the right and left with no change in gait speed and no evidence of imbalance; the patient will be able to achieve a safe, comfortable walking speed of 32 m/minute with the use of a cane and orthosis.

Short-Term Goals

Short-term goals for mobility retraining can be expressed in terms of the following:

1. Changing underlying impairments. One example is to decrease flexion contractures at the hip by 20 degrees, at the knee by 15 degrees, and at the ankle by 20 degrees.
2. Improving gait patterns. One example is to decrease forward trunk flexion by 20 degrees and thereby improve upright posture during the stance and swing phase of gait.
3. Accomplishing interim steps toward long-term goals. Examples include (*a*) to increase distance walked, with only standby assist, from 10 feet to 25 feet; (*b*) to increase speed—patient will be able to walk 200 feet, standby assist only, in 45 seconds; (*c*) to become independent in the use of a front-wheeled walker.

Short-term goals usually lead to treatment strategies aimed at resolving underlying impairments and improving the quality of gait strategies. Long-term goals often lead to treatment strategies related to improving the performance, such as increasing distance or speed. Often, the two are interrelated, as when the goal is to improve a particular aspect of the locomotor pattern to increase the velocity of gait. Finally, goals related to retraining mobility function can be defined in relation to the three requirements of gait.

Defining Goals Based on the Task Requirements of Gait

Progression

Treatment goals related to progression concern helping the patient develop the capacity to generate momentum to facilitate forward propulsion of the body. Specific examples include the following:

1. Improve the range and freedom of motion so that momentum can be transferred freely between body segments. This encompasses improving range of motion; decreasing contractures; reducing spasticity, which limits the velocity of motion; and reducing coactivation of muscles, which increases joint stiffness.
2. Increase the speed of walking, because generation of momentum requires a minimum speed of movement. This includes increasing the speed at which segments are moved. For example, increasing the speed and amplitude of hip flexion during the swing phase of gait advances the thigh segment quickly. This facilitates passive knee flexion for toe clearance and knee extension for foot placement. This goal requires facilitation of hip flexion in conjunction with knee extension, decreasing reliance on a flexor synergy pattern to accomplish the goals of swing.
3. Improve plantarflexor strength, since the plantarflexors generate the largest share of the forces necessary for forward propulsion.
4. Improve toe clearance during the swing phase of gait so that the swing leg is advanced without contacting the surface, since this decreases, or halts, forward momentum.

Stability
Treatment goals related to stability reflect the need for (*a*) good foot placement to facilitate weight bearing during initiation of stance, (*b*) sufficient extensor torque to support the body against gravity during single-limb stance, (*c*) facilitation of hip and trunk extensors to control the HAT segment, and (*d*) hip abductor strength and control to facilitate mediolateral stability. Thus, working toward postural support and stability during gait includes helping the patient to do the following:

1. Achieve a heel-first foot strike in the absence of coronal plane deviations. This position allows the body to move smoothly over the foot and to take advantage of the full weight-bearing surface of the foot, enhancing stability
2. Develop coordinated extension at the hip and knee to generate an extensor moment to support body weight during single-limb stance
3. Develop a vertical posture of the trunk with good hip and back extension to control the HAT segment and adequate activation of the abductors to control the pelvis
4. Facilitate extensor moments at the hip and knee while maintaining the capacity to dorsiflex the ankle, avoiding use of a total extensor synergy pattern during stance

Functional Adaptation
Treatment goals related to functional adaptation require the patient to modify movement and sensory strategies for locomotor control in response to changing task and environmental demands. Examples of functional adaptation goals include the following:

1. Integration of compensatory aspects of postural control into the ongoing gait cycle
2. Use of visual cues to identify upcoming disturbances to mobility and modify gait strategies to minimize their effect
3. The ability to change the speed and direction of gait safely, without loss of balance.
4. The ability to manage terrain changes, including curbs, ramps, steps, and uneven surfaces, safely and smoothly, with no loss of balance.

With comprehensive and realistic goals established, based on the patient's desires and problems, the clinician can move ahead to planning treatments designed to meet these goals.

⊘ TREATMENT OF GAIT

While most clinicians agree on the importance of retraining mobility function, including gait, there is no agreement on the best therapeutic approach. As a result, many approaches to retraining gait have been described. This chapter focuses on a task-oriented approach to retraining mobility function. In this book, task-oriented training is characterized by a range of therapeutic strategies that are organized around and specific to the task being retrained. For example, treatment of gait using a task-oriented approach is directed at: (*a*) minimizing or preventing specific impairments that constrain gait, (*b*) developing effective and efficient movement strategies that meet the essential requirements of gait, and (*c*) developing the ability to adapt gait strategies to changing task and environmental demands. Prior to discussing this approach in more detail, we consider some questions related to gait training in general.

The Question of Preambulation Skill Training

What is the role of preambulation skill training in recovery of gait? Some clinicians stress the importance of practicing preambulation skills as an essential part of retraining gait. Preambulation skills are activities that are considered precursors to ambulation and thus are preparatory to walking (Bobath, 1978; Davies, 1985; Voss et al., 1985; Schmitz, 1998).

Many of the preambulation gait training sequences are based on having the patient repeat activities that are part of a normal developmental sequence; extensive mat activities are often used prior to or in parallel with retraining gait (Schmitz, 1998; Charness, 1986). The sequence begins by having patients practice mobility and stability skills in prone and supine positions. This includes such activities as rolling, staying prone on elbows or hands, supine bridging, and practicing counterrotation trunk motions, that is, movements in which the shoulders rotate in

the opposite direction from the hips. As patients recover motor control in supine and prone positions, they begin to practice activities on all fours, then sitting, kneeling, half-kneeling, modified plantigrade position, and finally standing (Brunnstrom, 1970; Charness, 1986).

Do developmental skills learned through mat exercise transfer to gait? A growing number of researchers and clinicians question the requirement that patients regain mobility skills according to a developmental sequence (Forssberg, 1980; Mayston, 1992; Shumway-Cook, 1989; Carr and Shepherd, 1998). However, research examining this question is limited. Lord et al. (1998) compared the task-oriented and neurofacilitation approaches to retraining mobility function in 20 patients with multiple sclerosis. The neurofacilitation approach, as defined by Lord and colleagues, relied heavily on mat exercises and preambulation skill training. The task-oriented approach, as defined by these authors, focused on practicing goal-directed functional tasks, with no treatment aimed at underlying impairments. Results of this study showed that both approaches significantly improved all measures of mobility (10-m timed walk, RMI, stride length, RVGA, Berg Balance Test). In addition, they found no significant difference between the two approaches on any measure. In their discussion, the authors state that they were unsure whether the lack of significant difference in outcome measures between the two approaches suggested that they were equally effective or that despite the purported differences, the two treatment strategies used common interventions.

These authors raise an important point. In order to evaluate the effectiveness of an intervention or compare the relative effectiveness of two interventions, it is important to identify the essential components of each approach and to determine what elements the two approaches have in common and what elements are unique. Lord and colleagues explored the effectiveness of a task-oriented approach to retraining mobility. Their definition of a task-oriented approach differs markedly from the definition used in this text. Lord's definition of a task-oriented approach stressed the importance of practicing functional tasks while refraining from using interventions aimed at underlying impairments constraining function. In contrast, the task-oriented approach described in this book has at its focus the functional tasks being retrained but uses interventions aimed at underlying impairments constraining performance of the task, facilitating the development of effective and efficient task specific strategies and learning to adapt task performance to changes in environmental demands. Thus the term "task-oriented" is being used in different ways.

The Question of Whole Versus Part Practice

Should gait be practiced in its entirety or broken down into its component parts? A part practice approach to retraining gait involves breaking the gait cycle into component parts. These parts are practiced in isolation prior to assembling them into practice of the whole task. Techniques that require the patient to practice loading the hemiparetic leg during activities such as stepping up to a stool with the intact leg or stepping back and forth with the intact side are examples of part practice. They are done on the assumption that learning to load the leg under these conditions will transfer to improved control of the affected limb in stance during ongoing gait. In contrast to part practice, whole practice stresses practicing gait in its entirety, without working on individual component parts. In this approach to gait training, patients repeatedly practice walking with or without physical assistance and or assistive devices.

Treadmill and Partial Body Weight Support

The recent trend to retrain gait using a treadmill is an example of whole-task practice. In many instances the treadmill is combined with a supportive harness to provide partial body weight support (PWS), reducing the requirement for stability and en-

abling the patient to practice the entire gait pattern. As gait improves, support is decreased and the patient is required to control a greater and greater percentage of body weight (Finch et al., 1991; Waagfjord et al., 1990; Richards et al., 1993; Hesse et al., 1994, 1995). An example of a PWS harness system is shown in Figure 15-3.

Preliminary evidence comparing the harness treadmill approach to traditional physical therapy approaches in helping stroke patients learn to walk has found that use of the PWS systems helped patients achieve faster gait speed. However, the differences between the two groups disappeared after several months (Richards et al., 1993; Malouin et al., 1992; Harburn et al., 1993).

Hesse and colleagues have a group of studies comparing the effect of treadmill

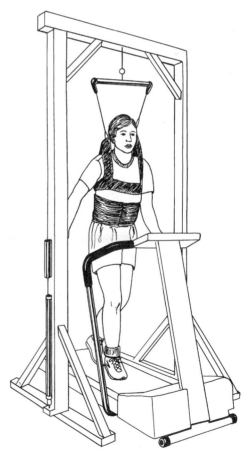

FIGURE 15-3. Gait retraining using a treadmill and harness system for partial support of body weight.

training with PWS to other forms of physical therapy (Hesse et al., 1994, 1995, 1999). In one study they compared treadmill training to neurofacilitation treatment in seven patients with hemiparesis following stroke. They used an applied behavioral analysis single case study with three weeks (15 sessions) of PWS treadmill training (A1), followed by three weeks (15 sessions) of neurofacilitation treatment (Bobath approach) (B), and finally three more weeks (15 sessions) of PWS treadmill training (A2). Treadmill training sessions lasted 30 minutes, PWS was progressively decreased from 70% to 0%, and gait was trained at velocities that ranged from initial speeds of 0.7 to 0.22 m/second to final speeds of 0.18 to 0.22 m/second. Manual assistance to advance and place the hemiparetic limb was provided as needed. Neurofacilitation training focused on preparation for walking using tone-inhibiting maneuvers, training of balance during sitting and standing, and practice on components of gait in isolation from the whole task. Gait significantly improved in all patients, with patients able to walk independently at the end of the study. Gait velocity, step and stride length, and cadence all significantly increased during the first treadmill training sessions (A1) but not during the neurofacilitation treatments (B). The authors conclude that practice of components of walking in isolation (the neurofacilitation approach) is not as effective as practicing the entire task of gait in the functional context of walking on a treadmill.

Hesse et al. (1999) have also compared gait characteristics in 18 patients with hemiparesis walking with PWS on a treadmill versus over ground. In general patients preferred a slower speed on the treadmill. Compared to over-ground walking, supported treadmill walking increased the single-stance period of the affected limb, decreased double-support time (the PWS enabled the patient to initiate swing with the unaffected leg earlier), and increased the symmetry of gait. During treadmill training there was a decrease in the premature activation of spastic plantarflexors during terminal swing, so patients were able to dorsiflex the ankle prior to initial

contact. Cocontraction of ankle antagonist muscles decreased, and a more appropriate phasic pattern of control emerged. Hip extension was significantly improved by the backward movement of the belt. The PWS system did have some disadvantages, however. The authors found a reduced level of activity in medial gastrocnemius and vastus lateralis when body weight was supported than with over-ground walking. Since these muscles are weak in hemiparesis, they advised that use of prolonged PWS should be avoided. Instead, PWS should be decreased as quickly as possible and patients allowed to bear maximal weight through the affected limb as soon as they are able to load the leg without collapse of the knee.

Richards et al. (1997) have begun exploring the use of PWS treadmill training with very young children who have cerebral palsy. Their preliminary work suggests that PWS treadmill training is feasible in children as young as 15 months and can be used in children who are not yet walking independently.

Thus there is growing evidence that supports the use of PWS support in conjunction with a treadmill as an effective and efficient form of gait retraining. This approach allows early task-specific training of gait in nonambulatory patients. Whether this approach results in significantly improved locomotor function in the long term remains to be determined.

The Question of Speed

What is the optimal walking speed at which to retrain gait? Several researchers have shown an association between walking speed and characteristics of gait. Olney et al. (1991, 1994) studied changes in gait associated with changes in gait speed in a group of patients with hemiparesis following stroke. Gait changes associated with increased walking velocity included greater hip extension at terminal stance and increased hip flexor moment at the initiation of swing. Wagenaar and Beek (1992) found that patients who have had a stroke, like healthy controls, modify gait characteristics (stride length and frequency) in response to changing gait velocities. Andriacchi et al. (1977) found that following a stroke, asymmetry in gait is highly dependent on walking speed: patients who walk faster tend to be less asymmetrical than those who walk slowly. This research suggests that one powerful way to improve gait is to increase the speed at which the patient is walking. This may seem counterintuitive to therapists who often work with patients at relatively slow walking speeds so as to improve the quality of the movement patterns used to achieve gait.

✑ TASK-ORIENTED APPROACH

This chapter discusses a task-oriented approach to retraining mobility function, with emphasis on gait retraining. As mentioned earlier, a task-oriented approach, as defined in this book, stresses therapeutic interventions that are specific to the task being trained. This includes treatments aimed at minimizing impairments, maximizing gait strategies that effectively and efficiently meet the requirements of gait, and accentuating the ability to adapt gait to changing task and environmental demands. While this approach does not use preambulation skill training, it does use both part and whole practice to retrain functional gait strategies. Finally, it lays considerable emphasis on practicing the skill of gait under varied task and environmental conditions.

Interventions at the Impairment Level

The goal of treatment aimed at the impairment level is to maximize the sensory-motor resources available for the performance of functional mobility skills. During retraining the task of walking, special emphasis is given to musculoskeletal impairments constraining the use of strategies that are effective in meeting the essential requirements of propulsion, postural control, and functional adaptation. For example, impairments that specifically impede the goal of propulsion include weakness of the ankle plantarflexors, which limits a forceful push-off in termi-

nal stance, and shortening of the hip flexors and/or ankle plantarflexors, which limits the ability to advance the body over the stance foot. Impairments that impede the goal of postural control include weakness of the ankle, knee, and hip extensors, limiting the generation of an extensor support moment, and weakness of the hip abductors, which impedes mediolateral stability.

Thus, therapeutic exercises that focus on strength and flexibility are used to correct or minimize impairments that can be changed and to prevent secondary impairments. Alleviating underlying impairments enables the patient to resume using previously developed strategies for gait. When permanent impairments make resumption of previously used strategies impossible, new strategies must be developed. In Chapter 6 we discussed treatment strategies aimed at resolving or preventing underlying musculoskeletal and neuromuscular impairments; this information will not be repeated in this chapter.

Does Changing Impairments Affect Functional Gait?

Though most clinicians use treatment strategies to remediate underlying impairments, the extent to which these types of improvements carry over to functional locomotion is still undetermined. For example, researchers have found that while therapeutic strategies were effective in significantly increasing hip flexion range of motion and improving trunk strength, improvements in these areas did not significantly improve gait speed (Godges et al., 1993). Judge et al. (1993) reported that gait measures did not change significantly in older adults following strengthening exercises. Krebs et al. (1998) examined the effect of moderate-intensity strength training on gait in 132 functionally limited elders. Following 6 months of progressive resistive exercises, strength improved by 17.6%. While gait velocity did not significantly change, mediolateral stability, as measured by mediolateral center of mass excursion and velocity, significantly improved. These authors suggest that previous studies showing no effect of strengthening exercise on gait have relied on time and distance measures and therefore inadvertently missed the most important contribution of strengthening exercises to gait: improvements in mediolateral stability (Krebs et al., 1998).

Damiano et al. (1998) examined the effect of a 6-week strengthening program on physical function in 11 children with cerebral palsy (6 with spastic diplegia, 5 with spastic hemiplegia). Results from this study showed that all children significantly improved strength in the targeted muscles. In addition, gait velocity improved as a result of increased cadence. An analysis of gait found no change in asymmetrical support times or joint motions as a result of increased strength.

Why does the research on the effects of strength training on gait velocity show conflicting results? Current research has shown that there is a nonlinear relationship between gait speed and strength in the lower extremity muscles (Buchner et al., 1996). This is shown in Figure 15-4*A*, which plots leg strength versus usual gait speed in a group of elderly subjects (Buchner et al., 1996). The regression curve plotting strength to speed is shown for the average age of 76 years and body weight of 71 kg. The hypothesized relationship between leg strength and gait speed is shown in Figure 15-4*B*. Since walking does not require maximum strength, normal walking speed can be maintained in the presence of a range of strength abilities (shown as a range of strength marked with an A in Fig. 15-4*B*). Thus, it is proposed that a patient who is already walking at this speed will not show further changes in gait in response to changes in strength. In contrast, the strength range marked by area B corresponds to the range where decrements in strength affect walking speed; thus, changes in strength will affect gait speed. Finally, the strength range marked as C illustrates the range of strength deficits in which walking is no longer permissible.

In summary, current research raises questions about the effect of retraining impairments on functional performance of gait,

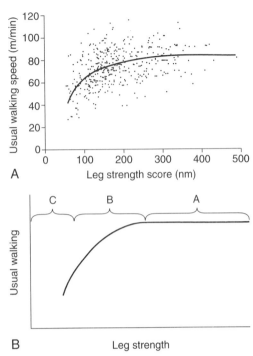

FIGURE 15-4. The relationship between strength and walking speed. **A.** A plot of leg strength scores versus usual gait speed in elderly subjects along with the regression curve plotting strength versus speed for the average age of 76 and body weight of 71kg. **B.** The hypothetical nonlinear relationship between gait speed and strength predicting the effect of changes in strength on gait speed. (Adapted with permission from Buchner DM, Larson EB, Wagner EH, et al. Evidence for a nonlinear relationship between leg strength and gait speed. Age Ageing 1996;25:387.)

suggesting that resolution of impairments **alone** may not be enough to ensure recovery of ambulation skills. In addition to treatments aimed at underlying impairments, interventions aimed at improving gait strategies and functional performance are required.

Intervention at the Strategy Level

The goal of retraining at the strategy level is to assist the patient in developing movement strategies that are effective and efficient in meeting the essential requirements of progression, postural support and stability, and functional adaptation. While much of gait retraining strives to assist patients in the recovery of previously used "normal" gait patterns, this may not be a realistic goal in the face of permanent sensory and motor impairments. Thus, a better standard for judging the efficacy of a patient's movement strategies, is to ask, "Are they meeting the demands of the task in the face of permanent impairments?"

The framework that follows presents therapeutic techniques used to achieve the specific requirements of gait. While techniques are organized around a single requirement, it should be recognized that many of the suggested therapeutic strategies are aimed at more than one requirement of gait. Therapeutic strategies are based on an understanding of normal and pathological gait and are drawn from our own efforts related to the application of a systems theory of motor control and motor learning as well as those of others (Carr and Shepherd, 1998) and from other sources, including the neurofacilitation approaches (Davies, 1985; Brunnstrom, 1970; Voss et al., 1985; Charness, 1986; Bobath and Bobath, 1984). It is important to remember that while these techniques are commonly used by clinicians to retrain gait, they have not necessarily been validated through controlled research studying patients with neurological impairments.

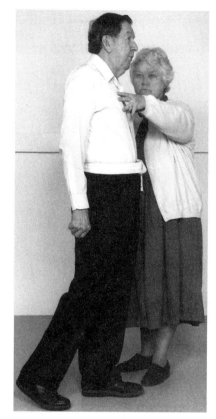

FIGURE 15-5.   Assisting a patient learning to maintain a vertical trunk posture during gait with manual cues.

Stability

Treatments aimed at improving stability include improving postural alignment of the HAT segment; effective generation of an extensor support moment in the stance limb; control of mediolateral stability, including placement of the foot at initial contact of stance; improving balance in single- and double-support phases of gait; and the use of assistive devices that broaden the base of support.

Control of the HAT Segment

Treatment of underlying impairments, such as weakness of the hip extensors and shortening of the hip flexors, will improve the capacity for vertical alignment of the HAT segment. During gait retraining, manual cues can be given to the patient at the shoulders (Fig. 15-5) or at the hips to facilitate a vertical posture and control of HAT

stability over the extended hips. Assistance can progress from light manual guidance to verbal cueing.

Often patients with poor balance look down while walking, bringing the neck and trunk into flexion. Verbal cues to look up in combination with a visual target at eye level can be used to facilitate extension of the neck and trunk and an upright position of the HAT segment. Finally, assistive devices such as long poles (Fig. 15-6) can be used to facilitate extension of the trunk and hips during walking.

Extensor Support Moment

Postural support requires the ability to load the stance limb without collapse. Treatment varies according to the underlying cause. When weakness of the hip and knee extensors is the cause, strengthening both concentrically and eccentrically is essential. Stretching of tight hip flexors and ankle

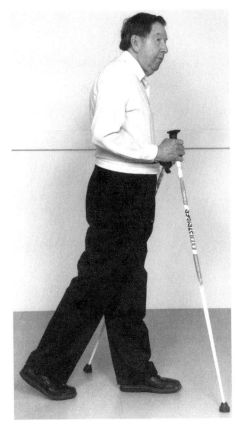

FIGURE 15-6.   During gait retraining, long poles can be used to facilitate extension of the HAT segment.

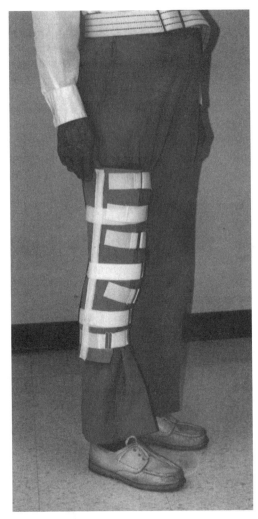

FIGURE 15-7.   External support with a knee brace for patients who do not have sufficient knee control to prevent collapse during loading.

plantarflexors, which limit the generation of extensor support, is indicated.

In patients who do not have sufficient knee control to prevent collapse during loading, the knee can be externally supported to prevent collapse, such as with a knee brace (Fig. 15-7). With the knee braced to prevent collapse, the patient can work on weight-bearing activities in stance and gait. For example, the patient can practice stepping with the unbraced leg, learning to advance the body over the stance foot, keeping the hip extended with the ankle dorsiflexed. Other activities that load the limb include stepping up onto a higher surface, such as a stool or taped newspapers (Fig. 15-8). The advantages of taped newspapers are that they are readily available and cheap and that the height can be varied according to the need of the patient. While the benefit of bracing the knee into extension is to facilitate weight bearing in the stance phase of gait, the benefit is lost during the swing phase, when the patient should flex the leg to advance the limb.

A common problem related to postural support involves hyperextension of the knee during loading at midstance. Treatment depends on whether the hyperextension is the primary impairment or compensatory to another problem elsewhere. If hyperextension is due to hyperactivity of the plantarflexors, an ankle–foot orthosis (AFO) with a plantarflexion stop can be used (Montgomery, 1987; Rosenthal et al., 1975). Alternatively, techniques to decrease muscle tone in the

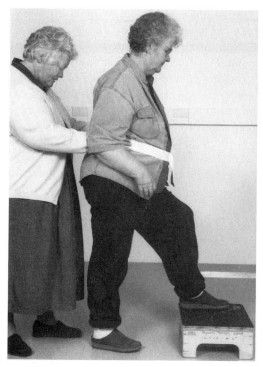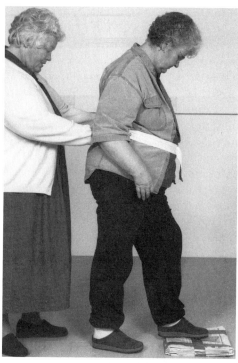

A   B

FIGURE 15-8.   Activities that increase weight bearing in a single-limb stance position include stepping up to a low stool (**A**) or to a taped stack of newspaper (**B**).

plantarflexors, such as having the patient practice weight bearing with the ankle dorsiflexed, lengthening the triceps surae, have been recommended (Montgomery, 1987; Carr and Shepherd, 1998).

When hyperextension of the knee is compensatory to weak quadriceps, strengthening exercises, electrical stimulation, and electromyographic (EMG) biofeedback have been recommended to facilitate activation of the quadriceps. Orthoses that block knee hyperextension have also been proposed to prevent hyperextension of the knee during gait.

In some patients with neurological dysfunction, problems related to support in midstance are due to excessive knee flexion rather than extension. When knee flexion results from weak quadriceps, functional electrical stimulation can be used to activate the quadriceps. Alternatively, or in combination, a positional feedback device such as an electric goniometer can be used to provide kinematic feedback. External devices can also be used to prevent knee flexion (Montgomery, 1987).

It has been recommended that patients practice generating an extensor support moment in other tasks, such as moving from sit to stand position or standing against a wall and flexing, then extending the knees and hips (Bobath and Bobath, 1975; Davies, 1985). Again, it is not known whether practicing an extensor support moment in a task other than gait will carry over to improvements in stability during the stance phase of gait.

Foot Placement at Initial Contact

Foot placement during initial contact and throughout the stance phase of gait is a major factor in determining stability; thus, improving movement and control of the ankle and foot at initial contact and during loading can significantly improve stability. Heel strike foot contact with a smooth transition to a stable foot-flat position facilitates **both** forward progression and a stable base of support important for stability. The treatment of problems impairing heel strike depends on the underlying cause.

Heel strike foot contact requires hip flexion in conjunction with knee extension and ankle dorsiflexion at terminal swing. Reducing musculoskeletal impairments that constrain a dorsiflexed position of the foot at initial contact is important. This includes stretching tight plantarflexors and hamstring muscles to allow knee extension and ankle dorsiflexion. The use of myofascial release techniques to reduce tightness in the intrinsic muscles and fascia of the foot can be helpful in preparing the foot to accept weight and in allowing motion at the foot as the shank moves forward over the stance foot.

When inadequate knee extension in late swing is the result of knee flexion contractures, manual stretching, casting, and splinting can be used to alter mechanical constraints. However, contractures simply recur if the underlying cause is chronic overactivity of the hamstring muscle during swing. Electrical stimulation of the quadriceps has been used reciprocally to inhibit an overactive hamstring muscle (Montgomery, 1987; Bogataj et al., 1989).

Inability to activate the tibialis anterior (TA) muscle is a common cause of impaired heel strike in the patient with neurological impairments. Strengthening exercises to increase force production of the TA are important in making sure the TA is capable of generating force in response to descending commands. Unfortunately, the capacity to generate force does not ensure that the muscle will be recruited automatically during gait. Nonetheless, strengthening is necessary to ensure that force generation capability is present.

Biofeedback and/or electrical stimulation of the TA in conjunction with a foot switch placed inside the patient's shoe has been used effectively to increase activation of the TA at heel strike (Basmajian et al., 1975; Takebe et al., 1975; Waters et al., 1975). Sensory stimulation of the TA, such as icing or tapping, during manually assisted step initiation has also been suggested as an approach to facilitate TA activation just prior to heel strike.

Use of an orthotic device that has motion at the ankle joint (hinge joint) but a posterior stop is an effective way to control foot drop in the patient who is unable to recruit the TA. The ankle joint motion of the orthotic device permits some dorsiflexion, allowing the tibia to advance over the supporting foot. Coronal-plane foot problems affecting foot strike can often be controlled with an AFO. A varus foot position during gait can be controlled with an AFO with a slight buildup of the lateral border of the foot. In addition, electrical stimulation of the toe extensors can reduce varus positioning during stance. A valgus foot position can be controlled with an AFO with a slight buildup of the medial border (Montgomery, 1987).

Manual cues to facilitate hip flexion, knee extension, and ankle dorsiflexion at terminal swing to ensure a heel-first foot strike pattern can be used; this is shown in Figure 15-9.

Improving foot placement by increasing step length can be assisted by making a grid on the floor, which helps to visually guide patients in establishing a better foot placement pattern. This is shown in Figure 15-10. Distance between horizontal stripes can be individualized to the patient's desired stride length (Jims, 1977).

Balance During Double- and Single-Limb Support

Postural stability (control of the center of mass in both the frontal and sagittal planes) is critical to functionally independent gait and emerges through the interaction of many sensory-motor systems. Therapeutic strategies focus on improving balance in single- and double-support phases of gait. Stability in the frontal plane is achieved through foot placement (step width) and depends to a large part on strength and coordination of the hip abductors (Patla, 1995). A common clinical practice used to help patients learn to improve control and movement of the center of mass involves having them practice voluntary lateral, anteroposterior, and diagonal movements of the center of mass in stance (Fig. 15-11). However, the degree to which practice of isolated weight

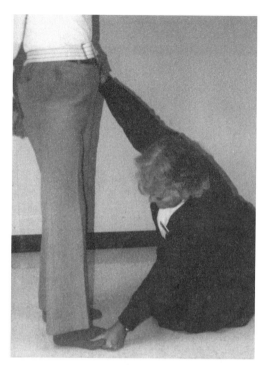

FIGURE 15-9. Helping the patient to accomplish a heel-first foot strike pattern. This position allows the body to move smoothly over the foot with good weight-bearing surface, enhancing both postural control and progression.

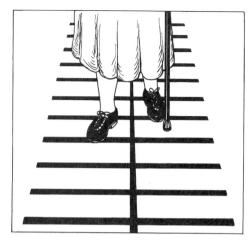

FIGURE 15-10. A floor grid that can visually guide patients toward better foot placement during gait. (Adapted with permission from Jims C. Foot placement pattern, an aid in gait training. Suggestions from the field. Phys Ther 1977;57:286.)

shift transfers to improved control of the center of mass in gait is unknown.

Use of Assistive Devices

Assistive devices contribute to postural stability by widening the base of support and providing additional support against gravity. A variety of assistive devices can be used to provide support, including walkers (standard and rolling), canes (quad, tripod and single point) and various types of crutches. A number of factors are to be considered when one is prescribing an assistive device for a patient with neurological impairments, including extent of physical disability, cognitive impairment, and the patient's personal motivations and desires (Schmitz, 1998).

Walkers provide the greatest degree of stability during ambulation, widening the base of support and improving both lateral and anterior stability. The variety of walkers includes straight walkers and rolling walkers with two or four casters. An advantage of rolling walkers is that they allow patients to maintain speed, facilitating the generation of momentum and thereby facilitating progression. However, the disadvantage of rolling walkers is that they have less stability than standard pickup walkers. Canes are usually held in the hand opposite the involved extremity, allowing a reciprocal gait pattern, with the opposite arm and involved leg moving together. Base of support can be further widened by choosing a cane with more points of contact with the floor, such as a small- or large-based quad cane.

A progression of assistive devices is often prescribed according to the amount of support required, such as walker, then quad or tripod cane, then single-point cane. Some treatment approaches discourage the use of assistive devices, particularly asymmetrical devices, such as canes, since it is believed that using such an aid encourages a patient to lean to the sound side to apply weight to the assistive device. This reinforces an asymmetrical gait pattern (Davies, 1985). To examine clinical assumptions regarding the amount of weight carried through various assistive devices, one study examined the effect of three types of walking aids (tripod cane, two high sticks, and a single-point cane) on gait in patients following stroke. This study found that the amount of support taken through an assistive device appears to be re-

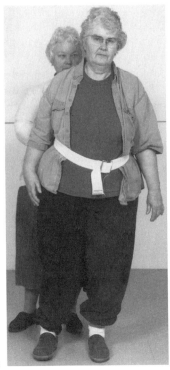 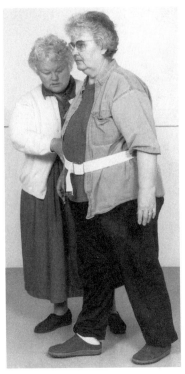

A   B

FIGURE 15-11.   To improve stability, patients practice controlled movement of the center of mass in lateral direction (**A**), in the anteroposterior direction (**B**), and in the diagonal direction (not shown).

lated to factors associated with severity of hemiplegia, such as ability to bear weight through the weak limb during stance, not features of the walking aid per se (Tyson, 1998).

It is important to consider the effects of using various assistive devices on factors other than gait skills, such as attentional resources. There appear to be attentional costs associated with using an assistive device. Attentional costs refer to the demand for attentional resources for information processing during the performance of a task. The attentional demands can vary depending on the type of assistive device used and the patient's familiarity with the device. One study examined the attentional demands associated with two types of walkers, a standard pickup walker and a rolling walker (Wright and Kemp, 1992). This study found that while both a rolling and a standard walker demand attention, a rolling walker is less demanding than a standard pickup walker.

Since there is some evidence that competing demands for attentional resources by postural and cognitive systems contribute to instability in the elderly (Shumway-Cook et al., 1997c), understanding the attentional requirements of the assistive devices we give patients is an important consideration during gait training. Further information describing types of assistive devices, procedures for measuring, and techniques for training gait with assistive devices on level surface, curbs, and steps may be found in detail in other sources (Schmitz, 1998).

Progression

Progression is affected by both the generation of energy through concentric contractions and the absorption of energy through eccentric contractions. Thus weakness limits the generation of forces necessary to progression, while impairments such as spasticity and muscle shortening may result in inefficient gait through excessive energy absorption.

Energy Generation

Much of the energy generated for gait comes from the gastrocnemius during push-off in terminal stance and secondarily through the hip flexors, which pull off during initial swing. Therefore, exercises to improve plantarflexor strength and reduce limitations in flexibility are critical, as are exercises to improve the strength of the hip flexors.

Patients can practice a forceful push-off (concentric contraction of the plantarflexors) while maintaining an extended leg posture: hip and knee extension coupled with plantarflexion of the ankle, as shown in Figure 15-12. This includes practicing lifting the

heel and moving the body weight anteriorly over the forefoot while the hip and knee are extended. Manual cues and assistance can be given by the clinician as needed to facilitate this component of gait.

To improve the ability of the hip flexors to participate in generation of power for progression, the patient can also practice pull-off (exaggerating hip flexion) during the initiation of swing. Manual cues and support of the leg can be provided by the therapist as needed. Other activities to facilitate hip flexion during swing include marching in place and practicing a high step gait, that is, bringing the knee up into an exaggerated flexed position (Fig. 15-13). Finally, as shown by Olney et al. (1991, 1994), increasing the speed of walking tends to increase the speed and amplitude of hip flexion during the initia-

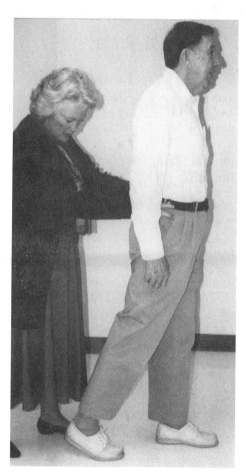

FIGURE 15-12. Patient practices a forceful push-off (concentric contraction) of the gastrocnemius in an extended leg posture.

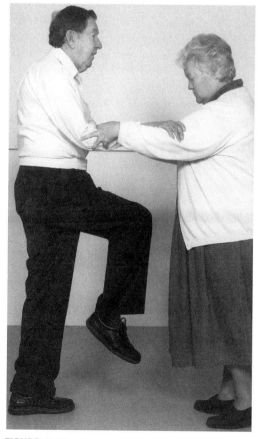

FIGURE 15-13. Improving use of the hip flexors to pull off the swing limb through practice of a high-steppage gait pattern.

tion of the swing phase of gait, and this facilitates passive knee flexion for toe clearance.

Treatments to reduce spasticity in the triceps surae improve forward movement of the shank over the foot. As discussed in the previous section, treatments to reduce the tone and tightness in intrinsic muscles of the foot ensure that the foot can roll off, lifting the heel and pushing onto the ball of the foot. Inability to advance the weight to the forefoot due to clawing of the toes can be treated with a shoe insert that spreads and extends the toes (Montgomery, 1987).

Advancement of the Swing Limb

To advance the swing limb, clearing the supporting surface with the foot, requires activation of the plantarflexors at push-off in conjunction with hip flexors at initiation of swing to draw the thigh segment forward with sufficient force to flex the knee passively. In addition, activation of the TA to dorsiflex the ankle is important to achieve foot clearance. Thus, loss of foot clearance can be caused by (*a*) weakness of the plantarflexors, hip flexors, or TA, (*b*) spasticity of the ankle plantarflexors and or hamstrings, or (*c*) neural control problems affecting the appropriate activation of muscles, such as the TA muscle, during swing.

Early in gait training, when the patient does not have sufficient control to advance the swing limb using hip and knee flexion, a towel can be placed under the patient's foot to facilitate advancement of the foot (Davies, 1985). This is shown in Figure 15-14. Alternatively, an elastic bandage (Fig. 15-15) can be used to prevent ankle plantarflexion, hence toe-drag, during the swing phase of gait (Davies, 1985).

Further suggestions to improve flexion of the swing limb were described earlier in this chapter.

Adaptation

The ability to adapt gait strategies to changes in task and environmental demands is the third essential requirement of gait. It is discussed in the following section, on treatment at the functional adaptation level.

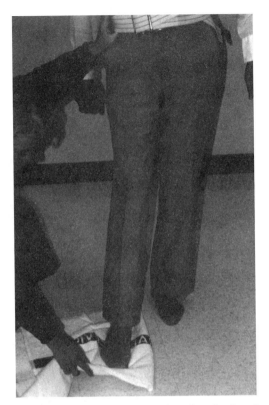

FIGURE 15-14.   Placing a towel under the hemiparetic leg to facilitate advancement of the swing limb without lateral trunk lean or hip hike.

Intervention for Functional Adaptation

The goal of retraining at this level focuses on helping patients develop the capacity to adapt gait to changing task and environmental contexts. As patients learn to develop strategies effective in meeting the task requirement of locomotion in relatively undemanding environments, such as on a level surface, training is broadened to include more complex and challenging conditions. So-called dynamic gait activities include walking at different speeds; on different surfaces, such as inclines, curbs, uneven surfaces, and carpeted surfaces; and in a variety of visual conditions, such as reduced lighting and in the presence of visual motion cues in the environment.

Collision avoidance is practiced in response to stationary and moving obstacles. This includes the ability to step over obstacles of various heights, such as those shown

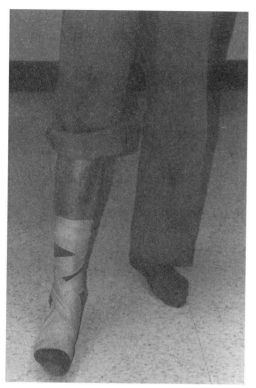

FIGURE 15-15.   Using an elastic bandage to maintain the ankle in dorsiflexion and to facilitate toe clearance.

No strategies to retrain compensatory responses to unexpected perturbations to gait have been identified. One possible approach might be to unexpectedly change the speed of a treadmill while the patient is walking. A harness system would be necessary to safely carry out perturbations to ongoing gait.

Finally, walking is practiced under conditions with varying attentional demands. This relatively new approach to retraining arises from the application of research examining the attentional demands of posture and gait in healthy people and those with neurological impairments. In order to vary attentional demands, a variety of secondary tasks (both cognitive and motor) are systematically introduced during the process of gait retraining (Shumway-Cook and Woollacott, 1997). The goals of this type of training are (*a*) to decrease the attentional demands of walking and (*b*) to improve the ability to allocate attentional resources effectively during the performance of multiple tasks, one of which is walking. Research comparing the effectiveness of dual- versus single-task gait retraining is under way in our lab.

in Figure 15-16*A*, and to step around obstacles (Figure 15-16*B*). Patients practice walking not just forward but sideways and backward, since many falls occur when individuals are required to step backward to get out of a closet or to avoid collision with a person who unexpectedly steps back while standing in line.

Dynamic gait activities also include the practice of walking under a variety of task conditions such as making abrupt stops, changing direction, and turning the head in the absence of steering changes. This is shown in Figure 15-17, in which a patient is practicing walking a straight path while turning the head from side to side to look for pictures posted at eye level on the walls. Patients also practice walking while interacting with an external physical load, such as carrying an object (Figure 15-18*A*) or opening a heavy door (15-18*B*). In this way patients learn to modify gait in **anticipation** of potentially destabilizing threats to balance during gait.

✌ RETRAINING STAIR WALKING AND OTHER MOBILITY SKILLS

Stair Walking

The patient with neurological impairments and decreased concentric control has primary problems climbing up stairs, while the patient with difficulty controlling eccentric forces has primary problems descending stairs. In addition, sensory impairments affect the patient's ability to clear the step during swing and place the foot appropriately for the next step. Published strategies for retraining stair walking have focused primarily on retraining patients who have had a stroke.

During stair ascent, the patient is taught to advance the uninvolved leg first. Manual assistance is given as needed to guide and control the involved leg (Bobath, 1978; Davies, 1985; Voss et al., 1985). This is shown in Figure 15-19. The clinician helps to con-

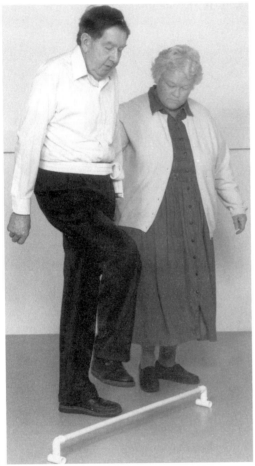
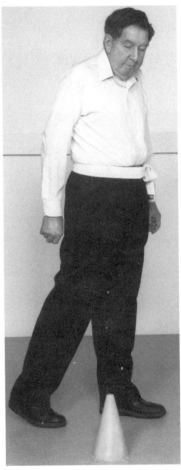

A   B

FIGURE 15-16.   Retraining dynamic gait skills. Practicing collision avoidance by stepping over (**A**) and around (**B**) obstacles.

trol the knee to prevent collapse during the single-limb stance phase and assists with knee and ankle flexion to ensure foot clearance in the swing leg (Fig. 15-20).

During stair descent, shown in Figure 15-21, the stroke patient is taught to advance the hemiplegic leg first. The therapist assists as needed with foot placement and knee control to prevent collapse of the leg when the uninvolved leg is advanced during swing.

Research has shown that certain stair features are critical in establishing effective movement strategies for stair walking. Thus, it is possible that accentuating stair features, such as the edge or height of the step, and drawing the patient's attention to these features, may enhance the patient's ability to develop effective stair-walking strategies.

Transfers and Bed Mobility

When retraining other types of mobility skills, such as transfers and bed mobility, it is important to remember that there is no single correct strategy for patients to learn. Research suggests that healthy young people perform such tasks as rising from a bed, standing up from the floor, or rolling, in many different ways. Variability characterizes the movement patterns used by neurologically intact individuals to perform everyday mobility skills. In fact, often the same exact strategy is never repeated. Instead, normal young adults seem to learn the rules for performing a task. This means that they learn what the essential or invariant requirements of a task are and develop a variety of strate-

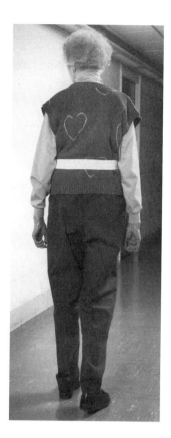

FIGURE 15-17. Retraining dynamic gait skills. Walking a straight path while practicing head turns.

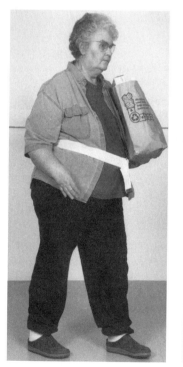
A

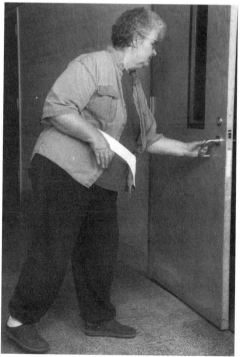
B

FIGURE 15-18.   Retraining dynamic gait skills. Practicing gait while interacting with external physical loads such as carrying an object (**A**) or opening a heavy door (**B**).

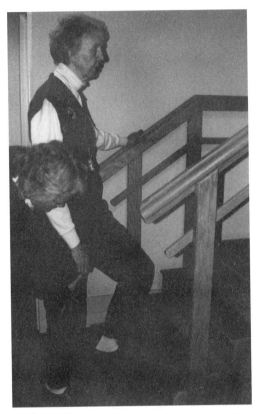

FIGURE 15-19.   Assisting stair walking, controlling the involved leg for single-limb stance in stair ascent.

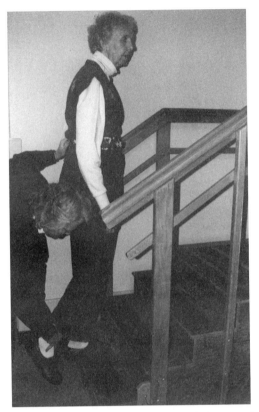

FIGURE 15-20.   Manual assistance with knee and ankle flexion to ensure foot clearance in the swing leg during stair ascent.

gies to accomplish these requirements. This suggests that the goal when retraining transfer skills in the patient with neurological disabilities is to help the patient develop sensory and motor strategies that are effective in meeting the task requirements despite persisting impairments.

Patients need to learn new rules for moving and sensing, given their impairments, rather than learning to use a "normal" pattern of movement. Research with neurologically intact subjects suggests that no single template for moving can be used to train patients. Instead, guided by the clinician, patients learn to explore the possibilities for performing a task. Patients learn the boundaries of what is possible, given the demands of the task and their constellation of impairments. Again, it is important to remember that the therapeutic strategies suggested in the following sections are attempts to apply a systems theory of motor control and current

research in motor learning to retraining mobility skills. These suggestions have not been validated through research. In addition, motor learning principles related to the acquisition of a learned skill are largely drawn from research with neurologically intact subjects. Research has not yet established the extent to which these principles can be applied to the patient with neurological dysfunction.

Sit to Stand

Remember from Chapter 12 that two basic strategies can be used separately or in combination to stand up: a momentum strategy and a force control strategy. A patient should be allowed to explore the possibilities for using momentum when performing a transfer task, since this strategy is most efficient and requires the least amount of muscular activity. Essential elements of teaching a momentum strategy include encouraging the pa-

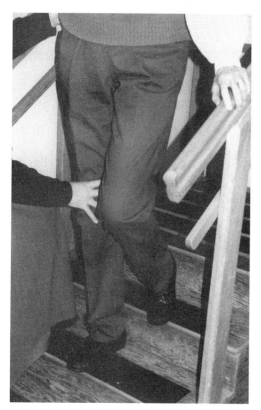

FIGURE 15-21.   Manually assisting control of the knee during stair descent.

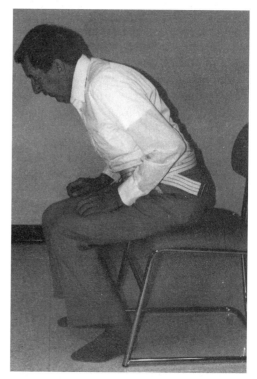

FIGURE 15-22.   Teaching a force control strategy for sit to stand entails asking the patient to move forward to the edge of the chair, incline trunk forward until the nose is over the toes, and then stand up.

tient to move quickly but safely and avoiding breaks in the motion. The clinician can verbally instruct the patient to move quickly, with no stops. An appropriate prompt might be, "Now try standing up again, but this time I want you to move quickly, with no stops." Manual cues can be used at the shoulders to set the pace. Patients who have trouble generating force quickly with the trunk can try swinging their arms freely while standing up, to increase momentum generated in upper body segments.

When teaching a momentum strategy, clinicians should be aware of the stringent stability requirements of this strategy and adequately safeguard a patient with poor postural control to prevent a fall. The risk of a backward fall is greatest at the beginning of the movement if the patient tries to transfer momentum from the trunk to the legs for a vertical lift before the center of mass is sufficiently forward over the feet. This is charac-

teristic of sit to stand in many hemiparetic patients. In contrast, the risk of a forward fall is greatest at the end of the movement in patients who are unable to control horizontal forces affecting the center of mass. When this occurs, the center of mass continues to accelerate forward of the base of support of the feet after the patient reaches a vertical position, resulting in a fall forward. This is characteristic of sit to stand in many patients with cerebellar pathology who have difficulty scaling forces for movement.

In contrast to the momentum strategy, a force control strategy is characterized by frequent stops. With force control strategy, the patient is taught to bring the buttocks forward to the edge of the chair. The trunk is brought forward, bringing the nose over the toes. This is shown in Figure 15-22. This brings the center of mass over the base of support of the feet. The patient is then cued to stand up. The patient can be encouraged to bring the arms forward, with or without a support, to assist in bringing the trunk mass forward; this is shown in Figure 15-23. Patients with weakness making it difficult to stand up from a normal-height chair can begin learning sit to stand from a raised chair, reducing the strength requirement for lifting the body (Fig. 15-24). As the patient improves, seat height can be lowered.

In patients with asymmetrical force production problems, facilitating symmetry is important when possible, since symmetrical weight bearing enhances both progression and stability during the task. A symmetrical weight-bearing posture is possible only for patients who can generate sufficient force to control the knee and prevent collapse of the body when the impaired limb is loaded. When this is not the case, the clinician must manually control the knee for the patient, for example as illustrated in Figure 15-25. It is important that manual assist of knee control not block forward motion of the knee as the patient stands up.

In patients with unilateral motor control problems such as hemiplegia, sensory stimulation techniques have been suggested as an approach to assisting the patient in learning

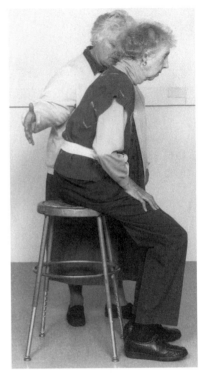

FIGURE 15-24.   Teaching sit to stand from a raised chair reduces the strength requirement for lifting the body and allows the weak patient to accomplish the task.

symmetrical weight bearing. Ideas include (*a*) pressure downward applied at the knee to increase the weight-bearing sensation of the foot in contact with the support surface (see Fig. 15-25), (*b*) lifting the patient's foot and rubbing the heel on the ground (Fig 15-26), (*c*) lightly pounding the heel on the ground, or (*d*) using pressure on the dorsum of the foot during the sit-to-stand movement.

It is often easier for a patient to learn to sit down than to stand up because eccentric force control is often gained prior to concentric force control (Carr and Shepherd, 1998; Duncan and Badke, 1987). When teaching patients to sit down, the therapist asks the patient to practice flexing the knees in preparation for sitting. This requires eccentric contraction of the quadriceps to control premature collapse of the knee.

The same principles for retraining sit to stand apply to retraining other types of transfers. For example, when learning to transfer

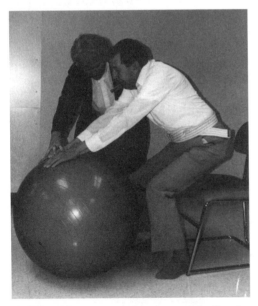

FIGURE 15-23.   Encouraging forward inclination of the trunk during sit to stand by bringing the arms forward.

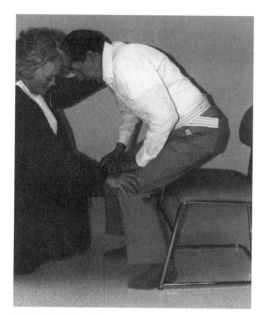

FIGURE 15-25. Manually controlling the knee when assisting a patient who is moving from sit to stand position.

from a chair to a chair (or bed, or mat), a patient can learn a standing pivot transfer, which is more consistent with a force control strategy, or a squat–pivot transfer, which is more consistent with a momentum strategy. In the standing pivot transfer, the patient moves from the seated position to a vertical stance position, then pivots around and sits down. Momentum is lost each time the patient stops to change position. In contrast, in a squat–pivot transfer, the patient positions the wheelchair at an angle to the bed or chair, moves to the edge of the chair, and in one motion moves the buttocks from one surface to another, keeping the hips, knees, and ankles flexed. This requires good eccentric control of the quadriceps and hip extensors.

It is often surprising to see the number of patients who find it easier to perform a squat–pivot transfer than a standing pivot transfer (often the preferred strategy taught in therapy). For example, a 24-year-old trau-

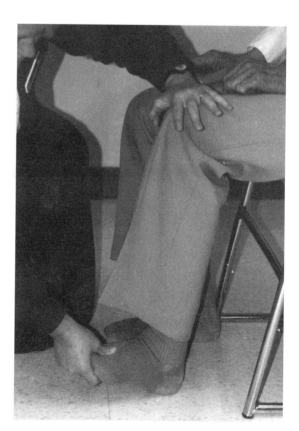

FIGURE 15-26. Facilitating weight bearing through the hemiplegic leg by providing downward pressure to the knee and lifting the patient's foot and rubbing the heel on the ground.

matic brain injury patient with cerebellar ataxia was being taught to transfer so that she could go home on leave from the rehabilitation center. She was being taught a standing pivot transfer and was unable to perform this independently because of instability on rising to a vertical position. As a result, she required moderate assistance to transfer safely. Since she had fairly good eccentric control of the knees but poor balance, it was decided to let her try experimenting with a momentum-driven squat–pivot transfer. To her surprise and ours, she learned to transfer from the bed to her wheelchair independently in one therapy session.

Bed Mobility Skills

Retraining bed mobility skills includes such tasks as changing position while in bed (for example, rolling from the supine position to side lying or prone), and getting out of bed, either to a chair or standing up. As noted earlier, researchers have found that normal young adults use a variety of momentum-related strategies when performing bed mobility skills. In contrast, force control movement strategies, characterized by frequent starts and stops, are frequently used by patients with neurological impairments.

Rolling

The most common approach to rolling in normal young adults involves reaching and lifting with the upper extremity, flexing the head and upper trunk, and lifting the leg to roll onto the side, then over to prone. However, there are many variations to this pattern. Most healthy young adults do not show rotation between the shoulders and pelvis, assumed by many clinicians to be an invariant feature of rolling.

There are at least two ways to teach a patient to roll over. The first relies mainly on the generation of momentum to propel the body from supine to prone. Motion is initiated with flexion of the head and trunk. At the same time, the patient reaches over the body with the upper extremity. In addition, to assist with the generation of momentum, the leg is lifted and rotated over the opposite leg to roll the body to side lying and on to prone.

An alternative to a momentum-based strategy is a force control (or combination) strategy. In this approach, the patient is taught to lift one leg and place the foot flat on the bed. Pressure downward by the leg propels the body to side lying and on to prone. Flexion of the head and trunk and reaching movements of the arms can assist in generating force to roll over (Davies, 1985, Voss et al., 1985; Carr and Shepherd, 1998).

Rising From a Bed

Research examining movement patterns used by normal adults to get out of bed suggests great variability in how this is accomplished. Still, momentum-based strategies are most often used. For example, the movement begins as the person pushes the trunk into flexion with the arms or grasps the side of the bed and pulls and pushes into flexion and immediately into a partial sitting position with the weight on one side of the buttocks. Without stopping, the person continues to roll off the bed into a standing position. This strategy has stringent stability requirements, but because there are no breaks in the movement, uses momentum to move the body efficiently. As noted in Chapter 14, there are many reasons this strategy is not appropriate for a patient with neurological dysfunction.

An alternative strategy involves teaching a patient to roll to side lying (with or without use of a bed rail when available) (Fig. 15-27A), then to push up to a sitting position (Fig. 15-27B). After the patient is stable in a symmetrical sitting position with the feet flat on the floor, he or she is taught to stand up (Fig. 15-27C) (Davies, 1985, Voss et al., 1985).

The Importance of Varying Task and Environmental Demands

Just as in gait, patients must learn to perform functional tasks, such as sit to stand and transfers, under varying task and environmental demands. To assist in the process of

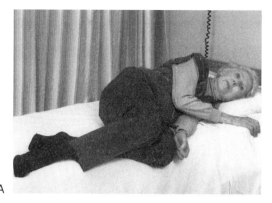

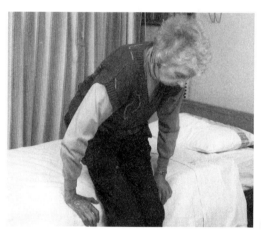

FIGURE 15-27. Learning to rise from a bed using a force control strategy breaks the movement into three stages: rolling to a side-lying position (**A**), then to a sitting position (**B**), and finally from sit to stand (**C**).

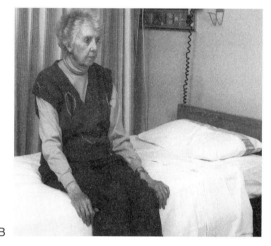

A

B

C

exploring movement strategies that are effective in meeting changing task and environmental demands, conditions of training are varied. For example, as shown in Figure 15-28, during the process of learning to move from sit-to-stand position, the patient may practice standing up from a wheelchair (Fig. 15-28*A*), from the bed (Fig. 15-28*B*), from a chair without arms (Fig. 15-28*C*), and from a low soft chair (Fig. 15-28*D*). In addition, patients may learn to embed sit to stand in a variety of other tasks, such as stand up and stop, stand up and walk, or stand up and lean over. This type of variability encourages the patient to modify strategies used to stand up in response to changes in task and the demands of the environment.

Often, as therapists, we are quick to guide patients toward the use of strategies that we know will be effective in meeting the demands of the task. Patients rarely have the time to experiment with a variety of solutions that are effective in meeting task demands. This concept of trial and error exploration in the learning of strategies that are effective in meeting task goals has a number of important implications for clinicians. Initial performance may be quite poor as patients learn to explore and to find their own solutions. Patients may not progress as fast as if they were taught a single solution to the task. If we value the importance of multiple solutions to task demands, short- and long-term therapy goals may have to be rewritten to reflect this. For example, the patient will demonstrate the ability to adapt motor responses by performing the sit-to-stand task in three ways.

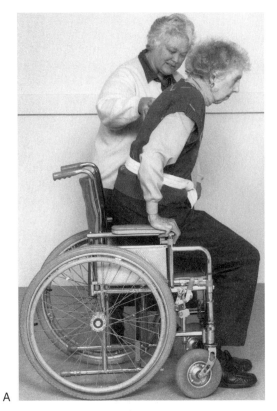

A

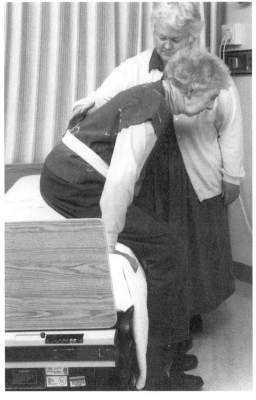

B

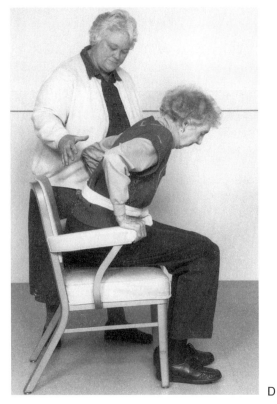

C

D

ⓔ SUMMARY

1. The key to recovery of mobility skills following neurological injury is learning to meet the task requirements of progression, stability, and adaptability despite persisting sensory, motor, and cognitive impairments. Research examining mobility strategies in neurologically intact subjects suggests that there is no one right strategy that can or should be used to meet these requirements.

2. Retraining the patient with impaired mobility skills begins with an examination of (*a*) functional mobility skills, (*b*) strategies used to accomplish stance and swing requirements of gait, and (*c*) underlying sensory, motor, and cognitive impairments that constrain the performance of functional mobility skills.

3. Visual gait analysis is the most commonly used clinical tool to aid therapists in systematically analyzing a patient's gait strategies.

4. A task-oriented approach to treatment, as defined in this book, focuses on helping patients to resolve specific impairments constraining the task, to develop strategies effective in meeting essential task requirements, and to learn how to adapt and modify these strategies so performance can be sustained in a wide variety of settings.

5. There are many approaches to retraining the patient with impaired mobility skills, particularly gait. Some approaches stress the importance of following a strict developmental sequence. This involves learning mobility and stability in developmental postures, such as all fours and upright kneel, prior to working on ambulation itself.

6. At the other end of the retraining spectrum are gait retraining approaches that focus solely on retraining the task of locomotion, with no emphasis on training possibly unrelated skills. Often, therapy is started with task-oriented gait training before the patient can sustain weight. Patients are supported by harnesses, and treadmills are used to facilitate walking.

7. Other approaches, such as the one presented in this chapter, stress a balance between therapeutic strategies focused on resolving impairments, retraining movement strategies for gait, and having the patient practice walking under various task and environmental conditions.

8. More research is needed to determine the comparative effectiveness of these approaches in retraining mobility skills in various types of patients with neurological impairments.

FIGURE 15-28.   Varying the environmental conditions while learning the task sit to stand. Practice conditions involve standing up from a wheelchair (**A**), from the bed (**B**), from a chair without arms (**C**), and from a low, soft chair (**D**).

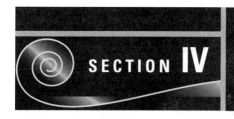

SECTION **IV**

Reach, Grasp, and Manipulation

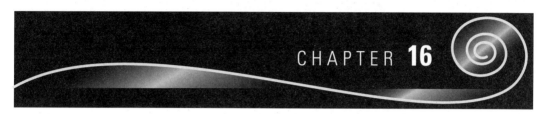

CHAPTER **16**

Normal Reach, Grasp, and Manipulation

⊘ INTRODUCTION

How important is upper extremity function to successfully moving through the activities of our day? Take a moment to scan the activities you completed within the first hour after waking up this morning. They probably included brushing your teeth, combing your

hair, buttoning your clothes as you dressed, and using your spoon as you stirred your coffee or ate your breakfast. In reviewing the typical activities of the day, it becomes apparent that upper extremity function is the basis for the fine motor skills important to activities such as feeding, dressing, and grooming.

In addition, though we may not be as consciously aware of it, upper extremity function plays an important role in gross motor skills such as crawling, walking, and the ability to recover balance and protect the body from injury when balance recovery is not possible.

Because of this interweaving of upper extremity control with both fine and gross motor skills, recovery of upper extremity function is an important aspect of retraining motor control and thus falls within the purview of most areas of rehabilitation, including both occupational and physical therapy.

In upper extremity control, as in balance and gait, three factors contribute to sensory-motor processing: (*a*) the constraints of the individual, including age, experience with the task, and presence or absence of pathology; (*b*) the type of task, for example, to point at an object, to grasp and manipulate an object, or to grasp and throw an object; and (*c*) the specific environmental constraints, including the properties of the objects to be grasped.

How does the nervous system accomplish the complex process of upper extremity control? Before we can answer this question, we need to understand the basic requirements of reaching, grasping, and manipulation. This will provide a framework for discussing normal control and the effect of neurological pathology on functional grasp and manipulatory skills. In addition, it will provide the structure for clinical management of upper extremity dysfunction in the patient with neurological impairments.

We suggest that the following components be considered key elements of upper extremity reach, grasp, and manipulation skills: (*a*) locating a target, also called visual regard, which requires the coordination of eye–head movements; (*b*) reaching, involving transportation of the arm and hand in space as well as postural support; (*c*) grasp, including grip formation, grasp, and release, and (*d*) hand manipulation skills.

As we mentioned in earlier chapters, the systems theory of motor control predicts that specific neural and musculoskeletal subsystems contribute to the control of the components of reaching, grasping, and manipulation. Musculoskeletal components include such things as joint range of motion, spinal flexibility, muscle properties, and biomechanical relationships among linked body segments. Neural components encompass (*a*) motor processes, including the coordination of the eye, head, trunk, and arm movements and coordination of both the transport and grasp phases of the reach; (*b*) sensory processes, including the coordination of visual, vestibular, and somatosensory systems; (*c*) internal representations important for the mapping of sensation to action; and (*d*) higher-level processes essential for adaptive and anticipatory aspects of manipulatory functions.

We begin our discussion of components of reach, grasp, and manipulation with visual regard, describing the manner in which the eyes and head are coupled during target location. We then discuss the components of reach and grasp, describing the role of the motor and sensory systems and higher-level adaptive abilities. Finally, we review some of the theories of the control of reaching movements.

ℯ LOCATING A TARGET

Eye–Head–Trunk Coordination

In order to reach for an object successfully, we must first locate the object in space. Normally, vision is used for object location. This typically involves movement of the eyes alone if the target is in our central visual field or of the eyes and head when the target is in the periphery.

How are reaching movements of the arm coordinated with the movements of the eye and head? Do we first move our eyes to a target, then our head, and finally our hand? Kinematic studies have shown that when an object to be grasped appears in the peripheral visual field, the following sequence of movements is normal. The eye movement onset has the shortest latency, so it begins first, even before the head. The eyes reach the target first because they move very quickly, so they focus on the target before the head stops moving (Jeannerod, 1990). However, electromyographic (EMG) studies have shown that activation of neck muscles usually occurs 20 to 40 msec prior to activation of the muscles controlling eye movements. However, because the eyes have less inertia than the head, the eyes move first, even though the neural signal occurs first in the neck muscles.

When head movement is necessary to look at an object, the amplitude of head movement is usually only about 60% to 75% of the distance to the target (Gresty, 1974; Biguer et al., 1984). However, when arm movements requiring great accuracy are performed, this behavior may be modified. It has been shown that people trained to throw with great accuracy make combined eye–head movements that go most of the distance to the target (Roll et al., 1986).

Some tasks require eye movements alone, while others require a combination of eye–head movement, and still other tasks require a combination of eye–head–trunk movements. Because of this variability, researchers have argued that eye–head coordination is not controlled by a unitary mechanism but rather emerges from an interaction of several neural mechanisms. These may include one neural mechanism that subserves the ability to locate objects in the near periphery, requiring primarily eye movements, with little head motion; a second mechanism to locate objects in the further periphery, controlling combined eye–head movements; and a third mechanism to locate objects in the far periphery, controlling the movements of eye–head and trunk together (Jeannerod, 1990).

What is the functional significance of this information to understanding and retraining a patient who has problems with functional grasp? Part of the patient's problems may relate to the coordination of eye–head movements needed for visual regard. Thus, when retraining, the clinician may focus on training the different control systems separately. For example, the clinician may begin by retraining eye movements to targets located within the central visual field, then

progress to retraining eye–head movements to targets located in the peripheral visual field. Finally, movements involving eye, head, and trunk motions can be practiced as patients learn to locate targets oriented in the far periphery.

Control of Eye Movements
Visual Pathways Related to Eye Movements

When we move our eyes to locate a stationary target we want to grasp, that object excites successive locations on the retina during the movement. In spite of this continual shift in input across the retina, we perceive a stable visual environment. How does the brain do this? Research has shown that neurons in the parietal cortex use information about the intended eye movement to update the brain's representation of visual space. The neurons anticipate the retinal consequences of the intended eye movement and shift the cortical representation first. Then the eye catches up.

These neurons thus send a corollary discharge of the output to the eye muscles to other areas of the brain, allowing the visual world to be remapped with each eye movement into the coordinates of the current gaze location. Goldberg and colleagues (Duhamel et al., 1992a,b) showed that these corollary discharge visual cells in the lateral intraparietal area start to increase their firing rate about 80 msec before a saccade occurs.

How are eye movements coordinated with arm movements? Fujii et al. (1998) found an area of premotor cortex that has neurons driving both saccadic eye movements and arm and neck movements. They noted that neurons in the ventral part of the premotor cortex evoked saccades when stimulated. This region was surrounded by neurons that activated muscles of the arms, shoulders, neck, and face; this led to the hypothesis that this area is involved in coordinating eye movements with movements of other body parts, including the eye–arm coordination necessary when reaching for targets.

Interactions Between Eye Movements and Hand Movements

There is evidence that eye and hand movements interact with and influence each other. For example, when accompanied by eye movement, hand movements are more accurate. In addition, during smooth-pursuit eye movements, there is an increase in gain if the hand is also following the target (Gauthier et al., 1988). Vercher et al. (1996) found that even in deafferented subjects, there was an increase in gain and reduction in latency for smooth pursuit when the hand was used to follow the target. Thus, they suggest it is the efference copy or corollary discharge about limb movement that helps the smooth-pursuit system rather than proprioceptive feedback from the hand movement.

Other research has shown that proprioceptive signals from the eye muscles do contribute to our ability to localize targets in extrapersonal space. Gauthier et al. (1990) performed an experiment in which they perturbed the movement of one eye so that it was deviated 30 degrees to the left while the subject was asked to point at a target located straight ahead. They found that the subjects mislocalized the targets to the left by 3 to 4 degrees.

❷ BEHAVIORAL CHARACTERISTICS (KINEMATICS) OF REACH AND GRASP

It is interesting to note that the control of arm movements changes depending on the goal of the task. For example, when the arm is used to point to an object, all segments of the arm are controlled as a unit. But when the arm is used to reach for and grasp an object, the hand appears to be controlled independently of the other arm segments, with the arm carrying out movements related to transport and the hand carrying out movements related to grasping the object. In this case, reaching for an object can be divided into two subcomponents, reach and grasp, which appear to be controlled by separate areas of the brain.

In the following section we first examine the kinematic characteristics of reaching movements and the way kinematics change with the task and the environment. We then discuss the contributions of specific neural and musculoskeletal subsystems to the control of both reach and grasp.

Studies have been performed to clarify the way reach and grasp movements are affected by both task and environment. As you will see, this research suggests that the ability to adapt how we reach is a critical part of upper extremity function, since reaching movements vary according to the goals and constraints of the task.

Researchers have shown that the velocity profiles and movement durations of a reach vary, depending on the goal of the task. If the subject was asked to grasp the object, the movement duration of the reach was much longer than if the subject pointed and hit the target. Also, when preparing to grasp an object, the acceleration phase of the reaching movement was much shorter than the deceleration phase, but if the subject was asked to hit the target with the index finger, the acceleration phase was longer than the deceleration phase, with the subject hitting the target at a relatively high velocity (Marteniuk et al., 1987). This is shown in Figure 16-1, which shows the different velocity profiles of the arm over time for grasping versus pointing movements.

In addition, if the subject grasped the target, then either fit it in a small box or threw it, movement times and velocity profiles were also different. Movement times were shorter for grasp and throw than for grasp and fit. In addition, the acceleration phase of the movement was longer for grasp and throw than for grasp and fit. Clearly, the task constraints and goals affect the reaching phase of the movement. This finding has implications for the clinician engaged in retraining the patient with problems related to reach and grasp. Since movements used during reaching for an object vary with the nature of the task, reaching movements for a variety of tasks must be practiced. For example, these tasks may include practicing reach during

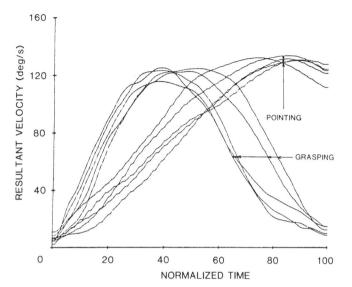

FIGURE 16-1. Velocity of the arm versus time (a velocity profile) for a number of individual trials of both pointing and grasping movements. In the grasp, the acceleration phase is shorter than the deceleration phase, while in the point, the reverse is true. (Reprinted with permission from Jeannerod M. The neural and behavioral organization of goal-directed movements, Oxford: Clarendon Press, 1990:19.)

reach and point; reach and grasp; reach, grasp, and throw; or reach, grasp, and manipulate.

⊘ SYSTEMS CONTRIBUTING TO REACH AND GRASP

Sensory Systems

What is the role of sensory information in controlling reach? You may recall that in Chapter 3, to clarify the function of the different levels of the nervous system, we took a specific upper extremity function task and walked through the pathways of the nervous system that contributed to its planning and execution. We gave the example of being thirsty and wanting to pour some milk from the milk carton in front of you into a glass.

Sensory inputs come in from the periphery to tell you what is happening around you, where you are in space, and where your joints are relative to each other: they give you a map of your body in space. Sensory inputs from the visual system go through two parallel pathways involved in goal-directed reaching: one related to what is being reached for (perception and object recognition) and the other related to where the object is in extrapersonal space (localization) and the action systems involved in object manipula-

tion. The perceptual pathway goes from visual cortex to temporal cortex, while the localization and action pathway goes from visual cortex to the parietal lobe.

Higher centers in the cortex take this information (possibly using the parietal lobes and premotor cortex) and make a plan to act on it in relation to the goal: reaching for the carton of milk. You make a specific movement plan: you're going to reach over the box of corn flakes in front of you. This plan is sent to the motor cortex, and muscle groups are specified. The plan is also sent to the cerebellum and basal ganglia, and they modify it to refine the movement.

The cerebellum sends an update of the movement output plan to the motor cortex and brainstem. Descending pathways from the motor cortex and brainstem then activate spinal cord networks; spinal motor neurons activate the muscles; and you reach for the milk. If the milk carton is full but you thought it was almost empty, spinal reflex pathways compensate for the unexpected extra weight and activate more motor neurons. Then the sensory consequences of your reach are evaluated, and the cerebellum updates the movement—in this case, to accommodate a heavier milk carton.

From this description, you can see that sensory information plays many roles during the control of reaching. Sensory information is used to correct errors during the execution of the movement itself, ensuring accuracy during the final portions of the movement. In addition, sensory information is used proactively in helping to make the movement plan.

In the following section we discuss recent research exploring the role of specific visual pathways involved in reach and grasp.

Visual Pathways Involved in Reach and Grasp

The two visual pathways involved in manipulation include the dorsal stream pathway, going from the visual to the parietal cortex, and the ventral stream pathway, going from the visual cortex to the temporal lobe. Research by Goodale and Milner (Goodale and Milner, 1992; Goodale et al., 1991) suggests that the dorsal stream projection to the parietal cortex provides action-relevant information about all phases of the reaching movement, including object position, structure, and orientation, while projections to the temporal lobe provide our conscious visual perceptual experience.

It is interesting to note that most neurons in the dorsal stream area show both sensory-related and movement-related activity (Andersen, 1987) and thus may be involved in sensory-motor transformation processes during the reaching movement. In addition, patients with lesions in these dorsal stream pathways that result in optic ataxia have problems not only with reaching in the right direction but also with positioning their fingers or adjusting the orientation of their hand when reaching toward an object and with adjusting their grasp to reflect the size of the object they are picking up.

Researchers have found that damage to the parietal lobe can impair the ability of patients to use information about the size, shape, and orientation of an object to control the hand and fingers during a grasping movement, even though this same information can be used to identify and describe objects (Goodale and Milner, 1992).

Goodale and Milner note that the two cortical pathways are different with respect to their access to consciousness. For example, a patient with ventral-stream lesions had no conscious perception of the orientation or dimension of objects, but she could pick them up with great adeptness. Thus it may be that information in the dorsal system can be processed without reaching conscious perception (Goodale and Milner, 1992).

Recent evidence supporting the concept of separate visual pathways for perception (ventral stream) and action (dorsal stream) in normal subjects comes from work by Haffenden and Goodale (1998). In this experiment they used a visual illusion to separate out perceptual judgments about an object's size and the ability to reach for it accurately. They used the Ebbinghous Illusion, in which two target circles of equal size are surrounded by an array of either smaller or larger circles. Subjects typically report that the circle surrounded by the smaller circles is larger than the one surrounded by larger circles. If the same pathway controlled perception and action, one would expect both perception and grasp to be equally affected by the illusion.

In this experiment subjects were asked either to manually estimate the size of a disc placed in the center of one of the two sets of circles (hypothesized ventral stream) or to reach for the disc (hypothesized dorsal stream), as shown in Figure 16-2*A*. Subjects manually estimated disc size as different, though they were the same. However, grip size was scaled to actual target size rather than apparent size. Figure 16-2*B* shows the difference in maximum grip aperture and manual estimation for the discs surrounded by either small or large circles. Note that maximum grip aperture is identical for the two situations, but manual estimation is significantly larger for the disc surrounded by the smaller circles than for the disc surrounded by the larger circles (Haffenden and Goodale, 1998).

Thus, it appears that the ventral stream of projections plays a major role in the perceptual identification of objects, while the dorsal stream mediates the required sensorimotor transformations for visually guided

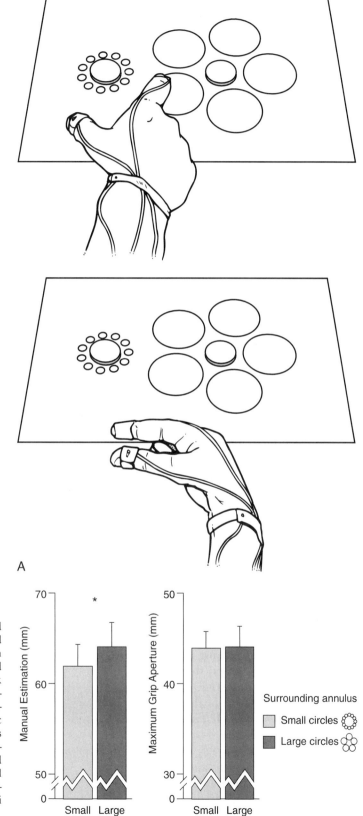

FIGURE 16-2. **A.** Reaching and manual estimation tasks. Hand is shown in the grasping task on the way to the target (*top*) and in the manual estimation task (*bottom*). **B.** Graphs of maximum grip aperture versus manual estimation size for the disc surrounded by small versus large circles. (Adapted with permission from Haffenden and Goodale. The effect of pictorial illusion on prehension and perception. J Cognit Neurosci 1998;10:127,128.)

actions directed at those objects (Goodale and Milner, 1992).

The Role of Visual Feedback in Reach and Grasp

The primary function of visual feedback in reaching appears to be related to the attainment of final accuracy. It has been hypothesized that the constancy of thumb position with relation to the wrist during reaching may be part of a strategy of providing clear visual feedback information regarding the end point of the limb (Wing and Frazer, 1983).

To determine the function of visual feedback in reaching, studies have been performed to compare reaches made with and without vision. Reaches with visual feedback showed a longer duration than those performed without feedback. Absence of visual feedback did not alter the grasp component of the reach (Jeannerod, 1990).

Can reaching occur in the absence of visual cortex function? It is usually accepted that destruction of the visual cortex in humans produces blindness except for very poor visual perception of illumination changes. However, research on monkeys with visual cortex lesions has shown some interesting results related to visual motor control. Though these monkeys appeared to be blind when their visual behavior was tested, they could still reach for objects that appeared in or moved across their visual field. It has been hypothesized that the superior colliculus in the midbrain contributes to this residual reaching behavior (Humphrey and Weiskrantz, 1969).

Since the monkey studies were performed, human studies have verified these results. In extending the monkey studies to humans, these researchers used a new experimental paradigm that had not been used before in humans. Instead of asking humans with visual cortex lesions if they could see an object, they asked them to try to point to where they "guessed" the target would be. It was shown that subjects did not point randomly; there was a significant correlation between pointing and target position. However, they did show larger constant errors

when reaching within their blind visual field. They typically overshot targets when they were within 30 degrees of midline and undershot them when they were beyond 30 degrees (Weiskrantz et al., 1974; Perenin and Jeannerod, 1975).

Visually Controlled Reaches Across the Midline

Is visual processing more complex when reaching to the contralateral side of the body? Yes. Researchers have consistently found that reaching movements across the midline (toward targets in the visual hemifield of the opposite arm) are slower and less accurate than movements to targets on the same side as the arm. Ipsilateral (uncrossed) reaches in these studies were shorter in latency, made with higher maximum velocity, completed more quickly, and made significantly more accurately than contralateral (crossed) reaches (Fisk and Goodale, 1985).

Thus, even normal adults show decrements when reaching to the contralateral side of the body. It is essential to remember this when evaluating patients with reaching problems. In addition, when structuring a training program, one may wish to begin with reaching to objects placed on the ipsilateral side prior to progressing to objects placed on the contralateral side.

Somatosensory Contributions to Reaching

Is somatosensory input essential for the production of reaching movements? Taub and Berman (1968) have shown that within 2 weeks of deafferentation, monkeys were able to perform adequate reach and grasp movements as long as vision was available. The researchers noted that the monkeys' movements were awkward at first, with animals only sweeping objects along the floor. Monkeys then developed a primitive grasp with four fingers together and no thumb and finally redeveloped a crude pincer grasp a few months after the lesion was made.

Other experiments discussed later in this chapter have shown that deafferented monkeys can make reasonably accurate single-joint pointing movements even when vision of the arm is occluded, when the pointing task was learned before deafferentation (Polit and Bizzi, 1979). In this case, even displacing the arm before the movement did not affect terminal accuracy, although the monkeys could not see or feel their arm position! Thus, it was concluded that the monkey is capable of using a central motor program to perform previously learned reaching movements and that kinesthetic feedback is not required for achieving reasonable accuracy when performing well-learned movements.

Experiments performed with humans with severe peripheral sensory neuropathy in all four limbs have shown similar results. One patient was able to perform a wide variety of hand movements, such as tapping movements and drawing figures in the air, even with the eyes closed. However, when he was asked to repeat the movement many times with the eyes closed, the performance deteriorated quickly. Thus, it appears that somatosensory information is not required for arm movement initiation or execution, as long as the movements are simple or non-repetitive. However, if subjects have to make complex movements requiring coordination of many joints or to repeat movements without visual feedback, they are unable to update their central representations of body space and show considerable movement "drift" and problems with coordination (Rothwell et al., 1982).

These experiments suggest that certain movements may be carried out without somatosensory feedback. Nevertheless, considerable work has also shown the important contributions of sensory feedback to the fine regulation of movement.

Researchers originally thought that it was mainly joint receptors that controlled position sense during reaching. However, more recent research suggests that joint receptors are active mainly at the extremes of joint motion but not at midposition. This would thus make it impossible for these receptors to signal limb position in the mid-working range of joints (Jeannerod, 1990).

More recent work has begun to build evidence for a strong role for muscle spindles in position sense. Experiments have been performed in which tendons were vibrated, specifically activating muscle spindle Ia afferents. Subjects consistently had the illusion that the joint was moving in the direction that it would have been moving if the muscle were being stretched. For example, when the biceps tendon was vibrated, it produced the illusion of elbow extension (Goodwin et al., 1972).

Cutaneous afferents are also important contributors to position sense. Mechanoreceptors in the glabrous area of the hand are strongly activated by isotonic movements of the fingers (Hulliger et al., 1979).

Interestingly, subjects who are recovering from paralysis report that when the muscle is still completely paralyzed, they have no feeling of heaviness in the limb. But as they begin to regain movement ability, they feel as if the limb is being held down by weights. These sensations of heaviness are reduced as movements become easier and strength increases. This may be due to an internal perception of the intensity of motor commands (Jeannerod, 1990).

Visual and Somatosensory Contributions to Anticipatory Control of Reaching

An essential component of all reaching movements is proactive visual and somatosensory control, which is responsible for the correct initial direction of the limb toward the target and the initial coordination between limb segments. In addition, visual information about the characteristics of the object to be grasped is used proactively to program the forces used in precision grip.

It has been hypothesized that visual and somatosensory information are also used to update proprioceptive and visual body maps that allow the accurate programming of reaching movements. To determine the influence of updated maps of the body workspace on the accuracy of a reaching movement, experiments were performed to manipulate visual information regarding hand and target positions prior to movement. It was shown that when a subject could not see the hand prior to movement, there were large errors in reaching the target. It was therefore concluded that a proprioceptive map of the hand by itself was not adequate to code the hand position in the reaching workspace. This suggests that somatosensory inputs must be calibrated by vision in order for the proprioceptive map and the visual map to be matched (Jeannerod, 1990). No experiments have yet been performed to determine how often the proprioceptive map must be updated by visual inputs to ensure accurate movements.

Motor Systems

Two Separate Descending Pathways for Reach and Grasp

During reaching, the arm movement carrying the hand to the target is performed in parallel with the preshaping of the fingers for grasping the object. Many experiments suggest that the respective motor systems contributing to reach and grasp involve separate descending motor pathways.

For example, reaching is observed in newborn infants, though grip formation develops later. Research has shown that infants of 1 week may reach for and intercept moving objects and contact them, but this is done with a hand that is wide open, without any grip formation. Grip formation appears to develop at about 10 to 22 weeks (Bruner and Koslowski, 1972).

In the monkey this is also the case. It has been shown that the appearance of the grasp component, at 8 months of age, is correlated with the maturation of connections between the corticospinal tract and the motor neurons (Kuypers, 1962). Children with pyramidal lesions also show similar problems with the grasp component of reaching, although the transport component may be normal (Jeannerod, 1990). This suggests that midbrain and brainstem pathways such as the red nucleus and reticular nuclei may control the more proximal muscles involved in reaching movements, while pyramidal pathways are required for the fine-control of grasping movements.

Experiments on monkeys performing a precision grip versus power grip task (Fig. 16-3) have shown that some neurons in the primary motor cortex fire only during the execution of a precision grip, not a power grip. This indicates that their connections are with intrinsic hand muscles rather than forearm muscles. These neurons show a short latency burst onset (about 11 msec) prior to muscle activation, which suggests they are monosynaptically connected to the motor neuron pools (Muir and Lemon, 1983; Lemon et al., 1986). Figure 16-3 shows the activity of a pyramidal tract neuron and an interosseus muscle during a precision grip task with light versus heavy force and during a power grip task (grasping a cylinder). Note that at both force levels, the pyramidal tract neuron is activated only during the precision grip task, not during the power grip task. However, the interosseus muscle showed activity in all three tasks.

Musculoskeletal Contributions

Reaching also involves a complex interaction of musculoskeletal and neural systems. Musculoskeletal components include such things as joint range of motion, spinal flexibility, muscle properties, and biomechanical relationships among linked body segments. In particular, it has been suggested that the following types of joint motion are essential to the ability to move the arm normally: scapular rotation, appropriate movement of the humeral head, the ability to supinate the forearm, shoulder and elbow flexion to approximately 100 to 120 degrees, the ability to extend the wrist slightly beyond neutral, and sufficient mobility in the hand to allow grasp and release (Charness, 1994).

Motor aspects of reaching include appropriate muscle tone, muscle strength, and coordination. More specifically, this involves appropriate activation of muscles to stabilize the scapula, rib cage, and humeral head during upper extremity reaching movements and activation of muscles at the shoulder, elbow, and wrist joint for transport of the arm.

The work of Kaminski et al. (1995) provides evidence for coupling between the trunk, scapula, and arm when one reaches toward targets. The authors found motion of the trunk to make a significant contribution

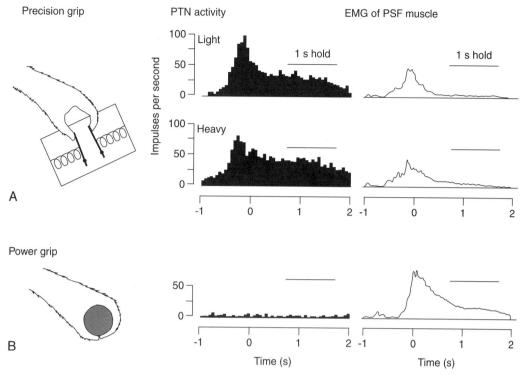

FIGURE 16-3.   Graph of activity (impulses/second) of a pyramidal tract neuron (PTN) and an interosseus muscle (PSF) during two tasks: **A.** A precision grip task executed with light versus heavy force (top two traces). **B.** A power grip task (bottom trace). (Adapted with permission from Muir and Lemon. Corticospinal neurons with a special role in precision grip. Brain Res 1983;261:312–316.)

during arm transport, affecting both the velocity and path of the hand. Specific evidence of coupling was documented during reaches for anteriorly placed targets, in that trunk rotation was countered by glenohumeral horizontal abduction and scapular retraction to keep the hand moving in a straight path.

In a patient with neurological deficits it is often not easy to determine the relative contribution of neural vs. musculoskeletal problems to abnormal reaching. Motor control problems that affect the inertial characteristics of the system will give rise to coordination problems even when the patterns of activation are normal. For example, an increase in stiffness will change the inertial characteristics of the head, arm, and/or trunk, making the initiation of motion more difficult. Thus, we see the important interaction between the biomechanics of movement and the neural control mechanisms.

Postural Support of Reaching

As was discussed in Chapter 7, postural control, defined as the ability to control the body's position in space for the purpose of stability and orientation, has a strong influence on upper extremity function. The ability to control the body's position in space is essential to moving one part of the body, in this case the arms, without destabilizing the rest of the body.

Just as manipulatory control is task dependent, postural requirements vary according to the task. For example, postural requirements involved in a seated reaching task are less stringent than those in a standing task and thus may require only muscles in the trunk. In contrast, postural demands during reaching while standing are greater, requiring more extensive activation of muscles in both the legs and trunk to prevent instability.

Postural demands can affect the speed

and accuracy of an upper extremity movement. When postural demands are decreased by external support, upper extremity movements are faster, since prior postural stabilization is not necessary (Cordo and Nashner, 1982).

Helping a patient to regain sufficient postural control to meet the postural requirements inherent in a reaching task is essential to retraining that task. The reader is urged to review Chapters 7 to 11, which discuss postural control, its relationship to reaching, and issues associated with retraining the patient with postural disorders.

☯ GRASPING

Classification of Grasping Patterns

Grasp patterns vary as a function of location, size, and shape of the object to be grasped (Johansson et al., 1992). In 1956 Napier classified human grasping movements as either power or precision grips. He found that precision and power grips could be used alternatively or in combination for almost every type of object. He also believed that it was not solely the shape or size of the object that determined the grip pattern, but the intended activity, since for example a cylindrical object could be used for writing (precision grip) or hammering (power grip) (Jeannerod, 1996; Napier, 1956).

The anatomical difference between the two grips involves the posture of both the thumb and the fingers. In a power grip the finger and thumb pads are directed toward the palm to transmit a force to an object. Power grips include the hook grasp (holding a handle of a suitcase), spherical grasp (holding a softball), and cylindrical grasp (holding a bottle). In contrast, during a precision grip, the forces are directed between the thumb and fingers. The two grips are used very differently in manipulative skills: the precision grip allows movements of the object relative to the hand and within the hand, while the power grip does not.

In addition to the power vs. precision distinction, researchers have shown that

subjects tend to classify objects into four broad categories according to prior knowledge about the object. These categories include four hand shapes: poke, pinch, clench, and palm. The boundaries between categories are determined by the pattern of hand movements used with these objects when they are grasped and manipulated. This differentiation of hand shape also appears during actual reaching in the preshaping of the grasp (Jeannerod, 1996; Klatzky et al., 1987).

Two important requirements are necessary for successfully grasping an object. First, the hand must be adapted to the shape, size, and use of the object. Second, the finger movements must be timed appropriately in relation to transport so that they close on the object just at the appropriate moment. If they close too early or too late, the grasp is inappropriate (Jeannerod, 1990). Most of the research related to grip formation has been on precision grip, and this will be discussed in the following section.

Anticipatory Control of Grasping Patterns: Precision Grip Formation

When reaching forward to grasp an object, the shaping of the hand for grasping occurs during the transportation component of the reach. Figure 16-4 shows changes in both hand movement velocity (16-4A, *left*) and grip size (16-4A, *right*) during a reach. This pregrasp hand shaping appears to be under visual control. What properties of an object affect anticipatory hand shaping? The application of this concept can be found in Lab Activity 16-1.

As you can see from this lab, there are two categories of properties of objects that affect pregrasp hand shaping: intrinsic properties, such as the object's size, shape, and texture, and extrinsic or contextual properties, such as the object's orientation, distance from the body, and location with respect to the body (Jeannerod, 1984).

Remember that grip formation takes place during the transportation phase and anticipates the characteristics of the object to be grasped. The size of the maximum grip

OBJECTIVE: To examine how properties of the task affect reach and grasp movements.

PROCEDURES: You will be working in pairs for this lab. You will need the following items for the lab: a pitcher of water, a glass, a quarter, a pencil, a block, and a plastic glass covered with oil. In the first part of the lab, observe the arm and hand movements of your partner while he or she picks up and sets down the glass, quarter, pencil, block and plastic glass coated with oil. Next, set the glass upright next to the water pitcher. Observe your partner while he or she reaches for the pitcher and pours a glass of water. Now, pour the water back into the pitcher and invert the glass next to the pitcher. Again observe your partner reaching for and pouring a glass of water.

ASSIGNMENT: Describe the properties of the objects that affected how your partner reached for and grasped the various objects. During the pouring task, how did changing the orientation of the glass affect the movement strategy used to pick up the glass? When during the reach for an object did the hand begin to shape in preparation for grasp? How did characteristics of the object affect anticipatory hand shaping?

opening is proportional to the size of the object. This relationship is shown in Figure 16-4B, with a subject reaching for a 2-mm rod versus a 10-cm cylinder. Each increase of 1 cm in object size is associated with a maximum grip size increase of 0.77 cm (Marteniuk et al., 1990). When subjects change the grip opening, they do it almost entirely with finger movements, while the thumb stays in one place. When reaching for an object, as the arm is transported forward, the fingers begin to stretch, and the grip size increases rapidly to a maximum and then is reduced to match the size of the object (Jeannerod, 1990).

Subjects show differential hand shaping for different shapes of objects as well. The distance between the thumb and index finger is usually largest during the final slow approach phase. It has been shown that adults with prosthetic hands show this same rela-

tionship between grasp and transport phases (Fraser and Wing, 1981). Apparently, this relationship is not due to neural constraints but may be the most efficient way to reach.

Grasp–Lift Tasks

The types of objects that are picked up during a given day may vary from a light pen to a heavy, slick bottle of oil. The nervous system is capable of adapting precision grip so that it adjusts to objects of many weights and surface characteristics. The control mechanisms underlying these abilities have been carefully investigated. It has been shown that there are discrete phases to any lifting task. These phases are associated with responses in sensory receptors of the hand.

The first phase of a lift starts with contact between the fingers and the object to be lifted. When contact has been established, the second phase begins, with the grip force and the load force (load on the fingers) starting to increase. The third phase begins when the load force has overcome the weight of the object and it starts to move. The fourth phase occurs at the end of the lifting task, when there is a decrease in the grip and load force shortly after the object makes contact with the table (Johansson and Edin, 1992).

This type of an organizational control scheme has many advantages. For example, it allows great flexibility in lifting objects of different weights. Thus, the duration of the loading phase depends on the object's weight: heavier objects require higher load forces before they move. This also ensures that proper grip forces are used during the load phase. This scheme also requires limited sensory processing, since the end of one phase serves as the trigger for the next.

To ensure a safe grip, the grip-to-load force ratio has to be above a certain level; otherwise, slipping will occur. One cannot assume that two objects of the same weight will require the same grip force, since one may be more slippery than the other. How does the nervous system choose the correct parameters for grip and load force? It appears to use both previous experience and

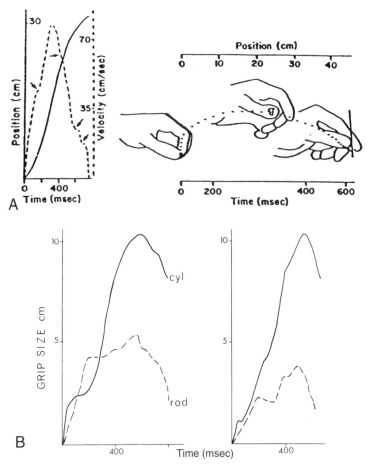

FIGURE 16-4. Characteristics of the transport phase of reaching. **A.** *Left.* Changes in hand movement velocity (broken line) and position (solid line) as a function of time during a reach. *Right:* Drawing of hand movement changes, including grip opening, during reach. **B.** Changes in grip size over time for two subjects reaching for a rod 2 mm in diameter and 10 cm long (dashed lines) versus a cylinder 55 mm in diameter and 10 cm long (solid lines). Note the different grip sizes but similar curve shapes. (**A.** Adapted with permission from Brooks VB. The neural basis of motor control. New York: Oxford University, 1986:133. **B.** Reprinted with permission from Jeannerod M. The neural and behavioural organization of goal-directed movements. Oxford: Clarendon, 1990:61.)

afferent information during the task. If there is a mismatch between the expected and actual properties of an object, receptors in the finger pads are activated. Pacinian corpuscles are very sensitive and easily capable of detecting that an object has started to move earlier than expected. In addition, visual and other types of cutaneous cues are important in determining the choice of grip parameters (Johansson and Edin, 1992).

◎ COORDINATION OF REACH AND GRASP

Though the neurophysiological and developmental research discussed earlier indicates that the two components, reach and grasp, are controlled by different motor systems, to be functionally effective they must be coordinated with each other. Thus transport of the hand must be coordinated with the shaping of the fingers to ensure that reaching ends when the fingers come in contact with the object.

Researchers have used kinematics to determine whether there are invariant relationships between reach and grasp components. It has been shown that there is a fixed ratio of maximum grip aperture to total movement time, such that it occurs at about 75% to 80% of movement time (Jeannerod, 1984; Wallace et al., 1990). This ratio was invariant across variations in movement time and speed and initial finger postures and was preserved even in pathological conditions. This is a strong indication of functional coupling of the two components (Jeannerod, 1996).

Invariance related to the coordination of reach and grasp has also been studied by examining the effect of a perturbation of one component on the second component. For example, to perturb the transport (reach) component, researchers displaced the object to be grasped and found that this perturbation to reach also affected grasp, since there was a brief interruption in grip aperture formation. In addition, when object size was changed to perturb the grip component, it affected the transport component. Thus, the two components were kinematically coupled during corrections for these perturbations (Paulignan et al., 1990). Though the two components are correlated, they appear to be only loosely time coupled. Thus, they appear to be functionally linked but without stereotyped structural relationships (Jeannerod, 1996).

Based on this research, we may hypothesize that in the case of a patient who has upper extremity paresis complicated by spasticity, both reach (transport) and grasp will be affected. We may predict, based on the neurophysiological research, that the patient will recover the reach phase earlier and more completely than the grasp phase (De Souza et al., 1980). While the two components are controlled separately, they require coordination to be functionally effective; thus, they must be trained both separately and together. For example, patients may be-

gin practicing the reach component by moving their hand toward an object but not actually grasping it. Because even the reach phase is task dependent, it is important to practice reaching in the context of many types of functional tasks, such as reach and point, reach in preparation for a grasp, reach in preparation for a grasp and lift, or grasp and move.

Patients may also work on grasp and release of an object close to their hand, alleviating the need for controlling reach. Finally, they may work on combining reach and grasp components.

❷ THEORIES OF NEURAL CONTROL OF REACH AND GRASP

Until now, we have described the biomechanical and neural contributions to the components of reach and grasp. However, another approach to studying the control of reaching has come from the field of psychology, where researchers have focused on describing basic characteristics of reaching and formulated theories about the neural control of reaching based on these characteristics.

Fitts' Law

Some basic characteristics of arm movements that you may find intuitively obvious are that whenever arm movement precision is increased or movement distance is increased, movement time becomes longer. In the 1950s, Fitts quantified these characteristics in the following experiments. He asked subjects to move a pointer back and forth between an initial position and a target position as quickly as possible. In the set of experiments, he systematically varied the movement distance and the width of the target. He found that he could create a simple equation relating movement time to the distance moved and the target width. This is the equation, which has become known as Fitts' law:

$$MT = a + b \log_2 2D/W$$

where a and b are empirically determined constants, MT is movement time, D is distance moved, and W is the width of the target. The term log₂ 2D/W has been called the index of difficulty. Movement time increases linearly with the index of difficulty, that is, the more difficult the task, the longer it takes to make the movement (Fitts, 1954; Keele, 1981).

This equation has come to be known as Fitts' law because its ability to relate movement time to movement accuracy and distance applies to many kinds of tasks, including discrete aiming movements, moving objects to insert them in a hole, moving a cursor on a screen, small finger movements under a microscope, and even throwing

darts. Fitts' law has proved accurate in describing movements made by subjects of all ages, from infants to older adults (Keele, 1981; Rosenbaum, 1991).

What are the constraints of the individual and the task that lead to this particular law regarding movement? It has been suggested that movement time increases with distance and accuracy in part because of the constraints of our visual system. It is difficult to translate our visual perception of the distance to be covered precisely into an actual movement; thus, as the hand approaches the target, time is needed to update the movement trajectory (Keele, 1981). The application of this concept can be found in Lab Activity 16-2.

 LAB ACTIVITY 16-2

OBJECTIVE: To examine the effect of task difficulty on reaching (Fitts' law). Remember, Fitts defined task difficulty in terms of target size (W, which is the width of the target) and the distance to move (D, which is the distance between targets). He thus quantified task difficulty (which he called index of difficulty, or ID) by using the following equation:

$$ID = log_2 (2D/W)$$

PROCEDURE: For this lab, you will work in pairs. Use a pencil and tap quickly and accurately between two targets that vary in width and distance. The objective is to make as many *accurate* tapping movements as possible in a 10-second period. Accuracy is important. Remember that there should be no more errors made in the most difficult task than in the easiest tasks. If the number of errors exceeds more than 5% of the pencil dots, the trial should be done again.

Two combinations of task difficulty will be used. In the first and easiest task, D = 2 cm and W = 2 cm. Solving the equation for ID, that would be log (base 2) of (2 × 2)/2. This works out to the log₂ of 2, which is 1 in the most difficult task. D = 16 cm and W = 1 cm. That is, the log₂ of (2 × 16)/1, which is 5.

Each person will perform three trials (10 seconds each) for the two task conditions. When you are the subject, your partner will time each trial and count and record the number of dots in each target. Your partner should verbally tell you to start and stop on each 10-second trial. The rest interval between trials should be the amount of time needed to count and record the taps. After the three trials you can switch jobs with your partner.

ASSIGNMENT: Make a table and record the number of taps on each of the three trials for both the easy and difficult task. Calculate the mean and standard deviation as well. For each task, calculate the average movement time in milliseconds for a single movement of the tapping task. Do this by dividing each number of taps by 10, which will give you the number of taps per second during the 10-second trial. Record this value in the table as well. Next, take the inverse of this number (1/x, where x is the average number of taps). Multiply this number by 1000 to obtain the average movement time in milliseconds. Record this average movement time in the table. How did the difficulty of the task affect movement time? If you tried to maintain the same speed on the difficult task as you used on the easy task, how would this affect your accuracy? Describe a functional task that has relatively low demands for accuracy and distance versus a functional task that has relatively high demands for accuracy. How will these differences in task difficulty impact your patient's performance?

How Does the Nervous System Plan Movements: Muscle Coordinate, Joint Angle Coordinate or End Point Coordinate Strategies?

In Chapter 1, when we discussed theories of motor control, we mentioned Bernstein's contributions to systems theory. He proposed that a given nervous system program will produce different outcomes in different situations because the response of the body will depend on the initial position of the limbs and on outside forces such as gravity and inertia. When body segments act together, the nervous system must also take into account the forces they generate with respect to each other. Bernstein hypothesized that the nervous system possessed a central representation of the movement that was in the form of a "motor image," representing the form of the movement to be achieved, not the impulses needed to achieve it. He believed that proprioception was important to the final achievement of the movement, not in a reflex-triggering sense but as it contributed to the central representation of the movement. He also suggested that one way to control the high number of degrees of freedom involved in any complex movement was to organize the actions in terms of synergies, or groups of muscles or joints that were constrained to act as a unit (Bernstein, 1967).

In fact, many researchers have now shown that hand movements are organized synergically or through coordinative structures. For example, it was shown that when subjects were asked to point at two targets, they moved the hands simultaneously, even if the reaching tasks were very different in difficulty (for example, one was near and large, and the other one was far away and small). Other researchers have noted this same tight bimanual coordination when subjects reached forward to manipulate an object with two hands. Thus, it has been suggested that independent body segments become functionally linked for the execution of a common task (Kelso et al., 1979; Jeannerod, 1990).

How does the nervous system control

complex arm movements to reach targets with speed and elegant precision? This is a complex problem that may be solved in various ways. For example, the nervous system may plan reaching movements with respect to the activation sequences of individual muscles; this has been referred to as a muscle coordinate strategy. Alternatively, reaching may be planned in relation to joint angle coordinates, that is, planning the movements of shoulder, elbow, and wrist joints to arrive at the target. This would mean that the nervous system was planning the movement around a set of intrinsic coordinates of the body, expressed in terms of the joint angles. Finally, the nervous system could plan arm movements in terms of the final end-point coordinates, using extrinsic coordinates in space (Hollerbach, 1990).

Levels of planning may also be considered in terms of a hierarchy, with for example both kinematic and kinetic levels of planning. Kinematic levels of planning would be organized around geometry, such as joint angle variables and end-point variables. Kinetic levels of planning would be organized around forces, such as the forces of muscle activation and joint torques.

On the one hand, it seems intuitively obvious that we would have to use some variation on end-point coordinate planning to do something like picking up a glass of water. If we plan a movement using intrinsic coordinates alone, without regard to the actual position of the object in space, the accuracy of the movement with respect to the end position needed is likely to be insufficient. But when the nervous system plans according to end-point coordinates, it has to make a complex mathematical transformation called an inverse kinematics transformation, which would transform end-point coordinates into joint angle coordinates. Then it has to create this trajectory by producing the appropriate muscle activation patterns (Hollerbach, 1990).

It has also been proposed that movements are planned in terms of joint angle coordinates, which has the advantage of not requiring an inverse kinematics transformation. This would mean that the organization of movement by the nervous system would be relatively simple. However, the nervous system would still have to do an inverse dynamics transformation that would transform joint angle coordinates into muscle torques and muscle activation patterns required to make the movement.

If trajectories were planned in terms of muscle activation patterns, it would have the advantage of simplifying the inverse kinematics and inverse dynamics problems, but we have also mentioned that muscle activation patterns are only indirectly related to final joint positions. Thus, programming movements in this manner could cause large inaccuracies (Hollerbach, 1990).

How does one go about determining how the nervous system plans movements? Hollerbach, in an excellent review of the research on arm movement planning, mentions that Bernstein (1967) actually made the following statement, which has guided modern physiologists in their experiments exploring the control of reaching movements: "If the spatial shape of a trajectory is invariant irrespective of the muscle scheme or the joint scheme, then the motor plan must be closely related to the topology of the trajectory and considerably removed from joints and muscles."

Thus, experimenters have begun to look for invariant characteristics in different variables related to the reach. If invariances are found across different conditions, this could be considered evidence that the nervous system uses this variable to plan movements. It has been shown that the path of the wrist in an arm movement is nonaffected by movement speed or load (weights held in the hand). The velocity profiles of a movement are also nonaffected by movement speed or load. These findings support the concept that the nervous system uses kinematic variables for planning (Atkeson and Hollerbach, 1985).

Remember that two types of kinematic variables may be used for movement planning: joint angle coordinates and end-point coordinates. If the nervous system controls movements in joint angle coordinates, the hand should move in a curved line, because

the movements will be about the axis of a joint, as you see in Figure 16-5A. However, if it plans movements with respect to extrapersonal space or end-point coordinates, the hand should be expected to move in a straight line (Fig. 16-5B) (Rosenbaum, 1991; Hollerbach, 1990).

To answer this question, Morasso (1981) asked subjects to point to targets in two-dimensional space (on a surface) and recorded their hand trajectories. They found that subjects tended to move the hand in straight lines, with their joints going through complex angular changes. Even when they were asked to draw curved lines, the subjects tended to draw a series of straight-line subunits. These results support the concept that the central nervous system programs movements according to end-point coordinates.

Other researchers have explored arm movement control further and have shown that the nervous system can directly control the joints and still produce straight-line movements. This is done by varying the onset times for the joint movements, with all joints stopping at the same time. This method of control gives movements with almost straight-line paths. This suggests that straight-line trajectories can occur even when the central nervous system is using joint angle coordinates to program movements. Thus, it is not clear whether the central nervous system programs movements exclusively by one method or the other (Hollerbach, 1990).

Russian researchers have shown that the elbow and wrist joints are controlled as a synergic unit. When subjects were asked to move the elbow and wrist joint congruently (flexing both together), the subjects could perform this task with ease, with joint motions starting and stopping as a unit. When asked to move the joints incongruently (flexing one and extending the other), they performed the task with considerable difficulty, moving the joints much less smoothly. This is additional evidence for joint-based planning (Kots and Syrovegin, 1966).

A number of additional theories on the control of reaching are described in the fol-

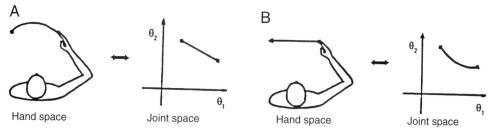

FIGURE 16-5. Variables that can be used for planning arm movements. **A.** If movements are controlled in joint coordinates, hand trajectories are curved. **B.** If movements are controlled in end point coordinates, joint space is curved (a complex elbow and shoulder movement is required). (Adapted with permission from Hollerbach JM. Planning of arm movements. In: Osherson DN, Kosslyn SM, Hollerbach JM, eds. Visual cognition and action: an invitation to cognitive science, vol 2. Cambridge, MA: MIT, 1990:187.)

lowing section. The first group of theories tends to assume that the nervous system is programming distance in making movements, while the second group of theories suggests that final location is the parameter being programmed.

Distance Versus Location Programming Theories

What do we mean by programming distance versus location? According to the distance programming theory, when making an arm movement toward a target, people visually perceive the distance to be covered, then activate a particular set of agonist muscles to propel the arm the proper distance to the target. At a particular point they turn off the agonist muscles and activate antagonist muscles at the joint to provide a braking force to stop the movement (Keele, 1986).

According to the location programming theory, the nervous system programs the relative balance of tensions (or stiffness) of two opposing (agonist and antagonist) muscle sets. According to this theory, every location in space corresponds to a family of stiffness relations between opposing muscles, as we explain later in the chapter. Let's first look at distance programming theories.

Distance Theories

Multiple Corrections Theory

It has been shown repeatedly that accuracy of arm movements decreases when vision is absent. For example, when subjects were asked to make arm movements of different durations to a target, movements of 190 msec or less were nonaffected by loss of vision, while movements of 260 msec or more were affected by loss of visual feedback (Keele and Posner, 1968). Thus, it appears that corrections of movement trajectories are based on visual feedback and that it takes about 200 to 250 msec for vision to be able to update a movement trajectory. Considering that some movement time must occur before the limb is close enough to the target to use visual feedback, one realizes that the visual processing time is slightly shorter. It has been shown (Carlton, 1981) that subjects need to see their hand for at least 135 msec during a movement to use vision to improve movement accuracy.

Researchers (Keele, 1968; Crossman and Goodeve, 1983) have proposed that aiming movements consisted of a series of submovements, each responding to and reducing visual error. Thus, an initial movement, before any visual correction takes place, covers most of the distance to a target and is independent of final precision. This model predicts a constant b for Fitts' law that is almost identical to the one that Fitts and Peterson calculated originally (Keele, 1981).

There are, however, some problems with this model. Typically, aiming movements to a target allows only one correction, if any, and when corrections are made, they do not have constant durations or proportions of the distance to the target (Rosenbaum, 1991).

How might this theory be used to explain problems related to inaccurate reaching movements commonly found in patients with neurological deficits? The multiple corrections theory stresses the importance of visual feedback when making corrections during a movement to increase accuracy. Thus, inaccurate movements could be the result of loss of visual feedback. When retraining a patient using a multiple corrections theory, the clinician could have the patient practice slow movements requiring a high degree of accuracy and draw the patient's attention to visual cues relating hand movement to target location.

Schmidt's Impulse Variability Model

Another way of explaining the characteristics of arm movement seen in Fitts' equation is to hypothesize that the initial phase of the movement, involving the generation of a force impulse, is more important than later phases of the movement, dealing with ongoing control. This would be true particularly when the movement is too fast for visual feedback to aid in accuracy.

Schmidt performed research in which subjects were asked to make fast movements over a fixed distance. These movements required large amounts of force, since high-velocity movements require large forces to generate the movement. He showed that the size of the subject's error increased in proportion to the magnitude of the force used. Thus, when he asked subjects to make a fast but accurate movement, the large forces required caused increased force variability. This increased variability resulted in a decreased movement accuracy (Schmidt et al., 1979). These movement characteristics are described in the following equation:

$$W_e = a + b\,D/MT$$

where W_e is variation in movement end point expressed in standard deviation units, D is distance moved, and MT is movement time. This equation is similar to Fitts' law. It indicates that simply taking into account the fact that faster movement requires more force can explain Fitts' law, without having to factor in a need for visual feedback for movement accuracy (Keele, 1981).

This theory alone cannot be used to explain aiming movements, since as we have seen earlier, many movements, particularly those lasting longer than 250 msec, do use visual feedback for accuracy.

Nonetheless, this theory does have relevance for the clinician involved in retraining upper extremity control. It suggests the importance of practicing fast movements of varying amplitudes during therapy sessions. In this way, the patient learns to program forces appropriately for quick and accurate movements.

Hybrid Model: Optimized Initial Impulse Model

The previous two models deal with two extremes of movement control, (*a*) the use of visual feedback to improve accuracy during ongoing portions of slower movements and (*b*) very fast movements that cannot easily use visual feedback, hence are controlled only through the amplitude of the initial impulse. In an attempt to create a model to explain the entire range of possible aiming movements, more recent studies (Meyer et al., 1988) have described a hybrid model that combines elements of both of these models. This hybrid model is referred to as the optimized initial impulse model.

Researchers studying this model hypothesized that a subject makes a first movement toward a target, which if successful, is the sole movement. However, if it is inaccurate, for example if it undershoots or overshoots the target, another movement will be required involving visual feedback during ongoing movement control. Clearly, the subject must find a balance between moving quickly, which requires a large initial force, and moving slowly enough to allow corrections to the ongoing movement, thereby ensuring accuracy.

It was found that an equation taking these issues into account was similar to Fitts' law:

$$T = a + b\,n(D/W)^{1/n}$$

where T is movement time, D is distance, W is width of the target, and n is the number of submovements used to reach the target (Rosenbaum, 1991).

Since functional activities require a variety of movements, both fast and slow, with varying degrees of accuracy, it is important to retrain a patient's ability to perform a continuum of movements that vary in both speed and accuracy.

Location Programming Theories

As we mentioned earlier, there are two ways that the nervous system may program arm movements, through distance programming or through programming the end-point location of the movement (Keele, 1981; Feldman, 1974). The example of a café door swinging on springs has sometimes been used to explain the location programming model (Keele, 1986). Figure 16-6*A* shows the door in a closed position. The movement of the café door is described as occurring when there is a reduction in length of one spring and the lengthening of the other spring. When the door is released, the imbalance between the springs causes the door to return to its closed position, with the springs at their resting length. If you want to keep the door open, you can simply change one spring for another of a different stiffness, and then it will have a new resting position (Fig. 16-6*B*).

It has been suggested that the agonist-antagonist muscle pairs at the joints are like the

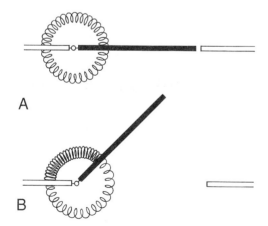

A

B

FIGURE 16-6.   The café door model. Simplified explanation of the mass–spring model of motor control. **A.** When a café door is at rest, it resembles a joint at midpoint, with both muscles at midlength. **B.** When one spring of a café door is shortened and the other is lengthened, the door is open, analogous to one muscle contracting and the other relaxing to allow the joint to flex.

springs of the café door. We can change the position of the joint simply by changing the relative stiffness of the two muscles, through higher or lower relative activation levels. Though this may sound like an unusual way for the nervous system to program reaching movements, experiments have shown that this occurs in many circumstances.

For example, experiments performed on monkeys (Polit and Bizzi, 1979) suggest that many movements may be controlled through location rather than distance programming. In these experiments, the monkeys were trained to make elbow movements to different targets whenever lights above those targets were turned on, as you see in Fig. 16-7*D*. The monkeys wore a large collar that blocked sight of the arm, eliminating visual feedback. In addition, in certain experiments, the dorsal roots of the spinal cord were severed, eliminating kinesthetic feedback from the arm. The accuracy of the monkeys' arm movements was measured with and without visual and kinesthetic feedback. Researchers found that the monkeys' reaching was normal, despite a loss of visual and kinesthetic feedback (Fig. 16-7*A*).

They then gave a perturbation to the deafferented monkey's arm, moving it from its original position just after the target light was turned on but before the monkey began to move. Remember that the monkeys could not feel or see their arm position when it was perturbed. Nevertheless, the monkeys reached for the target with reasonable accuracy (Fig. 16-7, *B* and *C*). If the monkeys were using distance programming for reaching, this would have been impossible, because they would have applied a fixed force pulse in the elbow muscles to move their arm to the new position. Since the arm had already been perturbed, they should have ended up in the wrong place.

The only way these results can be explained is through the use of end-point location programming. In this case, what the nervous system would program is the stiffness (or background activity level) settings on the agonist and antagonist muscles of the arm. For example, if the arm was originally in a flexed position, they would have high

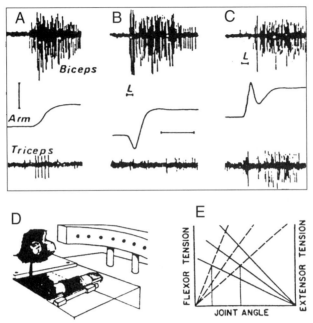

FIGURE 16-7. Experimental setup to test the mass–spring model of control. The deafferented monkey is pointing to a target but is unable to see its hand (**D**). **A.** The monkey flexes the arm to move to the target in a control trial. Biceps, triceps, and arm position traces are shown. The biceps muscle is predominantly active, with little activity in the triceps. **B.** The hand is moved by a torque motor to a new position farther from the target after the target is illuminated but before the hand starts to move. The biceps muscle is active and the triceps is silent. **C.** The hand is moved by a torque motor to a new position past the target after the target is illuminated but before the hand starts to move. The triceps muscle also shows considerable activity, since the monkey must extend the arm slightly. As you see from the movement traces, the monkey successfully pointed to the target, even when the unseen deafferented hand was perturbed. **E.** Flexor (broken lines) and extensor (solid lines) muscle tension levels that would move the arm to different joint angles. The intersection of two curves on the x-axis shows the joint angle produced by two combined tensions. (Reprinted with permission from Brooks VB. The neural basis of motor control. New York: Oxford University, 1986:138.)

background activity levels in the elbow flexors and low levels in the extensors. To move the arm precisely to the new location, they would simply change the background activity (stiffness) levels so that the spring constant of the elbow flexors was at a specific lower level and that of the extensors was at a predetermined higher level. This is shown graphically in Figure 16-7*E*. Once this new spring setting was made, it wouldn't matter where the limb was perturbed, because just like the café door, the limb would swing to its new spring setting. Thus, the monkey didn't have to know its starting point to go to the correct end point.

It is interesting that in these experiments, the monkeys were not able to continue to make accurate movements when the shoulder position was changed. It appears that without visual or somatosensory feedback from the arm, they could not update a central reference concerning shoulder position changes. These changes then threw off the elbow location programming (Polit and Bizzi, 1979).

More recent work (Kelso and Holt, 1980) with humans produced similar results. In this study, subjects were blindfolded and their fingers were anesthetized with a pressure cuff. Before testing began, they were trained to move their fingers to a specific position in space. They were then given brief finger perturbations during the course of their finger movement. With complete loss of finger sensation, there was very little difference in terminal error between the perturbed and unperturbed movements.

These results suggest that the nervous system is able to encode the location of body segments in space in relation to a base body position as varying activation levels of agonist and antagonist muscles. What does this mean? It has been suggested that this may explain why we can perform a skill (such as reaching for a cup or throwing a ball) hundreds of times without repeating exactly the same movement. According to classic programming theory, one would have to make a new program for each movement variation, but according to the mass–spring model, all one would have to do is program the appropriate muscle activity ratios, and the limb would move appropriately to its final position (Keele, 1986).

Do these results suggest that distance programming is wrong? No. Most likely, both strategies are used for arm movements, depending on the task and the context. For example, it has been shown that when humans make rapid elbow flexion movements (Hallett et al., 1975), they show a triphasic burst of contraction: first the biceps is activated, followed by the triceps (braking the movement), and then the biceps again. This same pattern was found in patients with loss of kinesthetic sensation. However, when subjects were asked to move more slowly and smoothly, they showed continuous biceps activity and no triceps activity. This has led some researchers to argue that the subjects are using mass–spring or location programming for slow movements and a combination of distance programming and location programming for faster movements.

There are also limitations to the mass–spring model. The model holds only with single-joint, one-plane movements. Most movements involve many joints, are carried out in three-dimensional space, and have to take into account gravity (Keele, 1981).

Ghez has also proposed a pulse–step model for arm movement control in which an initial pulse of force is followed by a step change in force levels. He states that the initial pulse component is required to overcome the constraints imposed by mechanical properties of the muscle and limb. This again could be considered a combined distance-and-location type of movement control (Ghez, 1979).

In summary, research studies appear to indicate that single-joint movements that are shorter than 0.25 seconds are too short to take advantage of visual feedback, while those longer than about 0.25 seconds involve visual feedback in the homing-in phase. Slower movements may involve location programming, while faster movements may involve a combination of distance and location programming. This model suggests that the capacity to modulate stiffness levels between the agonist and antagonist muscles is an important part of retraining accurate upper extremity movements.

☉ SUMMARY

1. From a kinematic perspective, coordination in reaching is characterized by the sequential activation of eye, head, and then hand movements. However, muscle responses in these segments tend to be activated synchronously, not sequentially. Thus, inertial characteristics play an important part in the final movement characteristics.

2. Reach and grasp are two distinct components that appear to be controlled by different neural mechanisms. Thus, patients with motor control problems can have difficulties in one or both aspects. This has implications for retraining.

3. Certain aspects of the grasp component, such as force of the grasp, are based on the person's perception of the characteristics of the object to be grasped and thus are programmed in advance.

4. Visual and somatosensory information is also used reactively for error correction during reaching and grasping.

5. Fitts' law expresses the relationship between movement time, distance, and accuracy, stating that when the demands

for accuracy increase, movement time will also increase.

6. There are two theories regarding the neural control of reaching: distance programming versus location theories.

7. According to the distance programming theory, when people make an arm movement toward a target, they visually perceive the distance to be covered, and then they activate a particular set of agonist muscles to propel the arm the proper distance to the target. At a particular point, they turn off the agonist muscles and activate antagonist muscles at the joint to provide a braking force to stop the movement.

8. According to the location programming theory, the nervous system programs the relative balance of tensions (or stiffness) of two opposing (agonist and antagonist) muscle sets. According to this theory, every location in space corresponds to a family of stiffness relations between opposing muscles.

9. Probably both strategies are used for arm movements, depending on the task and the context.

CHAPTER 17

Reach, Grasp, and Manipulation: Changes Across the Life Span

INTRODUCTION

The development of reaching and manipulation skills is complex and actually involves the development of many behaviors, each of which emerges progressively over time in association with maturation of different parts of the nervous and musculoskeletal systems and with experience. For example, the infant's ability to transport the arm toward an object precedes the ability to grasp. The ability to grasp emerges at 4 to 5 months, preceding the infant's ability to explore objects, which does not emerge until about the first year of life. Thus, the development of mature reaching and manipulation occurs gradually over the first few years of life.

This chapter explores the research on the development of reaching abilities in infants and children and the changes in reaching abilities that occur in older adults. We first discuss some of the early hypotheses concerning the development of reaching, which propose that reaching results from either the inhibition of primitive reflexes or the integration of those reflexes into voluntary movement (Twitchell, 1970). We also discuss the relative contributions of genetics and experience to the emergence of reaching in the neonate. We then review more recent studies that come from newer theories of motor control, such as the ecological, dynamic, and systems approaches.

Role of Reflexes in Development of Reaching Behaviors

Is early reaching reflexively controlled? This question has been debated in the developmental literature for many years. Early theories of the development of reaching argued that reflexes provide the physiological substrate for complex voluntary movements such as reaching (Twitchell, 1970). According to these theories, the transition from reflexes to voluntary reaching is a continuous process, with newborn reflexes gradually being incorporated into a hierarchy of complex coordinated actions (McDonnell, 1979). A review of eye–hand coordination development mentions that early developmental theoreticians may have overlooked another possibility regarding the development of reaching: that eye–hand coordination may emerge concurrently with the maturation of reflex function rather than emerging from the modification of reflex function (McDonnell, 1979). Thus, such reflexes as the grasp reflex may develop separately from the eye–hand coordination system, and may underlie different functions.

Reaching Behaviors: Innate or Learned?

A second question that has intrigued researchers concerns the extent to which the integration of sensory and motor systems underlying eye–hand coordination is genetically predetermined and/or experientially determined.

If the integration of eye–hand coordination were completely genetically predetermined, it would imply that the nervous system has a ready-made map of visual space and one of manipulative space laid out in a one-to-one correspondence. Thus, just by seeing an object, an infant would know exactly where to reach. In contrast, if eye–hand coordination were completely experientially determined, experience would be required to map visual space onto motor space or to learn to transform arm spatial coordinates into coordinates of the object.

The first hypothesis implies that once the nervous system's sensory and motor pathways for visually guided reaching have matured, the infant will be able to reach accurately for an object with little or no prior experience. The second hypothesis predicts a developmental learning period, during which the infant creates, through trial and error, the visual map or perceptual rules that overlie the motor map or actions required for reaching.

In the 1950s, Piaget's research on child development led him to believe that though nervous system maturation is a requirement for the appearance of a behavior, experience is responsible for its coordination with the senses. He believed that only through repeatedly and simultaneously looking at and touching an object would the visual and manipulative impressions be associated (Piaget, 1954).

Other researchers gave further support to this concept when they noted that neonates showed both visual and manual activity in the first few weeks after birth, but these movements were apparently unrelated (White et al., 1964). Thus, in the 1960s, many researchers in development supported the theory that visual and hand control systems are unrelated at birth.

In the 1970s, a group of scientists (Bower et al., 1970a,b) presented interesting evidence that they believed supported the opposite concept: that there was clear coordination of eye and hand in the newborn. They reported that infants between 7 and 14 days of age showed arm movements that were clearly directed toward the object in the visual field. They said a significant proportion of reaches were within 5 to 10 degrees of the object and that in 30% to 40% of the reaches, the hand closed around the object. They also observed that infants differentiated between objects that could be grasped (small object) from those that could not (large objects at large distances): they reached for the first but not the second.

Many researchers initially had difficulty replicating these experiments, and thus the findings were questioned (Dodwell et al., 1976). However, more recent studies indicate that an early form of eye–hand coordination does exist in the neonate, although reaching seems not to be as accurate or well coordinated as originally indicated (von Hofsten, 1982; Vinter, 1990).

In 1980, Amiel-Tison and Grenier, two researchers from France, wrote a surprising article on neonatal abilities. They reported that when the heads of neonates were stabilized, giving them postural support, amazing coordination of other behaviors was seen. For example, they reported that chaotic movements of the arms became still, and the infants appeared to be able to reach forward for objects, as you see in Figure 17-1. Their article is one example of recent research supporting the hypothesis that infants are born with certain innate abilities or behaviors, sometimes termed prereaching behaviors (Amiel-Tison and Grenier, 1980).

In the late 1970s and 1980s von Hofsten began exploring the development of eye–hand coordination in the neonate. He placed infants in an infant seat, moved an object in front of them, as you see in Figure 17-2, and carefully documented the number and accuracy of reaches that he observed. He observed the infants' arm movements with and without an object present. He showed that the number of extended movements performed when the infants were visually fixating on the object was twice as high as when the object was not fixated. The reaching movements were not very accurate.

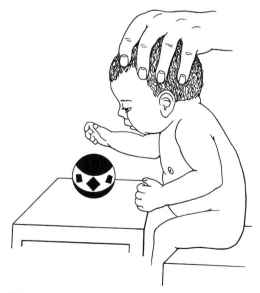

FIGURE 17-1. The release of reaching movements in a neonate by stabilizing the head. (Modified with permission from Amiel-Tison C, Grenier A. Evaluation neurologique du nouveau-né et du nourrisson. Paris: Masson, 1980:95.)

However, those that were made while the infants fixated on the target were aimed within an average of 32 degrees laterally and 25 degrees vertically toward the target, while those that were made without fixation were only within 52 degrees laterally and 37 degrees vertically. Though these reaching movements were less accurate than previously postulated, they were clearly aimed at the target, since they were significantly more accurate than the non–visually fixated movements. These results thus showed a clear effect of vision on forward-directed movements (von Hofsten 1984, 1993).

Von Hofsten noted that the system works from hand to eye as well. Several times the infant accidentally touched the object and immediately turned the eyes toward it. Neonates also have proprioceptive control of hand movements: they reach toward their mouth without vision in a goal-directed way. If they miss at first, they move to the mouth using proprioceptive feedback (von Hofsten 1984, 1993).

Thus, this research suggests that some aspects of reaching, in particular the ability to locate objects in space and transport the arm, may be present in rudimentary form (prereaching behaviors) at birth, while other components, such as grasp, develop later in the first year of life. These findings suggest support for the hypothesis that at least some aspects of reaching are innate.

In the next sections we follow the progression of the development of reaching and manipulation skills through infancy and childhood, exploring the emergence of various aspects of reaching and manipulation behaviors. We have already seen that location of an object in space is possible in the neonate and that the ability to move the arm toward the object in a rudimentary way is also available at birth. However, as you will see, more accurate reaching and the grasp component of reaching do not develop until 4 to 5 months of age, with pincer grasp developing at 9 to 13 months. Higher cognitive aspects of reaching begin to emerge at about 1 year of age. Throughout development, there appears to be a repetitive shift between visually triggered, or proactively guided,

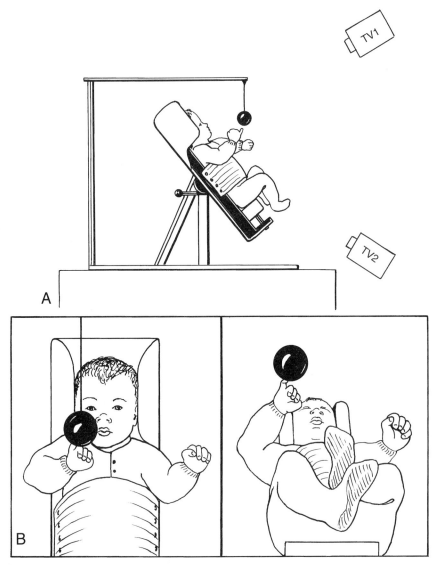

FIGURE 17-2.   **A.** Experimental setup used to study reaching in neonates. The infant is placed in an infant seat (50-degree angle) that has head support on the back and sides but allows the arms freedom to move. **B.** Outline of the infant as it touched the object, taken from single frames from the two video cameras seen in **A.** (Adapted with permission from von Hofsten C. Eye–hand coordination in the newborn. Devel Psychol 1982;18:452.)

reaching and visually guided, or feedback-controlled, reaching.

℮ LOCATING A TARGET: EYE–HEAD COORDINATION

In order to reach for a target the infant must first locate the target in space. If the target is moving, this requires that the infant stabilize gaze on the moving target and move the gaze at the same speed as the image of the target. This may involve eye movements alone or eye and head movements in combination. If the head is voluntarily moving at the same time, the eyes must compensate for the movement. When do infants develop the ability to track the movements of objects in space, and how does this ability improve with time?

Some smooth-pursuit tracking ability is present in the neonate, but only for objects covering a wide angle of visual space (about 16 degrees or more) moving slowly (10 degrees/second or less). For smaller objects there is typically only *saccadic* following of targets up to about 6 weeks of age (Shea and Aslin, 1990; Aslin, 1981). In addition, 1-month-olds show a substantial lag (180 msec) in following a moving stimulus (sinusoid), which is reduced with age. By about 3 months of age infants can keep the eyes on target most of the time, and by 5 months of age they show predictive abilities and thus are able to lead the sinusoidal motion of a target (von Hofsten and Rosander, 1996, 1997).

Is head motion involved in the early use of smooth pursuit? Yes, it is present even in 1-

month-olds and increases with age through at least 5 months. However, its lag is always large (250 msec). In spite of this lag, the infants finely coordinate head and eye movements to track moving targets accurately. Figure 17-3 shows the eye and head tracking ability of infants of 2 to 5 months of age. Note that head involvement is not substantial until 5 months. As its involvement increases, the contribution of eye movement naturally goes down. Note that gaze, which is the combination of head and eye movements, tracks the target almost perfectly, taking into account head movement lag and the relative contribution of eye and head movements to total gaze (von Hofsten and Rosander, 1997).

Are there similar neural mechanisms contributing to optokinetic reflexes (subcorti-

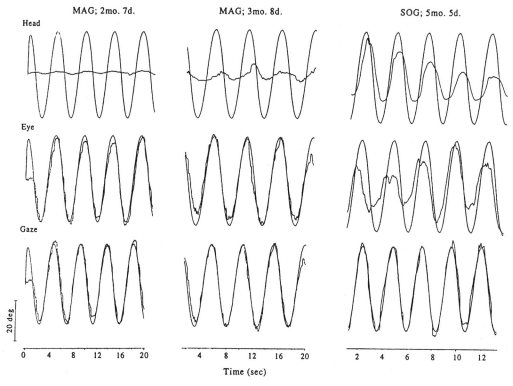

FIGURE 17-3.   Pursuit tracking of a sinusoidal motion by infants of 2 (*left*), 3 (*middle*) and 5 months of age (*right*); movement of the head (*upper trace*), eye (*middle trace*) and gaze (*lower trace*). Head involvement is not substantial until 5 months. As its involvement increases, the contribution of eye movement naturally goes down. Gaze, which is the combination of head and eye movements, tracks the target almost perfectly, taking into account head movement lag and the relative contribution of eye and head to total gaze. (Reprinted with permission from von Hofsten C, Rosander K. Development of smooth pursuit tracking in young infants. Vision Res 1997;13:1803.)

cal) and smooth pursuit (cortical) in young infants? It is possible that they have the same origin in young infants but differentiate into their different specialties with age and experience (von Hofsten and Rosander, 1997).

Eye–Head–Hand Coordination Development

In Chapter 16, we mentioned that when adults reach, the eye, head, and hand are coordinated so that the eyes move first, followed by the head and then the arm. How does eye, head, and hand coordination develop in children?

At 2 months, head–arm movements become coupled very strongly as the infant gains control over the neck muscles (von Hofsten 1984, 1993). Over the next 2 months, there is an increased uncoupling of head and arm movements, which allows more flexibility in eye–head–hand coordination. At about 4 months, infants begin to gain trunk stability, so they have a more stable base for reaching movements.

A number of developmental changes thus converge at about 4 months of age, all of which are essential for the emergence of successful reaching. This supports the concept that the emergence of successful reaching is due not to the maturation of a single system but to contributions of multiple maturing systems (von Hofsten 1984, 1993).

☑ REACH AND GRASP

Motor Components

Early Development

During the first year of life, there are a number of clear transitions in the infant's reach and grasp motor abilities. The first motor transformation in reaching skills appears to occur at about 2 months of age. Until this time, whenever the infant extends the arm, the hand opens in extension at the same time, so that it is difficult to grasp an object. At 2 months, the extension synergy is broken up, so that the fingers flex as the arm extends: the probability of seeing this behavior

goes from 10% to 70% of reaches from shortly after birth to 2 months (von Hofsten 1984, 1993).

At about 4 months, infants enter a new developmental phase involving integration of the newly developed skill of reaching. Reaches of 4-month-olds typically consist of several steps (often called movement units), and the final approach toward the object is crooked and awkward. In the next 2 months, the approach path straightens and the number of steps in the reach are reduced in number, with the first part of the reach getting longer and more powerful (von Hofsten 1984, 1993).

Konczak and Dichgans (1997) have performed a longitudinal study examining reaching in infants 4 months to 3 years of age. Figure 17-4 shows examples of sagittal hand paths of one infant reaching at four developmental times. They noted that most kinematic parameters did not assume adult-like levels before age 2 years. At this time 75% of the trials showed a velocity profile with a single peak. Between the second and third year improvements were minimal. They also noted that stable patterns of temporal coordination across arm segments, along with a unimodal end-point movement pattern (Fig. 17-4), emerged at about 12 to 15 months and continued to develop up to the third year. As mentioned earlier, probably a number of developmental changes contribute to this improvement, including development of trunk postural control.

Recently, laboratories have begun to use a dynamic systems approach to exploring the development of reaching. In one study the transition to the development of reaching was explored in infants aged 3 weeks to 1 year (Thelen et al., 1993). The researchers examined both spontaneous movements, without a toy, and task-directed movements, with a toy, recording kinematics (segment motions), kinetics (forces), and electromyography (EMG). Inverse dynamics calculations were used to determine joint torques. Torques were partitioned into net torques (net rotational forces), gravitational torques (force of gravity acting on the center of mass of the segment) and muscle torques (forces

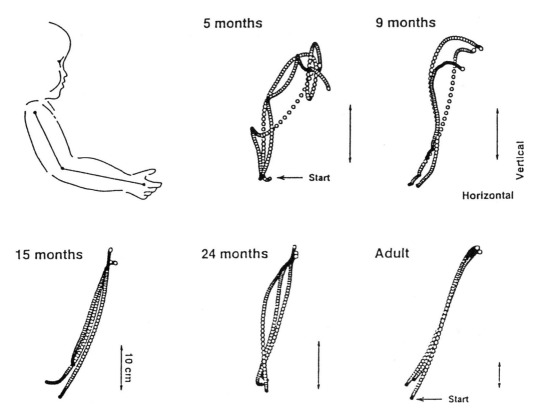

FIGURE 17-4. Hand paths used by one infant at four ages, recorded in the sagittal plane. Three reaches are shown for each age. Note the progression toward the smoothing of the end-point motion. Time between successive points is 10 msec. (Reprinted with permission from Konczak J, Dichgans J. The development toward stereotypic arm kinematics during reaching in the first 3 years of life. Exp Brain Res 1997;117:348.)

arising from active muscle contractions as well as passive tissue deformation).

Thelen and colleagues noted that the four infants studied entered the transition to reaching at different ages and with different activity levels and preferred movement patterns. They suggest that the process of learning to reach is one of discovering the match between intrinsic dynamics (the opportunities and constraints of their bodies) and their intention to bring the hand (using proprioceptive and/or visual cues) to the toy (using visual cues). They believe that the infants chose the patterns for executing a reach in a flexible way, in relation to their dynamic resources and the demands of the task rather than from a preexisting motor program.

For example, at the time of reach onset, each infant had characteristic intrinsic dynamics, including preferred postures, movements, and energy levels. They noted that two of the infants had higher energy levels and energized their muscles with large coactive phasic bursts, often rhythmically. Movements looked like bilateral flapping (described as similar to limit cycle oscillators). When they reached for the toy, they converted these oscillations into a task-specific movement (described as a point attractor) by damping down their oscillations and stiffening the arm with coactivation of the muscles.

The second two infants were quieter and thus had to lift their arms against gravity and move them forward. These movements were slow and sustained, with limbs relatively compliant and without perturbations from motion-dependent forces from connected segments. The authors conclude that smooth trajectories and coupling of joints were a byproduct of particular levels of force and arm stiffness or compliance (Thelen et al., 1993).

They also noted that infants acquired stable head control several weeks before reaching onset. Reaching onset involved a reorganization of muscle patterns in trapezius and deltoid muscles, serving to stabilize the head and shoulder and provide a stable base for reaching (Thelen and Spencer, 1998).

The authors note that their results support mass–spring (or equilibrium point) models of motor control in which the trajectory of the hand, joint angles, and muscle patterns are not explicitly planned. Instead, the central nervous system sets up new spring constants for the muscles at the involved joints that bring the joint to the desired position (Hogan et al., 1987).

Further research by Konczak et al. (1995, 1997), studying 9 infants 4 to 15 months of age, has shown that there are two developmental phases in hand trajectory formation: a first phase between 16 and 24 weeks involved rapid improvements, including reductions in movement time and number of movement units. This was followed by a second phase (28 to 64 weeks) involving fine-tuning of the sensorimotor system, in which there were more gradual changes in endpoint kinematics. They noted that early reaching was not limited by lack of ability to generate adequate levels of muscle torques. However, there were significant increases in their production of muscle flexor torque with time, with early reachers using a combination of flexion and extension torque and mature reachers using only adultlike flexor torques. These mature reachers, like adults, thus took advantage of motion dependent and gravitational forces to extend the arm.

In addition, relative timing of muscle- and motion-dependent torque peaks showed systematic development toward adult profiles with increasing age. They suggested that control problems of proximal joint torque generation could account for the segmented hand paths seen in early reaching. They concluded that the development of stable patterns of interjoint coordination does not oc-

cur simply by regulating torque amplitude but also by modulating the correct timing of force production and by the system's use of reactive forces (Konczak et al., 1995, 1997). Like Thelen and colleagues, they noted variability in the longitudinal profiles of each infant, indicating that each child followed his or her own strategy to explore the internal and external forces that are the basis of coordinated movements.

Sensory Components

Visually Triggered Versus Visually Guided Reaching

Development in the First Year of Life

Remember from Chapter 16 that reaching movements in adults have two phases, the transport phase and the grasp phase. It has been hypothesized that the beginning of the reach is visually triggered. That is, visual location of the target is used to initiate the movement. Thus, the position of the object is defined visually, while the position of the arm is defined proprioceptively. In contrast, the last part of the reach is considered visually guided. In this case, the position of the arm is defined visually with reference to the target, allowing precise adjustments to ensure the accuracy of the reach (Paillard, 1982).

Newborns seem able to use the visually triggered mode reasonably well, since they are able to initiate a reach aimed toward the target (von Hofsten, 1982). However, they do not appear to be proficient in the visually guided mode, since they are very inaccurate in their reaches. Visually guided reaching requires the ability to attend to the hand as it moves toward the object, as well as the ability to attend to the object. It also requires the ability to anticipate possible errors.

Research indicates that the visually guided mode of reaching emerges between the fourth and fifth months of life, just as trunk control and arm coordination are improving (McDonnell, 1979; von Hofsten, 1984).

In order to study the development of visually guided reaching in infants, researchers have fitted infants with special glasses with prism lenses to give an apparent lateral shift in the target position as the infants reached for small toys (McDonnell, 1979). By 5.5 months, when the infant's hand comes into view, he or she is able to perceive the discrepancy between hand position and target position and correct the trajectory. This suggests that by 5.5 months, visually guided reaching is evident in most infants.

Visually guided reaching, or the ability to make corrections to a trajectory based on visual information, peaks at around 7 months and then is gradually replaced by a ballistic style of reach, though infants can still use visual guidance when needed. In a ballistic style of reach, corrections are made at the end of the movement instead of during the ongoing movement. Once the movement is completed, the error between hand position and target position is used to correct the position of the hand in space.

Development in Childhood

To determine if there are continued developmental changes in children's use of visual feedback in making reaching movements, studies were performed in which children 4 to 11 years of age were asked to make movements with or without visual feedback. Hay has shown that there are interesting changes in the use of visual information by children between 4 and 11 years of age (Hay, 1978). Children between 4 and 6 years of age can make movements without visual feedback with reasonable accuracy, as you see in Figure 17-5. (Note that although 5-year-olds may appear to be more accurate than adults, there are no significant differences between these groups.) However, at age 7, there is an abrupt reduction in this ability, as seen in the increased errors made in reaching without visual feedback. The accuracy then begins to increase again, reach-

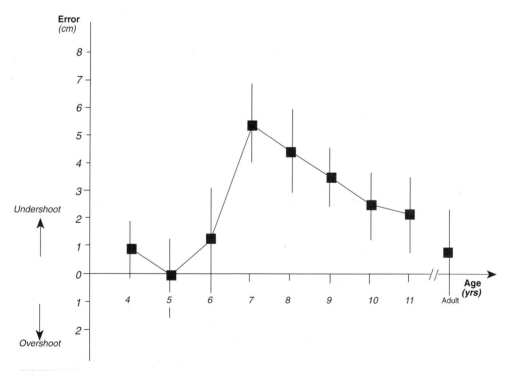

FIGURE 17-5. Pointing errors when visual feedback was not present for children 4 to 11 years of age, compared to adults. Large errors appear at 7 years of age, indicating reliance on visual feedback for reaching. These gradually are reduced in subsequent years, as children restrict feedback to the homing-in phase of the reach. (Adapted with permission from Hay L. Developmental changes in eye–hand coordination behaviors: preprogramming versus feedback control. In: Bard C, Fleury M, Hay L, eds. Development of eye–hand coordination across the life span. Columbia, SC: University of South Carolina, 1990:228.)

ing adult levels by 10 to 11 years of age. As we describe in the next section, this reduction in accuracy is reflected in an increased dependence on visual feedback at the age of 7 years. This is one piece of research to support the hypothesis that age 7 is a transition time in the development of reaching (Dellen and Kalverboer, 1984; Hay, 1990).

Other studies analyzing the kinematics of reaching movements without visual feedback in children 5 to 11 also support this hypothesis. Figure 17-6 shows that 5-year-olds produce mainly ballistic movements, with sharp decelerations at the end of the movement (*1, black bars*); this pattern shows a sharp decrease at age 7. At age 7, a ramp and step movement pattern increases (*3, gray bars*). At the same time, ballistic patterns with a smooth deceleration at the end of the movement increase, and they continue to increase through age 9 years (*2, striped bars*). It has been hypothesized that this may be due to the increased use of proprioceptive feedback control in 7-year-olds and the progres-

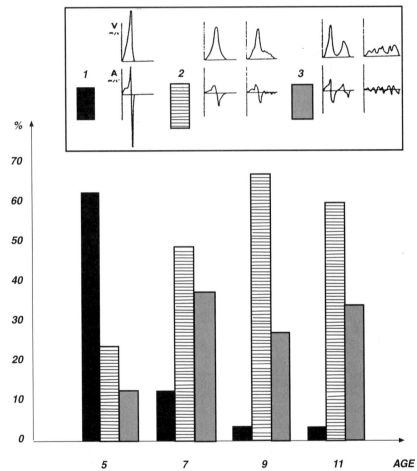

FIGURE 17-6. Percentage of time three reaching movement patterns were seen in children 5 to 11 years of age. 1, ballistic pattern with sharp accelerations and decelerations; 2, ballistic patterns with smooth decelerations; 3, step and ramp patterns. The 5-year-olds use the highest levels of ballistic patterns, while the 7-year-olds use high levels of step and ramp patterns, indicating increased reliance on vision. Children 9 to 11 use the highest levels of ballistic patterns with smooth decelerations, indicating primary use of visual feedback at the end of the movement (Adapted with permission from Hay L. Developmental changes in eye–hand coordination behaviors: preprogramming versus feedback control. In: Bard C, Fleury M, Hay L, eds. Development of eye–hand coordination across the life span. Columbia, SC: University of South Carolina, 1990:231.)

sive restriction of feedback control to the final homing-in phase in older children, possibly the result of increased efficiency of the movement braking system (Hay, 1979).

For a closer look at developmental changes in the use of visual feedback in reaching movements in children, experiments were performed in which children aged 5 to 11 were asked to make reaches while wearing prismatic lenses, which make an illusory shift in the image of the object. These experiments are similar to those described earlier, examining the use of visual feedback in reaching in neonates and infants. As you see in the upper part of Figure 17-7, as the children make a reach, the kinematics of the hand movement show a curved rather than a straight-line trajectory toward the object. This occurs as the hand shifts from an initially incorrect path, because of the shift in the visual image caused by the prismatic lenses, to a correct path when the hand comes into view, based on visual information of the relative hand and target positions. The length of the visually corrected path indicates the amount of visual feedback used in the movement (Hay, 1979).

As evident in the bottom half of Figure 17-7, 5-year-old children corrected the movement late in its trajectory, and in fact, the majority of these children did not make a correction until they reached the virtual target, indicating minimal use of visual feedback. Thus, in this age group, visual control occurs mainly after rather than during reaching movements. This is correlated with the highly stereotyped movement times seen in this age group.

The 7-year-old children corrected the movements earlier than any other group, indicating a strong use of visual feedback. While this gives rise to an increased flexibility in reaching behavior, it is coupled with increased variability in movement times and decreased accuracy when visual feedback is not present.

The 9- and 11-year-olds showed an intermediate level of trajectory correction, indicating a shift in the use of visual control toward the final phase of the movement trajectory. Thus, between 5 and 9 years of age there appears to be a reorganization in the programming of reaching movements from mainly feed-forward or anticipatory activation of reaching to predominant feedback control and finally to an integration of the feed-forward and feedback control, resulting in fast, accurate movements by 9 years of age.

Grasp Development
Emergence of Hand Orientation

When do infants begin to orient their hands to the position and shape of the object? To answer this question, researchers placed brightly colored rods either horizontally or vertically in front of the infant and recorded the characteristics of their reaching movements, as you see in Figure 17-8. Preparatory adjustments of hand orientation (vertical versus horizontal, depending on object orientation) occurred when infants first began to grasp objects, as early as 4.5 to 5 months of age (von Hofsten and Fazel-Zandy, 1984). However, the adjustments of the hand to the orientation of the object became more precise with age. Adjustments of the hand were often done before or during the early part of the reach, though they could also be seen during the approach phase.

To reach smoothly for an object, the infant must time the grasp appropriately with relation to encountering the object. If the hand closes too late, the object will bounce off the palm of the infant, and if the hand closes too early, the object will hit the knuckles. This type of planning requires visual control, since tactile control would not allow the hand to close until after touching the object (von Hofsten and Fazel-Zandy, 1984).

In experiments in which the kinematics of reaching of 5-, 6-, 9-, and 13-month-olds were compared to those of adults, it was shown that infant grasping was visually controlled as early as 5 to 6 months of age, with the hand starting to close in anticipation of reaching the object. Also, the opening of the hand was related to the size of the object for the 9- and 13-month-olds but not in the younger group. Finally, the 13-month-olds initiated the grasp farther from the target than the younger

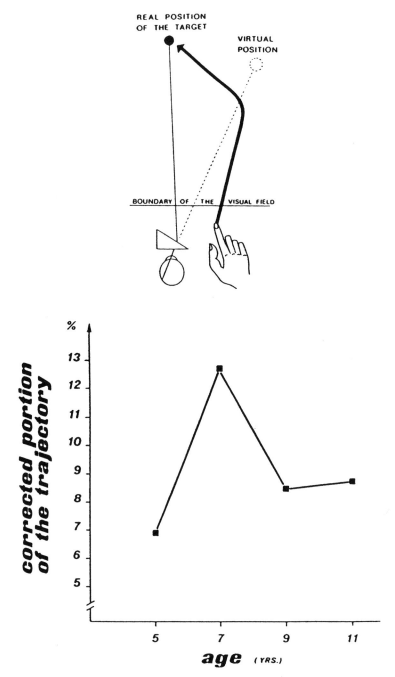

FIGURE 17-7.   *Top.* Diagram of reaching movements of children who wore prismatic lenses, displacing the apparent position of the target in the visual field. *Bottom.* Corrected portion of the reaching trajectory for 5-, 7-, 9-, and 11-year-olds. The 7-year-olds correct the reaching movement much earlier than the other age groups, indicating increased use of visual feedback. (Adapted with permission from Hay L. Spatial-temporal analysis of movements in children: motor programs versus feedback in the development of reaching. J Motor Behav 1979;11:196, 198.)

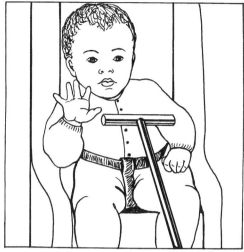

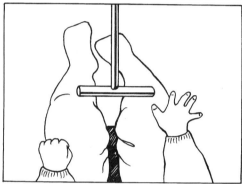

FIGURE 17-8.   Two video camera views of an infant reaching for a horizontal bar. The infant uses correct hand orientation for grasping the bar. (Adapted with permission from von Hofsten C, Fazel-Zandy S. Development of visually guided hand orientation in reaching. J Exp Child Psychol 1984;38:210.)

groups, with timing of the grasp similar to that seen in adults. The grasp component of the reach is still not mature in the 13-month-old, however, since unlike adults, they do not correlate the onset of closing of the hand with the size of the object to be grasped (von Hofsten and Ronnqvist, 1988).

Development of the Pincer Grasp

There are two ways that objects can be grasped. They can be grasped in a power grip, using the palm and palmar surface of the fingers, with the thumb reinforcing this grip, or they can be grasped in a precision grip, between the terminal pads of the finger

and the thumb. The precision grip requires that the fingers be moved independently and is a prerequisite for accurate and skilled movement of objects (Napier, 1956; Forssberg et al., 1991).

In the first months after birth, infant grasping movements are controlled by tactile and proprioceptive reflexes. Thus, when an object contacts the palm, the fingers close. Also, when the arm flexes, the hand closes as part of a flexor synergy. At about 4 months of age, with the onset of functional reaching, the palmar grasp is used exclusively by the infant. With subsequent development, first the thumb and then the fingers begin to operate independently, and at about 9 to 10 months of age, pincer grasp develops (Forssberg et al., 1991).

Developmental changes related to reaching and grasping skills correlate well with research performed on the anatomical development of the primate motor system. It has been shown that in primates, neural pathways controlling movements of the arm are different from those that control the fine movements of the fingers and hand. The two systems develop at different times. Arm control, which appears to be mainly coordinated at the brainstem level, develops earlier than hand and finger control, which appears to be coordinated at the cortical level (Kuypers, 1962, 1964).

Researchers found that infant monkeys show arm movements toward objects early in development but do not show independent finger and hand movements until they are 3 months old (Lawrence and Hopkins, 1972, 1976). It has also been shown that at about 9 to 13 months of age, with the development of the pyramidal tract, infants are able to control fractionated finger movements and thus develop more difficult grasping skills such as the pincer grasp (von Hofsten, 1984).

Recent experiments have followed the development and refinement of precision grasp in human infants and children ranging in age from 8 months to 15 years. Remember from Chapter 16 that when an adult is asked to lift an object, as soon as his or her fingers touch the object, cutaneous recep-

tors activate a centrally programmed response that consists of an increase in grip
forces and load forces designed to lift the object without letting it slip through the fingers. In adults, these two forces are always
programmed in parallel to prevent slips and
to avoid squeezing the object too hard
(Forssberg et al., 1991).

This parallel programming of grip and
load forces was not found in human infants.
In fact, until 5 years of age, the children
pushed the object into the table as they increased the grip force, showing a reversed
coordination between the two forces. In
these children, the grip force had to be very
high before the load force increased. In addition, the timing and sequence of the
phases of lifting were much longer in the infants. For example, the time between first
and second finger contact was three times as
long in 10-month-olds and twice as long in
children up to 3 years of age as in adults. It
was common for the younger children to
have several touches by the thumb and index
finger before the object was properly
gripped. Also, any finger could be the first to
contact the object (Forssberg et al., 1991).

When Do Children Start Using Anticipatory Control in Grasping and Lifting Objects?

In the study just discussed, it was noted
that children below 2 years of age did not increase grip and load forces in parallel but
used a sequential force activation with grip
force increases occurring prior to load force
increases. They also showed force increases
in steps, indicating a feedback strategy, since
the forces were not scaled in one force rate
pulse. In a second study Forssberg et al.
(1992) further examined the development
of this anticipatory control of precision grip,
exploring how weight from the previous lift
is used to scale current forces. They found
that anticipatory control of isometric force
output during lifts with precision grip
emerges during the second year. The children below 18 months of age showed no or
very small differences in force rates for lifts
using different weights, while children older

than 18 months showed this ability. This anticipatory control develops gradually, with
large changes occurring between 1 and 4
years of age, more gradual changes occurring between ages 4 and 11, and adult levels
being reached at about 11 years of age.

They also noted that the younger children used a high grip-to-load force ratio,
particularly in trials with nonslippery objects
(sandpaper) (Forssberg et al., 1995). This
showed their use of a large safety margin
against slips, indicating an immature capacity to adapt to the frictional condition. The
safety margin decreased during the first 5
years of life along with a lower variability in
the grip force and a better adaptation to the
current condition.

They found that by 18 months of age children could adapt grip forces to a surface
condition when the same surface was presented in blocks of trials but failed when the
surface was unexpectedly changed. They
suggest that this may indicate a poor capacity
to form a sensory-motor memory representation of the friction. These memory abilities
increased gradually with age, with older children requiring only a few lifts and adults
only one lift to update their force coordination to a new surface friction.

Learning to Grasp Moving Objects: Catching

Studies have also been performed to determine the emergence of the ability of infants
to reach for and grasp a moving object; this
can be considered a rudimentary form of
catching behavior. Researchers have shown
that by the time infants could reach successfully for unmoving objects, they were also
successful at reaching for moving objects. Infants as young as 18 weeks could catch objects moving at 30 cm/second. At 15 weeks
babies could intercept the object but were
not yet able to grasp it. These results suggest
that infants are able to predict where the object will be at a future point in time because
they must start reaching early to intercept it
in its path. It was noted that the infants did
not automatically reach toward every object
that passed by. Rather, they seemed to be
able to detect in advance whether they had a

reasonable chance to reach it (von Hofsten and Lindhagen, 1979).

Cognitive Components: Emergence of Object Exploration

When do infants first begin to change their manipulative activities in relation to the characteristics of the objects grasped? During the first year, the actions infants perform with objects tend to be mouthing, waving, shaking, or banging. Rigid objects tend to be banged, while spongy objects are squeezed or rubbed (Gibson and Walker, 1984). In studies of 6-, 9-, and 12-month-olds, it was noted that mouthing activity decreased with age and that object rotation, transferring the object between hands and looking at and fingering the object, increased (Corbetta and Mounoud 1990; Ruff, 1984).

At about 1 year of age, infants begin to understand how to use objects, but even before this age, they can discover simple functional relationships if these require little precision. Thus, an infant first uses a spoon for banging or shaking before using it for eating. The infant establishes the relationships between spoon and hand, spoon and mouth, and spoon and plate as subroutines before putting them together for the act of eating: the spoon is filled at the plate and transported to the mouth, which opens in anticipation (Connolly, 1979). At about 14 to 16 months of age, the infant develops the ability to adapt reaching to the weight of objects, using shape and size as indicators of weight (Corbetta and Mounoud, 1990).

At about 16 to 19 months of age, infants begin to understand that certain objects go together culturally, such as a cup in a saucer. Finally, at the end of the second year, they begin to perform symbolic actions, such as pretending to eat or drink (Corbetta and Mounoud, 1990).

After 1 year of age, infants begin to develop skills requiring more precision of movement and closer relationships between objects, such as fitting one object into another. At 13 to 15 months, infants begin piling two cubes on top of each other; at 18 months, three cubes; at 21 months, five

cubes; and at 23 to 24 months, six cubes. This shows that the infant is gradually developing coordinated reaching and manipulation, so that objects can be placed and released carefully (Corbetta and Mounoud, 1990; Bayley, 1969). The application of this concept can be found in Lab Activity 17-1.

 LAB ACTIVITY 17-1

OBJECTIVE: To examine how properties of the task affect reach and grasp movements in children of different ages.

PROCEDURES: For this lab, you will find in your community one child from at least two of the age groups 8 to 12 months, 12 to 18 months, 2 to 3 years, and 4 to 6 years. You will observe them performing certain tasks. Bring with you when you work with the children the following items (you can vary the size of the items so they are appropriate to the size of the child): two small plastic glasses (one with water in it and one empty), a small block (small square object), a crayon (something long and narrow), and a third small plastic glass or a cylinder that you have coated with oil. In the first part of the lab, observe the arm and hand movements of the children while they pick up the plastic glasses, block, crayon, and the plastic glass coated with oil. For the older children, place the two cups (one with water and one without) next to each other. Ask the child to pour you a cup of water. Then try it again, but invert the empty glass and place it near the glass with water.

ASSIGNMENT: Describe how the children of the different age groups reached for and grasped the various objects. When during reach did the hand begin to shape in preparation for grasp? How did characteristics of the object affect anticipatory hand shaping? For the older children, how did changing the orientation of the glass affect their hand orientation? Were they able to modify the orientation of the hand so they did not have to pour the water in multiple steps? Compare the data from the children to your own or other adult reach and grasp characteristics from Lab Activity 16.1. Do your results agree with those of von Hofsten and Forssberg on developmental changes in anticipatory hand shaping and in lifting objects?

℮ THE ROLE OF EXPERIENCE IN THE DEVELOPMENT OF EYE–HAND COORDINATION

Remember that in humans, reaching behavior has two aspects, a visually triggered portion and a visually guided portion. These two aspects of eye–limb coordination are also found in cats. Elegant studies on the development of these two aspects of eye–limb coordination have shown that movement-produced visual feedback experience is essential to the development of the visually guided portion of reaching (Hein and Held, 1967).

In these experiments, kittens were raised in the dark until they were 4 weeks of age and then allowed to move freely for 6 hours each day in a normal environment. But during this time, they wore lightweight opaque collars that kept them from seeing their limbs and torso. This is shown in Figure 17-9A. For the rest of the day, they remained in the dark. After 12 days of this treatment, the animals were tested for the presence of visually triggered versus visually guided placing reactions. This was accomplished by lowering the kitten toward a continuous surface (requires only visually triggered placing, since accuracy is not required) versus a discontinuous surface, made up of prongs (requires visually guided placing to hit the prong). All animals showed a visually triggered placing reaction, in which they automatically extended the forelimb toward a continuous surface. But they showed no greater than chance hits for a placing reaction to a pronged surface (Fig. 17-9B). However, after removal of the collar, the animals required only 18 hours in a normal environment before showing visually guided placing. It was thus concluded that visually triggered paw extension develops without sight, but visually guided paw placing requires prolonged viewing of the limbs (Hein and Held, 1967).

The researchers then asked what kind of contact with the environment is important for visually guided behavior. Is passive contact sufficient, or must it be active? To answer this question, they tested 10 pairs of kit-

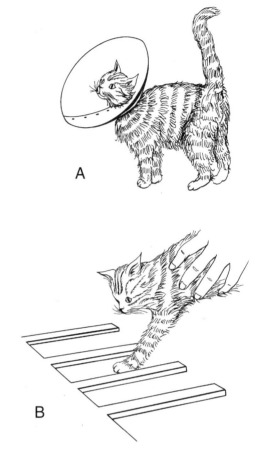

FIGURE 17-9.   A. Experimental collar worn by kittens to block their view of their paws during early development. **B.** Pronged apparatus for testing visually guided reaching. (Adapted with permission from Hein A, Held R. Dissociation of the visual placing response into elicited and guided components. Science 1967;158:391.)

tens. One kitten of each pair was able to walk freely in a circular room, pulling a gondola, and the other kitten was placed in the gondola and was passively pulled around the room. This is shown in Figure 17-10. Thus, both kittens had similar visual feedback and motion cues, but for the kittens who walked, the cues were active, and for the kittens who rode, they were passive.

The kittens had experience with the apparatus for 3 hours a day. At the end of the experiment, the active animals showed normal visually guided placing reactions and responses to a visual cliff test, in which a normal animal does not walk out over an illusory cliff, but the passive animals did not. Thus,

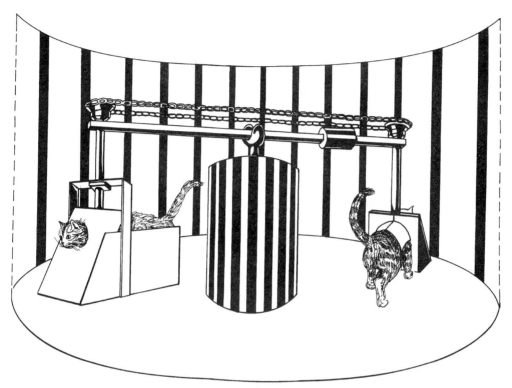

FIGURE 17-10.   Experimental apparatus in which one cat actively pulls the second cat, which is passively pulled in the gondola. (Adapted with permission from Held R, Hein A. Movement-produced stimulation in the development of visually guided behavior. J Compar Physiol Psychol 1963;56:873.)

the researchers concluded that self-produced movement is necessary for the development of visually guided behavior. However, once again, after 48 hours in a normal environment, the passive group of animals showed normal visually guided paw placement (Held and Hein, 1963).

✑ REACTION TIME REACHING TASKS

A great deal of research has been performed on developmental changes in reaction time tasks. In general, it has been shown that reaction times for simple tasks become faster as children mature. The greatest changes occur until about 8 to 9 years of age, with slower changes occurring subsequently, until reaction times reach adult levels at 16 to 17 years. However, when children are asked to perform more complex movements as

part of the reaction time task, these developmental changes vary according to the task. For example, in a study in which 2- to 8-year-old children were asked to make target aiming movements, a decrease in reaction time was observed from 2 to 5 years of age, followed by a stabilization in reaction time (Hay, 1990; Brown et al., 1986).

Movement time in these reaction time tasks also changes as a function of age. Remember from Chapter 16 that movement time depends on the accuracy and distance requirements of a task. Strategies for programming movements also vary, depending on whether the movement requires an accurate stop or not. If an accurate stop is required, the individual must use a braking action controlled by antagonist muscles. Alternatively, if the movement can be stopped automatically by hitting a target, antagonist muscle activation is not required.

Studies analyzing movement time for either type of movement in children 6 to 10 years of age have shown a reduction in movement time with increased age. As might be expected, movements that require an accurate stop are slower at all ages. However, the difference between the speed of the two types of movements is about three times as high at 6 years of age as at 8 to 10 years of age. It has been hypothesized that this is due to a difficulty experienced by the 6-year-olds in modulating the braking action of the antagonist muscle system (Hay et al., 1986).

Fitts' Law

Remember from Chapter 16 that Fitts' law shows a specific relationship between the time to make a movement and the amplitude

and accuracy of that movement. The difficulty of the task is related both to the accuracy and the amplitude requirements and is represented by the following equation:

$$ID = \log_2(2A/W)$$

where A = amplitude of the movement, W = width of the target, and ID = index of difficulty (Fitts, 1954).

Studies testing the extent to which Fitts' law applies to children have found that movement time decreases with age. This decrease is in general a linear change except for a regression that appears to occur at about 7 years of age. Remember that in the development of postural control there is also a regression, as indicated by an increase in postural response latencies, between 4 and 6 years of age. A study examin-

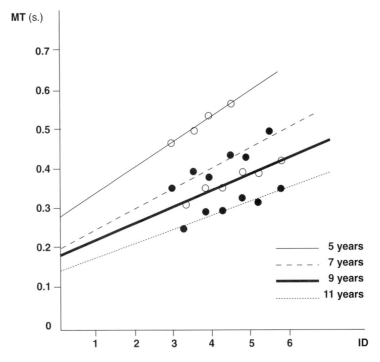

FIGURE 17-11. Relationship between movement time (MT, seconds) and the index of difficulty (ID) of a task, for four age groups of children. The intercept of the line with the y-axis reflects the general efficiency of the motor system, while the slope of the line reflects the amount of information per second that can be processed by the motor system. Almost all studies have shown that the y-intercept decreases with age, indicating increased efficiency. (Adapted with permission from Hay L. Developmental changes in eye–hand coordination behaviors: preprogramming versus feedback control. In: Bard C, Fleury M, Hay L, eds. Development of eye–hand coordination across the life span. Columbia, SC: University of South Carolina, 1990:227.)

LAB ACTIVITY 17-2

OBJECTIVE: To examine the effect of age on the ability of children to perform reciprocal tapping. Remember, Fitts defined task difficulty in terms of target size (W, the width of the target) and the distance to move (D, the distance between targets). He thus quantified task difficulty (which he called index of difficulty, or ID) by using the following equation: ID = $\log_2(2D/W)$.

PROCEDURE: For this lab you will find in your community a child from at least two of the age groups 5 years, 7 years, 9 years, and 11 years). You will observe them performing the following task. Bring with you when you work with the child a pencil and six pieces of paper, one for each of the three trials in each task. The papers should already be marked with appropriate target sizes and distances (see next paragraph). Ask the children to tap quickly and accurately between the two targets that vary in width and distance. The objective is to make as many *accurate* tapping movements as possible in a 10-second period. Accuracy is important. Remind them that there should be no more errors made in the more difficult task than in the easier one. If the number of errors exceeds more than 5% of the pencil dots, the trial should be done again.

Two combinations of task difficulty will be used. The first and easiest task has D = 2 cm and W = 2 cm. Solving the equation for ID, that would be log (base 2) of (2 × 2)/2. This works out to the $\log_2$ of 2, which is 1. The most difficult task has D = 16 cm and W = 1 cm. That is, the $\log_2$ of (2 × 16)/1, which is 5.

Each child will perform three trials (10 seconds each) for the two task conditions. You will time each trial and count and record the number of dots in each target. Tell the child when to start and stop on each 10-second trial (use a watch with a second hand). The rest interval between trials should be the amount of time needed to count and record the taps.

ASSIGNMENT: Make a table with a record of the number of taps on each of the three trials for both the easy and difficult task, for each child. Calculate the mean and standard deviation as well. For each task, calculate the average movement time in milliseconds for a single movement of the tapping task. Do this by dividing each number of taps by 10, which will give you the number of taps per second during the 10-second trial. Record this value in the table. Next, take the inverse of this number (1/x, where x is the average number of taps). Multiply this number by 1000 to obtain the average movement time in milliseconds. Record this average movement time in the table for each child. How did the difficulty of the task affect movement time for children in the different age groups? How did the children's performance change with increasing age? Compare your results with those of others in the class. Did you find a regression (slowing) in movement time for 7-year-olds compared to the younger and older children?

ing 5- to 9-year-olds has shown that these developmental decreases and regressions in movement time are not related to any changes in biomechanical factors, such as growth of the bones of the arm (Rey, 1968; Shumway-Cook and Woollacott, 1985a; Kerr, 1975).

Using Fitts' law, one can plot movement time as a function of index of difficulty for different age groups. This relationship is shown in Figure 17-11. The intercept of the line with the y-axis reflects the general efficiency of the motor system, while the slope of the line reflects the amount of information that can be processed per second by the motor system. Almost all studies have shown that the y-intercept decreases with age, indicating increased efficiency. However, age-related improvements in slope appear to depend on the task involved and appear to be more evident in discrete than in serial movements (Hay, 1990; Sugden, 1980). The application of this concept can be found in Lab Activity 17-2.

In summary, the emergence of reach, grasp, and manipulation occurs gradually during development and is characterized by changes in many systems. With the emergence and refinement of these skills, one sees changes in timing, coordination, and modulation of forces used for reach and grasp. We now examine age-related changes in reach, grasp, and manipulation.

@ CHANGES IN OLDER ADULTS

As we have noted in previous chapters on age-related changes in postural control and mobility skills, there are specific changes in these skills with age. These can be divided into (*a*) time-related changes, such as slowing of onset latencies for postural response or decreased movement speed in locomotion; (*b*) coordination factors related to changes in movement or muscle activation patterns; and (*c*) changes in the use of feedback and feed-forward control of both postural and mobility skills. We will find that these same factors are important to consider in examining age-related changes in reaching and grasping skills.

Reaching: Changes With Age

Changes in Reaching Movement Time With Age

A review of studies examining changes in the speed of reaching movements with age has shown that discrete reaching movements show a range of 30% to 90% reduction in velocity with aging, depending on the ages compared and the task performed. For example, one study examining changes in the speed of discrete arm movements showed a 32% reduction between ages 50 and 90 years, while another showed a reduction in movement speed of 90% comparing subjects aged 20 to 69 years performing a repetitive tapping task (Welford, 1982; Williams, 1990).

What are some of the age-related changes in different systems of the body that may contribute to this slowing in reaching movements? Different systems that may contribute to the slowing include (*a*) sensory and perceptual systems, such as the visual system's ability to detect the target; (*b*) central processing systems; (*c*) motor systems; and (*d*) arousal and motivational systems (Welford, 1982).

Welford performed an experiment to determine if changes in central mechanisms contribute to the slowing in reaching speed in older adults. In these experiments, subjects were asked to keep a pointer (which they could move with a handle) in line with a target that continuously moved from side to side in an irregular sinusoidal fashion, with the movement varying in both speed and extent. He found that as the speed of the

target movement increased, the subjects could follow it less easily until at some point it was impossible to follow.

However, there was a difference between the older and younger subjects. As you see in Figure 17-12, the older adults dropped off in their ability to follow the movements sooner than the young adults. Welford hypothesized that the limitation in the performance of the older adults was not due to problems with the motor system, because they could move faster if they were not following the target. He hypothesized that the limitation was not sensory, because the older adults could easily see the target. Therefore, he concluded that the limitation was in central processing abilities, that is, in the older adults' ability to match the target and pointer and react quickly to changes in target direction. This implies that the time spent in actual movement itself slows little compared to the time taken to make decisions about the next part of the movement sequence (Welford, 1977).

Changes in Reaching Coordination With Age

Motion analysis of the trajectories of older adults performing rapid aiming movements has indicated that they spend more time in the target approach or deceleration phase than do young adults. This is the period of sensory processing that ensures accuracy in reaching the target. A number of studies have explored possible contributing factors to this slowing in the target approach phase. A study by Pohl et al. (1996) compared the movements of young (mean age 25 years) and older (mean age 71 years) adults in a reciprocal tapping task with differing accuracy requirements (8-cm- versus 2-cm-wide targets 37 cm apart). They noted that the older adults showed significantly more movement adjustments coupled with a longer absolute adjustment time and a longer reversal time when moving between the two targets. The authors suggest that the young adults used more on-line and feed-forward processes in achieving the goals of speed and accuracy in movement, while the older adults relied more on slower feedback processes. The ap-

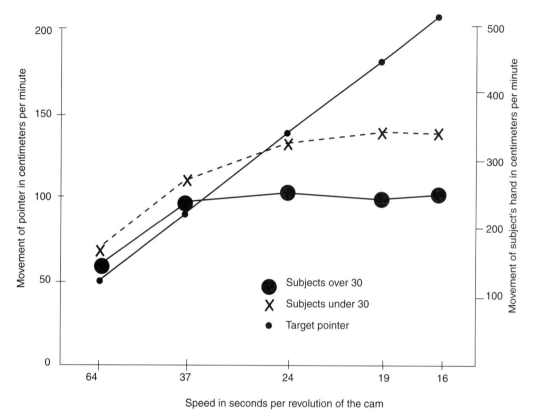

FIGURE 17-12.   Ability of young versus older adults to follow unpredictable target movements of different speeds. Older adults have more problems following the target movements at higher speeds. (Adapted with permission from Welford AT. Motor skills and aging. In: Mortimer JA, Pirozzolo FJ, Maletta GJ, eds. The aging motor system. New York: Praeger, 1982 : 159.)

plication of this concept can be found in Lab Activity 17-3.

Additional studies of movement kinematics in young versus older adults used a zigzag drawing task to three target sizes, 5, 10, and 20 mm (a digitizing tablet was used) and compared subjects at similar movement speeds (Morgan et al., 1994). Older adults showed comparable overall accuracy on the tasks but again showed more hesitancy and submovements, implying more reliance on visual guidance. The authors concluded that this indicates a central deficit in motor coordination. Other research has examined changes in force production during reaching movements in older adults and shown similar discontinuities in their movement trajectories (Vrtunski and Patterson, 1985). It is interesting to remember that increased

 LAB ACTIVITY 17-3

OBJECTIVE: To examine the effect of aging on the ability to perform a reciprocal tapping task.

PROCEDURE: Repeat the procedure from Lab 17-2, but with an older adult (70 years or older) from your community.

ASSIGNMENT: Repeat the assignment from Lab 17-2, with the following changes in questions. How did the difficulty of the task affect movement time for the older adult compared to your own or other young adult times from Lab 16-2? Did you notice any additional movement or hesitancy in making the movements? Do you think that the fitness level of the older adult would affect performance on the task?

submovements were characteristic of early reaching patterns in normal infants (von Hofsten, 1993). Like older adults, these submovements in infants are often associated with strong reliance on visual feedback during reaching (Hay, 1979).

It has also been shown that hand steadiness during reaching tasks decreases with age (Williams, 1990). When older adults were asked to insert a small stylus in slots of different diameters (half an inch to an eighth of an inch), steadiness dropped by 77% from the 50s to the 90s. Steadiness deteriorated faster in the nonpreferred hand than in the preferred hand.

Based on the literature, there appears to be little change with age in performance speed for reaching movements if subjects are asked to repeat the same simple action, such as tapping a pencil between two targets or performing a simple reaction time task (Welford 1977, 1982). In this case, the slowing may be as little as 16%. But if the complexity of the task is increased by making the target smaller, using successive targets, or using a choice reaction time task, slowing can range from 86% to 276%. Table 17-1 gives

examples of these differences in slowing of the performance of reaching movements with complexity of the task. The largest slowing in performance was in tasks involving symbolic translations (using a code to relate a stimulus to a response) or spatial transpositions (for example, a light cue on the left requiring a reach to the right). Though decrements have been found in performance on many reaction time tasks, a recent study has also shown that when older adults are not instructed to worry about accuracy on such a task, they demonstrate no decrease in reaching speed (Williamson et al., 1993).

The primary source of the slowing in complex reaction time tasks is in the first phase of performance, the time to observe the signals and relate them to action, rather than in the second phase, the time to execute the movement (Welford, 1977, 1982). When performing more continuous tasks, the second phase, that of movement execution, can overlap to some extent with the first. For example, a person may process the information relating to the next signal while making the first response. This type of task appears to be more difficult for older adults, possibly

---

TABLE 17-1.   Age-Related Slowing in the Performance of Reaching Movements as a Function of Task Complexity

Task	Age Groups Compared	Percentage Increase[a]
Simple key press or release to light or sound		
Average of 11 studies listed by Welford	20s, with 60s	16%
Ten-choice (Birren, Riegel, and Morrison, 1962)	18–33 with 65–72	
Straightforward relationship		27
With numerical code, mean of 5 studies		50
With verbal code, mean of two studies		45
With color code		94
With part color and part letter code		86
Ten-choice (Kay 1954, 1955)	25–34 with 65–72	
a. Signal lights immediately above response keys		−13 (no errors made)
b. Signal lights 3 ft from keys		26 (−43)
c. As b, but signal lights arranged so that leftmost responded to with rightmost key, and so forth		46 (−19)
d. With numerical code		56 (+138)
e. The difficulties of d and b combined		299 (+464)

[a] Percentage changes of errors are shown in parentheses.
Adapted with permission from Welford AT. Motor skills and aging. In: Mortimer JA, Pirozzolo FJ, Maletta GJ, eds. The aging motor system. NY: Praeger, 1962:163.

because they need more time to monitor their responses and thus have difficulty processing other signals simultaneously (Welford, 1982).

Adults 63 to 76 years old were compared to adults 19 to 29 years old on a task for which they moved as quickly as possible to one of two alternative end points, with one farther away than the other, in the same direction (Rabbit and Rogers, 1965). The younger subjects could overlap the time required to choose the end point with the initial stages of the movement itself, while the older subjects were less able to do this. Although there is no evidence that the time taken for monitoring increases with age, older adults seem less able to suppress monitoring.

What might be reasons for this lack of suppression? It has been hypothesized that suppression of monitoring occurs when the outcome of a task is certain; thus, if there is a possibility of error, monitoring is more probable. In addition, suppression of monitoring may be possible when movement subunits are coordinated into higher units of performance (Welford, 1982). However, to do this often requires that the subject hold the movement subunits together in working memory while performing the task.

A study tested this ability in older (ages 60 to 81) versus young (ages 17 to 28) adults. Subjects were asked to perform two serial key-pressing tasks, one that had few subunits (12, 12, 12, and so on) and one that was more complex (1234, 32, 1234, and so on). They found that the older adults were slower than the young adults, particularly with the second series (Rabbitt and Birren, 1967).

Grasping: Changes With Age

One of the problems faced by older adults is a decrease in their manual dexterity, which becomes apparent in such tasks as tying shoelaces and fastening buttons. For example, time required to manipulate a small object increases 25% to 40% by 70 years of age (Cole, 1991; Agnew et al., 1982) These age-related changes have been explored by measuring the fingertip forces used to grip and lift objects in experiments similar to those

performed with young children, described earlier. It is known that tactile sensation is reduced in older adults, which may affect their ability to detect how strongly they are holding an object.

Studies by Cole and colleagues (Cole, 1991; Cole et al., 1999) have shown that older adults (mean age 81 years) used grasp forces that were on average twice as large as those of young adults, with some older adults producing forces that were many times larger than the young adults' mean. Figure 17-13 shows examples of grasp force records for young versus older adults for their third trial picking up an object covered with sandpaper and their first and third trials picking up a slippery object (covered with rayon). Note that the older subject shows much larger grasp forces and takes longer to adapt to the final grasp force for the rayon object than the young adult. Variability of grip forces across trials was also much higher in the older than the young adults. A portion of the increased force was due to increased skin slipperiness. In addition, the older adults

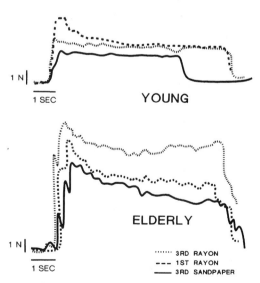

FIGURE 17-13. Grasp force traces from a young subject and an older adult showing typical grasp force patterns when lifting an object with a nonslippery (sandpaper) versus slippery (rayon) surface. Traces indicate the third lift with sandpaper, followed by the first and third rayon trials. N, newton. (Reprinted with permission from Cole KJ. Grasp force control in older adults. J Motor Behav 1991;23:255.)

LAB ACTIVITY 17-4

OBJECTIVE: To examine how properties of the task affect reach and grasp movements in older adults.

PROCEDURES: For this lab, you will repeat Lab Activity 17-1, but now you will find an adult 70 years or older in your community and observe him or her performing the tasks described in Lab Activity 17-1.

ASSIGNMENT: Describe how the older adult reached for and grasped the various objects. When during the reach for an object did the hand begin to shape in preparation for grasp? How did characteristics of the object affect anticipatory hand shaping? Compare the data from the older adult to young adult reach and grasp characteristics from Lab Activity 16.1. Do your results agree with those of Cole et al. (1991) regarding ability to change lift forces easily with changing object surface characteristics?

simply produced a higher margin of safety against object slippage (Cole, 1991).

Additional experiments have examined whether this increased safety margin is due to decreased tactile sensation or decreased ability to encode skin–object frictional properties (Cole et al., 1999). They argue that declining cutaneous afferent function contributes to safety margin increases after about 60 years of age. They noted that grip force adjustments in older adults to new surfaces were delayed about 100 msec compared to young adults. Previous research has shown that friction is signaled locally by fast-adapting afferents, which decrease in number with age, and this may account for the delays in force adjustments. The application of this concept can be found in Lab Activity 17-4.

Compensation and Reversibility of Decrements in Reaching Performance

Although decrements in reaching performance may be found in older adults in experimental conditions, they are often not observed in the workplace or in activities of daily living. It has been suggested that performance is preserved because many compensatory strategies are used to improve reach and grasp skills. Many compensatory strategies used by older adults appear to be unconscious, automatic processes. For example, older adults may increase the effort they put into the movement. In the workplace, they may work more continuously with fewer brief pauses. They may also prepare for movements that require speed and accuracy in advance, thus allowing anticipatory processes to aid in performance. In many tasks, they may also make a trade-off between speed and accuracy. Finally, it has also been shown that older adults set higher criteria for responding to reaction time signals in sensory discrimination tasks (Welford, 1982).

Can the changes in reaching skills that occur with aging be counteracted by practice or training? Yes! Clear improvement with practice has been reported for eye–hand coordination skills in older adults (Falduto and Baron, 1986). Greatest improvement is seen in complex tasks. Interestingly, older adults show more improvement with practice on performance of reaction time tasks than do younger adults (Jordan and Rabbitt, 1977). This may occur because young adults are closer to their ceiling of performance when starting to learn the task. However, practice does not eliminate the age differences in the performance of these tasks.

Practice in older adults also improves performance related to the perceptual processes involved in eye–hand coordination tasks, such as visual acuity, signal detection, and auditory discrimination. In addition, the effects of practice remain high, even 1 month after practice on eye–hand coordination tasks has ended. One study compared the performance of adults aged 19 to 27 with that of adults aged 62 to 73 on a task, called "Space Trek," that involved fine movements of the hands, signal detection, memory scanning, visual discrimination, and anticipation timing. Subjects were given 51 hour-long practice sessions over 2 to 5 months. One month after training ended, there was only a small decrease in performance levels (Welford, 1982).

In another study, adults aged 57 to 83 were given practice in eye–hand coordination skills by playing video games. These games involved making fast decisions about changes in the speed and direction of hand movements. Over a 7-week period, scores tripled on the task. In addition, practice on the video games transferred to other reaction time tasks that required subjects to quickly select a motor response (Clark et al., 1987).

These studies suggest that with practice older adults learn as much or more than young adults and that they retain the learned skills as well as young adults. In addition, the way subjects improved with practice was similar for the young and older adults; however, the older adults simply learned more slowly. This slower rate of learning of eye–hand coordination skills in older subjects may be due to material taking longer to register in long-term memory (Welford, 1982).

What does this mean in terms of determining the best strategies for teaching eye–hand coordination skills to older adults? Since the time required for registering information in long-term memory lengthens with age, learning must be unhurried. Otherwise extra information to be processed during the time required to register information in longer-term memory will simply disrupt the memory process.

In teaching eye–hand coordination skills, there are sometimes problems in translating verbal instruction into motor performance. To avoid this, one can use demonstrations. However, in this case, the pace of the demonstration should be under the learner's control. Thus, using slow-motion, self-paced videos in training may help (Welford, 1982).

Active decision making is also an important factor in learning at any age. In a maze study with adults, it was shown that learning took place much faster if the correct pathway was marked but the subject had to make an active choice. This helped subjects of all ages, but it especially helped older adults (von Wright, 1957). It was also shown that using a mixture of mental practice and physical practice when learning a pursuit rotor task was as good as physical practice alone

for 65- to 69- and 80- to 100-year-olds (Surberg, 1976).

Thus, learning of eye–hand coordination tasks by older adults can be facilitated by using a type of discovery learning employing demonstrations that can be self-paced, active learning, and a combination of physical and mental practice (Welford, 1982).

During development, the emergence of mature reach and grasp behavior is characterized by a reduction in reaction time, a decrease in safety margins during grip and lift, and a reduction in the number of subunits during the reaching movement, resulting in a smoother trajectory. Similarly, a decline in reach and grasp with aging is characterized by an increase in reaction time, an increase in safety margins, and an increase in the number of subunits contributing to a reaching movement. Multiple factors may be contributing to these characteristic changes across the life span. These include both primary deficits in the nervous and musculoskeletal systems and secondary strategies used to compensate for these deficits.

⊘ SUMMARY

1. Infants as young as a week old show prereaching behaviors, reaching toward objects that are in front of them. These reaches are not accurate, and the infants do not grasp the object, since an extension synergy controls the arm and hand movements. When the arm is extended, the hand is open. But the reaches are clearly aimed at the object, since they are significantly more accurate than arm movements when the eyes are not fixated on the object.

2. At about 2 months, the extension synergy is broken up, so that the fingers flex as the arm extends. At this time, head and arm movements become coupled as the infant gains control over the neck muscles.

3. At about 4 months, infants begin to gain trunk stability along with a progressive uncoupling of head, arm, and hand synergies. These changes allow the emer-

gence of functional reach and grasp behavior.

4. From 4 months onward, reaching becomes more refined, with the approach
path straightening and the number of
segments of the reach being reduced.

5. Visually triggered reaching is dominant
in the newborn, changing to visually
guided reaching at about 5 months of
age and returning to visually triggered
reaching by 1 year of age, though
guided reaching is still available.

6. The development of hand orientation
begins to occur at the onset of successful reaching, at about 5 months of age.

7. The pincer grasp develops at about 9 to
10 months of age, along with the development of the pyramidal tract.

8. Reaction time shows a progressive reduction with age, with sharper changes
occurring until 8 to 9 years, followed by
slower changes until 16 to 17 years.

9. Children aged 4 to 6 years make predominantly visually triggered (feed-forward) movements, using little visual
feedback. At 7 to 8 years, visual feedback is dominant, leading to poor
reaching in the dark but more accurate
reaching with vision present. By 9 to 11
years, feed-forward and feed-back
movements are integrated.

10. Older adults show a slowing in reaching
movements, with much of this due to
slowing of central processing. The slowing in performance on reaching movements is greater for complex tasks than
for simple ones.

11. Part of the slowing may result from an
inability to suppress monitoring of
movements because of either uncertainty concerning the accuracy of the
movement or inability to integrate
movement subunits into larger chunks
in working memory.

12. Most age-related decrements in reaching performance can be improved with
training. Training effects remain high
for at least a month after training has
ended and also transfer to other reaching tasks.

CHAPTER 18

Abnormal Reach, Grasp, and Manipulation

@ INTRODUCTION

Normal upper extremity function, including the ability to reach for, grasp, and manipulate objects, is the basis for fine motor skills important to activities such as feeding, dressing, grooming, and handwriting. In addition, upper extremity function plays an important role in gross motor skills, such as crawling, walking, recovering balance, and protecting the body from injury when recovery is not possible. Because upper extremity control is intertwined with both fine and gross motor skills, recovery of upper extremity function is an important aspect of retraining the patient with impaired motor control and falls within the purview of most areas of rehabilitation, including both occupational and physical therapy.

This chapter focuses on understanding problems related to reach, grasp, and manipulation in the patient with neurological pathology. We first review problems related to the key components of upper extremity control, incorporating a discussion of sensory, motor, and higher-level problems that affect the key components, including (*a*) locating a target, involving the coordinated movement of the eyes, head, and trunk; (*b*) reaching, involving transportation of the arm and hand in space as well as postural support; (*c*) grasp, including grip formation, grasp, and release; and (*d*) in-hand manipulation skills. We then use a case study approach to explore the types of upper extremity problems found in patients with specific types of neurological diagnoses.

✆ TARGET LOCATION PROBLEMS: EYE–HEAD COORDINATION

A critical aspect of manipulatory dysfunction is the inability to locate a target and maintain one's gaze on that target before a reach. Remember from Chapters 16 and 17 that some target location tasks require eye movements alone, while others require a combination of eye and head movement and still other tasks require a combination of eye, head, and trunk movements, depending on the eccentricity of the target in space. This has led researchers to suggest that eye–head coordination is not controlled by a single mechanism but rather emerges from an interaction of several different neural mechanisms (Jeannerod, 1990).

What types of problems affect the ability to locate a target in space, then maintain a stable gaze position during head movements toward it? Problems affecting target localization and gaze stabilization include (*a*) disruption of visually driven eye movements because of damage within the oculomotor system; (*b*) damage to the vestibular system, which disrupts vestibulo-ocular reflex control of eye movements in response to head movements; and (*c*) inability to adapt the vestibulo-ocular reflex to changes in task demands because of cerebellar damage (Martin et al., 1993). All of these types of problems affect the patient's ability to stabilize gaze on an object when moving the head. However, in this chapter we focus primarily on problems related to visually driven eye movements.

Visual Deficits and Object Localization

Central lesions affecting the processing of visual signals impair the ability to locate a target or object in space. Visual field deficits following a stroke, such as homonymous hemianopsia, restrict a patient's ability to see objects in half of the visual field, affecting reach and grasp in the contralesional hemifield (Jeannerod, 1990). Visual neglect and visual extinction are often the consequence of right cerebral hemisphere damage. Neglect patients show a profound lack of awareness of the contralesional side of personal and external space, while extinction patients fail to detect contralesional stimuli for the most part under conditions of bilateral stimulus. It is unclear whether neglect and extinction are related to sensory, attentional, or other factors.

In both visual neglect and extinction, the relative location of the target appears to influence the patient's ability to detect an object or target in space. Smania et al. (1998) examined the spatial distribution of visual attention in subjects with right hemispheric damage and either hemineglect or extinction. Subjects were required to press the space bar of a portable computer after the appearance of a light flash in one of four positions (10, 20, 30 or 40 degrees along the horizontal meridian) presented in either the left or right visual field. Both the neglect and the extinction group were less able to detect targets presented in their left hemifield. In addition, impairments in detecting targets increased with target eccentricity. This study reminds us that patients with right hemisphere damage who also have left unilateral neglect have difficulty reaching for objects presented on the left side of their body because of difficulty in locating objects presented in their left visual field. In addition, the more eccentric the target, the more difficulty the patient will have in reaching.

Until recently, pathology causing lesions in the visual cortex of humans was thought to cause total blindness except for a rudimentary ability to detect changes in illumination. However, recently it has been shown that monkeys with lesions in the striate cortex are still able to reach toward objects moving across their visual field (Humphrey and Weiskrantz, 1969). It has been hypothesized that these reaching movements may be due to visual processing in subcortical structures, such as the superior colliculus.

Research with humans has confirmed these findings. When patients were not asked whether they could see the object but simply to move their eyes toward where they thought the object might be, the direction and amplitude of their eye movements were significantly correlated with the position of the targets (Peoppel, 1973).

Experiments have been performed on subjects with hemianopia due to a hemispherectomy on one side (Perenin and Jeannerod, 1978). Patients with hemianopia were asked to point to the target when it appeared in either their normal visual field or their affected field. When it was in the affected field, they were asked to guess where it was and to point there, since patients said that they couldn't see it. Again, pointing positions in the hemianopic field were definitely correlated with the target positions.

Although subjects were initially very poor at reaching for objects in this manner, their performance improved with training. If they were simply told that the target would appear at a different location for each trial, with practice they showed a clear and rapid improvement in their abilities (Zihl and Werth, 1984).

Patients with parietal lesions also show problems with eye movements when these movements are a part of exploratory visual searches or reaching behavior. They may have problems breaking visual fixation (Balint's syndrome) or optic ataxia; they also may have slowed reaction time for saccades, with the saccades subdivided into staircase patterns (Balint, 1909; Waters et al., 1978).

Visual deficits affecting target localization also appear to affect hand motor function. Van Donkelaar and Lee (1994) tested the hypothesis that interactions between eye and hand movements occur when they are produced in conjunction with one another. They compared kinematic output of the eye and hand motor systems in both normal control subjects and subjects with cerebellar pathology during the performance of two tasks: (*a*) while tracking a moving target with the hand and (*b*) while performing a pointing movement to intercept a target. As one might expect, the subjects with cerebellar damage were slower to begin tracking the visual target and had less accurate and more variable hand movements than the control subjects. Interestingly, a large amount of the

increased variability in hand movements occurred just prior to and after each corrective eye movement (ocular saccade) made to track the object. The increased variability in hand movements could be decreased when vision of the hand was restricted. This can be seen in Figure 18-1. Figure 18-1*A* shows that in a normal control subject, variability of hand velocity does not change in the three visual conditions, normal, visual fixation and restricted vision (that is, the individual cannot see the hand). In contrast, Figure 18-1*B* indicates that hand velocity in a subject with cerebellar damage is greatest when under unrestricted visual conditions (*Normal*) and

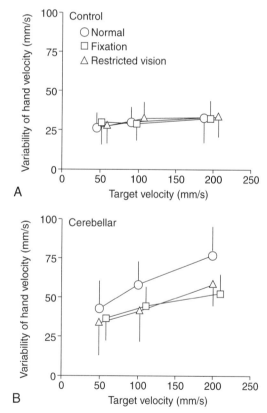

FIGURE 18-1.   A comparison of hand velocity variability produced in a tracking task during normal visual conditions (normal), when eye motion is restricted (fixation), and when vision of the hand is restricted (restricted vision) in a healthy control (**A**) and a subject with cerebellar pathology (**B**). (Adapted with permission from Van Donkelaar P, Lee RG. Interactions between the eye and hand motor systems: disruptions due to cerebellar dysfunction. J Neurophysiol 1994;72:1679.)

is reduced when vision is restricted. The authors conclude that there is a reciprocal interaction between the eye and hand motor systems. In addition, in cerebellar subjects, problems affecting the output of one system adversely affect the other, so that inaccuracies in hand movements are influenced by inaccuracies in eye movements and vice versa.

⊘ REACH AND GRASP PROBLEMS

As we mentioned earlier, reaching is controlled by a different neural mechanism from that of grasping; hence, patients can have impaired reach but intact grasp or vice-versa. For many patients who are neurologically impaired, however, both reach and grasp are affected, reflecting dysfunction in the multiple systems controlling upper extremity function. Separating the two, while artificial, makes it easier to analyze problems in each. However, it is important to remember that because of their close coordination and synchronization, pathology affecting one often disrupts the other.

Problems With Reach

Remember that during normal reaching, movement trajectories involving more than one joint tend to be straight and smooth and to have bell-shaped velocity profiles (Hogan et al., 1987). In contrast, movement trajectories in patients with neurological pathology are often characterized by loss of coordinated coupling between synergistic muscles and joints. Disruptions in the coordination of movements can affect the timing and trajectory of movements.

Motor Problems

Timing Problems

Studies on reach and grasp have consistently shown delayed movement times in most types of neural pathology. For example, studies examining reach in patients with hemiparesis following stroke found longer movement times in the involved arm than in nondisabled subjects. Prolonged movement times were associated with disruptions of interjoint coordination between the elbow and shoulder (Levin et al., 1993; Levin, 1996).

Steenbergen et al. (1998) studied children with hemiplegia secondary to cerebral palsy and found that total movement time, including both time to contact and time in contact with an object, was longer in the involved hand than in the noninvolved hand. They suggested that increased time to contact arose from problems in the reach or transport phase of the movement, while the increase in time in contact was probably the result of impaired sequencing of grip and lift forces.

Forsstrom and von Hofsten (1982) also studied children with cerebral palsy (either ataxic or athetoid) and found longer transport phases than in nondisabled children. Interestingly, despite their motor impairments, the disabled children were able to reach for and grasp even quickly moving targets. The researchers found that the children aimed their reaches well ahead of the moving targets. This suggests that when planning a reaching movement, the children were able to compensate for deficits that resulted in slowed movement times. They aimed their movements enough ahead of the target so they could sustain accuracy when reaching despite their movement impairments.

Reaching in patients with cerebellar dysfunction is also characterized by delayed movement times. Van Donkelaar and Lee (1994) found both response (reaction) and movement times were prolonged when reaching to moving targets. They suggest that delays in timing may be due to the patient's need for more time to determine target velocity information.

Delayed movement times, then, are a common feature of reaching in patients with a wide variety of neural pathologies. One factor implicated in prolonged movement times is a disruption to the coordination of multijoint movements.

Problems With Interjoint Coordination

Normally, elbow and shoulder joint angles change smoothly and at synchronized rates related to one another to produce a smooth reaching movement with a fairly straight trajectory. Children develop this coordination gradually during the first years of reaching (Konczak et al., 1995, 1997). In contrast, many studies have reported that in patients with a variety of neural pathologies, reaching movements are characterized by multijoint incoordination leading to abnormal movement trajectories.

For example, Bastian et al. (1996) studied movement trajectories in adult subjects with cerebellar pathology. Movement trajectories were characterized by either undershooting or overshooting the target (depending on whether the reach was fast or slow) and decomposition (moving one joint at a time). This can be seen in Figure 18-2. In Figure 18-2, *A* and *B*, the data from a normal control subject are shown. The wrist trajectories associated with a slow accurate (*A*) and a fast accurate (*B*) reach are smooth and straight. In addition the movements are quite accurate; this can be seen by comparing the position of the fingertip (*open circle*) to the target (*solid circle*). In contrast, the wrist trajectories and finger-point accuracy for a cerebellar pa-

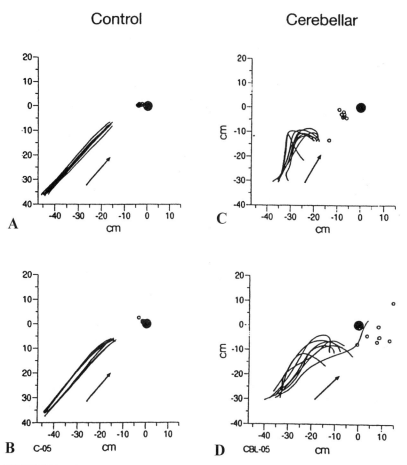

FIGURE 18-2.   A comparison of wrist path in a control (**A, B**) versus a subject with cerebellar pathology (**C, D**) moving in slow accurate (**A, C**) and fast accurate (**B, D**) conditions. *Arrows,* direction of movement. *Shaded circle,* location of target. *Open circles,* position of the tip of the index finger at the end of the movement. (Redrawn with permission from Bastian AJ, Martin TA, Keating JG, Thach WT. Cerebellar ataxia: abnormal control of interaction torques across multiple joints. J Neurophysiol 1996;76:497.)

tient are shown in Figure 18-2, *C* (slow accurate conditions) and *D* (fast accurate conditions). For both slow (*C*) and fast (*D*) movements, wrist trajectories show decomposition, that is, an initial vertical movement primarily related to shoulder flexion, followed by a horizontal movement related to elbow extension during the latter half of the reach. In addition, slow movements were associated with hypometric reaches (undershooting), while the fast movements were hypermetric (overshooting). Control subjects initiated shoulder and elbow motion within 73 msec of one another. In contrast, the subjects with cerebellar pathology initiated shoulder flexion approximately 296 msec before the onset of elbow extension (Bastian et al., 1996).

Bastian et al. (1996) also used kinetics to examine the torque profiles in individuals with cerebellar pathology and found that subjects with cerebellar damage produced very different torque profiles from those of healthy controls. During the slow accurate reaches, excessive activation of the elbow flexors prevented normal elbow extension early in the reach. In the fast movement condition, the subjects with cerebellar damage produced inappropriate shoulder muscle torques and were not able to vary elbow muscle torques in response to changes in interaction torques produced by movements in adjacent body joints. These abnormalities in torque resulted in dyscoordination and decomposition of multijoint movements. Interestingly, the authors suggest that many of the movement abnormalities demonstrated by individuals with cerebellar pathology may be compensatory. For example, decomposition may be a strategy used to compensate for impaired multijoint control. Since single-joint control appears to be better than multijoint control, patients with cerebellar lesions may decompose movements into sequential movement at individual joints as a strategy to minimize the effects of multijoint dyscoordination. Slowed movement time may be a strategy used to maximize accuracy, while undershooting may compensate for poor end-point control.

Impaired multijoint coordination has also been reported in several studies examining upper extremity movements in subjects with Parkinson's disease. Tuelings et al. (1997) used tasks similar to handwriting to study upper extremity control in individuals with Parkinson's disease. They found that many of the fine motor control problems (as shown by these tasks) in Parkinson's disease patients were caused by a reduced ability to coordinate wrist and finger movements and by a reduced ability to control wrist flexion.

Levin (1996) used pointing movements to study upper extremity control in 10 hemiparetic and 6 control subjects to determine the relationship between functional upper extremity limitations and underlying impairments such as abnormal synergies and spasticity.

Subjects were seated in front of a horizontal surface and made reaching movements to four targets in front of them (200 and 400 mm) and in the ipsilateral and contralateral workspace. This is shown in Figure 18-3. The targets were arranged so that (*a*) moving toward the ipsilateral target required an out-of-synergy movement, such as a combination of shoulder horizontal abduction and elbow extension; (*b*) movement to the contralateral target could be performed with an extensor synergy, such as shoulder adduction and elbow extension; and (*c*) move-

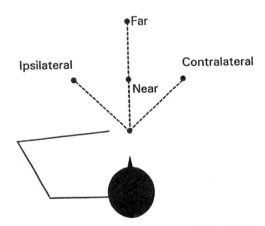

FIGURE 18-3. Target positions (*solid circles*) for reaching movements made on a horizontal surface. (Reprinted with permission from Levin MF. Interjoint coordination during pointing movements is disrupted in spastic hemiparesis. Brain 1996;119: 283.)

ment to the near and far targets required a combination of flexor and extensor synergies to move the arm forward. Kinematic data were used to study coordination of finger, wrist, elbow, and shoulder joints. In addition, subjects underwent clinical evaluation to assess spasticity (modified Ashworth scale) and sensory-motor function (Fugl-Meyer scale).

For all hemiparetic subjects, movement times were significantly longer and movement amplitudes smaller in the affected arm than in the nonaffected arm. In the affected arm, trajectories were characterized by segmented movements, increased variability, and disrupted interjoint coordination. This can be seen in Figure 18-4, which compares end-point trajectory and interjoint coordination between all four targets in the nonaffected arm and the affected arm of one of the hemiparetic subjects. As the figure shows, in the nonaffected arm the trajectories are smooth and continuous, with good coordination of movement in the elbow and shoulder joints. In contrast, the subject could not produce smooth end-point trajectories in the affected arm (*left*), and movement to the contralateral target is segmented and poorly coordinated. Movement segmentation resulted from a lack of coordination between shoulder and elbow joint movements, reminiscent of the findings from studies on reaching in subjects with cerebellar pathology. This disruption of interjoint coordination led to a limitation in active range of elbow and shoulder joint motion, resulting in hypometric movements that undershot the target.

Poor coordination was obvious for both movements made within the extensor synergy (to the contralateral target) and those requiring out of synergy movements (to near and far targets). Thus the disruption to movements was not strictly linked to the presence of pathological movement synergies. Finally, severity of spasticity was correlated with both movement time and amplitude but not with interjoint coordination measures. The author suggests that regardless of the location of the lesion, following a stroke, the central nervous system may not

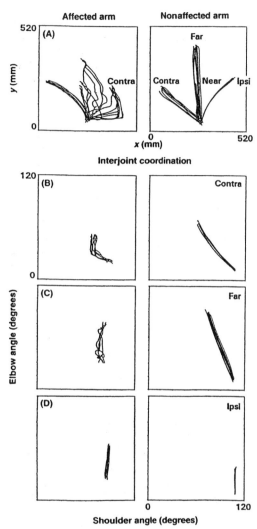

FIGURE 18-4. A comparison of end-point trajectories (**A**) in spatial coordinates and interjoint coordination (**B-D**) in angular coordinates for the affected left arm (*left panels*) and the nonaffected arm (*right panels*) for a subject with hemiparesis and severe spasticity. Diagrams show movements made from the starting position to the target positions. Trajectories shown in **A** are for movements made to the contralateral (contra), far, near and ipsilateral (ipsi) targets. Interjoint coordination (elbow versus shoulder angle diagrams) for the movements in **A** are shown for the contralateral (**B**), far (**C**), and ipsilateral (**D**) targets. (Adapted with permission from Levin MF. Interjoint coordination during pointing movements is disrupted in spastic hemiparesis. Brain 1996;119: 285.)

be able to determine the optimal set of relationships between muscles and segments to perform smooth coordinated reaching movements (Levin, 1996).

The Role of Spasticity in Impaired Reach. Many clinicians view spasticity or disorders of tone to be the most significant impairment constraining function in the patient with central nervous system pathology (Davies, 1985; Bobath, 1978). However, the extent to which spasticity impairs upper extremity function is still unclear. Results from a study examining the extent to which abnormal stretch reflexes in antagonist muscles impair arm movements in stroke patients raises questions about the extent to which velocity-dependent spasticity limits upper extremity control (Sahrmann and Norton, 1977). For example, it has been hypothesized that flexor spasticity in the biceps may prevent effective activation of the triceps and extension of the arm. Results from studies examining upper extremity reaching movements in patients with hemiplegia do not support the hypothesis that the primary constraint on upper extremity reaching is spasticity of the biceps, but rather suggest that weakness and inability to recruit motor neurons in the triceps are the main constraints (Sahrmann and Norton, 1977).

Other studies examining reaching and other types of movements have found inappropriate shortening reactions that constrain upper extremity movements. A shortening reaction is the inappropriate activation of the stretch reflex during shortening contractions of a muscle, which impairs a patient's ability to move the arm. Inappropriate shortening reactions have been reported in patients following stroke (Sahrmann and Norton, 1977) and in patients with Parkinson's disease (Johnson, 1991).

It is important to note that none of these studies denies the fact that spasticity impairs motor control in the patient with neurological deficits. These studies do, however, challenge the assumption that spasticity is the primary impairment to normal motor control (Katz and Rymer, 1989; Gordon, 1987).

Sensory Problems

The ability to adapt reaching movements to changes in task and environmental demands is an essential component of normal upper extremity control. Sensory information is critical to adapting movements and is used to correct errors during the execution of upper extremity movement, ensuring accuracy during the final portions of the movement.

The Effect of Visual Deficits on Visually Guided Reach

The primary function of visual feedback in reaching appears to be related to the attainment of final accuracy. It has been hypothesized that the constancy of thumb position with relation to the wrist during reaching may be part of a strategy of providing clear visual feedback regarding the end point of the limb (Wing and Frazer, 1983).

Lesions on either side of the posterior parietal area in humans can cause marked eye–hand coordination impairment, or optic ataxia. Optic ataxia is defined as the inability to reach for objects in extrapersonal space in the absence of extensive motor, visual, or somatosensory deficits (Jeannerod, 1990). Patients with optic ataxia typically misreach for objects within the visual field that is contralateral to their lesion.

This disorder was first described by Balint (1909) using the term visual disorientation. He noted that the patient could reach normally with his left hand, but when asked to reach with his right hand, he made mistakes in all directions, until he eventually bumped into the object with his hand. He found that the problem was related to visual control of that hand, because if he asked the patient first to point to the object with his left hand, then he could reach accurately with his right hand. On autopsy, it was found that the patient had a lesion in the posterior parietal areas, including the angular gyrus and the anterior occipital lobe on both sides of the brain (Jeannerod, 1990).

These patients also have specific motor disorganization problems. It has been hypothesized that their problems relate to programming visually guided goal-directed movements. It has been shown that the deceleration phase of reaching is much longer than that in the normal hand, with many small peaks. In addition, these patients have problems with grasp formation. Figure 18-5 shows a reach of a patient with optic ataxia with his normal hand (*A*), affected hand with visual feedback (*B*), and without vision (*C*). Even with visual feedback, the affected hand did not begin to close until the last moment, and the terminal grip was too big. Without visual feedback, grasp formation did not occur (Jeannerod, 1990). Thus, it has been suggested that optic ataxia results from a specific problem with eye–hand coordination mechanisms responsible for adjusting finger posture to the shape of the object (Jeannerod, 1990).

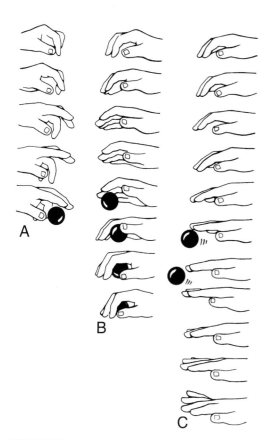

FIGURE 18-5. Grip patterns of a patient with optic ataxia. **A.** Normal hand. **B.** Affected hand, visual feedback. **C.** Affected hand, no visual feedback. (Reprinted with permission from Jeannerod M. The neural and behavioral organization of goal-directed movements. Oxford: Oxford University, 1990:225.)

The Effect of Somatosensory Deficits on Reach

Is somatosensory input essential for the production of reaching movements? As noted in earlier chapters, experiments by Sherrington in the late 1800s showed that monkeys that were deafferented on one side of the spinal cord stopped using the affected limb. He thus concluded that sensory feedback was critical to movement control. In contrast, researchers who deafferented both limbs of animals showed that the animals recovered motor function. Movements were initially awkward but improved within as little as 2 weeks, as long as visual feedback was available (Taub and Berman, 1968).

Interestingly, recovery starts with the animals only being able to sweep the object across the floor. Then a coarse grasp with all four fingers develops, and then a pincer grasp reappears (Taub, 1976). It has been suggested that when unilateral deafferentation occurs, the animals may learn not to use the deafferented limb or may even develop inhibition of the deafferented arm (Taub, 1976). This learned disuse hypothesis is supported by the fact that unilaterally deafferented animals recover movement coordination as well as bilaterally deafferented animals if their normal limb remains immobilized so that they have to use the deafferented limb (Jeannerod, 1990).

Also, remember from Chapter 16 that experiments on deafferented monkeys showed that when making single-joint movements, they could reach targets with relative accuracy even when they could not see the hand. Displacing the forearm just prior to movement onset during a reach also did not significantly disturb pointing accuracy in these deafferented animals. It was thus concluded that single-joint movements depend on changes in muscle activation levels that are programmed prior to movement onset and that no feedback is required for reasonably accurate execution of these movements (Polit and Bizzi, 1978).

In addition, recent experiments on humans after pathological deafferentation have confirmed the results of experiments on monkeys (Rothwell et al., 1982). One patient had suffered a severe peripheral sensory neuropathy, so that there was loss of sensation in both the arms and the legs. Light touch, vibration, and temperature sensation were impaired or absent in both hands. Tests showed that in spite of these problems, the patient could perform many motor tasks even without vision. For example, the patient could tap, do fast alternating flexion and extension movements, and draw figures in the air, using only the wrist and fingers (Jeannerod, 1990; Rothwell et al., 1982).

It was also noted that electromyographic (EMG) activity during flexion and extension of the thumb was similar to that seen in normal subjects. The subject could also learn new thumb positions with vision and then reproduce those positions without vision. Thus, motor learning was also possible. However, the patient's performance rapidly deteriorated when asked to repeat the movement many times with the eyes closed.

In a second study on patients with periph-eral sensory neuropathy, patients could perform repetitive flexion and extension movements of the wrist, with normal EMG activity, as long as the movements were not too fast. At a certain point, however, the intervals between the EMG bursts tended to disappear. It was hypothesized that this was due to the high level of cocontraction of agonist and antagonist muscles seen in these patients (Sanes et al., 1985). Patients could also hold a steady posture with their deafferented limb as long as they had visual feedback. However, without visual feedback, large errors were made, and the limb drifted back to its initial position, as shown in Figure 18-6 (Sanes et al., 1985).

What does this information tell us about the role of kinesthetic feedback in reaching? It appears that it is not required for movement initiation and execution. However, it is still important for accurate reaching involving multiple joints. Researchers testing humans with peripheral sensory neuropathy

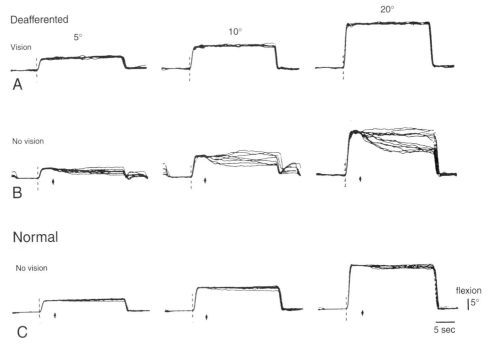

FIGURE 18-6.   Wrist position of a patient with peripheral sensory neuropathy. The patient was asked to rotate the wrist to reach positions of 5, 10, and 20 degrees against an elastic load. **A.** With vision the patient had no problems. **B.** Without vision the position drifted back in the direction of the load. **C.** A normal subject's performance without vision. (Adapted with permission from Sanes JN, Mauritz KH, Dalakas MC, Evarts EV. Motor control in humans with large-fiber sensory neuropathy. Hum Neurobiol 1985;4:101.)

found that patients were able to make accurate movements only if they involved single joints. They showed great problems in performing natural movements used in normal life (Sanes et al., 1985).

Problems With Grasp

Studies have examined the reach and grasp behavior of developmentally disabled children, including those with hemiplegia or Down syndrome (Jeannerod, 1986; Eliasson et al., 1991; Cole et al., 1988). In some cases of mild impairment, hemiplegia is not readily identified until about 40 weeks, when the infant first begins to use the pincer grasp and manipulate objects (Jeannerod, 1990). One child of 23 months used the hand with hemiplegia only when the normal hand was immobilized, and even then, it was with great difficulty that the child grasped objects. Figure 18-7, adapted from film records, illustrates the child reaching for a prong from a pegboard with the normal hand and the affected hand, with visual feedback. Note that the normal hand did not anticipate the shape of the object well, but a finger extension–flexion pattern was used. Also, contact of the hand with the object caused the fingers to close around the object, giving an accurate grasp. However, the hemiplegic hand showed an exaggerated opening during the entire movement, with no anticipatory grasp formation. There was a very slight closing of the hand after contact with the object, giving a very clumsy grasp (Jeannerod, 1990).

In a second child 5 years of age, the hemiplegic hand showed more nearly normal reach and grasp movements. The authors suggest that more normal movement patterns may be the result of many years of rehabilitation training (Jeannerod, 1990). Figure 18-8 depicts film records of her reaching movements with her normal hand (*A*) and her hemiplegic hand (*B–D*). Note that reaching in the hemiplegic hand was affected only in relation to the pattern of grip formation. Finger shaping was abnormal, with the index finger extended in an exaggerated manner and then flexing only slightly if at all before contacting the object.

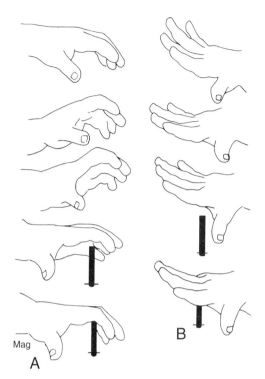

FIGURE 18-7. Drawing from film records of the reaches of a 23-month-old child with hemiplegia reaching for a prong from a pegboard with the nonaffected hand (**A**) and the affected hand (**B**). (Adapted with permission from Jeannerod M. The neural and behavioral organization of goal-directed movements. Oxford: Oxford University, 1990:72.)

Because of these problems, the objects were sometimes dropped during the grasp (Jeannerod, 1990).

Some experiments addressed the reach and grasp skills of patients with lesions in the somatosensory pathways at brainstem levels and at parietal cortex levels. In the patient with the lesion at the brainstem level, the hand ipsilateral to the lesion was affected. When vision was present, grasp formation was normal, as shown in Figure 18-9*A*, except that it lasted longer than in the normal hand. However, without vision, the grasping movements were critically changed (Fig. 18-9, *B* and *C*). Finger grip was either absent altogether or incomplete. In the first reach the patient made with no visual feedback, there was no grip formation at all, while in the second reach, there was incomplete grip formation (Jeannerod, 1990).

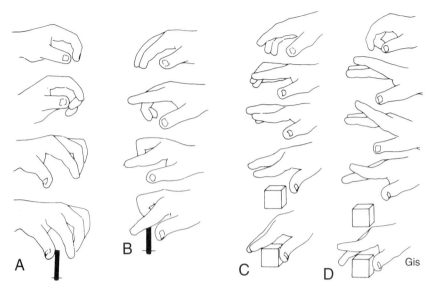

FIGURE 18-8. Drawing from film records of the reaches of a 5-year-old child with hemiplegia after many years of rehabilitation reaching for a prong from a pegboard with the nonaffected hand **(A)** and the affected hand **(B–D)**. (Adapted with permission from Jeannerod M. The neural and behavioral organization of goal-directed movements. Oxford: Oxford University, 1990:73.)

Patients with lesions to the parietal lobe, particularly the postcentral gyrus and the supramarginal gyrus, show patterns for reach and grasp similar to those of patients with peripheral sensory problems. In a detailed study on the recovery of reach and grasp in a patient with a parietal lobe lesion, researchers found that the patient did not use her right hand spontaneously immediately following her lesion but later used it in many actions as long as she had visual feedback. Without visual control, her movements were very awkward. For example, she was unable to sustain repetitive tapping movements unless she could see or hear her fingers moving (Jeannerod, 1990).

In contrast to patients with peripheral deafferentation, who could grip normally as long as visual feedback was present, grip formation was impaired in the patient with a

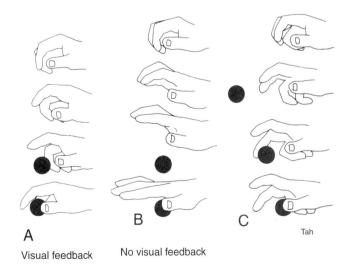

A
Visual feedback

B   C

No visual feedback

FIGURE 18-9. Drawing from film records of the grip patterns of a patient with a lesion of the somatosensory pathway at the brainstem level. **A.** With vision, grasp was normal. **B, C.** Without vision, it was absent or incomplete. (Adapted with permission from Jeannerod M. The neural and behavioral organization of goal-directed movements. Oxford: Oxford University, 1990:205.)

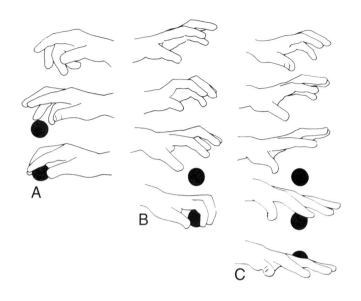

FIGURE 18-10.   Grip patterns of a patient with a parietal lobe lesion. **A.** Normal hand, visual feedback. **B.** Affected hand, visual feedback. **C.** Affected hand, no visual feedback. (Adapted with permission from Jeannerod M. The neural and behavioral organization of goal-directed movements. Oxford: Oxford University, 1990:208.)

parietal lesion, even with visual feedback (Jeannerod, 1990). Figure 18-10*A* shows the grasp component of a reach with the patient's normal hand, while Figure 18-10, *B* and *C* show the grasp of the affected hand both with and without visual feedback. When she reached with the affected hand with vision, the patient made grasps using the whole palm of the hand. Without visual feedback, only the initial part of the transportation phase was normal. Then the hand seemed to "wander above the object, without a grasp" (Jeannerod, 1990, p. 207). Thus, loss of sensory information results in abnormal grip and lift forces and problems in the control of fine movements of the hand.

Problems With Grip and Lift

The ability to produce and regulate force is an important aspect of tasks in which an object has to be grasped and lifted. Tactile sensation from the fingertips is particularly important when lifting objects with a precision grip to adjust the amplitude of forces used to grip and lift. If grip force is too tight, the object cannot be manipulated; if it is too loose, the object is dropped. In a precision grip, forces for gripping and lifting are generated simultaneously and appear to depend on cutaneous input.

Impairments in the regulation of forces for precision grip and lift tasks have been reported in a wide variety of patients with neural pathology. For example, disruptions to the initiation and sequencing of grip and lift forces have been reported in patients with Parkinson's disease. Ingvarsson et al. (1997) reported frequent oscillations and fluctuations in the force profiles associated with grip and lift movements in subjects with Parkinson's disease who were not taking medication. The amplitude of oscillations decreased when subjects were taking medication, suggesting that the oscillations were due to action tremor superimposed on the force trajectories.

Additional research (Fellows et al., 1998) investigated force development in 16 individuals with Parkinson's disease and 12 age-matched controls. Subjects performed a grip and lift task under conditions in which the weight of the object was altered both with and without warning. Results for the grip and lift task under the four conditions are shown in Figure 18-11. The subjects with Parkinson's disease, like the control subjects, lifted the unpredictable load using grip force parameters they had used in the preceding lift. Both groups were able to modulate grip forces to the new load during the lift. However, subjects with Parkinson's disease required a significantly longer time to develop grip force than the healthy controls

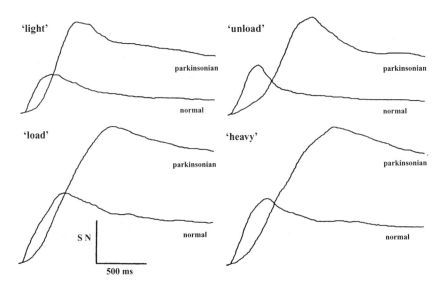

FIGURE 18-11.   Mean grip force curves for a patient with Parkinson's disease and an age-matched healthy control obtained from five lifts performed under four conditions (expecting and lifting a light load (*light*), expecting and lifting a heavy load (*heavy*), expecting a heavy load and lifting a light load (*unload*), and expecting a light load and lifting a heavy load (*load*). As expected, for both the patient with Parkinson's disease and normal control subjects, peak grip force values were higher for the heavier loads than for lighter loads (compare traces labeled *heavy* to those labeled *light*). Subjects with Parkinson's disease tended to produce inappropriately high grip forces compared to normal controls in all conditions. (Adapted with permission from Fellows SJ, Noth J, Schwarz M. Precision grip and Parkinson's disease. Brain 1998;121: 1176.)

in all conditions. In addition, they showed significantly higher levels of grip force during the lift phase of the movement, indicating a higher safety margin than seen in control subjects. However, individuals with Parkinson's disease were capable of modulating grip forces to match changes in the object's weight.

A study examining grasp and lift in children with cerebral palsy documented the presence of excessive and oscillatory grip forces (Eliasson et al., 1991). Elliason also found that in contrast to healthy control children, children with cerebral palsy coordinated grip and load force not simultaneously but sequentially. The authors suggest that these excessive grip forces, establishing a high safety margin against slips, may be compensatory to unstable motor output. This type of safety margin has been reported in older adults and in healthy children under age 5, who also show oscillations in force control.

What are some of the factors that contribute to impairments in force regulation during grip and lift tasks? A number of studies suggest sensory deficits as a primary cause.

Sensory Deficits and Precision Grip

How does loss of somatosensation affect precision grip? Robertson and Jones (1994) evaluated the relationship between somatosensory impairments and prehensile function, including precision grip, in 10 subjects with left-hemisphere cerebrovascular accidents and 14 control subjects. They found that in the subjects with hemiparesis, impaired somatosensation (pressure sensitivity and two-point discrimination) was correlated to the subject's poor performance on object recognition tests but did not predict performance on functional hand tests, such as the Jebsen Hand Function test. They also found that loss of somatosensation significantly affected the regulation of grip and lift forces. Subjects showed marked fluctuations in force during grasping, suggesting impairments in the ability to regulate forces. Surprisingly, despite impaired somatosensation, the subjects continued to be able to adapt forces to changes in the weight and surface properties of the object being held.

Lesions of the anterior parietal lobe result in somatosensory deficits that limit precision grip and in-hand manipulation skills (Jeannerod, 1996). Pause et al. (1989) referred to these motor impairments due to central sensory deficits as tactile apraxia. Lesions of the posterior parietal area produce spatial disorientation and misreaching. Lesions in this area affect the ability to shape the hand according to object size and configuration. Deficits are more severe in the absence of visual feedback from the limb (Jeannerod, 1996). Damage to posterior parietal areas produces a disconnection between visual and proprioceptive inputs, so that limb and object positions in space are no longer be matched with each other. Thus the importance of the posterior parietal lobe is in organizing object-oriented action. Sakata et al. (1985) suggest that neurons in this area are able to integrate visual and motor signals related to object oriented action, thus linking sensory information on object properties with corresponding motor commands.

Impaired Anticipatory Control of Precision Grip

As discussed in Chapters 16 and 17, the development of precision grip and manipulation depends on the availability of both tactile information from both slow and fast adapting afferents, which convey information on texture, and weight-related information from muscles spindles and tactile afferents (Johansson, 1996). During an ongoing lift, small slips between the skin and the object result in activation of cutaneous receptors, which cause the grip force to be in-

creased. Sensory information is also used in the development of internal representations about an object's physical characteristics. During subsequent lifts, expectations based on internal representations of the object are used to preprogram grip and lift forces. Thus, scaling of forces is performed prior to the lift and is dependent on both sensorimotor memory (internal representations) and current sensory (visual and tactile) information (Gordon et al., 1997). Anticipatory control emerges with development. By age 6 to 8 years, anticipatory control of fingertip forces (both pinch and vertical lift) is adultlike (Gordon et al., 1997).

Gordon and Duff (1999) studied anticipatory grip and lift forces in 15 children aged 8 to 14 years who have the spastic hemiplegia type of cerebral palsy. Their study found that children with cerebral palsy were initially impaired in their ability to scale forces during the first few trials of a grip and lift task. However, they eventually learned to use anticipatory control of load forces based on the texture and weight of an object, but only after extended practice with the object.

What is the basis for deficits in initial ability to scale the rate of force to the weight of the object to be lifted in children with cerebral palsy? Gordon and Duff (1999) report no clear relationship between degree of spasticity and anticipatory control of grip and lift in children with cerebral palsy, suggesting that spasticity, while present, was not the major factor related to impaired grip and lift. In addition, they found that sensory information from the **noninvolved** hand could transfer to improve anticipatory scaling of forces by the contralateral (involved) hand in subsequent manipulations (Gordon et al., 1999). These two findings suggest that sensory deficits account for many problems related to precision grip and lift.

The assumption that sensory deficits are a major factor in impaired precision grip in children with cerebral palsy is supported by results from a study by Eliasson et al. (1991), who found impaired tactile regulation of isometric fingertip forces during grasping in these children. They suggest that children with cerebral palsy who have sensory impairments may not be able to extract enough information during initial manipulatory experiences to form internal representations of the object's properties. Instead they appear to require considerable practice to form accurate internal representations of objects.

Gordon et al. (1997) also studied anticipatory control of manipulative forces in individuals with Parkinson's disease. Subjects performed a grip and release task under three conditions. The subject's ability to use anticipatory control to scale force output in response to both predictable and unpredictable changes in weight was assessed. The authors conclude that subjects with Parkinson's disease do not appear to have problems using stored internal representations when regulating force output (Gordon et al., 1997).

Problems With Release

Gordon also studied task-dependent problems during release of an object in subjects with Parkinson's disease, both on and off medication. Release was studied under three task conditions: object replacement and release at preferred speed, object replacement and release at fastest speed, and object squeeze and release (object remained stationary on the supporting surface, so there was no replacement phase). Results showed that impairments in grasp and release depended on the task condition. Coordination of grip and load forces in subjects with Parkinson's disease approximated those of normal subjects during object replacement and release at preferred speeds. In contrast, when instructed to move as quickly as possible, release was significantly slower than for age matched controls (Gordon et al., 1997). These findings were consistent with those of Kunesch et al. (1995), who also found that impaired release of an isotonic force was impaired in subjects with Parkinson's disease.

Eliasson and Gordon (in press) examined release in children with hemiplegic cerebral palsy. The found that these children tended to replace objects more quickly than controls yet took a longer time to release objects from finger contact.

Hemispheric Specialization in Reach and Grasp

It appears that each hemisphere has a specialized role in the control of goal directed voluntary movements. Winstein and Pohl (1995) studied control of a reciprocal aiming task in 20 individuals with unilateral brain damage (10 with left hemisphere damage and 10 with right hemisphere damage) and 10 age-matched controls. Seated subjects moved the stylus for 10 seconds as fast and accurately as possible to one target and back or between two targets under three conditions of difficulty. The low-difficulty task required subjects just to tap repetitively on a single disc; the medium-difficulty task required subjects to alternate taps between two 8-cm wide targets; the high-difficulty task required alternate tapping between two 2-cm discs. Both the low- and medium-difficulty tasks required primarily open-loop control, while the high-difficulty task required closed-loop control.

This study showed that while all subjects with brain damage had slowed movement times, there were distinct differences between the two groups. Subjects with a right-sided stroke showed deficits primarily in the closed-loop portion of the movement (high-difficulty task), specifically just prior to target impact, when visual information was necessary for accuracy. In contrast, the subjects with left-sided stroke showed more deficits during the open-loop portion of the movement (the low- and medium-difficulty tasks). Differences between the two groups of patients suggest that the right hemisphere has a role in processing visual feedback for movement adjustments affecting control of aiming movements in tasks with high demands for accuracy. In contrast, the left hemisphere has a preferential role in some aspects of motor programming, including the timing and sequencing of movement phases specifically related to the ballistic components of the reaching movement (Winstein and Pohl, 1995).

Other researchers have examined reaching abilities in patients with unilateral damage of the left or right cerebral hemispheres

(Fisk and Goodale, 1988; Smutok et al., 1989). These studies too have shown that during a task requiring fast and accurate reaches, both groups of subjects with hemiplegia were less accurate than controls and required more time to complete the reach after the target was illuminated. In addition, like Winstein and Pohl (1995), they found a significant difference between the performance of subjects with right- and left-hemisphere lesions. While the group with lesions of the right hemisphere took longer to initiate a reach, the movements themselves were similar to those of the control group. In contrast, the group with lesions of the left hemisphere did not have problems in the time required to initiate the reach but took much longer to execute the reach itself.

Thus, reach was impaired in both groups but for apparently different reasons. These authors suggest that a lesion in the right hemisphere affects the patient's ability to quickly detect the spatial position of the target (higher-level visual processing). In contrast, a lesion in the left hemisphere appears to affect the patient's ability to select an appropriate program (higher-level motor processing) to achieve the target position and/or to modify that program as it is being executed (Fisk and Goodale, 1988; Smutok et al., 1989).

Reach and Grasp in the Nonhemiparetic Limb

Traditionally, researchers have maintained that unilateral cerebral lesions manifest in the limb contralateral to the lesions. Now researchers are also finding subtle deficits affecting the ability to reach on the nonhemiparetic side (Giulliani et al., 1993; Gordon et al., 1999; Sunderland, 2000). For example, a study examining motor problems in the nonhemiparetic limb has suggested that weakness is a contributing factor in reaching problems in this limb as well as the hemiparetic limb (Giulliani et al., 1993). Other studies have found that problems in reaching with the nonhemiparetic arm following unilateral hemispheric lesion may involve other factors as well. In addition, Gordon et

al. (1999) studied the coordination of fingertip forces during object manipulation in both involved and noninvolved hands in children with hemiplegic cerebral palsy. They found subtle deficits in sequencing of grip–lift movements in the noninvolved hand. Sunderland (2000) studied dexterity and apraxia in the ipsilateral hand in 24 patients with an acute stroke. All patients showed initial deficits in the ipsilateral hand on tests of dexterity and apraxia; however, most had recovered by 6 months post stroke. Seven patients, all of whom had left-hemisphere damage, continued to show persisting problems related to dexterity and apraxia in the ipsilateral hand.

Bilateral impairments in hand function found in both children with cerebral palsy and in adult patients following unilateral stroke are not surprising, considering that 10% to 30% of fibers in the lateral corticospinal tract are uncrossed. These data support an anatomical substrate for bilateral impairment in hand function in individuals with lesions affecting one hemisphere.

℮ APRAXIA

In the preceding sections, our discussion of abnormal reach and grasp has related to the examination of problems in each of the constituent components, visual regard, reach, grasp, manipulation and release. However, the use of the upper extremity in the performance of simple everyday tasks is more than the simple summation of these components. It requires the integration of these components into an action plan. An action plan specifies the conceptual content of the action along with its hierarchical and sequential organization (Poizner et al., 1990). The left cerebral cortex includes structures specialized for higher-order motor programming or the formation of action plans (Schwartz et al., 1991).

One way researchers have studied the nature of these motor programs is by analyzing the types of errors made by patients with left-hemisphere damage. Disorders that result from dysfunction of this specialized left hemisphere have been termed apraxias. One type of apraxia that has been studied extensively is ideational apraxia, or frontal apraxia (Luria, 1966), or frontal lobe executive disorder (Norman and Shallice, 1986). This is a disorder of the execution of movement that cannot be attributed to weakness, to incoordination or sensory loss, or to poor language comprehension or inattention to commands.

To understand this disorder, it is helpful to appreciate what occurs when a normal adult decides to perform a task. It is hypothesized that the first step is formulating the intention to perform the task and then formulating an action plan. The essential requirement of an action plan is that it specifies the goal of the action along with the hierarchical and sequential organization of nested actions that are required to achieve the ultimate goal. Intentions, as defined by activated action plans, are an integral feature of all purposeful behavior. It has been hypothesized that the core of the intentional disorder of frontal apraxia is a weakening of the top-down formulation of action plans, that is, an inability to sustain the intent to the completion of the action plan (Schwartz et al., 1991).

As a result, irrelevant objects exert a strong influence on the action plan, and this leads to numerous performance errors. Researchers have begun to develop a system for coding performance errors based on this concept of hierarchically organized units of action within an action plan. These studies have enumerated examples of errors during the performance of common activities of daily living, including buttering hot coffee, putting clothes on backward or inside-out, drinking from an empty cup, skipping key steps during activities such as shaving, toothbrushing, or hairbrushing, using a fork to eat cereal, putting toothpaste on a razor, scrubbing the upper lip and chin with a toothbrush, eating toothpaste, and applying arm deodorant over a shirt (Schwartz et al., 1991). In a classic paper, Luria (1966) describes the behavior of a frontal apraxia patient who would light a candle and put it in his mouth to perform the habitual movements of smoking a cigarette.

A CASE STUDY APPROACH TO UNDERSTANDING REACH AND GRASP PROBLEMS

Phoebe J.: Reach and Grasp Problems Following Cerebral Vascular Accident

Impairments in reach and grasp, particularly precision grip, are common following stroke. However, the type of problem depends on the location of the lesion. In the case of Phoebe J., it is likely that reach and grasp movements in her affected arm will be characterized by decreased movement speed and a lack of smoothness and coordination in movement trajectories because of abnormal patterns of muscle activity. Deficits in coordinated arm movements will be most evident in the limb contralateral to her lesion and will occur together with spasticity, muscle weakness, and stereotyped movement patterns. When Phoebe J. reaches with her affected arm, the movement trajectory is likely to be quite segmented, with increased variability due to impaired interjoint coordination. During grasp, she will likely show marked fluctuations in force due to impairments in the ability to regulate forces.

In addition to her neuromotor impairments, she is likely to have visual problems such as field deficits (homonymous hemianopsia), neglect, and extinction, which will affect her ability to reach and grasp objects presented in the contralesional hemifield. Other impairments within the somatosensory system are likely to impair precision grip significantly.

A complication that may interfere with her recovery of upper extremity function following her stroke is pain and/or swelling in her hemiparetic arm. In addition to shoulder pain, she may develop a shoulder–hand syndrome, which occurs in approximately 15% of all stroke patients. The shoulder–hand syndrome includes pain when moving and loss of range of motion in both the shoulder and the hand. In severe cases, there is pain at rest. If the shoulder–hand syndrome is prolonged, it can lead to a frozen shoulder.

There is no agreement concerning the underlying cause of shoulder pain following stroke, nor is there agreement on methods for treatment (Davies, 1985; Partridge et al., 1990; Roy, 1988, Cailliet, 1980).

Laurence W.: Reach and Grasp Problems in Parkinson's Disease

Poor manual dexterity and resting tremor in the extremities are common symptoms associated with Parkinson's disease and are thus likely to impair upper extremity function in Laurence W. It is important to remember that his impairments in reach and grasp are likely to be task dependent. For example, when he is performing fast, accurate movements, reaching impairments related to force regulation may be most apparent. In contrast, in simple motor tasks or during slow movements for which speed and accuracy are not important, he may show much better control of both reach and grasp.

Laurence W. is likely to show relatively little impairment when performing a reach and grasp movement at his preferred speed or when the movement amplitude is small. In addition, his ability to adjust to external perturbations during reach and grasp will be less impaired than adjustments to self-generated perturbations. Across all tasks, however, he will show a reduced capability to coordinate multiple joints. In addition, tremor may result in a disrupted force trajectory. He may take longer to develop grip force and may use excessive force when lifting an object to ensure that it does not slip. However, surprisingly, Laurence W. may retain the ability to modulate forces to match changes in object weight. Finally, he may have difficulty releasing an object.

Zach C.: Reach and Grasp Problems Following Traumatic Cerebellar Injury

Cerebellar damage results in dysmetria, which is characterized by errors in the direction, amplitude, velocity, and force of movement. Zach C. is ataxic, so during reach and grasp tasks, movements are slow and inaccurate, with increased variability in the movement trajectory. When reaching for an object or pointing to a target, he produces movement trajectories that may either undershoot a target if he is moving slowly or overshoot the target if he is moving quickly. In addition, movements are segmented (decomposition of movement), with movements at multiple joints occurring sequentially rather than synchronously. Most likely both eye and hand movements are inaccurate when Zach C. is reaching for a stationary object. In addition, when reaching for moving objects, he may be unable to match the target velocity and thus demonstrate inaccuracies when reaching or tracking.

Sara L.: Reach and Grasp Problems in Spastic Diplegia Forms of Cerebral Palsy

Sara L., the 3-year-old child with spastic diplegia, is likely to have impaired upper extremity function, which is common in individuals with cerebral palsy. In a study of children with cerebral palsy by Van Heest et al. (1993), only 42% had a normal grasp, 40% had normal release, and 36% had a persistent grasp reflex. What kind of problems with reach and grasp can we expect in Sara L.? We expect movement times to be delayed during reach and grasp. However, slowed movement times may be less of a problem when reaching for a moving target, since many children with cerebral palsy appear to be able to compensate and aim their movements enough ahead of the target so they can make accurate reaches.

We expect poor anticipatory grasp formation during reaches with the involved arm. In addition, grip and load forces are likely to be uncoordinated. She probably uses excessive grip forces when lifting an object to compensate for poor motor control. We may expect to see that initially Sara L. will be impaired when learning to perform a task that requires precision grip. However, with practice this should improve significantly, as the child develops better internal representations of the object.

Both sensory and motor impairments contribute to impaired reach, grasp, and manipulation in Sara L., as in other children with cerebral palsy. Neuromuscular impairments include weakness, spasticity, abnormal synergies, muscle imbalance, and incoordination. Sensory problems include impaired stereognosis, two-point discrimination, and position sense and an inability to distinguish rough and smooth.

⊘ SUMMARY

1. Problems with reach, grasp, and manipulation are a finding in most patients with neural pathology.
2. Understanding the cause of these problems is complex because of the many interactions between neural substrates involved in reach, grasp, and manipulation skills.
3. A critical aspect of reach and grasp is the ability to locate a target and maintain one's gaze on that target preceding a reach. Problems affecting target localization and gaze stabilization include (*a*) disruption of visually driven eye movements due to damage within the oculomotor system; (*b*) damage to the vestibular system, which disrupts vestibulo-ocular reflex control of eye movements in response to head movements; and (*c*) inability to adapt the vestibulo-ocular reflex to changes in task demands because of cerebellar damage.
4. Visual deficits affecting target localization also appear to affect hand motor function because of the reciprocal interaction between the eye and hand motor systems.
5. Impaired interjoint coordination is common in many types of neural pathology and affects both the timing and trajectory of movements made dur-

ing reach and grasp. In addition, most patients with neural pathology show delayed movement times.

7. Sensory impairments can also affect reach, grasp, and manipulation. Sensory impairments can affect the regulation of forces in response to slips during an ongoing grip and lift task. In addition, sensory impairments can affect the formation of internal representations, important to regulating forces in subsequent lifts.
8. It appears that each hemisphere has a specialized role in the control of goal-directed voluntary movements. The right hemisphere appears to have a role in processing visual feedback for movement adjustments affecting control of aiming movements in tasks with high demands for accuracy. In contrast, left hemisphere appears to have a role in some aspects of motor programming, including the timing and sequencing of movement phases specifically related to the ballistic components of the reaching movement.
9. Traditionally, researchers have maintained that unilateral cerebral lesions manifest in the limb contralateral to the lesions. Now researchers are also finding subtle deficits affecting the ability to reach on the nonhemiparetic side.
10. Damage to the left hemisphere may cause apraxia, a disorder of the execution of movement that cannot be accounted for by weakness, incoordination, sensory loss, poor language comprehension, or inattention to commands. The core of this disorder may be a weakening of the top-down formulation of action plans, that is, an inability to sustain the intention to the completion of the action plan. As a result, irrelevant objects exert a strong influence on the action plan, leading to performance errors.

CHAPTER 19

Clinical Management of the Patient With Reach, Grasp, and Manipulation Disorders

Susan Duff, Anne Shumway-Cook, and Marjorie Woollacott*

℮ INTRODUCTION

Problems with reach, grasp, and manipulation affect many of the activities performed

*Susan V. Duff, MA, PT, OT, BCP, CHT.
Clinical Coordinator for the Upper Extremity Center of Excellence, Shriners Hospital for Children, Philadelphia, Pennsylvania

in daily life, such as dressing, eating, and grooming. As such, they are a major focus of intervention for clinicians involved in the rehabilitation of patients with neurological pathology. Upper extremity dysfunction manifests in different ways as seen in the following case studies. The first case illustrates loss of function in an adult patient following a stroke, while the second case exemplifies a child with insufficient development of prehensile skill.

CASE #1

Phoebe J., our patient who sustained a stroke in the right hemisphere, has been referred for therapy secondary to activities of daily living (ADL) deficits and inadequate use of her left upper extremity. Initially after her stroke, her left arm movements were confined to flexion synergy. Now she is beginning to develop isolated movement, although her arm movements appear weak and uncoordinated. Pheobe J. demonstrates crude grasp and release of large objects but has tremendous difficulty attaching small fasteners on clothing. She appears to have subtle but distinct problems coordinating reach and grasp in her noninvolved arm. In addition, she is showing ADL performance errors and has difficulty sequencing tasks.

CASE #2

Tim R. is a 4.5-year-old boy mainstreamed to a regular preschool whose teacher has referred him to therapy because of her concerns about his fine motor skills. Tim R. was born prematurely at 28 weeks' gestation and had an early history of retinopathy of prematurity. He wears glasses and has frequent absences due to illness. On observation in the classroom, he is markedly smaller than the other children, yet he easily engages with them socially. Tim R. prefers his right hand for fine motor tasks and holds a crayon with a cross-thumb grasp. He has difficulty tracing shapes, and while he has begun to copy letters and numbers from a visual model, he often reverses letters and uses varying size proportions. He also has difficulty using fasteners, tying his shoes, and performing other functional tasks that require a range of prehension patterns and dexterity.

This chapter focuses on the clinical management of problems related to reach, grasp, and manipulation in clients like Phoebe J. and Tim R. A task-oriented approach will be used to review examination methods pertinent to upper extremity control of reach, grasp, and manipulation. Our case studies will be used to illustrate how behavior is examined at three levels of performance, including 1) functional independence, 2) key movement strategies and components used during functional tasks; it also addresses 3) impairments that restrict and resources that enhance movement and function. All three levels can affect the execution of life roles. The three-level examination attempts to answer the following questions:

1. To what degree can the patient consistently perform functional tasks that engage one or both upper limbs? What is the extent and quality of use of one or both limbs as they are engaged in functional tasks?
2. What strategies and movement components does the patient take advantage of during task performance? Can the patient adapt these strategies to changing task conditions, and are the movements efficient?
3. What cognitive, visual-perceptual, musculoskeletal, sensory, or other impairments constrain how the patient performs the task? Can these impairments be changed through intervention, thereby enhancing the patient's functional ability?

The second half of the chapter uses a task-oriented approach to review intervention options aimed at the underlying impairments constraining function, the key components of movement used to perform functional tasks, and the ability to adapt performance of functional tasks to changing task and environmental demands.

⊘ A TASK-ORIENTED APPROACH TO EXAMINATION

Upper extremity control can significantly affect one's ability to take part in life roles. Trombly (1995) suggests that when examining individuals referred for rehabilitation, the clinician should first consider factors that limit successful execution of life roles, because of the personal importance they hold. Furthermore, if one cannot engage in age-appropriate self-care, work or school, and leisure activities or play, further examination is indicated.

Beginning with an interview will ensure that intervention is directed toward primary areas of concern expressed by the patient. Symptoms and concerns should be reviewed and medical and social history obtained. Within the interview you may be able to obtain information about tasks that the individual has difficulty performing and the person's opinion on why this may be so (for example, pain or weakness). In addition, information on family and cultural values that influence the performance of skills may be investigated, since these will directly impact treatment outcome. For example, a child who is able to tie his or her own shoes at school may not carry this over at home because of time constraints when getting ready for school or parental values related to functional independence. Through an interview the clinician can gain a general sense of an individual's cognitive status and where to begin the examination.

Examination at the Functional Level

Once it has been determined that an individual is unable to meet role expectations, a functional examination can help determine how well he or she can perform a variety of daily tasks pertinent to roles that depend on control of the upper extremity. Some functional tasks may be relevant to more than one life role (Dunn et al., 1994). Also, it is important to remember that the ability to perform any functional task is dependent on one's skill in relation to the task demands and the environment or context in which it is performed.

Observation

Prior to initiating a standardized functional examination, it is helpful, when possible, to observe the individual performing tasks in context. For example, it would be useful to observe Phoebe J. in the morning, while she is attempting to perform self-care tasks, or during a meal. Tim R. could be observed in the classroom during art activities, snack time, and when the class is getting ready to go out to the playground. During an observation one can gain insight into underlying impairments that may be constraining performance of functional tasks. Thus, an observation can help the therapist focus the examination appropriately.

Functional Scales

Functional tests incorporating upper extremity skills such as reach and grasp vary from merely checklists to ordinal or interval scales. Standardized assessments using ordinal scales, such as 1 to 4, have been criticized because the intervals between the scores are not necessarily equal (Fisher, 1994; Keith, 1984; Merbitz et al., 1989). However, statistical methods, such as the Rasch technique, can be used to convert ordinal data to interval scales through logarithmic transformations (McHorney et al., 1997). Scales that incorporate the Rasch Item Response Theory scaling model include the Functional Independence Measure (FIM) (Granger et al., 1986), the Patient Evaluation and Conference System and the Assessment of Motor and Process Skills (AMPS) (Fisher, 1994).

Functional Scales for Adults

Numerous adult ADL assessments (checklists or scales) primarily address self-care capabilities (Feinstein et al., 1997). Areas of primary concern in adults include bathing, dressing, grooming, toileting, feeding, mobility, and continence. Two popular ADL scales that were developed on a disability basis include the FIM (Keith et al., 1987) and the Barthel Index (Mahoney and Barthel, 1965). The content of the FIM was developed in part using the framework established by the World Health Organization's international classification of impairments, disabilities, and handicaps (1980). It measures function in the areas of self-care, sphincter control, mobility, locomotion, communication, and social cognition. Although it is an ordinal scale, it can be transformed to an interval scale using the Rasch analysis (Heniemann et al., 1993). The FIM is best used to evaluate rehabilitation progress. It has been found be a good predictor of burden of care (Granger et al., 1979) and of disability in individuals who have sustained strokes (Oszkowski and Barreca, 1993).

An older yet broadly used test is the Barthel Index, developed to evaluate function during rehabilitation. It involves 10 tasks that are rated on a two- or three-point ordinal scale and weighted to achieve a maximum score of 100. Rasch analysis has not yet been used to transform this test from an ordinal to interval scale, which is one area of criticism. However, Granger et al. (1979) determined that a score of 60 or below indicated dependence in self-care.

Standardized instrumental activities of daily living (IADL) scales also offer an approach to assessing upper extremity function by examining skills that require environmental interactions, such as telephone usage, traveling, shopping, preparing meals, housework, and management of finances. The AMPS (Fisher, 1994) is an IADL assessment. This scale can be used to identify deficits in functional performance and examine underlying causes based on observation. Sample areas of assessment include meal preparation and home management. Individuals perform two to three familiar tasks among a range of 50 and are rated in two areas of skill, IADL motor and IADL process. This interval scale has been found to have both reliability and validity.

Pediatric Functional Scales

Haley and colleagues have designed two standardized pediatric functional scales that allow data to be collected by either observation or interview (Haley et al., 1992; Costner et al., 1998). The Pediatric Evaluation of Disability Inventory (Haley et al., 1992) is standardized for children 6 months to 7.5 years. It provides an assessment of the skills children can perform independently and those for which they need assistance. Areas of assessment include self-care, mobility, and social functioning as measured through three separate scales: functional skills, caregiver assistance, and modifications required for function.

The School Functional Assessment (Costner et al., 1998) is normed for children kindergarten to sixth grade. It was designed to identify strengths and limitations related to performance of school-related functional tasks. It is divided into three parts, which are rated separately: participation, task supports, and activity performance. Part three includes both physical activity performance and cognitive/behavioral activity performance and rates execution of tasks on a scale of 1 to 4 (1, does not perform task; 2, partial performance; 3, inconsistent performance; 4, consistent performance). Part three is the most pertinent to use for an evaluation of functional performance involving the upper extremity (Table 19-1).

Another functional scale tailored for children is the WeeFIM (Guide for the Functional Independence Measure for Children, 1993). The WeeFIM (based on the adult FIM) was designed to measure function over time and to measure burden of care (Braun and Granger, 1991). It can be administered by interview of a primary caregiver (parent or teacher) or by direct observation (Sperle et al., 1997). Normative data on the WeeFIM is available for infants and children 6 months to 7 years of age (Msall et al., 1994). The six subscales, scored on a seven-point ordinal scale (1, total assistance, to 7, complete independence) focus on self-care, sphincter control, transfers, locomotion, and cognition.

Amount and Quality of Upper Extremity Use

As discussed in early chapters, following a unilateral central nervous system (CNS) lesion, the patient may be unwilling to use an involved upper extremity when the less affected extremity is available, and this can be a major limitation to the development or recovery of arm function. Since functional assessments may fail to capture the amount

TABLE 19-1.   School Function Assessment (SFA)

Three Parts of Assessment With Adaptations Checklist
1. Participation
2. Task supports
3. Activity performance
   a. Physical Tasks
   b. Cognitive/behavioral tasks

Sample: Activity Performance: Physical Tasks
1. Travel
2. Maintaining and changing positions
3. Recreational movement
4. Using materials
5. Setup and cleanup
6. Eating and drinking
7. Hygiene
8. Clothing management
9. Up and down stairs
10. Written work
    1. *Does not perform*
    2. *Partial performance*
    3. *Inconsistent performance*
    4. *Consistent performance*

Tasks within clothing management

1. Removes hat	1	2	3	4
2. Removes front-opening garment top (e.g., coat)	1	2	3	4
3. Puts on hat	1	2	3	4
4. Puts on front-opening garment top (e.g., coat)	1	2	3	4
5. Lowers garment bottoms from waist to knees and pulls up from knees to waist (e.g., for toileting)	1	2	3	4
6. Zips and unzips, not including separating and hooking zipper	1	2	3	4
7. Removes pullover top (e.g., sweatshirt)	1	2	3	4
8. Removes shoes or boots	1	2	3	4
9. Hangs clothing on hook or hanger	1	2	3	4
10. Puts on pullover top (e.g., sweater)	1	2	3	4
11. Puts on and removes socks	1	2	3	4
12. Puts on shoes or boots (do not consider tying or closures)	1	2	3	4
13. Secures shoes by tying or using Velcro	1	2	3	4
14. Separates and hooks zippers	1	2	3	4
15. Buttons a row of buttons with one-to-one correspondence	1	2	3	4
16. Fastens a belt buckle	1	2	3	4
17. Buttons small buttons (less than 1 inch)	1	2	3	4

Reprinted with permission from Coster W, Deeney T, Haltiwanger J, Haley S. School Function Assessment (SFA). San Antonio: The Psychological Corporation of Harcourt Brace & Co., 1998.

and quality of upper extremity usage, it may be valuable to document this separately. Taub and Wolf (1997) used a motor activity log with individuals recovering from stroke to document the amount and quality of use these individuals had with the hemiparetic arm at baseline and throughout constraint-induced treatment, involving constraint of the nonaffected arm. This assessment incorporates two separate Likert scales that range from 1 to 5 and measure the amount of use and quality of use in the involved limb. A motor activity log can be tailored to the activities most pertinent to the daily life of each individual, as has been done for research purposes with adult stroke patients (Blanton and Wolf, 1999) and children with hemiplegic cerebral palsy (Charles and Lavender, 1997). (Table 19-2 lists sample activities examined in children.) The log can be used to document baseline and progressive use of the limb. This information can be obtained via observation or interview with the patient or a relative (parent, spouse) or other caregiver.

Standardized Tests of Hand Function

Although Trombly (1995) has made a clear argument for context-based examination, it is not always feasible to test function in this manner within the clinical setting. Therefore, a number of commercially available standardized tests have been designed to examine upper extremity function during simulation of functional tasks.

Work Simulation

Two tests commonly used as work simulation tools for adults include the Valpar Work Samples (Valpar Corporation, Tucson), and the BTE Work Simulator (Baltimore Therapeutic Equipment Co., Baltimore). The Valpar Work Samples is a standardized assessment that uses 19 work samples to evaluate reaching, handling, manipulating, and feeding (Baxter-Petralia et al., 1990). The BTE Work Simulator also measures upper extremity function through the use of a mechanical device with 18 tool attachments. These assessments allow one to quantify the individual's ability to handle and manipulate

tools, and performance is compared to normative data (Curtis and Engalitcheff, 1981). If needed, a functional capacity evaluation (FCI), which is an objective measure of one's ability to meet specific vocational and avocational demands based on current status, can be conducted (Rivet, 1992). This test is often done to facilitate return to work and can be quite extensive. Therefore the reader is referred to other sources for a full review (Rivet, 1992; Schultz-Johnson, 1987).

A few tests of hand function can be used to simulate work and tool usage and may be incorporated into an FCI (Apfel and Carranza, 1992). They include the Bennet Hand Tool Dexterity Test (Psychological Corporation, New York), the Crawford Small Parts Dexterity Test (Psychological Corporation, New York), the Purdue Pegboard (Lafayette Instrument Company, Lafayette, IN) and the Stromberg Dexterity Test (Psychological Corporation, New York). These tests can also be used to measure other aspects of dexterity, as reviewed under assessment at level two (manipulation subsection).

ADL Simulation

The Jebsen-Taylor Test of Hand Function Test was designed to simulate hand function common to many ADL tasks (Jebsen et al., 1969). It contains seven timed subtests: writing, card turning, picking up small items, simulated feeding, stacking checkers, picking up light cans, and picking up heavy cans (Figure 19-1) and requires that both hands be tested (nondominant hand tested first). The test takes 10 to 15 minutes to administer. In addition, it has established norms against which a patient's performance can be compared for both adults (Jebsen et al., 1969) and children (Taylor et al., 1973). The Jebsen-Taylor generally has excellent test–retest reliability, with the exception of writing and feeding subtests, which tend to show practice effects (Stern, 1992). Studies have found a moderate correlation between scores on the Jebsen-Taylor test and ADL ability as measured by the Klein-Bell ADL Scale (Lynch and Bridle, 1989). However, the correlations have not been high enough to warrant substitution of the Jebsen for an ADL test.

	TABLE 19-2.	Motor Activity Log

Instructions

I am going to read a list of activities to you. After each activity, I would like you to use the scales that I have placed in front of you to tell me about the use that your son or daughter (or you) has in his or her involved arm for each activity that is listed. I will ask you to think about both the quality of movement and the amount of use of the involved arm. Let's take a moment to go over the scales to make sure that you are clear about what each item on the scale means. If you don't have any further questions, let's begin going over the activities that are listed. We will begin by going over the activities list twice. I will ask you first to think about the amount of use of your son or daughter's involved arm 1 year ago, and then we will go through the list again, thinking about use of the involved arm 1 week ago.

Amount of Use (AOU) Scale
0. Did (does) not use the involved arm.
1. Occasionally tried (tries) to use the involved arm.
2. Used (uses) the involved arm but did (does) most of the activity with the noninvolved arm.
3. Used (uses) the involved arm about half as much as normal or half as often as the noninvolved arm.
4. Used (uses) the involved arm almost as much as normal.
5. Used (uses) the involved arm as much as normal.

Quality of Movement (QOM) Scale
0. The involved arm was (is) never used for that (this) activity.
1. The involved arm moved (moves) during the activity but was (is) of little use (very poor).
2. The involved arm was (is) of some use during that (this) activity but needed (needs) some help from the stronger arm. It moved (moves) very slowly or with difficulty (poor).
3. The involved arm was (is) used for the purpose indicated, but movements were (are) slow or were (are) made only with some effort (fair).
4. The movements made by the involved arm were (are) almost normal but not quite as fast or accurate as normal.
5. The ability to use the involved arm for that (this) activity was equal to the ability to use the noninvolved arm (normal).

Sample Activities	Yes/No/Not Applicable	AOU	QOM
1. Holds a book for reading using two hands			
2. Uses both hands to towel dry face or other body part			
3. Carries an object in the involved hand while using the noninvolved hand to perform a task			
4. Uses both hands for dressing (e.g., holds shirt or trousers with both hands, pulls garments over head or hips using both hands.			
5. Carries an object in the noninvolved hand while using the involved hand to perform a task such as opening the refrigerator			
6. Eats finger food, such as popcorn or potato chips, with the involved hand			
7. Uses both hands to play video games that require both hands			
8. Uses both hands to button or zip an article of clothing			
9. Uses both hands in sports such as baseball, basketball, stickball			

This scale is intended for use with the parents of children with hemiplegia (Charles, Lavender and Taub, 1997).
Adapted with permission from Taub and Wolf (1997).

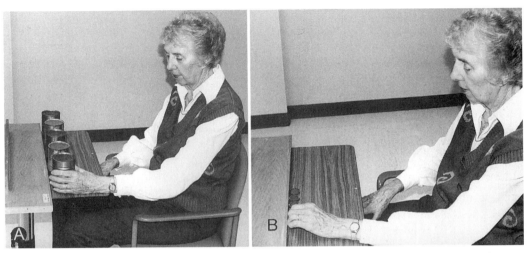

FIGURE 19-1.   Two items from the Jebsen Taylor Hand Function Test. **A.** Lifting light cans. **B.** Stacking checkers.

Handwriting

Analysis of separate functional tasks is sometimes warranted. For example, if a child is having difficulty meeting role expectations as a student due to poor handwriting, task performance could be examined separately. Sample assessment tools include the Developmental Skill Observations of the "K" and "1" Child and Observations for Cursive Writing Skills Training by Mary Benbow, MS, OTR (1992). Another commonly used test is the Evaluation Tool of Children's Handwriting (ETCH) by Susan Amundson, OTR (1995). Dysfunctional behaviors observed during writing may include poor wrist stabilization in extension or failure to steady the paper when writing. Formal assessments, such as the ETCH, typically include measures of global legibility, writing speed, pencil management, and specific handwriting tasks, such as near and far point copying and number and alphabet writing. Some formal tests have normative data available, while others compare the children against themselves and progress is documented accordingly. Formal assessments may highlight problems that can be addressed through further evaluation. For example, if a child seems to have difficulty with copying from the blackboard, one may wish to investigate visual-motor or visual-perceptual function or visual memory.

The advantage of functional performance-based tests and measures is their ability to quantify functional performance and compare it to established norms. Two limitations of this type of testing are that (*a*) the tests do not always examine the quality of movement used and (*b*) the tests do not provide insight into why a patient is unable to perform a functional skill. Thus, formal tests and measures should be coupled with analysis of motor components and strategies as well as underlying impairments or resources such as hand strength.

Examination at the Strategy Level

Examination at the strategy level involves the evaluation of key elements of upper extremity movement, including one's planning ability (anticipatory control). Although an individual may perform a functional task successfully, the repertoire of movement strategies may be limited, which can restrict performance over a range of conditions. Deficits in any one of these areas can significantly limit one's function even if the individual has adequate resources, such as strength and range of motion.

The key elements of upper extremity control include (*a*) visual regard, (*b*) reach and grasp formation, (*c*) grasp, (*d*) manipulation, and (*e*) release. Ideally, examination of upper extremity control would evaluate these key elements separately. In addition, tests can examine the patient's ability to adapt these components to changes in task and environmental demands.

Visual Regard

Examination of eye–head coordination, which underlies localization of an object to be grasped, requires the assessment of three components (Jeannerod, 1984, 1990; Herdman, 1999; Shumway-Cook and Horak, 1990). First, the patient's ability to locate and maintain a stable gaze on either a fixed or moving target, presented in the *central and/or near peripheral* visual field is examined and graded on a three-point scale; intact, impaired, or unable. The patient is asked to keep the head still and move only the eyes. Both saccadic eye movements to fixed targets and smooth pursuit eye movements used to track moving targets are tested. Figure 19-2 shows a patient making saccadic eye movements to a still target located in the near peripheral field. Subjective complaints related to blurred or unstable vision, dizziness or nausea reported by the patient are recorded. In examining our patient, Phoebe J., you might note that she has difficulty making accurate eye movements to targets that are presented in her left visual field. She also has difficulty tracking moving targets.

Next, the patient's ability to locate and stabilize gaze on targets presented in the *far peripheral* visual field is examined (Fig. 19-3) and graded as previously described. Patients should be able to localize a target with the eyes and maintain a stable gaze on that target while the head is moving. Finally, the patient's ability to make eye–head–trunk movements necessary to locate targets oriented in the far periphery is examined. Patients are tested initially in the seated position; however, depending on the patient's abilities, eye–head coordination may be tested in standing and during walking as well (Shumway-Cook and Horak, 1990).

Reach and Grasp

Reach and grasp formation before the object is touched have distinct features that may reveal underlying problems with planning and anticipatory control. Grasp formation begins during transport in anticipation of the object's size and contour (Jeannerod, 1986) (Figure 19-4). Examination of reach and grasp in the clinic can occur during the per-

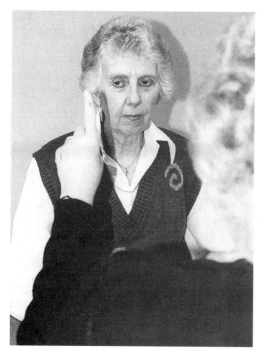

FIGURE 19-2. Testing eye–head coordination: the patient's ability to make saccadic eye movements to locate and maintain gaze on a target in the near peripheral field.

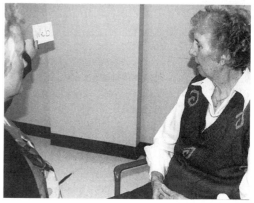

FIGURE 19-3. Testing eye–head coordination: the patient's ability to make coordinated eye–head movements to locate a target in the far peripheral visual field.

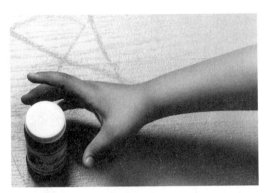

FIGURE 19-4.   Grip formation during transport in anticipation of object size and contour.

formance of functional tasks. Observation and description of the characteristics of reach and grasp can be improved by videotaping and/or using a stopwatch to time movements. Videotaping allows the clinician to analyze movement components by repeated viewing and pausing at segments of interest. However, since videotaping is time consuming and not often available in the clinic, a stopwatch may be a simple way to capture the temporal components of the movement, such as total movement time (initiation of reach to contact with the object) and general timing between reach and grip formation.

Since the movement characteristics of transport and grasp depend on the task and environment (Wu et al., 1998), the clinician is advised to use a variety of activities to assess performance. Tasks that incorporate pointing at various targets or reaching and grasping objects in different portions of the workspace demand that the individual employ a variety of movement strategies. To assess reach and grasp adaptability, targets or objects can be placed ipsilateral and contralateral to the reaching arm, close to the trunk (within arm's reach) and/or at the extreme ends of the workspace (requiring trunk motion). In addition, when examining reach to grasp, it is important to remember Fitt's law (Fitts, 1954), defined as the relationship between movement speed and accuracy. If accuracy demands are high (object to be lifted is fragile or unstable), subjects typically slow down during the final phase of

transport. The relationship between movement speed and accuracy can be examined clinically by altering the type of objects to be lifted.

Two problems you can expect to see in patients who have impaired or underdeveloped reach are extended movement time and an awkward hand path. Problems with grip formation may involve (*a*) impaired anticipatory hand shaping during reaching, resulting in inaccurate hand closure around the target object, as when web space contacts the object before the fingers; (*b*) premature finger closure, resulting in unstable grasp points on the object; or (*c*) inadequate finger aperture for objects of different shapes and sizes because of impairment, such as weak finger extension). Therefore, during the reach it is important to observe the trajectory (path and speed) of the reach, the orientation of the hand, and the shape of the fingers relative to the thumb so as to determine at what point in the movement trajectory the hand opens maximally and then begins to close in anticipation of the object and whether the thumb remains in a stable position during the course of the movement, serving as a reference point for the reach and grasp.

Since anticipatory control of grip formation and final object contact depend on accurate identification of object location and properties, the clinician is reminded to examine the patient's ability to use visual information for this end. Inaccurate grip formation may also be due to poor visual stabilization on the target.

The contribution of the trunk during reach to grasp movements should be analyzed not only for its role as a postural stabilizer (Massion, 1992, for review) but also for its role in the terminal stage of hand transport. As shown by Kaminski et al. (1995), when reaching for anteriorly placed targets, the necessary trunk rotation is countered by glenohumeral horizontal abduction and scapular retraction to keep the hand moving in a straight path. This is demonstrated in Figure 19-5.

Because of its importance, movement of the trunk should be incorporated into the

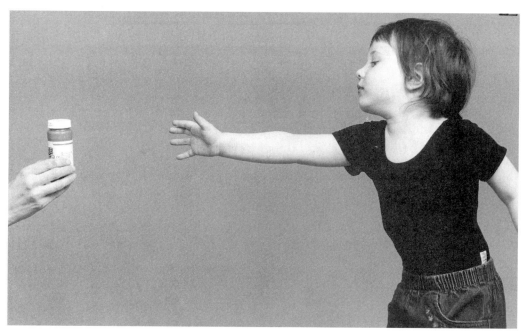

FIGURE 19-5.   The importance of coupling movements between the trunk, glenohumeral joint, and scapula during reaching for anteriorly placed targets.

analysis of reach to grasp movements to targets, especially those placed at the terminal end of the workspace. The clinician can use clinical observations to ascertain the extent of trunk usage during reaches in various locations in the workspace. If available, an overhead video camera can be used during analysis to capture the coordination of the trunk and arm. More realistically, observations from various viewpoints (lateral, posterior, and anterior) can provide a general estimate of trunk involvement.

Anticipatory Control of Grasp

In preparation for grasp, relevant features of the object, such as location, size, shape, texture, and weight, are identified. We draw upon previously formed internal representations and body awareness to plan movements and forces. If anticipatory force scaling is impaired, one must wait for sensory feedback to make modifications in the grip or fingertip forces, which is often too late and can result in object slippage or crushes unless compensatory strategies are employed.

In the clinic impaired anticipatory control may be inferred by visually observing motor behaviors. Behavioral signs of impaired anticipatory control include (*a*) repeatedly knocking over or missing objects when the hand is not open wide enough to grasp them (underestimated width of grip aperture) (*b*) contacting objects with the web space first instead of the fingertips (delay in finger closure prior to contact), (*c*) denting or crushing lightweight objects after grasping (exaggerated grip force) or (*d*) difficulty raising heavy but liftable objects off a table (underestimated load force rate). If one or more signs are evident, the clinician must determine the reason for the lack of anticipatory control, for example impaired sensibility, which can distort the internal representation of an object.

Grasp Stabilization

Prehension patterns vary with the configuration of the object to be grasped. The repertoire of grasp patterns available to an individual can easily be examined by using a simple grasp and lift test designed by Sollerman (1984). The nine items in this test require the use of various patterns: a spherical grip to open a jar, a three-jaw chuck to open a tube of toothpaste, and a cylindrical grip to grasp and lift a glass, among others. Following each lift the examiner rates the pattern on a scale of 1 to 4 (1, unable to complete task; 2, completes task with significantly altered pattern; 3, completes task with a slightly deviant pattern; 4, completes task with normal pattern). Performance can be rated during an observation or review of a videotaped session. This assessment, shown in Table 19-3, can be used to establish a baseline and document progress in recovery of prehension patterns.

Numerous tasks require a sustained grip on a utensil or tool. For instance, handwriting requires a sustained grip on a writing implement. Given the incidence of dystonia (writer's cramp) and fatigue following sustained writing tasks, grip position on writing implements warrants close examination. Ten pencil and crayon grips typically observed during development and compiled from various authors are shown in Figure

19-6 (Schneck and Henderson, 1990). These grip postures can be useful when analyzing pencil grip in children and adults.

Although children younger than 4 years use a variety of grip patterns, the most common ones found among nondysfunctional children older than 6.6 years were the dynamic tripod and lateral tripod (Schneck and Henderson, 1990). In a study of adult grip patterns Bergmann (1990) found that 88% of them used the dynamic tripod, while 9% used a lateral tripod grip. Once a consistent grip pattern has been identified, its efficiency during the performance of functional tasks can be determined through the use of timed copying tests at close and far points (see Handwriting under Examination at the Functional Level).

Manipulation and Release

Once an object is secured, it can be either stabilized or manipulated. Stabilization re-

---

TABLE 19-3.   Sollerman's Grips

Each activity listed is videotaped and scored using the following criteria:
0. Cannot grip the object
1. Grips the object but cannot complete the task
2. Uses an awkward grip and motion but completes the task
3. Uses a slightly deviant grip and motion but completes the task
4. Uses a normal grip and motion and completes the task

Grip	Activity	Score
Transverse grip	Grasp a 2.5-cm-diameter horizontal bar in midair and place it on the table	
Transverse grip	Move a 2.5-cm-diameter vertical bar from one pegboard position to another	
Transverse grip	Lift a glass and pretend to drink	
Diagonal grip	Hold a knife and cut paste into pieces	
Five-finger pinch (modified spherical grip)	Pull a sleeve on and off the unaffected arm	
Tripod pinch (3-jaw chuck)	Unscrew a 2-cm cylindrical cap from a toothpaste tube	
Tripod pinch (3-jaw chuck)	Unscrew a 7-cm cylindrical lid from a jar	
Lateral pinch	Grasp a vertically oriented plate ($5 \times 5 \times 1$ cm)	
Palmar pinch (pad to pad)	Pick up a small cube and touch the chin with it	

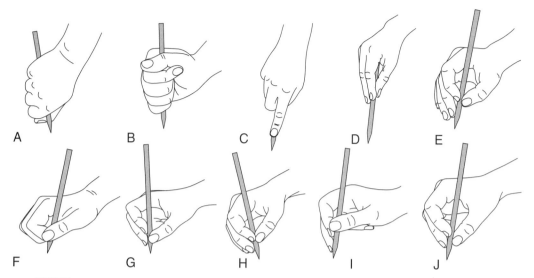

A   B   C   D   E

F   G   H   I   J

FIGURE 19-6. Ten pencil and crayon grips typically observed during development. (Adapted with permission from Schneck CM, Henderson A. Descriptive analysis of the developmental progression of grip position for pencil and crayon control in nondysfunctional children. Am J Occup Ther 1990;44:895.)

quires the use of isometric fingertip forces over a sustained period to prevent slippage of the object. Manipulation is the movement of an object in space or with reference to another object. It requires adaptation to the physical and spatial properties of objects (Corbetta and Mounoud, 1990) and includes several categories of tasks, such as use of tools, including pencils, pens, and scissors); dressing, including tying shoes and buttoning; eating, including use of a knife and opening containers), and other tasks, such as money handling (Swanson et al., 1978). Performance of these skills requires a variety of hand movements with reference to an object, including pushing, pulling, shaking, throwing, transferring, and releasing.

In order to examine the ability of individuals to manipulate objects and adequately regulate fingertip forces, the clinician may ask them to grasp, lift, and release objects of varying sizes, shapes, weights, and textures (Figure 19-7). In addition, patients can be observed while performing a variety of tasks. For example, they may be asked to grasp and lift, grasp and throw, or grasp and place (into small holes). Questions that can be asked relating to the patient's performance during observations: Does the individual

vary the grip pattern used according to the weight, size, and shape of the target object? Does the patient show errors in anticipatory force scaling as evidenced by a consistently excessive squeeze (grip) force for objects of varying weight, slips when lifting heavy and/or large objects, or overshoot during successive lifts with lightweight objects? How much voluntary control and range does the individual demonstrate through the wrist, finger, and thumb extensors to allow them to release large objects? What is the pattern used for release (for example, wrist flexion

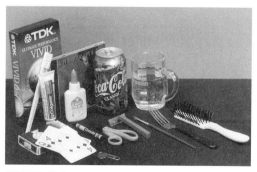

FIGURE 19-7. Objects of varying size, shape, weight, and texture that can be used to roughly estimate the ability of an individual to form an adequate anticipatory grip pattern and scale the fingertip forces used during object manipulation.

used to extend the fingers)? Can the individual place one object on top of another, demonstrating graded control? Observations can also be made during functional tasks, dexterity testing, or assessments of in-hand manipulation, since many of those components require variable grasp, manipulation, and release.

Our patient, Phoebe J., makes frequent errors in programming grip and lift forces, and objects frequently slip from her grasp when she is trying to lift them. She typically uses too much force when grasping and lifting a paper cup, compressing the sides of the cup and spilling the liquid inside. This suggests errors in the anticipatory scaling of the grip and load force.

Standardized Dexterity and Fine Motor Tests

Dexterity is the ability to manipulate various objects using different prehension patterns quickly. Examination of dexterity allows one to determine not only the prehension patterns available but also the efficiency of prehensile movements during object manipulation. Examinations employed differ between adults and children and between diagnoses. It is important to keep in mind that patients with apparent unilateral involvement often exhibit upper extremity control problems on both sides of the body (Gordon et. al, 1999; Pohl and Winstein, 1999). Hence, the clinician should examine both sides. Some commonly used tests of hand dexterity and manipulation skills for adults and children are detailed next.

Purdue Pegboard Test. The Purdue Pegboard Test addresses finger manipulation and hand dexterity (Tiffin, 1968). This time-based measure of dexterity requires placement of pins into holes or assembly of a group of pins, washers, and collars. The four subtests examine prehension in the right hand, left hand, and both hands and performance on a bimanual assembly task. The patient's performance is compared against standardized normative data. Like all timed tests, the Purdue does not evaluate the cause of impaired prehension; it documents only that impairment exists. Normative data are

also available for adolescents 14 to 19 years of age (Mathiowetz et al., 1986).

Minnesota Rate of Manipulation Test. The Minnesota Rate of Manipulation Test (MRMT) (American Guidance Service) is a standardized test of manual dexterity containing five subtests: the placing test, turning test, displacing test, one-hand turning and placing test, and two-hand turning and placing test (AGS, 1969). These are timed tests of dexterity that require the subject to manipulate blocks and place them in a series of holes. The placing and turning tests are the most commonly administered of the five subtests. The MRMT is standardized, and norms are available.

Developmental Fine Motor Tests

The fine motor component of developmental tests is often used to evaluate prehensile skill. Commonly used tests normed for infants and young children include the Peabody Fine Motor Scale (up to 7 years) (Folio and Fewell, 1983), the Gesell Developmental Schedules (up to 2.5 years) (Gesell et al., 1940), The Bayley Scale of Infant Development (0-30 months) (Bayley, 1969), and the Erhardt Developmental Prehension Assessment (up to 6 years) (Erhardt, 1984). The fine motor section of the Bruininks-Oseretsky Motor Development Scale (Bruinicks, 1978) contains both unimanual and bimanual items and is suitable for older children. Normative data are available for children 4.5 to 14.5 years of age. The fine motor section of this assessment has four subtests, including upper limb coordination, speed, and dexterity; response speed; and visual-motor control. Although most items are timed, a few are scored on the number of repetitions or errors performed or by a point score (0, 1, 2). If possible, it may be useful to videotape performance during a fine motor assessment, which may provide greater insight into dexterity, bimanual control, and underlying movement strategies.

In-Hand Manipulation

In-hand manipulation is defined as the process of adjusting an object within one hand after grasping it (Exner, 1989; Pehoski, 1995). As depicted in Figure 19-8, elements

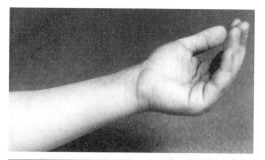

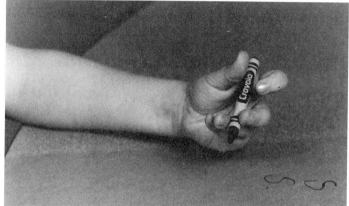

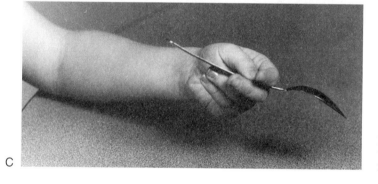

FIGURE 19-8. Elements of in-hand manipulation include (**A**) translation, (**B**) shift, and (**C**) rotation (simple or complex).

of in-hand manipulation include (A) *translation,* moving an object from the fingers to the palm and back, as when picking up a coin and moving it to the palm; (B) *shift,* defined as adjusting the position of an object held near the distal interphalangeal joints of the fingers with the thumb opposed, for example moving a pen so it is held closer to the point for easier writing; and (C) *rotation* (simple or complex), involving turning an object, stabilizing it, and then moving it, such as turning a paper clip or a spoon so it can be used after it has been picked up off the table.

Given its strong association with fine motor coordination and handwriting (Case-

Smith, 1996; Cornhill and Case-Smith, 1996), evaluation of in-hand manipulation may provide greater insight into dexterity problems and serve as a method to document improvement. Case-Smith (1995) modified the nine-hole peg test to examine in-hand manipulation during their study of prehensile skill in children. In that study, the children turned five pegs 180 degrees one at a time and replaced them in their respective holes, while being timed. The task was performed twice and the scores added for a total score. Based on observation, this method seems to incorporate primarily the rotation component of in-hand manipulation. Translation from fingertips to the palm can be evaluated by asking subjects to lift five pegs, holding all of them in one hand simultaneously while being timed.

Other methods for quick examination of translation, shift, and rotation include (*a*) placing a pencil in the individual's palm and asking the individual to adjust it for use and (*b*) placing a quarter in the palm and asking the individual to use the fingers to insert it into a vending machine. The In-Hand Manipulation Test designed by Exner and colleagues (Breslin and Exner, 1999) objectively examines all three components of in-hand manipulation and has been found to have construct validity. However, further validity testing is indicated before it is ready for clinical use.

Examination at the Impairment Level

The third level of examination identifies factors that limit or enhance an individual's performance and strategic planning of task-specific movements. Therefore, it includes an examination of perception (cognition, visual perception), musculoskeletal and neuromuscular factors (range of motion, strength, spasticity, mass patterns), and kinesthetic sensibility. An examination of these underlying systems has been discussed in detail in Chapter 6, so only a brief review of strategies for examining impairments specific to upper extremity control is presented here.

Perception and Cognition

According to Abreu and Toglia (1987), perceptual assessment incorporates both cognitive and visual perceptual capabilities. Typically clinicians vary in the depth of focus they place on these two measures. Furthermore, the amount of time spent on this portion of the assessment is dependent on one's observation and clinical judgment of its relevance to an individual's upper extremity performance. During an observation of functional performance one may suspect deficits that require further examination and possibly attention during treatment.

Cognition

Cognition is defined as one's ability to acquire, organize, and use knowledge. Key cognitive skills inherent in fine motor tasks include problem solving, selective attention, planning, memory, and intention, among others. While one can reach, grasp, and manipulate objects despite cognitive limitations, one's ability to acquire a range of solutions for difficult tasks and correctly identify the usefulness of objects is affected by cognition. Although it is difficult to fully isolate cognitive and motor skills, some evaluations attempt to make clear distinctions (Abreu and Toglia, 1987; Exner and Henderson, 1995). If one observes Phoebe J. having difficulty sequencing a self-care task, it may be that her intention and problem-solving abilities are limited. She also may have poor selective attention, which limits how well she can extract relevant cues regarding the task and the environment. It is important to distinguish whether your client has a cognitive or visual perceptual problem that is limiting function. In addition to formal tests, assessment may be done through observation and videotaping and by conducting an interview immediately following task performance.

Problem Solving. The ability to use a range of solutions to a particular movement problem is key to adaptability or flexibility. An individual who can perform a functional task only one way may have difficulty problem solving. Adolph (1994) has done convincing research examining how infants and toddlers navigate *slopes* from early crawling to late walking. She found that the most significant behavioral features of success were their approach to the problem (risk taker, cautious, or fearful) and their ability to figure out the movement problem (approach to the slope). Compensatory strategies can be deceiving. Although a patient may appear to figure out how to get around an upper extremity movement problem through the use of a compensatory strategy, it is also possible that the inflexible use of a single compensatory strategy is indicative of difficulty arriving at new solutions as well as difficulty with the movements themselves.

There is no easy way to evaluate problem-solving ability. Most often it is inferred from observation. However, one can assess whether or not individuals can solve movement problems by giving them an action or movement goal and observing how they accomplish it over repeated trials and in various contexts. When observing, one should ask a few questions, such as these: Did the individual come up with a range of solutions to the action (or movement) goal or fix on one solution (successful or not)? Did the individual require verbal or manual coaching to enhance successful achievement of the goal? Is the individual persistent in making attempts? It may take a few treatment sessions before one can feel generally confident about an individual's problem-solving ability.

Selective Attention.   The ability to attend to relevant cues in the environment has been found to be a prerequisite to upper extremity control (Jeannerod, 1984, Gordon et al., 1991). When one is first learning or relearning a skill, one must pay close attention to salient (regulatory) cues inherent in the task and the environment (Gentile, 1987). (Regulatory cues are environmental cues that do not change, yet are important to the task.) Inattention to regulatory cues can detract from performance and lead to accidents. For example, Phoebe J.'s left visual neglect most likely affects her upper extremity function. She may inaccurately anticipate the location, size, and shape of an object and either close her hand too soon or wait until she reaches the object before closing her hand around it. Tim R. may not closely attend to the line of a circle drawn on paper and repeatedly move the scissors off the line when cutting it out.

Selective attention requires behavioral monitoring during simulated and real functional tasks to gain an appreciation of an individual's ability. Typical questions during observations include these: Does the individual require cueing to focus attention on important task features? How much cueing is needed? How long can the person focus attention following manual or verbal cueing? Which type of cueing works best? Can the environment be set up differently to enhance selective attention?

Planning.   In order to perform functional tasks appropriately, one must be able to plan and execute movement efficiently. Planning overlaps with the strategy level of assessment. It requires that one extract relevant information from the environment and integrate it with experience and sensory (tactile and proprioceptive) and perceptual (cognitive and visual) cues. Impairments in planning that impact upper extremity control are sequencing and praxis (among others).

Apraxia or Developmental Dyspraxia   As discussed in Chapter 6, there are many forms of apraxia. Since the few tests available used to examine apraxia are similar, the clinician must tease out through clinical reasoning the form of apraxia they are observing. One test is the Goodglass Test for Apraxia (Goodglass and Kaplan, 1972), which requires motor performance of an action in response to a command or demonstration. Actions are subjectively scored as intact, impaired, or severely impaired. This test seems usable for both adults and children.

Somatosensory dyspraxia is the association of poor motor function with diminished tactile and kinesthetic perception. Two subtests extracted from the Sensory Integration and Praxis Tests (Ayres, 1989) are suitable for testing dyspraxia. In one, Imitation of Postures, the child must imitate the mirror image for 12 positions; the other is Praxis on Verbal Command. A score of intact or not is given. Although this test is normed for children 4 to 8.11 years, adolescents and adults with apraxia can be rated subjectively on test items to acquire a general idea of their ability.

Based on the definition of apraxia, many individuals with neurological deficits who have sensory and musculoskeletal deficits cannot be considered to have pure apraxia. However, most clinicians agree that difficulty executing motor behaviors upon command or imitation warrants further assessment that may be accomplished using the tests we have listed.

Visual Perception
This broad category encompasses a range of skills that should be identified separately from eye–head coordination described ear-

lier. Although a number of tests claim to assess visual perception, one is cautioned against making strong assumptions about their relationship to function. It is always advisable to follow up or precede any formal visual perceptual assessment with a contextual observation. Also, since there is a vast number of tests for adults and children, the reader is referred elsewhere for a full review (Cermack and Lin, 1997; Decker and Foss, 1997). Only a few tests are reviewed here.

The choice one makes in assessment is clearly directed by the functional deficit. For example, in a child with reported handwriting difficulties, one can gain insight into visual-motor capabilities by using the Beery-Buktenica Test of Visual-Motor Integration (Beery, 1997). In an earlier manual, Beery (1989) reported that a child who can accurately draw a cross should be ready to begin handwriting instruction.

The Test of Visual-Perceptual Skills, Revised (TVPS-R) (Gardner, 1996) is a pediatric nonmotor assessment of visual perception normed on children 4 years to 12 years, 11 months of age. This test is also normed on children 12 to 18 years (TVPS-UL-R) (Gardner, 1996). The seven subtests included in this assessment are discrimination, memory, spatial relationships, form constancy, sequential memory, figure ground, and closure. Age-specific standardized scoring is available. Other nonmotor assessments are the Motor Free Visual Perceptual Test, Revised (MVPT-R) (Colarusso and Hammill, 1996) and the MVPT (Bouska and Kwatny, 1983). The MVPT-R is standardized on children 4 to 11 years of age and the MVPT, on adults. It includes five categories: spatial relationships, visual discrimination, figure ground, visual closure, and visual memory. Many tests of visual perception, such as the MVPT, are accompanied by screens for acuity and size of visual fields that may have a significant impact on performance.

Musculoskeletal and Neuromuscular Factors

One's ability to move may be restricted by available joint motion, weakness, or the ability to make isolated movements with or without spasticity. In order to obtain a clear picture of musculoskeletal impairments, it is important to assess all three areas.

Range of Motion

The American Society of Hand Therapists has established procedure guidelines aimed at enhancing reliability of range-of-motion measures (Adams et al., 1992, for details). Factors that affect reliability include the size and placement of the goniometer or ruler, the amount of passive force used during measurement, and the method of documentation. Normative data associated with upper extremity function are available from the American Society of Orthopedic Surgeons (1965). Normative data compiled across various authors are also available (Gilliam and Barstow, 1997).

Since measurements of hand motion differ somewhat from standard procedure, we briefly review them for clarity. A composite measure of total active motion or total passive motion through a single digit (finger or thumb) can be made following guidelines published by the American Society of Hand Therapists (ASHT) (Adams et al., 1992). Total motion is the sum of active flexion measurements of the metacarpophalangeal, proximal, and distal interphalangeal joints, minus the extension deficits of the same joints. A ruler can be used to measure finger flexion and thumb movements. Composite finger flexion and hook fist flexion are typically measured with the centimeter ruler of a finger goniometer taken as the distance between the fingertip and the proximal palmar crease (composite) and the fingertip and the distal palmar crease (hook) (Gilliam and Barstow, 1997). Thumb carpometacarpal joint opposition can also be measured with a ruler from the volar interphalangeal (IP) joint of the thumb to the third metacarpal.

Strength

The ability to generate sufficient force (strength) is essential to active upper limb movement and function. However, as described in previous chapters, strength testing in the individual with a neurological lesion is controversial. The primary methods used to evaluate strength are manual muscle testing and commercially available dynamometers. Commercially available dynamometers provide an objective strength measure of grip and pinch strength as well as the strength of larger muscle groups (Wadsworth and Krishman, 1987). The grip dynamometer adjusts for various hand widths, shown in Figure 19-9 (Jamar Dynamometer, Asimow Engineering Company, Los Angeles) (Bechtol, 1954; Fess, 1992). The ASHT has established guidelines for use of a calibrated grip dynamometer, which include 90 degrees of elbow flexion with the forearm and wrist in neutral with the mean of three trials recorded in kilograms or pounds (Fess, 1987, 1992). Use of all five-handle positions should reveal a skewed bell curve (when plotted) with maximal strength in the second or third handle position.

In cases of weak grip or an inability to grasp the handle, a bulb dynamometer or a blood pressure cuff rolled to 5 cm and inflated to 5 mm Hg can be used to document grip strength. Change in the millimeters of mercury is recorded as the power of grip (Fess, 1990). Pinch strength can be evaluated using electronic pinch meters (Pinch Gauge, B and L Engineering, Santa Fe Springs, California) (Fess, 1990). Usually three types of pinch are assessed: (*a*) *tip-to-tip* (thumb tip to index finger tip), (*b*) *three-jaw chuck* (thumb pulp to index and long finger

pulp), and (*c*) *key or lateral pinch* (thumb pulp to lateral aspect of index finger). The use of a pinch meter to assess these patterns of pinch is shown in Figure 19-10. Typically three trials are taken and compared to normative data or against baseline measures. Normative tables for grip and pinch strength are available (Mathiowetz et al., 1985, 1986b).

Coordination

Determining available isolated movement or the degree to which a patient is constrained by abnormal synergies is still considered by many clinicians an important part of assessing upper extremity control (Gowland, 1990). Signe Brunnstrom (1966) proposed stages of recovery, which indicated the degree to which voluntary control was constrained by abnormal synergistic movement.

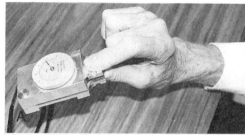

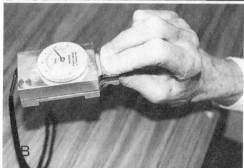

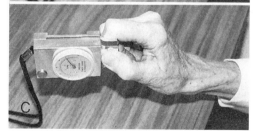

FIGURE 19-10. Use of a pinch meter to measure precision grip strength. Three types of pinch are examined. **A.** Tip-to-tip. **B.** Three-jaw chuck. **C.** key or lateral grip.

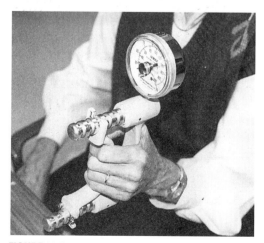

FIGURE 19-9. A Jamar dynamometer can be used to objectively measure grip strength.

This approach to assessment is the basis for the more recent test, the Fugl Meyer Measurement of Physical Performance. This test quantifies movement disorders in the patient who has had a stroke (Fugl-Meyer et al., 1975) and has a subsection that specifically addresses upper extremity motor function. This ordinal scale (0, cannot perform; 1, partially performed; 2, fully performed) incorporates coordination and speed during selected movement tasks.

Another test, which has a separate subsection on upper limb function, is the Motor Assessment Scale (MAS) by Carr and Shephard (Carr et al., 1985) (Table 19-4). For this assessment three upper limb items are scored on a scale arranged in increasing difficulty from zero (unable to complete) to six (high level performance). Test–retest reliability of 0.98 was determined from pilot work (Carr et al., 1985). Other studies have determined that the MAS has high interrater reliability and concurrent validity (Poole and Whitney, 1988).

Edema

Upper extremity edema affects many patients with neurological deficits and can be attributed to an inadequate pumping mechanism acting on the venous and lymphatic systems and a disruption in the normal physiology of tissue (Zarro, 1986). Since edema expands the size of the wrist and hand, active motion can be significantly limited, which leads to disuse during functional tasks. Edema can be evaluated by measuring limb or hand circumference at reproducible anatomical landmarks or through volumetric measurement (Waters et al., 1978). Volumetric assessment measures the water displaced when a limb is immersed. One commercially available hand volumeter consists of a plastic tank with a dowel centered in the lower third of the container to control the depth of hand immersion. A spout at the top of the container allows the displaced water to collect in a 500- to 800-mL-capacity graduated cylinder (Jaffee and Farney-Mokris, 1992). Since there are significant differences between dominant and nondominant hands, clinicians should not compare volume measurement of the affected and unaffected arms in those with hemiplegia. Instead, volume of the impaired extremity should be compared to itself over time (Waters et al., 1978). Since volumes are lower in sitting than in standing, it is important to maintain a consistent testing position. Baseline measurements of edema can be compared against subsequent change.

Sensibility

Sensibility has been shown to be a valid predictor of hand function (Bell-Krotoski et al., 1993; Dellon and Kallaman, 1983; Gordon and Duff, 1999b). For example, static and moving two-point discrimination have been found to correlate highly with haptic gnosis or functional sensibility (Dellon and Kallaman, 1983). Furthermore, Gordon and Duff (1999b) found static two-point discrimination to strongly predict whether children with hemiplegic cerebral palsy could adapt their fingertip force to texture during object manipulation. Since sensibility strongly affects movement, it is advisable to assess its integrity. Sensibility tests performed in the upper extremities primarily focus on the hands, in particular the fingertips. The most valid and reliable measures of sensibility currently available are touch pressure tests, two-point discrimination tests, and haptic gnosis (stereognosis) tests. A detailed description of sensory testing and norms may be found in an evaluation manual published by the ASHT (Stone, 1992).

Touch pressure sensitivity reflects the integrity of the nerve fiber and can be tested using the Semmes-Weinstein monofilaments (Semmes and Weinstein, 1960) or the Weinstein Enhanced Sensory Testing. The use of graduated nylon monofilaments (Fig. 19-11) is considered one of the most reliable and valid tests of sensory capacity and its relationship to functional abilities (Bell-Krotoski, 1990). Following perpendicular placement (vision occluded) of a nylon filament along the finger pulp, the individual reports when he or she feels the pressure of the tip (the filament bends when the peak force threshold is reached) (Bell-Krotoski, 1990).

TABLE 19-4. Motor Assessment Scale

Upper Arm Function	Details	Score
1. Supine, protract scapula with arm in 90 degrees of flexion.	1. Therapist places arm in position and supports elbow in extension.	
2. Supine, hold arm in 90 degrees shoulder flexion for 2 seconds.	2. Therapist places arm and patient must maintain the position with some external rotation. Elbow within 20 degrees of full extension.	
3. Supine, hold arm in 90 degrees of shoulder flexion, flex and extend elbow to take palm to forehead.	3. Therapist may assist supination of forearm.	
4. Sitting, hold extended arm in forward flexion at 90 degrees to body for 2 seconds.	4. Therapist places arm and patient maintains position without excess scapular elevation. Forearm held in midposition.	
5. Sitting, patient lifts arm to above position in item 4, holds for 10 seconds, then lowers it.	5. Patient must maintain position with some external rotation without pronation.	
6. Standing, hand on wall. Maintain hand position while turning body toward wall.	6. Arm is abducted to 90 degrees with palm flat against the wall.	

Hand Movements	Details	Score
1. Sitting, extension of wrist. Patient is asked to lift object off the table by extending the wrist.	1. Patient rests forearm on table while sitting. Therapist places cylindrical object in palm of patient's hand. No elbow flexion.	
2. Sitting, radial deviation of wrist. Patient is asked to lift hand off the table (from mid-position).	2. Therapist places forearm in midposition (resting on ulnar side, thumb in line with forearm, and wrist in extension).	
3. Sitting with elbow at side, pronate and supinate forearm.	3. Elbow unsupported and at a right angle; three-quarters range is acceptable.	
4. Sitting, reach forward, pick up ball of 14 cm (5 inches) diameter with both hands and put it down.	4. Balls placed on table at a distance that requires elbow extension. Palms should be kept in contact with the ball.	
5. Sitting, pick up a polystyrene cup from the table and replace it from one side of the body to the other.	5. Do not allow alteration in shape of cup.	
6. Sitting, continuous opposition of thumb and each finger more than 14 times in 10 seconds.	6. Each finger taps the thumb, starting with index. Do not allow thumb to slide from one finger to the other or to go backward.	

Advanced Hand Activities	Details	Score
1. Pick up the top of a pen and put it down.	1. Patient reaches to arm's length, picks up and releases pen top on table close to body.	
2. Pick up one jellybean from a cup and place it in another cup.	2. Teacup (arm's length) contains eight jellybeans. Left hand takes jellybean from cup on right and releases it in cup on left.	
3. Draw horizontal lines to stop at a vertical line 10 times in 20 seconds.	3. At least 5 lines must touch and stop at the vertical line. Lines should be about 10 cm.	
4. Hold a pen, make rapid consecutive dots on a sheet of paper.	4. Patient must make at least 2 dots per second for 5 seconds. Patient picks pen up and positions it without assistance. Pen must be held as for writing. Dots, not dashes.	
5. Take a dessert spoon of liquid to the mouth.	5. Do not allow head to lower toward spoon. Liquid must not spill.	
6. Hold a comb and comb hair at back of head.	6. Shoulder external rotation, abducted 90 degrees, head erect.	

Reprinted with permission from Carr JH, Shepherd RB, Nordholm L, Lynne D.
Investigation of a new motor assessment scale for stroke patients. Phys Ther 1985;65:175–180.

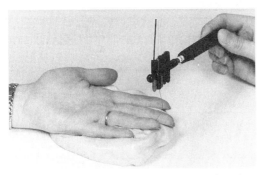

FIGURE 19-11. The use of graduated nylon monofilaments to test touch and pressure sensibility. The Semmes-Weinstein monofilament test.

Static or moving two-point discrimination (Stone, 1992) examines one's ability to detect two stimuli simultaneously applied at varying distances. However, it is difficult to duplicate the amount of pressure used during testing and the rate of moving two-point discrimination from one trial to the next. Reliability during two-point discrimination can be increased by using a commercial testing instrument such as the DiskCriminator (Figure 19-12).

Proprioception, or position sense, is typically tested by holding the involved part laterally and passively moving the joint to be tested (Carey et al., 1993; Dannenbaum and Jones, 1993; Trombly and Scott, 1989). Although proprioception does play a significant role in grasp and lift tasks, most measures of proprioception remain somewhat limited, since the amount of force used to hold the part during testing and the rate of passive movement cannot be controlled.

Stereognosis, or haptic perception, is a measure of active sensibility and represents the most complex of the sensory-perceptual skills (Fess, 1990). The Modified Picking-Up Test (Dellon, 1981; Dellon and Munger, 1983) is a method of testing haptic perception in which the individual must perform a timed placement test prior to an object recognition test with vision occluded. The objects require increasing levels of discrimination. A variation of this test requires visual matching of various plastic shapes against a visible picture card (Manual Form Perception Test from Sensory Integration and Praxis Test, Los Angeles, California).

Pain

Another complication that interferes with the recovery of upper extremity function is pain, because of its unpleasant sensory and emotional experience (Merskey et al., 1986). Subjective pain information can be obtained through history, interviews and questionnaires, body diagrams, or pain rating scales (Maurer and Jezek, 1992). Through an interview and a questionnaire one can obtain information about the location and extent of pain and determine whether pain is constant or intermittent, present at rest or present only when the person moves. The McGill Pain Questionnaire (Melzack, 1975) provides a descriptive word list from which patients can choose the quality and intensity of pain. Body diagrams let the individual visually describe the location and type of pain, but it requires sincere interpretation on the part of the patient. Rating scales such as the Visual Analog Scale have been found to have good predictive validity and high concurrent validity in children (Jedlinsky et al., 1999) and adults (Price et al., 1983). A patient is given a 10-cm line drawn vertically or horizontally on paper. The end of each line is labeled; on one end it says, "Pain as bad as it can be," and the other end, "No pain." To obtain an objective measure, the clinician divides the 10-cm line into 20 increments from which the distance from no pain to the mark

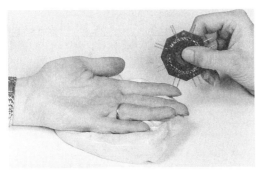

FIGURE 19-12. The DiskCriminator, a commercially available two-point discriminator testing instrument.

TABLE 19-5. Summary of Evaluation Profile for Phoebe J.

Level 1: Function	Level 2: Strategies and Key Components of Movement	Level 3: Impairments
1. Self-care: Dressing with grooming, bathing, toileting	Planning and sequence of selfcare tasks	Perception: cognition and visual perception (Mini Mental Status Exam, MVPT)
2. Cooking and self-feeding	Movement: Eye-head coordination, anticipatory control of reach to grasp stationary objects, prehension patterns available.	Musculoskeletal: range of motion, strength, isolated movement available and degree of spasticity in LUE (left upper extremity)
3. Mobility using assistive devices	Manipulation ability	Sensibility present in LUE; edema present in LUE; pain at rest and with movement

can be measured. Another rating scale that appeals to children is the Faces Pain Rating Scale (Wong and Baker, 1988).

Case Studies

Tables 19-5 and 19-6 summarize evaluation profiles for Phoebe J. and Tim R. Although the list is not exhaustive, it does highlight key areas of function and specific tests that should be considered during an evaluation.

In summary, when examining the impact of upper extremity dyscontrol on function, it is necessary for the clinician to examine per-

formance at all three levels: impairment, strategy and function. However, since the list of possible tests and measures is extensive, it is important to focus on areas that seem to restrict upper extremity function as relevant to the execution of life roles.

⌨ TRANSITION TO INTERVENTION

Developing therapeutic strategies to retrain upper extremity control in the patient with neurological dysfunction begins with the

TABLE 19-6. Summary of Evaluation Profile for Tim R.

Level 1: Function	Level 2: Strategies and Key Components of Movement	Level 3: Impairments
Self-help: Use of fasteners on coats, shoe tying and untying, hand washing, toileting	Sequencing of classroom projects	Cognition: Visual and auditory memory for ABCs and numbers Perception: VMI (Beery and Butenica, 1997), TVPS (Gardner, 1996)
Manipulation of materials: Pencils, scissors, glue, tape, other supplies	Manipulation skills: prehension patterns frequently used, pencil grip, in-hand manipulation skill	Musculoskeletal: Strength and isolated movement of fingers and thumb, proximal muscular control
Functional handwriting	Observation of visual motor strategies used for copying; method used to hold paper steady	Sensibility through both hands; pain following extensive use of hands (may be endurance issue)

TABLE 19-7. A Summary of Problems, Goals, and Methods Appropriate for Phoebe J.

Level	Problems	Long-Term Goals	Short-Term Goals	Methods
Level 1: Function	1. Phoebe J. is unable to prepare meals for herself.	1. Phoebe J. will be able to prepare three simple meals without assistance.	1. Phoebe J. will prepare a simple three-step meal without assistance.	1. Written three-step directions to follow with practice; informational cues on sequencing as needed.
	2. Phoebe J. is unable to perform self-grooming.	2. Phoebe J. will be able to groom herself in preparation for guests or outings.	2. Phoebe J. will be able to manage a hairbrush, toothbrush, and toothpaste tube without assistance or with assistive devices.	2. Modeling, task-specific practice, and problem solving through solutions. 3. Assistive devices may be needed for each short-term goal, such as built-up foam on hairbrush to facilitate use of gross grasp.
Level 2: Strategies and Key Movements	1. Phoebe J. is unable to sequence tasks with more than 2 steps.		1. Phoebe J. will follow step-by-step verbal directions and/or written instructions for simple meal preparation.	1. Written directions will be available to her during task-specific practice. Steps will be added to simple meal preparation per tolerance.
	2. Phoebe J. can achieve only a gross grasp with her left hand.		2. Phoebe J. will grasp objects of various sizes and shapes using a gross grasp and other patterns as available such as a lateral pinch.	2. Practice reaching for objects that initially require a gross grasp and progress to those requiring a lateral pinch.
	3. Phoebe J. seems to wait until she contacts objects before closing her fingers (poor anticipatory control).		3. Phoebe J. will prepare for object contact during reaches by opening and closing her hand in advance.	3. During reaches, provide verbal cue to open, then close fingers in preparation for object contact. Replay videotaped practice and talk through performance.
Level 3: Impairments	1. Phoebe J. has visual and auditory memory deficits.		1. Phoebe J. will be able to state the sequence of written directions following one reading.	1. Verbal rehearsal prior to practice. Replay of videotaped sessions, discussing steps taken during performance.
	2. Phoebe J. has incomplete isolated movement of thumb and finger flexors.		2. Phoebe J. will be able to isolate her thumb to achieve a lateral pinch.	2. Active practice of thumb movement in various planes with light manual resistance.
	3. Phoebe J. has weak wrist and finger extensors.		3. Phoebe J. will increase active wrist extension to 25 degrees and MCP extension to -10 degrees.	3. Biofeedback and resistive activities, such as 1- to 3-pound weights, Theraputty and Velcro boards (pushing for finger extension).
	4. Sensibility is impaired through her fingers and thumb.		4. Phoebe J. will identify two objects without vision.	4. Identification of various textures and objects with and without vision.

MCP, metacarpophalangeal.

identification of a comprehensive list of the patient's strengths and weaknesses at all three levels. These levels include functional ability, available strategies, and movement components, as well as specific impairments and available resources.

Long-Term Goals

As proposed in Chapter 5, long-term goals should be objective and measurable and in terms of recovery of upper extremity function expressed in terms of self-care, work, or leisure activities executed to fulfill role expectations. For example a long-term goal for Phoebe J. could be, "Phoebe J. will be able to prepare a morning meal independently (to fulfill her role as a homemaker)." A long-term goal for Tim R. could be "Tim R. will be able to independently dress himself for playground activities (to fulfill his role as a student)."

TABLE 19-8.   A Summary of Problems, Goals, and Methods Appropriate for Tim R.

Level	Problems	Long-Term Goals	Short-Term Goals	Methods
Level 1: Function	1. Tim R. cannot secure fasteners on his coat in preparation for recess.	1. Tim R. will don and doff his coat, including fasteners, prior to and following recess.	1. Tim R. will secure and undo the small buttons on his coat within 2 minutes, prior to and following recess.	1. Teacher or therapist modeling and task specific practice with verbal and manual cues.
	2. Tim R. requires moderate assistance to complete art projects that require the use of scissors.	2. Tim R. will complete art projects, requiring the use of scissors, independently.	2. Tim R. will trace a circle, cut it out and paste it on the paper as described in the directions.	2. Introduce scissors adapted with smaller finger openings to enhance stability. Verbal and manual cueing during execution of task. Peer modeling.
Level 2: Strategies	1. Tim R. cannot adapt to new fasteners if he wears a new jacket. He is unable to problem-solve without becoming frustrated.		1. Tim R. will be able to don and doff a range of coats with varying fasteners (zippers, snaps, buttons), demonstrating a range of solutions.	1. Modeling and task-specific practice. Informational feedback on solutions used.
	2. Tim R.'s in-hand manipulation skill is limited.		2. Tim R. will be able to shift objects among his fingers as needed to button.	2. Modeling and practice with a host of materials which must be manipulated in one hand.
Level 3: Impairments	1. Tim R. has weak intrinsic muscles, which may contribute to his weak pinch/grip and difficulty with in-hand manipulation.		1. Tim R. will increase the strength of his lateral pinch and 3-jaw chuck pinch by 0.5 pounds in 2 months.	1. Theraputty exercises at school and with home exercise program. 2. Construction of objects using Legos or similar materials.

Short-Term Goals

Short-term goals should also be objective and measurable. They may be described with regard to resolving impairments and recovery of key components of upper extremity control. Short-term goals may also include movement planning, sequencing, and the capacity to adapt strategies so that functional tasks can be performed in changing environmental contexts. In addition, they may be described as interim steps to achieving independence in a functional task. Table 19-7 provides examples of problems, goals, and methods that might be useful for Phoebe J. Table 19-8 summarizes problems, goals, and methods that might be useful for Tim R.

☉ A TASK-ORIENTED APPROACH TO INTERVENTION

Whether aiming for improvement in a range of functional skills or just one task in particular, a task-oriented approach to intervention focuses on all levels in which deficits are exposed. For example, in the case of Phoebe J., interventions within a single treatment session could include strengthening her wrist and finger extensors (impairment level), grasp and release of various objects requiring different prehension patterns (strategy level), and practice of a task that incorporates all features (functional level), such as stacking plastic glasses on a shelf in a cabinet.

The relationship between underlying impairments and hand function may be task dependent (Gordon and Duff, 1999b). In addition, if one does not consider the context in which the individual performs, treatment may focus on impairments irrelevant to function. Conversely, if impairments are not addressed, deficits may persist in limiting function unnecessarily.

General Issues

Before beginning a discussion of a task-oriented approach to retraining reach, grasp,

and manipulation, we consider some important general issues related to treatment of upper extremity function.

Proximal Versus Distal Control

Since, as researchers have shown, control over proximal body segments is not a necessary precursor to working on distal hand function, the two can be addressed simultaneously rather than sequentially. In essence, one should not wait for proximal control to emerge before working on hand function. The degree to which recovery occurs is dependent on plasticity within the system. It is possible that select areas of the CNS can substitute for injured regions (see Chapter 4) (Merzenich and Jenkins, 1993; Merzenich et al., 1983). Proximal functions involving the transport phase and/or shoulder stability may be easily substituted by the use of alternative neural pathways. In contrast, cortical motor neuronal lesions often result in profound loss of precision movements of the hand because alternative pathways are not readily available (Rothwell, 1994). Therefore, recovery of isolated hand movement and prehensile function may be limited.

Motor Learning and Practice Schedules

How individuals learn motor skills depends on many factors that must be considered when the clinician treats clients with upper extremity dyscontrol. As reviewed in Chapter 2, factors impacting motor learning, such as conditions of practice, modeling, and verbal and mental rehearsal are important considerations when establishing a treatment program.

Therapists frequently vary practice by changing the order of tasks practiced (for example, day 1, buttoning first, then zippering; day 2, zippering first, then buttoning), altering the context (natural versus simulated environment), and emphasizing different subcomponents of a task, such as speed of execution and target distance. The practice of tasks in natural contexts with multidimensional goal-oriented purpose embedded in it, elicits higher success in acquisition and transfer than simulated contexts (Ferguson and Trombly, 1997). Again, it is best to verify that your client has actually retained the tasks practiced and can generalize them to related situations.

Therapists should take advantage of the powerful effect both modeling and verbal and mental rehearsal have on motor skill learning. These techniques may be valuable at both the strategy and functional level of treatment and are highlighted periodically in the remainder of this chapter.

Special Considerations Related to Children

The therapeutic techniques used to train and retrain upper extremity control vary according to the particular problems facing each patient. Specific techniques may be suitable for adults but controversial or contraindicated for use with children. For example, to treat joint capsule tightness that is limiting motion in an adult patient, therapists often employ ultrasound prior to passive mobilization or exercise. However, in children, the appropriateness of the use of ultrasound over growing bone remains controversial (Michlovitz and Zarro, 1986). In contrast, biofeedback and electrical stimulation have been shown to be beneficial in both adults and children. With these considerations in mind, we now turn to discussing a task-oriented approach to training reach, grasp, and manipulation skills.

Intervention at the Impairment Level

Treatment strategies aimed at modifying sensory and motor impairments were presented in detail in Chapter 6; therefore, only a brief discussion of some treatment suggestions often used in modifying impairments in the upper extremity is presented here.

Cognition and Perception

As emphasized in Chapter 6, cognitive and perceptual impairments can significantly restrict functional movement and are a major factor in lack of progress in those with neurological insults (Warburg, 1994; Bernspang et al. 1989; Titus et al., 1991; Sea et al., 1993).

Table 6-3 reviews perceptual and cognitive impairments. This section reviews interventions aimed at addressing select cognitive and perceptual impairments crucial to upper limb motor control and related function (see Chapter 6 for greater detail).

Attention and Unilateral Neglect

Identification of an object's properties allows us to use anticipatory control for grip formation during transport as well as for fingertip force regulation. Therefore, an essential part of training reach and grasp is helping patients learn to identify and attend to relevant perceptual cues and object properties. These cues are critical to shaping the hand prior to contact and scaling fingertip forces during manipulation. For the stroke patient who has unilateral neglect (neglect of one side of the body or extrapersonal space) the clinician may place target objects in the area of the workspace that the patient tends to neglect and ask the patient to find the target objects. To promote identification of an object's physical properties, patients can be encouraged to explore objects both visually and haptically (with their hands), drawing their attention to characteristics that are important in correctly shaping their hand and scaling fingertip forces. Before a patient grasps and lifts an object, he or she can be asked about perceptions regarding its essential characteristics. This helps patients to attend to relevant perceptual cues related to the task. For example, the clinician could ask, "Do you think that object is heavy or light? Is it slippery or not?" "Can you open your hand wide enough to secure the object?" Although research suggests that retraining perceptual aspects of grip is important to the recovery of control, strategies for such retraining are just emerging and have yet to be tested experimentally.

Musculoskeletal and Neuromuscular Impairments

A number of methods are available to enhance range of motion and strength and to reduce the effects of spasticity and increase isolated movement. For example, passive and active exercises, myofascial release

(Manheim and Lavett, 1989), the Felden-krais method (Apel, 1992) or related approaches (Wanning, 1993) can be employed to mobilize structures essential to upper extremity control. Many sources describe in detail approaches to mobilizing the trunk, scapula, and shoulder structures and enhancing movement in the patient with a neurological impairment (Bobath,1970; Boehme, 1988; Carr and Shepard, 1986; Davies, 1985; Duncan and Badke, 1987; Voss et al., 1985).

Although many techniques are used clinically, they have yet to be validated through controlled research. Hemiplegic patients (adults or children) who habitually hold the involved upper extremity in mass flexion typically develop tightness of the hand and wrist flexors, which limits the development or return of active movement. Within treatment active movement should follow any attempt at passive stretching. For instance, after stretching the finger, wrist, and elbow flexors, one may ask the patient to attempt to tap or grasp (depending on prehension) a stable object from the table within reach and at the distal end of the workspace.

Figure 19-13 shows one approach to active mobilization of musculoskeletal structures in the trunk, arm, and hand (Carr and Shephard, 1986). In this approach, the patient, in the supine position, rotates the shoulders and hips in the opposite direction to lengthen the trunk, arm, and hand muscles

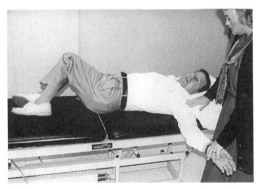

FIGURE 19-13. Counterrotation between the shoulders and hips results in elongation of the trunk and is used to reduce muscle tightness in the trunk and arm muscles.

that have shortened because of paresis or spasticity. Other approaches to remediating musculoskeletal constraints include the use of plaster casts, splints, and orthoses to increase range of motion and mobility of arm and hand structures (Cannon, 1985; Cruick-shank and O'Neill, 1990; Fess et al., 1981; Law et al., 1991; Lindholm, 1985; Malick, 1980; Neuhaus et al., 1981; Smith and Harris, 1985; Yasukawa, 1992; Zizlis, 1964).

Splints and Functional Electrical Stimulation

Fabricating splints that minimize joint restrictions and allow functional use of the hand is optimal. However, in cases of flaccidity or inactive hand movement, positions that reduce the chance of undesirable contractures associated with immobility are preferred. An example of this is the *intrinsic plus* position of the hand (Figure 19-14*A*) in which the thumb rests in partial abduction, and the fingers are positioned to ensure that the ligaments are taut and the joints adequately positioned (MP flexion and IP extension). If a patient demonstrates excessive wrist flexion that interferes with the achievement of active prehension, a semiflexible splint (see Figure 19-14*B*) may be suitable; this allows partial wrist movement within the active range yet prevents extreme wrist flexion, which can be limiting. Sustained low-load stretch to muscle and joint structures, accomplished through splinting, has been found to increase the number of muscle sarcomeres and alter the noncontractile tissue (joint capsule, ligaments) (Blanchard et al., 1985; Tardieu et al., 1988). It is important to remember that although hand splinting does provide support and prevent contractures, nonaffected musculoskeletal structures should be allowed to move freely to prevent secondary impairments due to immobility.

Studies have shown that glenohumeral subluxations often found in adult stroke patients may be successfully reduced by functional electrical stimulation (FES) with surface electrodes (Faghri et al., 1994), removing the need for trays and slings, which may impede active movement of the

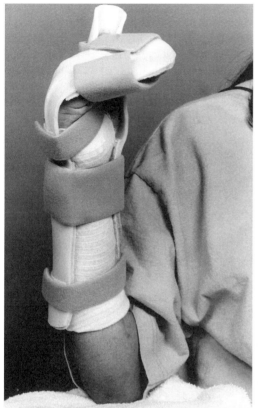

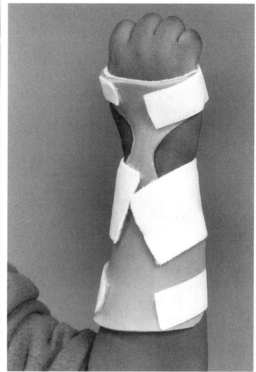

A

B

FIGURE 19-14.   Splints used to position the hand include the *intrinsic plus* splint (**A**) and a semiflexible wrist splint (**B**).

hemiparetic limb. Another study done on children with hemiplegic cerebral palsy (Scheker et al., 1999) combined FES 1 hour a day (to triceps and wrist–finger extensors) with dynamic bracing (assisted metacarpophalangeal extension, biceps strengthening aimed at supination) during two 30-minute sessions per day or three 20-minute sessions. Static bracing was done at night to stretch the contracted extrinsic finger, wrist, and elbow flexors. Results demonstrated a reduction in spasticity based on the Zancolli classification (Zancolli et al., 1983) and improved hand function. Based on these findings, a clinician may wish to combine FES with splinting for maximum benefit. Since time lines for treatment vary with the nature of the dysfunction, clinical judgment must guide schedules for FES use and splint wear. Given the positive effects of the work on FES, it may be possible either to replace splints or

slings or reduce their use, affording greater opportunity to develop or regain active upper limb control.

Sensory Reeducation

It is uncertain just how much functional sensibility can be improved following a peripheral or central lesion. Does sensory reeducation teach patients how to use the remaining sensibility to their advantage, or does it actually alter the physiological basis for sensation? Investigators involved in training and retraining of sensory function report that improvement is highly dependent on the individual's motivation as well as training. Patients who were willing to use the impaired limb were better able to recover function.

A number of published reports recount sensory retraining methods for patients who have sustained peripheral and central neural injuries resulting in decreased sensibility (Maynard, 1978; Dellon et al., 1974; Callahan, 1990). Several authors have recommended that sensory reeducation programs focus on both protective and discriminative sensory functions (Bell-Krotoski et al., 1993; Dellon et al., 1974; Callahan, 1990; Brand, 1980; Vinogrand et al., 1962).

A safe guideline to follow is related to the level of performance on the Semmes-Weinstein monofilaments test (see Chapter 6 for a discussion of this test of sensory function). If individuals are unable to detect 4.83 pressure rating, they are considered to have absent or significantly impaired protective sensation. In those cases, treatment should focus on teaching strategies to protect the limb from harmful stimuli (Brand, 1980). Table 19-9 summarizes a series of guidelines aimed at protecting the hand and arm from injury. As dictated by returning or developing sensibility (once protective sensation is intact or touch pressure is above a rating of 4.83), treatment can focus on the detection and localization of moving and stationary light touch stimuli. As patients learn to perceive constant and moving touch, sensory

reeducation can shift to stereognosis (size and shape discrimination, object recognition).

A large part of sensory reeducation makes use of higher cortical functions, including attention, learning, and memory, to facilitate sensory detection, recognition, and localization (Dellon et al., 1974). Tactile retraining generally is done with and without vision. For example, since it is known that moving stimuli are more detectable than stationary stimuli, the patient can be taught to move the hand to achieve a moving stimulus and thus improve the chances for sensory awareness. Vision can be used to compensate for deficits in tactile sensation; thus, the patient can be taught to look at the hand when reaching or grasping an object (Bell-Krotoski et al., 1993). For a more complete discussion of methods for sensory reeducation, the reader is referred to articles by Callahan (1990) and Bell-Krotoski et al. (1993).

Edema and Pain

In order to reduce hand edema one or more of the following strategies can be used: compression (through the use of Isotoner gloves, finger sleeves, or Coban wrap), ice, elevation above the heart level, and active muscle pumping. Effectiveness of any method can be verified using volume or circumference measurement. Reduction in edema with an increase in active movement may assist in pain reduction. Other methods to reduce pain include the use of heat or cold modalities or transcutaneous electrical nerve stimulation (TENS) (Mannheimer and Lampe, 1984). Depending on the characteristics of the pain, TENS may be appropriate for rest periods after exercise or during active movement.

Intervention at the Strategy Level

A task-oriented approach to retraining involves more than just the resolution of impairments constraining performance of functional tasks. Alleviating underlying impairments allows the possibility of using previously developed strategies for upper ex-

---

TABLE 19-9.   Protective Strategies for Patients With Decreased Sensibility in the Upper Extremity

1. Avoid exposure to thermal extremes and sharp objects.
2. Do not use excessive force when gripping a tool or object.
3. Build up small handles to distribute force and avoid localized increase in pressure.
4. Avoid tasks that require the use of a uniform grip over long periods.
5. Change tools frequently to alter grip and to rest tissues.
6. Observe skin for signs of stress.
7. Treat blisters and lacerations quickly and with care to avoid infection.
8. Maintain daily skin care, including soaking and oil massage to maintain optimal skin condition.

Adapted with permission from Brand PW. Management of sensory loss in the extremities. In: Omer E, Spinner M, eds. Management of peripheral nerve problems. Philadelphia: WB Saunders, 1980:262–272.

tremity control. When permanent impairments make the resumption of previously used strategies impossible, patients must be guided in the recovery or development of sensory and motor strategies that are effective in performing the key components of upper extremity control. Key movement components such as a smooth hand path and anticipatory grip formation may be best elicited if real tasks are used instead of simulated ones (Wu et al., 1998). Since research has shown that development of key components such as reach and grasp are driven by the nature and context of the activity, retraining these key components must be done within the context of purposeful tasks.

Eye–Head Coordination

An important part of upper extremity control is training or retraining eye–head coordination, which is essential to locating and stabilizing gaze on a target or an object to be grasped. Problems that affect the ability to locate objects and stabilize gaze can affect the accuracy and precision of reaching movements. Since different control mechanisms underlie the movements of eyes, head, and trunk, these systems need to be trained separately and in combination.

A progression of exercises for retraining eye–head coordination and gaze stabilization in patients with vestibular dysfunction has been proposed by Susan Herdman, a physical therapist, and David Zee, M.D., at Johns Hopkins University Medical School (Herdman, 1999; Zee, 1985). These exercises have been used successfully to retrain eye–head coordination problems in patients with central neurological disorders (Herdman, 1999; Zee, 1985).

This approach is reviewed in Table 19-10 and begins with exercises to retrain saccadic and smooth-pursuit eye movements while the head is still. Exercises are progressively given to retrain coordinated eye movements in conjunction with head movements to targets in the peripheral visual field. Also practiced are exercises to maintain a stable gaze on an object moving in phase with the head. Finally, movements of the eye, head, and

trunk are practiced as patients learn to locate targets in the far periphery. Exercises are practiced with the patients sitting, standing, and walking (Herdman, 1999; Zee, 1985).

Research in the field of training and retraining visual perception in patients with central neural lesions is just beginning. Strategies to assist patients with visual field deficits, such as homonymous hemianopsia, involve teaching them to consciously scan the space represented by the impaired visual field (see earlier suggestions regarding treatment strategies for visual neglect).

Reach and Grasp

Reaching requires the ability to move the arm in a coordinated way in all directions. It involves transporting the hand to an object to be grasped, forming the grip appropriately, stabilizing or manipulating the object, and moving the grasped object to a new location.

Training or retraining upper extremity movement control, in cases of congenital or acquired paresis, often begins with therapeutic strategies used to facilitate active motion by the patient. Several authors have laid out a progression of activities for retraining arm function, which includes training or retraining control of arm movements underlying the transport phase of upper extremity function (Duncan and Badke, 1987; Bobath, 1970; Carr and Shepard, 1986; Davies, 1985; Boehme, 1988; Voss et al., 1985). Most of the suggestions are directed toward practicing control of isolated joint movements with the patient supine, sitting, and standing. These exercises are based on the assumption that practicing activation of isolated muscles will carry over to functional tasks. For example, retraining active control of arm movements is often begun with the patient in the supine position with the shoulder flexed and the elbow extended (Fig. 19-15*A*). This position minimizes the amount of force the patient must generate to move the arm actively against gravity. However, based on what we know about difficulty transferring learning of tasks performed in isolation to improving

TABLE 19-10.   Eye–Head Coordination Exercises for Gaze Stabilization

Stage I. Eye Exercises

A. Exercises to improve visual following (smooth pursuit)
1. Sit in a comfortable position; do not move your head.
2. Hold a small target (about 2 × 2 inches, like a matchbook cover) containing written material at arm's length in front of you.
3. Keep your head still.
4. Move your arm slowly from side to side about 45 degrees. Try to keep the words in focus as you move.
5. Move your arm to the left, then right, then center. Rest for 3 seconds. Repeat 5 times.
6. Move your arm up and down about 30 degrees. Move your arm up, then down, then center. Rest for 3 seconds. Repeat 5 times.

B. Exercises to improve gaze redirection (saccade)
1. Sit in a comfortable position; do not move your head.
2. Hold two small targets (2 inches × 2 inches), one in each hand, about 12 inches apart in front of you.
3. Move your eyes only from one target to the other.
4. Move right; move left. Stop and rest.
5. Repeat 5 times.
6. Hold the two targets in front of you vertically, above and below the midline. Keep your head still; move your eyes only from one target to the other.
7. Move eyes up, eyes down. Stop and rest.
8. Repeat 5 times.

Stage II. Head Exercises

A. Move head, object still
1. Side-to-side movements: Hold at arm's length a small target, such as a matchbook. Try to keep the words in clear focus; move your head slowly from side to side. Move head to the right, move head left, move head to the center. Rest. Repeat 5 times.
2. Up and down movements: Repeat, but move your head up and down while keeping your eyes on the target held in front of you. Move head up; move head down; come to the center. Stop and rest. Repeat 5 times.
3. To progress, move your head faster and faster until you can no longer read the words. Repeat using a target that is attached to the wall 6 feet away.
4. Practice steps 1 and 2 with your eyes closed. Try to visualize the target in your mind and focus on it as if your eyes were open.

Stage III. Eye–Head Exercises

A. Move eyes and head to stationary objects
1. Side-to-side movements: Hold two small targets (2 inches × 2 inches), one in each hand, about 36 inches apart in front of you. Move your head and eyes to look at first one target, then the other. Try to clearly focus on the words on each target each time you move your head and eyes. Look left; look right; then rest. Repeat 5 times.
2. Up-and-down movements: Hold the two targets in front of you vertically, above and below the midline, about 36 inches apart. Move your head and eyes to look at first one target, then the other. Try to clearly focus on the words on each target each time you move your head and eyes. Look left; look right; then rest. Repeat 5 times.
3. To progress, repeat steps 1 and 2, moving your head at faster and faster speeds until you can no longer read the words. Repeat using a target that is attached to the wall 6 feet away.

B. Move eyes, head, and object in phase together
1. Side-to-side movements: Hold a small target (about 2 inches × 2 inches, like a matchbook cover) containing written material at arm's length in front of you. Move your arm and head together from side to side. Try to keep the words in clear focus while you move your arm and head together slowly from side to side (about 45 degrees). Move left; move right; move center; rest. Repeat 5 times.
2. Up-and-down movements: Hold a small target (about 2 inches × 2 inches, like a matchbook cover) containing written material at arm's length in front of you. Move your arm and head together up and down. Try to keep the words in clear focus while you move your arm and head together slowly up and down about 30 degrees. Move up; move down; move center; rest. Repeat 5 times.
3. To progress, repeat steps 1 and 2, moving your head at faster and faster speeds until you can no longer read the words. Repeat using a target which is attached to the wall 6 feet away.

Reprinted with permission from Zee DS. Vertigo. Curr Ther Neurol Dis 1985:1–13.

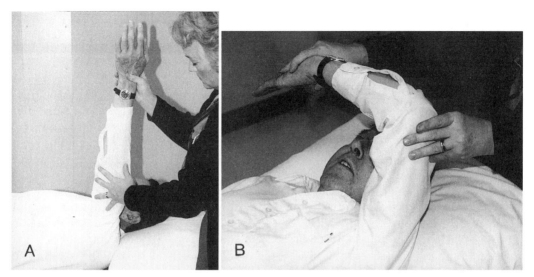

FIGURE 19-15.   Exercises to assist active movement in the upper extremity. The supine position can make use of gravity to assist movement. In this case the patient is asked to touch his nose. Gravity assists elbow flexion while the triceps work eccentrically to slow the descent of the hand.

performance in context, these suggestions must be examined more closely.

The inclusion of target objects into upper extremity movement activities often engages the patient more successfully than movement alone, since it makes the task more goal directed. The target objects used vary depending on grasp function. For example, in those without grasp, simply pointing to pictures and tasks involving knocking down blocks or pushing balls will suffice. As grasp improves, so can the complexity of the task and objects used.

In cases of weakness, it may be best to require movement in the gravity-eliminated plane. For example, shoulder horizontal abduction and elbow extension can be practiced in sitting by asking the individual to knock over a series of cardboard blocks with the dorsum of the hand, given table support provided under the elbow initially. This task can progress to performance of the same movement without elbow support.

In some cases, gravity can assist motion. For example, as shown in Figure 19-15*B*, when the supine patient is asked to touch his hand to his nose (or shoulder or head), gravity assists elbow flexion, while the patient ec-

centrically activates the triceps to slow the descent of the hand (this may be combined with FES). As isolated control improves transport, activities that activate the triceps both concentrically and eccentrically (possibly in conjunction with FES), such as tapping a suspended ball or throwing a beanbag toward the feet after retrieving it from the ipsilateral shoulder, may be used.

Biofeedback and Functional Electrical Stimulation

Biofeedback and FES using surface electrodes have been used successfully to facilitate active motion in the paretic upper extremity of adults following stroke and in children with cerebral palsy (Carmick, 1993, 1997; Chae et al., 1998; Kraft et al., 1992; Scheker et al., 1999; Wolf et al., 1989a). More recently, researchers have begun to examine the clinical outcomes of implantable and percutaneous FES in children with tetraplegia following spinal cord injury (Mulcahey et al., 1997; Davis et al., 1997) and in children with diplegic cerebral palsy (Finson et al., 1998, 1999).

How effective is biofeedback and FES in the recovery of upper extremity function, and do outcomes differ between adults and children? Wolf et al. (1989a) compared two biofeedback approaches to retraining functional upper limb control in 20 chronic stroke and 6 head-injured patients 1 to 7 years post injury. Inclusion criteria required that participating patients have the ability to initiate some voluntary wrist and finger extension and thumb abduction. During training, one group of 10 subjects used a motor copy approach, in which they attempted muscle activation on the involved side using movement from the noninvolved extremity as a reference. The other group of 10 subjects used targeted training, which required that they reduce activity in the spastic muscle and recruit activity in the antagonist muscle. The study found that the two approaches were equally effective in making changes in upper extremity function in patients with a chronic neurological lesion; however, the motor copy group tended to show their improvements later than did the targeted training group (Wolf et al., 1989a).

The positive outcomes from these research studies suggest support for the integration of both biofeedback and FES into clinical practices related to the development and recovery of active movement of upper limbs in both adults and children. Since implantable FES is still relatively new, surface electrodes targeted appropriately can be used for practice of single-joint or multijoint movement (pointing to targets) or within the context of functional tasks such as reaching into cupboards. For example, if a child with hemiplegic cerebral palsy tends to flex the wrist both to grasp and release objects, treatment could be directed at the wrist and finger extensors. Within a single treatment session surface FES could initially be placed appropriately and active wrist and finger extension movements practiced. This could be followed by pointing; by reach, grasp, and release of different objects; and by a game for children, such as stacking blocks. Difficulties encountered with surface FES include inaccurate timing of muscle onset for select tasks, cross-talk between nearby muscles, and skin intolerance to electrode adhesive. Once

an individual gains active control of the movements without FES input, it may be wise to transfer to biofeedback or eliminate both modalities altogether.

Adaptive Positioning

Adaptive seating is a frequently used therapeutic intervention designed to improve upper extremity function, including reach and grasp. Adaptive seating programs are based on three assumptions: (*a*) adaptive seats will reduce abnormal muscle tone; (*b*) improved muscle tone will improve postural stability; and (*c*) increased postural stability will enhance upper extremity control (McPherson et al., 1991; Shellenkens et al., 1983; Kluzik et al., 1990; Waksvik and Levy, 1979).

Several studies have examined the effect of altered seat angles on arm movements in children with and without cerebral palsy. While one study reported faster arm movements in children with cerebral palsy with a backrest set at 90 degrees (Nwaobi et al., 1983), most studies have not found seating posture to make a difference on immediate reaching movements as measured through kinematic analysis (McPherson et al., 1991; Seeger et al., 1984). These results do not rule out a long-term effect of altered seating posture on reaching. Quite possibly the effects of positioning are specific to the type of upper extremity task being performed. For example, Noronha et al. (1989) compared the effects of seating and prone standing in subjects with cerebral palsy on the time to complete eight subtests on the Jebsen-Taylor Hand Function Test (Jebsen et al., 1969). They found that some subtests were performed faster while the subjects were seated (small objects subtest), while other subtests were performed faster with the subjects in the prone standing position (simulated feeding). The authors report that the most atypical grasping patterns occurred during the simulated feeding subtest, which requires subjects to use sustained grip on a spoon and employ forearm rotation. These results suggest that the effects of positioning may be task specific (Noronha et al., 1989).

Retraining Task-Dependent Characteristics of Reach

Since the characteristics of the transport phase vary according to the task to be performed, it is important to structure training or retraining so that the patient learns to modify the movements used to transport the arm and hand in space in a task-dependent way. The following list offers various possible ways to train and retrain reaching based on research examining the characteristics of transport movements during upper extremity tasks. It is important to remember that these suggestions, like other suggestions made throughout this chapter, have yet to be validated through experimental testing.

1. Since the transport phase of movements such as pointing, reaching, grasping, and manipulating an object have very different movement characteristics, one cannot train a patient in one task and expect that the performance skills will automatically carry over to the transport phase of the other reaching tasks. Therefore, we suggest that training should be specific to each of these task types.

2. It has been shown that visual feedback is important for anticipatory control and to make corrections during a movement to enhance accuracy. Therefore, training patients to become proficient in scanning for relevant cues before the movement and using visual information to correct ongoing movements is essential to upper extremity control. To do this, the clinician may have to provide informational cues on target location and characteristics of the object to be grasped. It may be advantageous to have patients practice slower movements, drawing their attention to visual cues relating to hand movement, particularly thumb position in relation to target location.

3. In order to facilitate the modulation of force, the clinician could ask the patient to reach slowly then quickly to targets placed at various distances and locations in the workspace. In this way, the patient learns to program forces appropriately for slow and fast and movements requiring increased accuracy.

4. Research also suggests that the ability to move to a new position in space without the use of visual feedback is important when making reaching movements. This can be accomplished through modulation of stiffness in the agonist and antagonist muscles around the joints (see the discussion of location programming in Chapter 15). By giving patients tasks requiring location programming, the clinician can assist the patient in learning to modulate levels of stiffness in the upper extremity. One approach might be to place the patient at a table where he or she could locate the target visually but not be allowed to see his or her hands. The clinician would determine if they could still be accurate in locating the target in space, based on programming stiffness of the agonist and antagonist muscles.

5. Pohl and Winstein (1999) provide evidence of improved aiming performance in the less affected upper limb of adult stroke patients following a single 1-day practice session. Although further study is needed to evaluate the permanency and generality of these practice effects, this study reinforces the need to include the less affected extremity in reach and grasp training.

Retraining Anticipatory Aspects of Reach and Grasp

Despite the importance of planning movement and forces, it is difficult to teach anticipatory control. However, therapists can encourage its development by enhancing underlying resources and by providing opportunities to grasp and manipulate diverse objects in a variety of locations and contexts with and without informational preparation and feedback.

What can be done to assist patients who seem to underestimate or overestimate the location and size of targets? First, it is necessary to examine related components, such as vision and sensibility in the hand. Typically, we rely on sensory feedback to develop and strengthen our internal representations of object properties and distances, which we use for anticipatory control of grip formation and force scaling during object manipulation. If there are deficits in either vision or sensation in the hand, the potential for development or recovery of these components should first be determined. With an estimate of the potential, visual and/or sensory reeducation techniques may be conducted (reviewed earlier in the chapter). Until sensibility in the hand improves or if the potential for development or recovery is low, patients should be allowed extended practice or be taught compensatory techniques if current strategies are inefficient. With extended practice, patients with underdeveloped or impaired anticipatory control demonstrate significant improvement (Gordon and Duff, 1999a). Furthermore, modeling or mental rehearsal (self-initiated or verbalized through the therapist) prior to movements may allow longer processing and preparation time.

Grasp and Manipulation

Hand function requires the ability to grasp, release, and manipulate objects, as well as the capacity to adapt how we grasp in response to characteristics of the target object. Training and retraining grasp function in the patient with paresis and dyscontrol often begins with the establishment of a power grip, then moves to progressively more precise grip patterns (Erhardt, 1982). The power grip uses simultaneous finger flexion and allows for a cylindrical hold on objects. It may be easier to retrain this pattern first for a few reasons. First, finger fractionation (used with precision grips) may be limited. Second, power grip plays an important role in holding and manipulating assistive mobil-

ity devices. When retraining power grasp, patients are often assisted in molding the hand to the shape of variously sized cylindrical objects in a finger flexion pattern, with the thumb opposed. Once achieved, the power grasp can be practiced in both the vertical and horizontal planes to allow practice employing various forearm and wrist positions. This is shown in Figure 19-16. It has been recommended that grasp retraining progress to teaching patients a succession of more precise grips (as cortical motor neuronal connections and subsequent isolation of the fingers will allow). A lateral pinch often is encouraged along with a three-jaw chuck pattern involving the thumb opposed to two fingers (Erhardt, 1984) and a pincer grasp (either tip to tip or pad to pad), which involves index finger and thumb opposition. Figure 19-17 depicts a child with hemiplegic cerebral palsy attempting a precision grip (pincer grasp).

As discussed earlier, research has shown that many of the elements of grasp, including how we orient and shape our hand and the amount of force we use to grip, are planned, that is, determined before we even touch the object to be grasped. Hand orientation, shape, and force characteristics are determined by our previous experience with grasping objects in conjunction with our ability to perceive relevant cues about the target object. These two factors are used to program hand shape and the force characteristics of grasp and manipulation (Jeannerod 1986; Fisk, 1990; Forssberg et al., 1991; Westling and Johansson, 1984).

An important part of gaining or regaining functional upper extremity control requires learning to modify grasp strategies for changing task demands. Retraining the ability to adapt grasp should address both motor and perceptual aspects of the task, since recovery of effective grip requires (*a*) control over extrinsic and intrinsic muscles of the hand and (*b*) the ability to discriminate perceptual cues critical to anticipatory hand shaping and force scaling.

Errors in grasp, including gripping too loosely and letting objects slip or gripping too tightly and crushing objects, result from

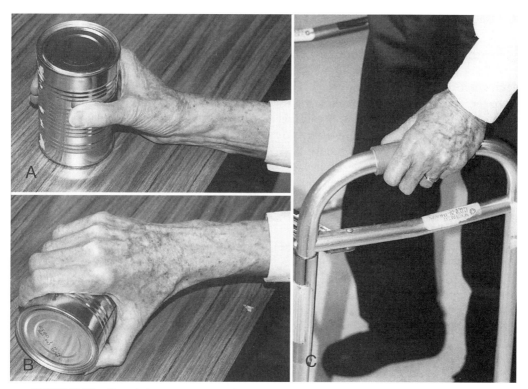

FIGURE 19-16.   Retraining power grasp. Power grasp used to pick up an object according to orientation. **A.** Vertical. **B.** Horizontal. **C.** To hold an assistive device used for gait.

impairments in force scaling. However, it is not always easy to determine whether errors are the result of poor control over muscles or are due to problems in correctly perceiving characteristics of the object to be gripped and thus scaling the forces incorrectly.

The power (ulnar) and skill (radial) sides of the hand can be encouraged to develop separate roles through practice of tasks that require the power side to stabilize and the skill side to manipulate. One sample task requires patients to roll Silly Putty between their thumb and index finger while the ring and small fingers hold a small object. Alternatively, they can practice squeezing the trigger of a spray bottle with the index and long fingers while the ring and small fingers hold the neck of the bottle. One can also train fingertip force control by having the child drop a selected number of water drops from an eye dropper or pick up and place fragile objects such as foam without denting them. Training and strengthening the intrinsic muscles is best accomplished with resistive Theraputty. However, other activities may include lacing cardboard or leather with pipe cleaners or plastic laces.

In-Hand Manipulation

An important part of the development or recovery of hand function is helping patients

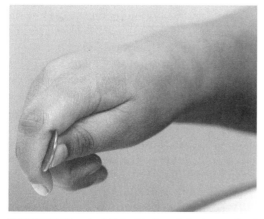

FIGURE 19-17.   A child with hemiplegic cerebral palsy attempting a precision pincer grasp.

regain the ability to manipulate an object within the hand itself, without setting it down or transferring it to the opposite hand, termed in-hand manipulation. Inadequate finger fractionation (isolated finger and thumb movements) makes it difficult to manipulate objects in one hand. Many individuals with neurological deficits have lost or never had intact cortical motor neuronal mechanisms (Rothwell, 1994). Therefore, one's expectations for the development of in-hand manipulation skills must be realistic. However, many individuals with hemiplegia have developed learned disuse of their impaired limb (Taub et al., 1975, 1993). Based on the concept of constraint-induced therapy, or forced use (Taub and Wolf, 1997) (reviewed later in the chapter), these individuals may benefit from massed practice. In-hand manipulation practice with individuals with hemiplegia can be graded from objects of high friction and multiple points of contact to slippery objects with minimal points of contact. The size and shape of the objects can also be varied.

According to Exner (1989) children are candidates for in-hand manipulation training if they exhibit basic grasp and release patterns, can grasp objects with the fingers and/or the pads of the fingers, and can isolate at least some finger movement. Activities that often coincide with in-hand manipulation training include sensory reeducation and intrinsic muscle strengthening. The effectiveness of practice conditions (cues, task difficulty) to enhance skill must be considered. For example, one child may benefit from verbal and visual cueing (demonstration), while another only needs verbal cues. Furthermore, one child may be able to begin training at the level of object rotation, while another must begin with finger-to-palm translation.

Treatment over multiple sessions could focus on all three forms of in-hand manipulation, translation, rotation, and shift (Exner, 1990). Activities using small items, such as coins, may prove beneficial. For example, one could have a child pick up pennies one at a time, translate them to the palm, and hold them in the ulnar side of the

hand. In addition, pennies can be placed one at a time in a child's palm with the instruction for each penny to be translated to the fingertips and shifted to the thumb and index pads. Rotation and shift can be practiced by placing a pencil in the palm of a child's hand with the instruction for the child to rotate it and adjust it to rest between the pads of the thumb, index, and long fingers. Numerous other games can incorporate in-hand manipulation components. The key is to begin at the appropriate level of difficulty, keeping expectations for improvement realistic.

You can see how we use in-hand manipulation for yourself. Pick up a pencil, shift your fingers closer to the tip, and begin to write. Now, alter the position of the pencil so you can erase. This is a demonstration of rotation. Your in-hand manipulation skills enabled you to change the position of the pencil in your hand without using the other hand or setting the pencil down to alter your grip.

Release

To achieve a functional grasp, patients must be able not only to grasp but to release objects. For many patients with neurological lesions, a power grasp is accomplished by using a mass pattern of flexion. While this pattern is successful in creating grasp, the patient may be unable to extend the fingers actively and release the object without the assistance of the other hand. Alternatively, a patient may use wrist flexion to extend the fingers passively and thus accomplish release (Boehme, 1988; Erhardt, 1982).

Rhoda Erhardt, an occupational therapist, has published an extensive assessment form that describes a developmental sequence for releasing objects (Erhardt, 1982). This sequence has been used as the basis for a program to train or retrain release in the individual with a neurological impairment (Boehme, 1988), although deviations from the sequence are likely and acceptable. The suggested sequence begins with learning to release an object that is externally stabilized. This approach is based on the observation that children learn to release an object externally stabilized on a supporting surface prior to learning to release objects in space (Boehme, 1988). Thus, patients are taught to release objects that are stabilized by the patient's other hand, by the therapist's hand, or by a supporting surface. This is followed by learning to release objects that are not supported. Patients practice releasing an object using a pattern of finger extension with the wrist in neutral, as opposed to release resulting from wrist flexion, producing a mechanical extension of the fingers via tenodesis. As release improves, practice can include the release of objects into a container and progress to graded release needed to stack objects.

Intervention at the Functional Level

A task-oriented approach to intervention requires that gains made in resolving impairments and improving key components of movement be extended into improvements in performance of functional tasks. Treatment at all levels (impairment, strategies, and function) is organized around the specific set of functional tasks being trained. In addition, since the ability to adapt to changing environmental conditions is an important therapeutic goal, the context under which functional tasks are practiced is controlled and modified.

Context Considerations

Dunn et al. (1994) have put together a therapeutic framework for practice, *The Ecology of Human Performance (EHP)*, which considers the effect of context. This model stems from the theory that ecology, or the interaction between person(s) and the environment, affects human behavior and performance. In order to use this framework in practice the authors have established five approaches to intervention (Table 19-11).

These categories can be defined and applied to develop upper extremity control: (*a*) *Establish or restore* (remediate) the person's skills and abilities in context; for example, in the case of Phoebe J., increase active

shoulder strength for reaching above chest level during kitchen tasks. (*b*) *Alter* the context in which the person performs to ensure a match between skills and abilities versus changing the setting to meet the needs; for example, in the case of Phoebe J., discuss with her having a family member perform some of the more complex kitchen duties. (*c*) *Adapt* the contextual features and task demands to provide support to person's performance; for example, in the case of Phoebe J., place items on low shelves in the kitchen to minimize high reaches. (*d*) *Prevent* barriers to performance in context; for example, again in the case of Phoebe J., gradually move items to levels that demand reaching to higher levels. (*e*) *Create* circumstances that promote more adaptable performance in context; for example, Phoebe J. will plan a lunch for family members (Dunn et al., 1994).

Handwriting

Aside from the act of handwriting itself, training or retraining any manipulative skill encompasses key underlying components, a few of which have been reviewed under grasp and manipulation (Benbow et al., 1992). These components include the enhancement of wrist stabilization and hand arches, development of the power and skill sides of the hand, training in fingertip force control, and strength training of the intrinsic muscles of the hand.

Well-designed handwriting programs, available to enhance both manuscript and cursive writing, can be used within most school-based therapy programs and/or carried out by classroom teachers. Two such programs are Mary Benbow's "Loops and Other Groups," (1991) and "Handwriting Without Tears" by Jan Olsen (1998). Benbow's program is aimed at teaching cursive handwriting from a kinesiological perspective through creative clustering of letters into "kites" and other subgroups and practicing them. Its success lies in the ease of instruction and ample practice time allotted for each grouping. Olsen's program is also used successfully. It emphasizes multisensory

---

TABLE 19-11.   Ecology of Human Performance

This framework considers the interaction between the person and the environment and its effect on human task performance. This framework can be applied to the development of upper extremity control in Phoebe J. and her role as a homemaker. The activities used during treatment depend on the goal of the intervention and the status of the person's recovery. Note the different example activities used below.

Goal of Intervention	Interpretation	Activity Example
Establish or restore (remediate)	Improve person's skills and experiences.	Introduce tasks and exercises that strengthen finger flexors and wrist extensors. With greater strength Phoebe J. may be able to expand the use of her *involved* hand during bimanual tasks (e.g., hold a bowl with her *involved* hand while stirring the contents with the *noninvolved* hand).
Alter	Select context that enables performance. Place person in different setting.	Have Phoebe J. assist in meal preparation by setting the dining room table in her own home, using her *involved* hand and arm to hold extra items while placing them strategically on the table with her *noninvolved* hand.
Adapt	Change aspects of context and/or tasks to allow person to perform task.	Introduce adapted tools with large handles that allow Phoebe J. to hold onto them with her involved hand (e.g., stir the contents of a bowl using her *involved* hand while the *noninvolved* hand holds the bowl).
Prevent	Change course of events based on predictions of barriers to performance.	Since Phoebe J.'s *involved* upper limb tends to fatigue and her balance is fair, have her prepare meals while sitting at a table with her elbows supported.
Create	Provide enriched contextual and task experiences to enhance performance.	Have Phoebe J. prepare a lunch for her family members that requires the use of her *involved* hand to manipulate a range of pots, pans, and tools unimanually and bimanually. The items could be retrieved from their original locations in cupboards and shelves to expand reach and grasp demands and trunk and balance requirements.

---

experiences to prepare the child for handwriting and features gray blocks and simple line structure to visually guide manuscript printing and progress to writing in cursive. Use of assistive devices, such as pencil grips and support for the fingers and writing utensil, may also facilitate handwriting (Fig. 19-18).

Sequencing Functional Tasks

Modeling and verbal and mental rehearsal may be the best strategies to enhance sequencing (McCullagh et al., 1989). For example, Phoebe J. has difficulty sequencing the steps associated with simple meal preparation. During therapy sessions throughout a given week, the therapist could model the sequence of a multistep process, such as making a peanut butter sandwich and preparing a cup of tea, while giving simple verbal cues

along the way (minimal words used). Before Phoebe J. attempts to repeat the same task, she could be asked to repeat the sequence (declarative or explicit learning), then imagine herself performing the sequence (mental rehearsal). During practice the therapist may initially coach the patient through the sequence as needed, verbally and/or manually. Treatment could progress to practice from a written list (given intact vision) to practice without verbal or written cues.

Tim R.'s sequencing problems may center on classroom art projects. In those situations peer modeling may be effective only if the child is able to filter out irrelevant cues and focus only on those that are important to sequence the task correctly (Exner, 1995; Vygotsky, 1978). It is possible that Tim R. is unable to carry out task sequences for a number of reasons (impaired visual perception, distractibility when given verbal in-

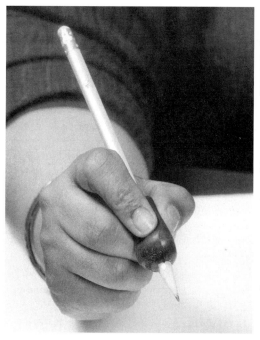

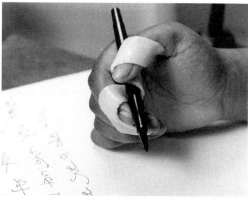

FIGURE 19-18. Assistive devices such as pencil grips (**A**) and a custom-made support for the fingers and writing utensil (design by Bobbie Ciocco, OTR) (**B**) used to facilitate handwriting.

structions or visual demonstrations, and/or constructional apraxia, among others).

If peer modeling of task sequences is ineffective, Tim R. may need individual coaching on sequencing, as in the case of Phoebe J., and this coaching may include visual modeling and verbal rehearsal prior to the task (Vygotsky, 1978). For example, during the construction of an art project, one could begin by showing him the end product and have him verbally state how to complete it step by step. If he fails to give a correct response, the therapist can verbally interject, reviewing the correct step(s). Once the project is complete, the therapist may have to model the task sequence. It may be reinforcing for Tim R. to repeat the task sequence to the therapist or to teach a fellow student how to complete it by demonstration and verbal cueing.

Problem Solving and Apraxia

Learning to solve movement problems is a major step toward the development or recovery of motor skills (Adolph, 1994). To promote this, the clinician can facilitate problem solving by asking the patient to demonstrate, for example, how to hold the

fork to get the potatoes on it, or offer a verbal solution to the problem. For clients without perceptual deficits, modeling of an alternative strategy that can be copied may allow for easy success. If they have perceptual problems, such as poor spatial relations, one may have to model the task and then provide verbal or manual cues to initiate or guide them through the appropriate movement(s). Whenever manual assistance is given, the therapist (or helper) becomes part of the movement solution. Therefore, any manual assistance should be immediately followed by practice of the task independently to give patients the opportunity to plan and carry out the movement themselves.

Constraint-Induced Movement Therapy

Researchers have known for many years that restraining the intact limb in monkeys will force the animal to use the impaired arm (Knapp et al., 1963). This knowledge has led to the development of constraint-induced, or forced-use, paradigms in adults and children with hemiplegia, designed to restrain the use of the unaffected limb and encourage the use of the affected upper extremity through massed practice (Wolf et al., 1989b; Taub et al., 1993; Charles, 1999; Crocker et al., 1997; Lavender and Gentile, 1998; Yasukawa, 1990).

Wolf et al. (1989b) had 25 adult hemiplegic stroke and head-injured subjects wear slings, restraining the nonimpaired arm during waking hours for 14 days. In follow-up, they found the speed of task execution improved for most functional tasks for up to a year following intervention. Taub et al. (1993) compared constraint-induced therapy (treatment group) against an attention comparison group (controls) in chronic hemiplegic stroke patients. The treatment group had their unaffected limb restrained during the waking hours for 14 days. For 10 weekdays of those 14 days the treatment group spent 6 hours a day practicing tasks that required upper extremity function with the affected limb (eating, throwing a ball, writing, pushing a broom, manipulating checkers and pegs), while the control group was instructed to focus attention on the affected limb and received placebo and range-of-motion exercises. Results suggested that motor ability and ADL skills were significantly improved following restraint of the noninvolved arm compared to the control group, and improvements were sustained 1 to 2 years post intervention (Taub et al., 1993).

Other studies have supported the use of constraint-induced therapy for both adults (Kunkel et al., 1999; Miltner et al., 1999) and children with hemiplegia (Charles, 1999; Crocker et al., 1997; Yasukawa, 1990). Research has also begun to correlate functional recovery following constraint-induced therapy with cortical changes (enlarged motor cortex representations and increased levels of excitability) (Liepert et al., 1998).

Constraint-induced and forced-use paradigms are still at a research stage of development. Therefore, it is not clear if and how they may be used in retraining upper extremity control in the patient with an upper motor neuron lesion. Criteria must be established for patients for whom this approach may be appropriate. Many patients are excluded from this type of treatment because

of imbalance and the need to use the unimpaired upper extremity for balance control and to prevent falls. One important and encouraging aspect of these constraint-induced training studies is the awareness that motor improvements are possible even in chronically impaired patients who are 1 to 5 years post onset and in those with congenital hemiplegia.

Bilateral Isokinematic Training

Mudie and Matyas (2000) have developed an approach to retraining upper extremity function following stroke using bilateral isokinematic training (BIT). This approach was developed from their clinical observations that functional recovery in the hemiparetic limb was better when patients practiced a reach-to-target task with both upper limbs simultaneously than when practice was limited to the hemiparetic limb in isolation. They hypothesized that retraining the hemiparetic arm with bilateral isokinematic movements (identical movements performed bilaterally but with each limb independently) might help to reorganize cortical motor neuronal networks via mechanisms that are inaccessible to training based on unilateral actions alone. Their rationale for this approach is based on the work by Turton et al. (1996) and Kelso et al. (1979).

Turton et al. (1996) reported that a cerebrovascular accident results in the depletion of neuronal pools and a disruption of the unique temporal and spatial organization of cortical motor neuronal excitability necessary for the execution of a skilled movement task. Recovery requires both the recruitment of additional cortical motor neuronal cells into task-appropriate motor neuronal pools and the reorganization of appropriate firing patterns in the reconstructed networks.

The studies by Kelso et al. (1979) on interlimb coordination during the simultaneous performance of bimanual tasks suggest that when both limbs are performing identical actions, the same movement organization occurs in both hemispheres. In fact, there may be a single command or central mechanisms applied to both limbs. When the two hands perform identical tasks, there is a tight phasic relationship observed in which one limb entrains the other, causing them to function together as a unit. Based on these studies Mudie and Matyas developed a therapeutic approach to retraining upper extremity function that uses simultaneous performance of movement tasks in the impaired and nonimpaired limbs.

Mudie and Matyas (2000) report data from 12 controlled single-case experiments (patients with hemiparesis secondary to stroke) using multiple baseline design across three separate reach and grasp activities. All 12 patients showed significant improvements in the hemiplegic arm following bilateral training compared to either unilateral movement training or use of the nonhemiplegic arm to guide the hemiplegic arm. The improvements were specific to the task trained and were well maintained even 6 months following the training period. The authors suggest that following stroke, the undamaged hemisphere may provide a template of appropriate firing for a restored neural network. The template is available through transcortical communications that are no longer inhibited during bilateral simultaneous isokinematic performance.

The BIT approach is in direct contrast to constraint-induced therapy, which actively restrains use of the intact arm, forcing the use of the involved extremity in functional tasks. It is possible that BIT is an appropriate approach early in recovery, when rapid reorganization of the cortex following stroke is occurring and new networks controlling movement are being formed. Constraint-induced therapy may then be appropriate in ensuring that new networks are used and in avoiding learned disuse.

Case Studies

Tables 19-8 and 19-9 illustrate how the identification of problems leads to the formation of goals and treatment planning in our two case studies. The examples are not considered all inclusive, yet they allow the concepts to be examined more closely.

SUMMARY

1. Retraining control of the upper extremity is important to most areas of rehabilitation, including physical and occupational therapy. While both areas of therapy retrain upper extremity control, physical therapists tend to focus on postural and mobility aspects of upper extremity function and occupational therapists tend to focus on ADL aspects, including the recovery of fine motor skills.

2. A task-oriented approach to assessment of upper extremity function requires a battery of tests that measure (*a*) functional performance, either ADL or work related; (*b*) key components of control, including eye–head coordination, transport, grasp, release, and manipulation; and (*c*) underlying sensory, motor, and cognitive impairments, including range of motion, strength, sensation, volume, and pain.

3. Preparing treatment plans to retrain upper extremity control requires the identification of a comprehensive list of the patient's problems, including the functional limitations or disabilities, as well as the specific impairments that constrain function. From this list, short- and long-term treatment goals are established and therapeutic strategies are developed to meet those goals.

4. A task-oriented approach to retraining upper extremity control seeks to minimize impairments while maximizing the patient's capacity for function. Retraining involves the development of therapeutic strategies (*a*) to remediate as many sensory, motor, and cognitive impairments as possible, (*b*) to generate strategies to achieve the key components of upper extremity control, and (*c*) to develop the capacity to perform functional tasks under a variety of environmental contexts.

5. Research suggests that the development of control over proximal body segments is not a necessary precursor to the emer-

gence of distal hand function. Proximal and distal segments of the upper extremity appear to be controlled separately and therefore can be retrained simultaneously rather than sequentially.

6. Hand function requires the ability to grasp, release, and manipulate objects, as well as the capacity to adapt how we grasp in response to characteristics of the object to be grasped. Many elements of grasp, including hand shape and force characteristics, use our internal representation of an object's physical properties. Thus, retraining hand function requires attention to both motor and perceptual aspects of the task.

7. Sensory reeducation programs focus on several aspects of sensibility, including protective and discriminative sensory functions. It is unclear whether sensory reeducation teaches patients how to use the remaining sensibility to their advantage or it actually alters the physiologi-cal basis for sensation. It is certain, however, that the capacity to adapt to impaired sensibility is dependent on the patient's motivation as well as training. Studies have shown that patients who were willing to use the impaired limb were better able to recover function.

8. A major constraint on recovery of arm function may be the unwillingness of patients to use an impaired upper extremity when the less affected extremity is available. Results of studies examining constraint-induced, or forced-use, paradigms suggest that motor ability can be significantly improved by restricting the hemiplegic patient's use of the noninvolved arm. One important and encouraging aspect of these studies is the awareness that motor improvements are possible even in chronically impaired patients who are 1 to 5 years post onset of injury and in those with congenital conditions such as hemiplegic cerebral palsy.

Abel MF, Damiano DL. Strategies for increasing walking speed in diplegic cerebral palsy. J Pediatr Ortho 1996; 16:753–758.

Abrams TW, Kandel ER. Is contiguity detection in classical conditioning a system or a cellular property? Learning in Aplysia suggests a possible molecular site. Trends Neurosci 1988; 11:128–135.

Abreu BC. The effect of environmental regulations on postural control after stroke. Am J Occup Ther 1995; 49:517–525.

Abreu BC, Toglia JP. Cognitive rehabilitation: A model for occupational therapy. Am J of Occup Ther 1987; 41(7):439–448.

Adams JA. A closed-loop theory of motor learning. J Motor Behav 1971; 3:111–150.

Adams LS, Greene LW, Topoozian E. Range of Motion. In: Casanova JS, ed. Clinical Assessment Recommendations. 2nd ed. Chicago, IL: American Society of Hand Therapists, 1992:55–70.

Adolph KE. Learning to solve the problem of moving: Exploration, experience, and control. Paper presented at; Development of Skill in Infancy and Early Childhood. The Annual Conference in The Movement Sciences, Teacher's College, Columbia University, New York, NY, 1994.

Agnew PJ, Dip OT, Maas F. Hand function related to age and sex. Arch Phys Med Rehabil 1982; 63:269–271.

AGS. The Minnesota Rate of Manipulation Tests, Examiner's Manual. Circle Pines, MN, Western Psychological Services, 1969.

Aguayo AD, Clarke DB, Jelsma TN, et al. Effects of neurotrophins on the survival and regrowth of injured retinal neurons. In: Growth Factors As Drugs for Neurological and Sensory Disorders. Ciba Foundation Symposium, 1996:135–148.

Alexander GE, Crutcher MD. Functional architecture of basal ganglia circuits: neural substrates of parallel processing. Trends Neurosci 1990; 13:266–271.

Alexander NB, Mollo JM, Giordani B, et al. Maintenance of balance, gait patterns and obstacle clearance in Alzheimer's disease. Neurology 1995: 45:908–914.

Alexander NB, Schultz AB, Warwick DN. Rising from a chair: effect of age and functional ability on performance biomechanics. J Gerontol 1991; 46: M91–M98.

Alexander RM. Optimization and gaits in the locomotion of vertebrates. Physiol Rev 1989; 69:1199–1227.

Allum JHJ, Honegger F, Schicks H. The influence of a bilateral vestibular deficit on postural synergies. J Vestib Res 1994; 4:49–70.

Allum JHJ, Pfaltz CR. Visual and vestibular contributions to pitch sway stabilization in the ankle muscles of normals and patients with bilateral peripheral vestibular deficits. Exp Brain Res 1985; 58:82–94.

Almli RB, Finger S. Toward a definition of recovery of function. In: Le Vere TE, Almli RB, Stein DG, eds. Brain injury and recovery: theoretical and controversial issues. New York: Plenum, 1988:1–4.

American Academy of Orthopedic Surgeons. Joint Motion: Method of Measuring and Recording. Chicago, IL: The Academy, 1965.

American Society of Hand Therapists. Clinical Assessment Recommendations. 2nd ed. Chicago, IL: American Society of Hand Therapists, 1992.

Amiel-Tison C, Grenier A. Evaluation neurologique du nouveau-né et du nourrisson. (Neurological evaluation of the human infant.) New York: Masson, 1980:81–102.

Amundson S. Evaluation Tool of Children's Handwriting (ETCH). Morganville, NJ: ETCH Adm., 1995.

Andersen RA. In: Mountcastle VB, Plum F, Geiger SR, eds. Higher Functions of the Brain, Part 2: The Nervous System, vol 5, Handbook of Physiology, Section 1. American Physiological Association, 1987: 483–518.

Anderson JB, Sinkjaer T. Stretch reflex variations during gait. In: A Pedotti, Mcferrairin, J Quintern, R Riener, eds. Neuroprosthetics. Berlin, Springer, 1996:45–50.

Anderson ME, Binder MD. Spinal and supraspinal control of movement and posture. In: Patton HD, Fuchs AF, Hille B, et al., eds. Textbook of physiology, vol. 1: Excitable cells and neurophysiology. Philadelphia: WB Saunders, 1989:563–581.

Andrews AW, Bohannon RW. Distribution of muscle strength impairments following stroke. Clin Rehabil 2000; 14:79–87.

Andriacchi TP, Oagle, JA, Galante JO. Walking speed as basis for normal and abnormal gait measurements. J Biomechanics 1977; 10:261–268.

Aniansson A, Grimby F, Gedberg A. Muscle function in old age. Scan J Rehabil Med 1978; 6(Suppl):43–49.

Aniansson A, Hedberg M, Henning G, et al. Muscle morphology, enzymatic activity and muscle strength in elderly men: a follow up study. Muscle Nerve 1986; 9:585–591.

Aniansson A, Ljungberg P, Rundgren A, et al. Effect of a training programme for pensioners on condition and muscular strength. Arch Gerontol Geriatr 1984; 3:229–241.

Apel U. The Feldenkrais method: Awareness through movement. WHO Reg Publ Eur Ser 1992; 44:324–7.

Apfel ER, Carranza J. Dexterity. In: Cassanova J, ed. Clinical Assessment Recommendations. Chicago, IL: American Society of Hand Therapists, 1992.

APTA. Guide to Physical Therapy Practice. Phys Ther 1997; 77:1163–1650.

Arshavsky Yu I, Berkinblit MB, Fukson OI, et al. Recordings of neurones of the dorsal spinocerebellar tract during evoked locomotion. Brain Res 1972a; 43:272–275.

Arshavsky Yu I, Berkinblit MB, Gelfand IM, et al. Activity of the neurones of the ventral spino-cerebellar tract during locomotion. Biophysics 1972b;17: 926–935.

Asanuma H, Keller A. Neuronal mechanisms of motor learning in mammals. NeuroReport 1991; 2:217–224.

Ashmead DH, Hill EW, Talor CR. Obstacle perception by congenitally blind children. Percept Psychophysiol 1989; 46:425–433.

Aslin R. Development of smooth pursuit in human infants. In: Fischer DF, Monty RA, Senders EJ, eds. Eye movements: cognition and vision perception. Hillsdale, NJ: Erlbaum, 1981:31–51.

Assaiante C, Amblard B. Ontogenesis of head stabilization in space during locomotion in children: influence of visual cues. Exp Brain Res 1993; 93:499–515.

Assaiante C, Amblard B. An ontogenetic model for the sensorimotor organization of balance control in humans. Hum Movement Sci 1995; 14:13–43.

Assaiante C, Woollacott M, Amblard B. Development of postural adjustment during gait initiation: kinematic and EMG analysis. J Motor Behavior (in press).

Atkeson CG, Hollerbach JM. Kinematic features of unrestrained vertical arm movements. J Neurosci 1985; 5:2318–2330.

Ayres AJ. Sensory Integration and Praxis Tests. Torrence CA: Sensory Integration International, 1989.

Ayres J. Sensory Integration and Learning Disorders. Los Angeles: Western Psychological Services, 1972.

Bach-y-Rita P, Balliet R. Recovery from stroke. In: Duncan P, Badke MB, eds. Stroke rehabilitation: the recovery of motor control. Chicago: Year Book, 1987:79–107.

Badke MB, DiFabio RP. Balance deficits in patients with hemiplegia: considerations for assessment and treatment. In: Duncan P, ed. Balance: proceedings of the APTA Forum. Alexandria, VA: APTA, 1990:73–78.

Badke M, Duncan P. Patterns of rapid motor responses during postural adjustments when standing in healthy subjects and hemiplegic patients. Phys Ther 1983; 63:13–20.

Bailey CH, Chen M. Morphological basis of long-term habituation and sensitization in Aplysia. Science 1983; 220:91–93.

Baker M, Regenos E, Wolf SL, Basmajian JV. Developing strategies for biofeedback: applications in neurologically handicapped patients. Phys Ther 1977; 57:402–408.

Baker MP, Hudson JE, Wolf SL. A "feedback" cane to improve the hemiplegic patient's gait. Phys Ther 1979; 59:170–171.

Balint R. Seelenhamung des "Schauens," optische Ataxie, raumlische Storung des Aufmersamkeit. Monatshr Psychiatr Neurol 1909; 25:51–81.

Baloh RW: Dizziness, Hearing Loss and Tinnitus: The Essentials of Neurotology. Philadelphia: FA Davis, 1984.

Barnes MR, Crutchfield CA, Heriza CB. The neurophysiological basis of patient treatment. Vol II: Reflexes in motor development. Morgantown, WV: Stokesville, 1978.

Barton S, Wolf SL. An application of upper-extremity constraint-induced movement therapy in a patient with subacute stroke. Phys Ther 1999; 79(9):847–53.

Basmajian JV, De Luca CJ. Muscles alive: their functions revealed by electromyography. 5th ed. Baltimore: Williams & Wilkins, 1985.

Basmajian JV, Kukulka CG, Narayan MD, Takebe K. Biofeedback treatment of foot-drop after stroke compared with standard rehabilitation technique: effects on voluntary control and strength. Arch Phys Med Rehabil 1975; 56:231–236.

Bastian AJ, Martin TA, Keating JG, Thach WT. Cerebellar ataxia: Abnormal control of interaction torques across multiple joints. J Neurophysiol 1996; 76:492–509.

Baxter-Petralia P, Bruening LA, Blackmore SM, McEntee PM. Physical capacity evaluation. In: Hunter JM, et al., eds. Rehabilitation of the Hand. St Louis: CV Mosby, 1990:93–108.

Bayley N. Bayley Scales of Infant Development. San Antonio, TX: Psychological, 1969.

Bechtol CO. Grip test use of dynamometer with adjustable hand spacing. JAMA 1954; 36:820–824.

Beery KE. The Beery-Butenika Test of Visual-Motor Integration, 4th Revision. Cleveland: Modern Curriculum Press, 1997.

Beery KE. The Test of Visual Motor Integration. Parsippany, NJ: Modern Curriculum Press, 1989.

Belen'kii VY, Gurfinkel VS, Paltsev YI. Elements of control of voluntary movements. Biofizika 1967; 12:135–141.

Bell-Krotoski J. Light touch-deep pressure testing using Semmes-Weinstein monofilaments. In: Hunter JM, Schneider LH, Mackin EM, Callahan AD, eds. Rehabilitation of the Hand. 3rd ed. St. Louis: Mosby, 1990:585–593.

Bell-Krotoski J, Weinstein S, Weinstein C. Testing sensibility, including touch-pressure, two-point discrimination, point localization, and vibration. J Hand Therapy 1993; 2:114–123.

Benbow M. Loops and Other Groups: A Kinesthetic Writing System, Instructor's ed. Randolph, NJ: OT Ideas, 1991.

Benbow M, Hanft B, Marsh D. Handwriting in the classroom: Improving written communication. In: Royeen C., ed. Classroom Applications for School-Based Practice from The American Occupational Therapy Association Self Study Series. Rockville, MD: The American Occupational Therapy Press, 1992.

Berardelli A, Sabra AF, Hallett M. Physiological mechanisms of rigidity in Parkinson's disease. J Neurol Neurosurg Psychiatry 1983; 46:45–53.

Berg K. Measuring balance in the elderly: validation of an instrument. Dissertation. Montreal: McGill University, 1993.

Berg K, Wood-Dauphinee SL, Willimans JT. Measuring balance in the elderly: validation of an instrument. Can J Public Health 1992; 83:S9–11.

Berg K, Wood-Dauphinee S, Williams J, Gayton D. Measuring balance in the elderly: preliminary development of an instrument. Physiother Canada 1989; 41:304–308.

Berger W, Altenmueller E, Dietz V. Normal and impaired development of children's gait. Hum Neurobiol 1984a;3:163–170.

Berger W, Dietz V, Quintern J. Corrective reactions to stumbling in man: neuronal coordination of bilateral leg muscle activity during gait. J Physiol Lond 1984b;357:109–125.

Berger W, Horstmann GA, Dietz VL. Tension development and muscle activation in the leg during gait in spastic hemiparesis: the independence of muscle hypertonia and exaggerated stretch reflexes. J Neurol Neurosurg Psychiatry 1984c;47:1029–1033.

Berger W, Quintern J, Dietz V. Pathophysiology of gait in children with cerebral palsy. Electroencephalogr Clin Neurophysiol 1982; 53:538–548.

Berger W, Quintern J, Dietz V. Stance and gait perturbations in children: developmental aspects of compensatory mechanisms. Electroencephalogr Clin Neurophysiol 1985; 61:385–395.

Bergmann K. Incidence of atypical pencil grasps among nondysfunctional adults. Am J Occup Ther 1990; 44:736–740.

Bernardi M, Macaluso A, Sproviero E, et al. Cost of walking and locomotor impairment. J Electromyogr Kinesiol 1999; 9:149–157.

Bernspang B, Vitanin M, Eriksson S. Impairments of perception and motor functions: Their influence on self care ability 4 to 6 years after a stroke. Occup Ther J Res 1989; 9:27–37.

Bernstein, N. The coordination and regulation of movement. London: Pergamon, 1967.

Bertenthal BI, Rose JL, Bai DL. Perception-action coupling in the development of visual control of posture. J Exper Psychol 1997; 23:1631–1643.

Berthoz A, Pozzo T. Intermittent head stabilization during postural and locomotory tasks in humans. In: Posture and gait: development, adaptation and modulation. Amblard B, Berthoz A, Clarac F, eds. Amsterdam: Elsevier, 1988; 189–198.

Berthoz A, Pozzo T. Head and body coordination during locomotion and complex movements. In: Swinnen SP, Heuer H, Massion J, Casaer P, eds. Interlimb coordination: neural, dynamical and cognitive constraints. San Diego: Academic, 1994:147–165.

Biguer B, Prablanc C, Jeannerod M. The contribution of coordinated eye and head movements in hand pointing accuracy. Exp Brain Res 1984; 55:462–469.

Bilodeau EA, Bilodeau IM, Schumsky DA. Some effects of introducing and withdrawing knowledge of results early and late in practice. J Exper Psych 1959; 58:142–144.

Binder S, Moll CB, Wolf SL. Evaluation of electromyographic biofeedback as an adjunct to therapeutic exercise in treating the lower extremities of hemiplegic patients. Phys Ther 1981; 61:886–893.

Birren JE, Cunningham W. Research on the psychology of aging: principles, concepts and theory. In: Birren JE, Schaie KW, eds. Handbook of the psychology of aging. 2nd ed. New York: Van Nostrand & Reinholdt, 1985:3–34.

Bjorklund, A. Long distance axonal growth in the adult central nervous system. J Neurol 1994; 241:S33-S35.

Black FO, Nashner LM. Vestibulo-spinal control differs in patients with reduced versus distorted vestibular function. Acta Otolaryngol (Stockholm) Suppl 1984; 406:110–114.

Black FO, Nashner LM. Postural control in four classes of vestibular abnormalities. In: Igarashi M, Black FO, eds. Vestibular and visual control of posture and locomotor equilibrium. Basel: Karger, 1985:271–281.

Black FO, Shupert C, Horak FB, Nashner LM. Abnormal postural control associated with peripheral vestibular disorders. In: Pompeiano O, Allum J, eds. Vestibulo-spinal control of posture and movement. Progress in brain research. Amsterdam: Elsevier Science Publishers 1988; 76:263–275.

Black P, Markowitz RS, Cianci SN. Recovery of motor function after lesions in motor cortex of monkeys. Ciba Found Symp 1975; 34:65–83.

Blanchard O, Cohen-Solal L, Tardieu C, Allain JC, Tabary C, Le Lous M. Tendon adaptation to different long term stresses and collagen reticulation in soleus muscle. Connect Tissue Res 1985; 13(3): 261–267.

Blanton S, Wolf AL. An application of upper-extremity constraint-induced movement therapy in a patient with subacute stroke. Phys Ther 1999; 79(9): 847–853.

Bleck EE. Locomotor prognosis in cerebral palsy. Dev Med Child Neurol 1975; 17:18–25.

Blin O, Ferrandez AM, Pailhouse J, Serratrice G. Dopa-sensitive and dopa-resistant gait parameters in Parkinson's disease. J Neurol Sci 1991; 103:51–54.

Blin O, Ferrandez AM, Serratrice G. Quantitative analysis of gait in Parkinson patients: Increased variability of stride length. J Neuro Sci 1990; 98:91–97.

Bliss TVP, Lomo T. Long-lasting potentiation of synaptic transmission in the dentate area of the anaesthetized rabbit following stimulation of the perforant path. J Physiol (Lond) 1973; 232:331–356.

Bobath B. Abnormal postural reflex activity caused by brain lesions. London: Heinemann, 1965:8.

Bobath B. Adult Hemiplegia: Evaluation and Treatment. London: Wm Heinemann Medical Books, 1970.

Bobath B. Adult Hemiplegia: Evaluation and Treatment. London: William Heinemann Medical Books, 1978.

Bobath B, Bobath K. Motor development in different types of cerebral palsy. London: Heinemann, 1976.

Bobath K, Bobath B. The neurodevelopmental treatment. In: Scrutton D, ed. Management of the motor disorders of cerebral palsy. Clinics in Developmental Medicine, no. 90. London, Heinemann Medical, 1984.

Boehme R. Improving Upper Body Control. Tucson, AZ: Therapy Skill Builders, 1988.

Boenig DD. Evaluation of a clinical method of gait analysis. Phys Ther 1977; 7:795–798.

Bogataj U, Gros N, Malezic M, et al. Restoration of gait during two to three weeks of therapy with multichannel electrical stimulation. Phys Ther 1989; 69:319–327.

Bohannon RW. Comfortable and maximum walking speed of adults aged 20–79 years: reference values and determinants. Age Ageing 1997; 26:15–19.

Bohannon RW, Andrews AW. Relationships between impairments in strength of limb muscle actions following stroke. Percept Mot Skills 1998; 87: 1327–1330.

Bohannon RW, Smith MB. Inter-rater reliability of a modified Ashworth scale of muscle spasticity. Phys Ther 1987; 67:206–207.

Bohannon RW, Walsh S. Nature, reliability, and predictive value of muscle performance measures in patients with hemiparesis following stroke. Arch Phys Med Rehabil 1992; 73:721–725.

Borst MJ, Peterson CQ. Overcoming topographical orientation deficits in an elderly woman with right cerebrovascular accident. Am J Occup Ther 1993; 47:551–554.

Bouisset S, Zattara M. A sequence of postural movements precedes voluntary movement. Neuroscience Letters 1981; 22:263–270.

Bourne LE, Dominowski RL, Loftus EF. Cognitive Processes. Englewood Cliffs, NJ: Prentice Hall, 1979.

Bouska MJ, Kwatny E. Manual for Application of the Motor Free Visual Perceptual Test to the Adult Population. Philadelphia: Temple University Rehabilitation Research Training Center, No. 8, 1983.

Bower TGR, Broughton JM, Moore MK. The coordination of visual and tactual input in infants. Perception Psychophysics 1970a;8:51–53.

Bower TGR, Broughton JM, Moore MK. Demonstration of intention in the reaching behavior of neonate humans. Nature 1970b;228:679–681.

Bradley NS, Bekoff A. Development of locomotion: animal models. In: Woollacott MH, Shumway-Cook A, eds. Development of posture and gait across the lifespan. Columbia: University of South Carolina, 1989:48–73.

Bradley NS, Smith JL. Neuromuscular patterns of stereotypic hindlimb behaviors in the first two postnatal months. I. Stepping in normal kittens. Dev Brain Res 1988; 38:37–52.

Brand PW. Management of sensory loss in the extremities. In: Omer E, Spinner M, eds. Management of Peripheral Nerve Problems. Philadelphia: WB Saunders, 1980:862–872.

Brandstater M, deBruin H, Gowland C, et al.: Hemiplegic gait: analysis of temporal variables. Arch Phys Med Rehabil 1983; 64:583–587.

Brandt EN, Pope AM (eds.). Enabling America. Washington DC, National Academy, 1997.

Brandt T, Daroff RB. The multisensory physiological and pathological vertigo syndromes. Ann Neurol 1979;7:195–197.

Brandt T, Wenzel D, Dichgans J. Die Entwicklung der visuellen Stabilisation des aufrechten Standes bein Kind: Ein Refezeichen in der Kinderneurologie (Visual stabilization of free stance in infants: a sign of maturity). Arch Psychiatr Nervenkr 1976; 223:1–13.

Brauer S. Mediolateral postural stability: changes with age and prediction of fallers. Doctoral Dissertation, University of Queensland, June 1998.

Brauer S, Burns Y, Galley P. Lateral reach: A clinical measure of medio-lateral postural stability. Physio Res Int 1999; 4:81–88.

Braun JJ, Meyer PM, Meyer DR. Sparing of a brightness habit in rats following visual decortication. J Comp Physiol Psychol 1986; 61:79–82.

Breniere Y, Bril B. Development of postural control of gravity forces in children during the first 5 years of walking. Exp Brain Res 1998; 121:255–262.

Breniere Y, Do MC. When and how does steady state gait movement induced from upright posture begin? J Biomech 1986; 19:1035–1040.

Breniere Y, Do MC, Sanchez J. A biomechanical study of the gait initiation process. Journal de Biophysique et de Medecine Nucleaire 1981; 5:197–205.

Breslin DM, Exner CE. Construct validity of the In-Hand Manipulation Test: A discriminant analysis with children without disability and children with spastic diplegia. Am J Occup Ther 1999; 53(4):381–386.

Bril B, Breniere Y. Posture and independent locomotion in childhood: learning to walk or learning dynamic postural control? In: Savelsbergh GJP, ed. The development of coordination in infancy. Amsterdam: North-Holland, 1993, 337–358.

Brogren E, Hadders-Algra M, Forssberg H. Postural control in children with spastic diplegia: Muscle activity during perturbations in sitting. Dev Med Child Neuro 1998; 38:379–388.

Bronstein AM, Hood JD, Gresty MA, Panagi C. Visual control of balance in cerebellar and Parkinsonian syndromes. Brain 1990; 113:767–779.

Brooks VB. The neural basis of motor control. New York: Oxford University, 1986.

Brooks VB, Thatch WT. Cerebellar control of posture and movement. In: Brooks VB, ed. Handbook of physiology, section 1: Nervous system, Vol II Motor Control, Part 2.

Brown JE, Frank JS. Influence of event anticipation on postural actions accompanying voluntary movement. Exp Br Res 1987; 67:645–650.

Brown JV, Sepehr MM, Ettlinger G, Skreczek W. The accuracy of aimed movements to visual targets during development: the role of visual information. J Exp Child Psychol 1986; 41:443–460.

Brown LA, Shumway-Cook A, Woollacott MH. Attentional demands and postural recovery: the effects of aging. J Gerontology 1999; 54a;M165–171.

Brown P, Steiger MJ. Basal ganglia gait disorders. In: AM Bronstein, Th Brandt, MH Woollacott, eds. Clinical disorders of balance, posture and gait. Arnold, London, 1996; 156–167.

Brown TG. The intrinsic factors in the act of progression in the mammal. Proc R Soc Lond (Biol) 1911; 84:308–319.

Bruce MF. The relation of tactile thresholds to histology in the fingers of the elderly. J Neurol Neurosurg Psychiatry 1980; 43:730.

Bruininks R, Woodcock R, Weatherman R, Hill B. Scales of Independent Behavior. Allen TX, Teaching Resources, DLM, 1984.

Bruininks RH. Bruininks-Oseretsky Test of Motor Proficiency. Circle Pine, Minn.: American Guidance Service, 1978.

Bruner JS, Koslowski B. Visually pre-adapted constituents of manipulatory action. Perception 1972; 1:3–14.

Brunnstrom S. Motor testing procedures in hemiplegia: based on sequential recovery stages. Phys Ther 1966; 46:357–375.

Brunnstrom S. Movement therapy in hemiplegia: a neurophysiological approach. New York: Harper & Row, 1970.

Buchner DM, DeLateur BJ. The importance of skeletal muscle strength to physical function in older adults. Annals of Behavioral Medicine 1991; 13:1–12.

Buchner DM, Larson EB, Wagner EH, Koepsell TD, DeLateur BJ. Evidence for a non-linear relationship between leg strength and gait speed. Age Ageing 1996; 25:386–391.

Bullinger A. Cognitive elaboration of sensorimotor behaviour. In: Butterworth G, ed. Infancy and epistemology: an evaluation of Piaget's theory. London: Harvester, 1981:173–199.

Bullinger A, Jouen F. Sensibilite du champ de detection peripherique aux variations posturales chez le bebe. Arch Psychol 1983; 51:41–48.

Burgess PR and Clark FJ. Characteristics of knee-joint receptors in the cat. J Physiol Lond 1969; 203:317–325.

Burtner PA, Qualls C, Woollacott MH. Muscle activation characteristics of stance balance control in children with spastic cerebral palsy. Gait Posture 1998; 8:163–174

Burtner PA, Woollacott MH, Qualls C. Stance balance control with orthoses in a select group of children with and without spasticity. Dev Med Child 1999; 41:748–757.

Butland RJA, Pang J, Gross ER, Woodcock AA, Geddes DM. Two-, six-, and 12-minute walking tests in respiratory disease. Br Med J 1982; 284:1607–1608.

Butterworth G, Cicchetti D. Visual calibration of posture in normal and motor retarded Down's syndrome infants. Perception 1978; 7:513–525.

Butterworth G, Hicks L. Visual proprioception and postural stability in infancy: a developmental study. Perception 1977; 6: 255–262.

Butterworth G, Pope M. Origine et fonction de la proprioception visuelle chez l'enfant. In: de Schonen S, ed. Le developpement dans la premiere année. Paris: Presses Universitaires de France, 1983: 107–128.

Chae J, Bethoux F, Bohine T, Dobos L, Davis T, Friedl A. Neuromuscular stimulation for upper extremity motor and functional recovery in acute hemiplegia. Stroke 1998; 29:975–979.

Cailliet R. The shoulder in hemiplegia. Philadelphia: FA Davis, 1980.

Callahan AD. Sensibility testing: clinical methods. In: Hunter JM, Schneider LH, Mackin EJ, Callahan AD, eds. Rehabilitation of the Hand. St. Louis: CV Mosby, 1990:600–602.

Campbell AJ, Borrie MJ, Spears GF. Risk factors for falls in a community-based prospective study of people 70 years and older. J Gerontol 1989; 44:M112-M117.

Campbell AJ, Reinken J, Allen BC, Martiniz GS. Falls in old age: A study of frequency and related clinical factors. Age & Aging 1981;10:264–279.

Campbell SK, Wilhelm IJ. Development from birth to 3 years of age of 15 children at high risk for central nervous system dysfunction. Phys Ther 1985; 65:463–469.

Campbell SK. Measurement of motor performance in cerebral palsy. In: Forssberg H. Hirschfeld H, eds. Movement disorders in children. Basel: Karger, 1991; 264–271.

Cannon N. Manual of Hand Splinting. New York: Churchill Livingstone, 1985.

Capute AJ, Accardo PJ, Vining EPG, et al. Primitive reflex profile. Baltimore: University Park, 1978.

Capute AJ, Wachtel RC, Palmer FB, Shapiro BK, Accardo PJ. A prospective study of three postural reactions. Dev Med Child Neurol 1982; 24:314–320.

Carey L, Matyas T, Oke L. Sensory loss in stroke patients: Effective training of tactile and proprioceptive discrimination. Arch Phys Med Rehabil 1993; 74:602–611.

Carmick J. Clinical use of neuromuscular electrical stimulation for children with cerebral palsy, Part 2: Upper extremity. Phys Ther 1993; 73(8):514–526.

Carmick J. Use of neuromuscular electrical stimulation and [corrected] dorsal wrist splint to improve the hand function of a child with spastic hemiplegia. Phys Ther 1997; 6:661–671.

Carlsoo, A. The initiation of walking. Acta Anat 1966; 65:1–9.

Carlton LG. Processing visual feedback information for movement control. J Exp Psychol Hum Percept;1981; 7:1019–1030.

Carr JH, Shepherd RB. Motor relearning programme for stroke. Rockville, MD: Aspen Publications, 1983.

Carr JH, Shepherd RB. Motor relearning programme for stroke. Rockville, MD: Aspen, 1986.

Carr JH, Shepherd RB, Nordholm L, Lynne D. Investigation of a new motor assessment scale for stroke patients. Phys Ther 1985; 65:175–180.

Carr JH, Shepherd RB. Neurologic Rehabilitation: Optimizing Motor Performance. Oxford: Butterworth and Heinemann, 1998.

Case-Smith J. The relationship among sensorimotor components, fine motor skill, and functional performance in preschool children. Am J Occup Ther 1995; 49(7):645–52.

Case-Smith J. Fine motor outcomes in preschool children who receive occupational therapy services. Am J Occup Ther 1996; 50(1):52–61.

Castle ME, Reyman TA, Schneider M. Pathology of spastic muscle in cerebral palsy. Clin Orthop 1979; 142:223–233.

Catalano JF, Kleiner BM. Distant transfer and practice variability. Percept Mot Skills 1984; 58:851–856.

Cavagna GA, Franzetti P. The determinants of the step frequency in walking in humans. J Physiol (Lond) 1986; 373:235–242.

Cavanagh PR, Gregor RJ. Knee joint torques during the swing phase of normal treadmill walking. J Biomech 1975; 8:337–344.

Cermack S, Lin KC. Assessment of unilateral neglect in individuals with right cerebral vascular accident. Topics in Geriatric Rehabilitation 1997; 10:42–55.

Chambers HG. The surgical treatment of spasticity. Muscle Nerve 1997:Supp 6: S121-S125.

Chandler LS, Skillen M, Swanson MW: Movement Assessment of Infants, A Manual. Authors, Rolling Bay, WA, 1980.

Chandler JM, Hadley EC. Exercise to improve physiologic and functional performance in old age. In: Studenski S. Clinics in Geriatric Medicine: Gait and Balance Disorders, 1996 Vol 12, pp. 761–784. Philadelphia: Saunders.

Chang HA, Krebs DE. Dynamic balance control in elders: gait initiation assessment as a screening tool. Arch Phys Med Rehabil 1999; 80:490–494.

Charles J, Lavender G. Modification of the motor Activity Log for Children with Hemiplegia, Personal Communication, 1997, Teachers College, Columbia University.

Charles J. Constraint-induced therapy in children with hemiplegic cerebral palsy. Poster presention made at The Combined Sections Meeting of The American Physical Therapy Association, Seattle, WA., 1999.

Charles J, Gordon AM. Constraint-induced therapy in children with hemiplegic cerebral palsy. Poster presentation made at The Combined Sections Meeting of The American Physical Therapy Association. Seattle WA, 1999.

Charness A. Stroke/head injury: a guide to functional outcomes in physical therapy management. Rockville, MD: Aspen Systems, 1986.

Charness AL. Management of the upper extremity in the patient with hemiplegia. Course syllabus, Annual Meeting, Washington Physical Therapy Association, 1994.

Chen HC. Factors underlying balance restoration after tripping: Biomechanical model analyses. Doctoral Dissertation, University of Michigan, 1993.

Chen H, Ashton-Miller JA, Alexander NB, Schultz AB. Stepping over obstacles: gait patterns of healthy young and old adults. J Gerontol 1991; 46:M196-M203.

Chen HC, Schultz AB, Ashton-Miller JA et al. Stepping over obstacles: Dividing attention impairs performance of old more than young adults. J Gerontol 1996; 51A:M116–122.

Chong R, Horak F, Woollacott M. Parkinson's disease impairs the ability to change set quickly. J Neurol Sci 2000;175:57–70.

Clark J, Lanphear A, Riddick C. The effects of videogame playing on the response selection processing of elderly adults. J Gerontol 1987; 42:82–85.

Clark JE, Whitall J. Changing patterns of locomotion: from walking to skipping. In: Woollacott MH, Shumway-Cook A, eds. Development of posture and gait across the lifespan. Columbia: University of South Carolina, 1989:128–151.

Clark SA, Allard T, Jenkins WM, Merzenich MM. Receptive fields in the body-surface map in adult cortex defined by temporally correlated inputs. Nature 1988; 332:444–445.

Claverie P, Alexandre F, Nichol J, Bonnet F, Cahuzac M. L'activité tonique reflexe du nourisson. Pediatrie 1973; 28:661–679.

Cohen H, Blatchly C, Gombash L. A study of the clinical test of sensory interaction and balance. Phys Ther 1993a;73:346–354.

Cohen LG, Bandinelli S, Findlay TW, Hallett M. Motor reorganization after upper limb amputation in man: a study with focal magnetic stimulation. Brain 1991; 114:615–627.

Cohen LG, Brasil-Neto JP, Pascual-Leone A, Hallett M. Plasticity of cortical motor output organization following deafferentation, cerebral lesions, and skill acquisition. In: O Devinsky, A Beric, M Dogali, eds. Electrical and Magnetic Stimulation of the Brain and Spinal Cord. New York: Raven, 1993B:187–200.

Colarusso RP, Hamill DD. Motor Free Visual Perceptual Test-Revised. Western Psychological Services, Los Angeles, CA, 1996(5).

Cole KJ. Grasp force control in older adults. J Motor Behav 1991; 23:251–258.

Cole KJ, Abbs JH, Tuner GS. Deficits in the production of grip forces in Down's syndrome. Dev Med Child Neurol 1988; 30:752–758.

Cole KJ, Rotella DL, Harper JG. Mechanisms for age-related changes of fingertip forces during precision gripping and lifting in adults. J Neurosci 1999; 19:3228–3247.

Collen FM, Wade DT, Bradshaw CM. Mobility after stroke: Reliability of measures of impairment and disability. Int Disabil Studies 1990; 12:6–9.

Collen FM, Wade DT, Robb GF, Bradshaw CM. The Rivermead Mobility Index: a further development of the Rivermead Motor Assessment. Int Disabil Studies 1991; 13:50–54.

Connolly KJ. The development of competence in motor skills. In: Nadeau CH, Halliwell WR, Newell KM, Roberts GC, eds. Psychology of motor behavior and sport. Champaign, IL: Human Kinetics, 1979: 229–250.

Cook T, Cozzens B. Human solutions for locomotion: 3. The initiation of gait. In: Herman RM, Grillner S, Stein PSG, Stuart DG, eds. Neural control of locomotion. New York: Plenum, 1976:65–76.

Corbetta D, Mounoud P. Early development of grasping and manipulation. In: Bard C, Fleury M, Hay L, eds. Development of Eye-hand Coordination Across the Lifespan. Columbia, SC: University of South Carolina Press, 1990:188–216.

Corbetta D, Mounoud P. Early development of grasping and manipulation. In: Bard C, Fleury M, Hay L, eds. Development of eye-hand coordination across the lifespan. Columbia: University of South Carolina, 1990:189–213.

Cordo P, Nashner L. Properties of postural adjustments associated with rapid arm movements. J Neurophysiol 1982; 47:287–302.

Cornhill H, Case-Smith J. Factors that relate to good and poor handwriting. Am J Occup Ther 1996; 50(9):732–9.

Corry IS, Cosgrove AP, Wailsh EG, McClean D, Graham HK. Botulinum toxin A in the hemiplegic upper limb: A double-blind trial. Dev Med Child Neurol 1997; 39:185–193.

Coryell J, Henderson A. Role of the asymmetrical tonic neck reflex in hand visualization in normal infants. Am J Occup Ther 1979; 33:255–260.

Coster W, Deeney T, Haltiwanger J, Haley S. School Function Assessment (SFA). San Antonio: The Psychological Corporation of Harcourt Brace & Co., 1998.

Cote L, Crutcher MD. The basal ganglia. In: Kandel E, Schwartz JH, Jessell TM, eds. Principles of neuroscience. 3rd ed. New York: Elsevier, 1991:647–659.

Cowie RJ, Robinson DL. Subcortical contributions to head movements in macaques: 1. Contrasting effects of electrical stimulation of a medial pontomedullary region and the superior colliculus. J Neurophysiol 1994; 72:2648–2664.

Cozean CD, Pease SW, Hubbell SL. Biofeedback and functional electric stimulation in stroke rehabilitation. Arch Phys Med Rehabil 1988; 69:401–405.

Craik R. Changes in locomotion in the aging adult. In: Woollacott MH, Shumway-Cook A, eds. Development of posture and gait across the lifespan. Columbia: University of South Carolina, 1989:176–201.

Craik RL. Recovery processes: maximizing function. In: Contemporary management of motor control problems. Proceedings of the II Step Conference. Alexandria, VA: APTA, 1992:165–173.

Craik RL, Cozzens BA, Freedman W. The role of sensory conflict on stair descent performance in humans. Exp Brain Res 1982; 45:399–409.

Crenna P. Spasticity and "spastic" gait in children with cerebral palsy. Neurosci Biobehav Rev 1998; 22:571–578.

Crenna P, Inverno M. Objective detection of pathophysiological factors contributing to gait disturbance in supraspinal lesions. In: Fedrizzi E, Avanzini G, Crenna P. Motor development in children. New York: John Libbey, 1994: 103–118.

Crisostomo EA. Duncan PW, Propst MA, et al. Evidence that amphetamine with physical therapy promotes recovery of motor function in stroke patients. Ann Neurol 1988; 23:94–97.

Crocker MD, Mackay-Lyons M, McDonnell E. Forced use of the upper extremity in cerebral palsy: A single case design. Am J Occup Ther 1997; 51(10):824–33.

Crocker M. Forced use of the upper extremity in cerebral palsy: a single case design. Am J Occup Ther 1997; 51:10.

Crossman ERFW, Goodeve PJ. Feedback control of hand-movement and Fitts' law. Q J Exp Psychol 1983; 35A:251–278.

Cruickshank DA, O'Neill DL. Upper extremity inhibitive casting in a boy with spastic quadriplegia. Am J Occup Ther 1990; 6:552–555.

Cupps C, Plescia MG, Houser C. The Landau reaction: a clinical and electromyographic analysis. Dev Med Child Neurol 1976; 18:41–53.

Curtis RM, Engalitcheff J Jr. A work simulator for rehabilitating the upper extremity—preliminary report. J Hand Surg 1981; 6:499–510.

Damiano DL, Abel MF. Relation of gait analysis to gross motor function in cerebral palsy. Dev Med Child Neurol 1996; 38:389–396.

Damiano DL, Abel MF. Functional outcomes of strength training in spastic cerebral palsy. Arch Phys Med Rehabil 1998; 79:119–125.

Dannenbaum R, Dykes R. Sensory loss in the hand after sensory stroke: Therapeutic rationale. Arch Phys Med Rehabil 1988; 69:833–839.

Dannenbaum R, Jones L. The assessment and treatment of patients who have sensory loss following cortical lesions. J Hand Ther 1993; 6:130–138.

Das P, McCollum G. Invariant structure in locomotion. Neuroscience 1988; 25:1023–1034.

Davies P. Aging and Alzheimer's disease: new light on old problems. Paper presented at Neuroscience Society Annual Meeting, New Orleans, 1987.

Davies PM. Steps to follow. New York: Springer-Verlag, 1985.

Davis SE, Mulcahey MJ, Betz RR, Smith BT, Weiss AA. Outcomes of upper extremity tendon transfers and functional electrical stimulation in an adolescent with C-5 tetraplegia. Am J Occup Ther 1997; 51(4):307–312.

Day BL, Steiger MJ, Thompson PD, Marsden CD. Effect of vision and stance width on human body motion when standing: Implications for afferent control of lateral sway. J Physiol 1993; 469:479–499.

Decety J, Sjoholm H, Ryding E, et al. The cerebellum participates in mental activity: tomographic measurements of regional cerebral blood flow. Brain Res 1990; 535, 313–317.

DeFabio R, Badke MB. Relationship of sensory organization to balance function in patients with hemiplegia. Phys Ther 1990; 70:542–560.

DeJersey MC Report on a sensory programme for patients with sensory deficits. Aust J Phyiother 1979; 25:165–70.

DeKleijn A. Experimental physiology of the labyrinth. J Laryngol Otol 1923; 38:646–663.

Dellen T Van, Kalverboer AF. Single movement control and information processing, a developmental study. Behav Brain Res 1984; 12:237–238.

Dellon AL, Curtis RM, Edgerton MT. Reeducation of sensation in the hand following nerve injury. Plast Reconstr Surg 1974; 53:297–305.

Dellon AL. Clinical use of vibratory stimuli to evaluate peripheral nerve injury and compression neuropathy. Plast Reconstr Surg 1980; 65(4):466–76.

Dellon AL. Evaluation of Sensibility and Re-education of Sensation in the Hand. Baltimore: Williams & Wilkins, 1981.

Dellon A, Kallman C. Evaluation of functional sensation in the hand. J Hand Surgery 1983; 8:865–870.

Dellon AL, Munger BL. Correlation of histology and sensibility after nerve repair. J Hand Surg 1983; 8(6):871–5.

Del Rey P, Whitehurst M, Wood J. Effects of experience and contextual interference on learning and transfer. Percept Motor Skills 1983; 56:581–582.

DeLuca PA, Perry JP, Ounpuu S. The fundamentals of normal walking and pathological gait. AACP & DM Inst. Course 2. 1992.

DeQuervain IAK, Simon SR, Leurgans S, et al. Gait pattern in the early recovery period after stroke. J Bone Joint Surg 1996; 78A:1506–1514.

De Souza LH, Hewer RL, Miller S. Assessment of recovery of arm control in hemiplegic stroke patients. 1. Arm function tests. Int Rehab Med 1980;2:3–9.

Dettman MA, Linder MT, Sepic SB. Relationships among walking performance, postural stability, and functional assessments of the hemiplegic patient. Am J Phys Med 1987; 66:77–90.

Deuschl G, Bain P, Brin M. Consensus statement of the Movement Disorder Society on tremor. Mov Disord 1998; 13:2–23.

De Vries JIP, Visser GHA, Prechtl HFR. The emergence of fetal behavior: 1. Qualitative aspects. Early Human Dev 1982; 7:301–322.

Diener HC, Dichgans J, Bruzek W, Selinka H. Stabilization of human posture during induced oscillations of the body. Exp Brain Res 1982; 45:126–132.

Diener HC, Dichgans J, Guschlbauer B, Bacher M. Role of visual and static vestibular influences on dynamic posture control. Hum Neurobiol 1986; 5:105–113.

Diener HC, Dichgans J, Guschlbauer B, Mau H. The significance of proprioception on postural stabilization as assessed by ischemia. Brain Res 1984; 296: 103–109.

Dietz V, Quintern J, Berger W. Electrophysiological studies of gait in spasticity and rigidity: evidence that altered mechanical properties of muscle contribute to hypertonia. Brain 1981; 104:431–439.

Dietz V, Schubert M, Discher M, Trippel M. Influence of visuoproprioceptive mismatch on postural adjustments. Gait Posture 1994; 2:147–155.

Dietz V, Schmidtbleicher D, Noth J. Neuronal mechanisms of human locomotion. J Neurophysiol 1979; 42:1212–1222.

Dietz V, Trippel M, Horstmann GA. Significance of proprioceptive and vestibulo-spinal reflexes in the control of stance and gait. In: Patla AE, ed. Adaptability of human gait. Elsevier: Amsterdam, 1991:37–52.

DiFabio R, Badke MB. Relationship of sensory organization to balance function in patients with hemiplegia. Phys Ther 1990; 70:543–552.

DiFabio RP, Badke MB. Stance duration under sensory conflict conditions in patients with hemiplegia. Arch Phys Med Rehabil 1991; 72:292–295.

DiFabio FP, Badke MB, Duncan PW. Adapting human postural reflexes following a localized cerebrovascular lesion: analysis of bilateral long latency responses. Brain Res 1986; 363:257–264.

Dobkin BH. Neurologic rehabilitation. Philadelphia: FA Davis, 1996.

Dodwell PC, Muir D, Difranco D. Responses of infants to visual presented objects. Science 1976; 194:209–211.

Dombovy MI, Basford JR, Whisnant JP, Bergstralh EJ. Disability and use of rehabilitation services following stroke in Rochester, Minn, 1975–1979. Stroke 1987; 18:830–836.

Donoghue JP, Suner S, Sanes JN. Dynamic organization of primary motor cortexant put to target muscles in adult rats. II. Rapid reorganization following motor nerve lesion. Exp Brain Res 1990;79:492–503.

Dowling JE. The retina: an approachable part of the brain. Cambridge, MA: Belknap, 1987.

Drillis R. The influence of aging on the kinematics of gait: the geriatric amputee. Pub 919. National Academy of Science, National Research Council, 1961.

Duffy CJ, Wurtz RH. Medial superior temporal area neurons respond to speed patterns in optic flow. J Neurosci 1997; 17:2839–2851.

Duhamel JR, Colby CL, Goldberg ME. The updating of the representation of visual space in parietal cortex by intended eye movements. Science 1992a;255:90–92.

Duhamel JR, Goldberg ME, Fitzgibbon EJ, et al. Saccadic dysmetria in a patient with a right frontoparietal lesion. Brain 1992b;115:1387–1402.

Duncan P. Balance dysfunction and motor control theory. Syllabus from a talk. Washington State APTA annual conference, 1993.

Duncan PW. Stroke: physical therapy assessment and treatment. In: Contemporary management of motor control problems. Proceedings of the II Step Conference. Alexandria, VA: APTA, 1991:209–217.

Duncan P, Badke MB. Stroke rehabilitation: the recovery of motor control. Chicago: Year Book, 1987.

Duncan P, Badke MB. Determinants of abnormal motor control. In: Duncan P, Badke MB, eds. Stroke Rehabilitation: The Recovery of Motor Control. Chicago: Year Book Medical Publishers, 1987:135–159.

Duncan PW, Chandler J, Studenski S, et al. How do physiological components of balance affect mobility in elderly men? Arch Phys Med Rehabil 1993; 74:1343–1349.

Duncan P, Richards L, Wallace D, et al. A randomized, controlled pilot study of a home-based exercise program for individuals with mild and moderate stroke. Stroke 1998; 29:2055–2060.

Duncan P, Studenski S, Chandler J, Prescott B. Functional reach: a new clinical measure of balance. J Gerontol 1990; 45:M192–M197.

Dunn W, Brown C, McGuigan A. The ecology of human performance: A framework for considering the effect of contex. Am J Occ Ther 1994; 48:595–607.

Edstrom L. Selective changes in the sizes of red and white muscle fibers in upper motor lesions and parkinsonism. J Neurol Sci 1970; 11:537–550.

Edstrom L, Grimby L, Hannerz J. Correlation between recruitment order of motor units and muscle atrophy patterns of upper motor neuron lesions: significance of spasticity. Experientia 1973; 29:560–561.

Edwards AS. Body sway and vision. J Exper Psychol 1946; 36:526–535.

Edwards JM, Elliott D, Lee TD. Contextual interference effects during skill acquisition and transfer in Down's syndrome adolescents. Adapt Physical Activity Q 1986; 3:250–258.

Eichhorn J, Orner J, Rickard K, Craik R. Aging effects on dual-task methodology using walking and verbal reaction time. Issues Aging 1998; 21:8–12.

Eliasson A-C, Gordon AM. Release in children with hemiplegic cerebral palsy. (in press). Dev Med Child Neurol.

Eliasson AC, Gordon AM, Forssberg H. Basic coordination of manipulative forces in children with cerebral palsy. Dev Med Child Neurol 1991; 134:126–154.

Eng JJ, Winter DA, Patla AE. Strategies for recovery from a trip in early and late swing during human walking. Exp Brain Res 1994; 102:339–349.

Eng JJ, Winter DA, Patla AE. Intralimb dynamics simplify reactive control strategies during locomotion. J Biomechanics 1997; 30:581–588.

Engardt M, Knutsson E, Jonsson M, Sternhag M. Dynamic muscle strength training in stroke patients: effects on knee extension torque, electromyographic activity, and motor function. Arch Phys Med Rehabil 1995; 76:419–25.

Erhardt RP. Developmental hand dysfunction: theory, assessment, treatment. Laurel, MD: Ramsco, 1982.

Erhardt RP. Developmental hand dysfunction: theory, assessment and treatment. Tucson, AZ: Therapy Skill Builders, 1982.

Erhardt RP. Erhardt Developmental Prehension Assessment. Laurel, MD: Ramsco, 1984.

Evans RW, Gualtieri CT, Patterson D. Treatment of closed head injury with psychostimulant drugs: a controlled case study as an appropriate evaluation procedure. J Nerv Ment Dis 1987; 175:106–110.

Evarts EV. Relation of pyramidal tract activity to force exerted during voluntary movement. J Neurophysiol 1968; 31:14–27.

Eyring EJ, Murray W. The effect of joint position on the pressure of intra-articular effusion. J Bone Joint Surg 1965; 47A:313–322.

Exner CE. Development of hand functions. In: Pratt PN, Allen AS, eds. Occupational Therapy for Children. St Louis: CV Mosby, 1989.

Exner C. In-hand manipulation skills in normal young children: A pilot study. Occ Ther Pract 1990; 1(4):63–72.

Exner CE, Henderson A. Cognition and motor skill. In: Henderson A, Pehoski C, eds. Hand Function in the Child: Foundations for Remediation. Philadelphia: Mosby, 1995.

Faghri PD, Rodgers MM, Glaser RM, Bors JG, Ho C, Akuthota P. The effects of functional electrical stimulation on shoulder subluxation, arm function recovery, and shoulder pain in hemiplegic stroke patients. Arch Phys Med Rehabil 1994; 75:73–79.

Fahn S. The freezing phenomenon in parkinsonism Adv Neurol 1995; 65:53–63.

Fahn S, Marsden CD. The treatment of dystonia. In: Marsden CD and Fahn S, eds. Movement Disorders 2. Butterworth, London, 1987.

Fahn S, Marsden DC, Caine DB. Classification and investigation of dystonia. In: Marsden CD and Fahn S, eds. Movement Disorders 2. London: Butterworth, 1987.

Falduto L, Baron A. Age-related effects of practice and task complexity on card sorting. J Gerontol 1986; 41:659–661.

Farley CT, Taylor CR. A mechanical trigger for the trot-gallop transition in horses. Science 1991; 253:306–308.

Feeney DM, Gonzalez A, Law WA. Amphetamine restores locomotor function after motor cortex injury in the rat. Proc West Pharmacol Soc 1981; 24:15–17.

Feeney DM, Gonzalez A, Law WA. Amphetamine haloperidol and experience interact to affect the rate of recovery after motor cortex injury. Science 1982; 217:855–857.

Feeney DM, Sutton RL. Pharmacology for recovery of function after brain injury. Crit Rev Neurobiol 1987; 3:135–185.

Feeney DM, Sutton RL, Boyeson MG, et al. The locus-coeruleus and cerebral metabolism: recovery of function after cortical injury. Physiol Psych 1985; 13:197–203.

Feinstein AR, Josephy MS, Wells CK. Scientific and clinical problems in indexes of functional disability. Annals of Internal Medicine 1986; 105:413–420.

Feldman AG. Change in the length of the muscle as a consequence of a shift in equilibrium in the muscle-load system. Biofizika 1974; 19:534–538.

Fellows SJ, Noth J, Schwarz M. Precision grip and Parkinson's disease. Brain 1998; 121:1171–1184.

Fentress JC. Development of grooming in mice with amputated forelimbs. Science 1973; 179:704.

Ferguson JM, Trombly CA. The effect of added-purpose and meaningful occupation on motor learning. Am J Occup Ther 1998; 51(7):508–15.

Fernie GR, Gryfe CI, Holliday PJ, Llewellyn A. The relationship of postural sway in standing: the incidence of falls in geriatric subjects. Age Ageing 1982; 11:11–16.

Ferris DP, Louie M, Farley CT. Running in the real world: adjusting leg stiffness for different surfaces. Proceedings of the Royal Society, London B, 1998; 265:989–994.

Fess EE. A method for checking Jamar dynamometer calibration. J Hand Ther 1987; 1:28–32.

Fess E. Assessment of the upper extremity: Instrumentation criteria. Occup Thery Pract 1990; 1:1–11.

Fess EE. Documentation: essential elements of an upper extremity assessment battery. In: Hunter JM, ed. Rehabilitation of the Hand. 2nd ed. St. Louis: CV Mosby, 1990:53–81.

Fess EE. Grip Strength. In: Casanova JS, ed. Clinical Assessment Recommendations, 2nd ed. Chicago, IL: American Society of Hand Therapists, 1992:41–45.

Fetter M. Vestibular system disorders. In: Herdman S, ed. Vestibular Rehabilitation, 2nd edition. Philadelphia: FA Davis, 2000: 91–102.

Fiatarone MA, Marks EC, Ryan ND, Meredith CN, Lipsitz LA, Evans WJ. High-intensity strength training in nonagenarians: effects on skeletal muscle. JAMA 1990; 263:3029–3034.

Fiatarone M, O'Neill E, Doyle R, et al. Exercise training and nutritional supplementation for physical frailty in very elderly people. N Engl J Med 1994; 339:1769–1775.

Fiez, JA, Petersen SE, Cheney, MK, Raichle, ME. Impaired non-motor learning and error detection associated with cerebellar damage. Brain 1992; 115, 155–178.

Finch L, Barbeau H, Arsenault B. Influence of body weight support on normal human gait: development of a gait retraining strategy. Phys Ther 1991; 71:842–856.

Finley FR, Cody KA. Locomotive characteristics of urban pedestrians. Arch Phys Med Rehabil 1970; 51:423–426.

Finley FR, Cody KA, Finizie RV. Locomotion patterns in elderly women. Arch Phys Med 1969; 50:140–146.

Finley FR, Cody KA, Sepic SB. Walking patterns of normal women. Arch Phys Med Rehabil 1970; 51:637–650.

Finson R, Smith B, McCarthy J, Betz R, Mulcahey MJ. Intramuscular functional electrical stimulation (FES) to augment walking in children with cerebral palsy. RESNA June 25–29, 1998:143.

Finson R, Akers, Mulcahey MJ, Betz R. The effects of percutaneous functional electrical stimulation (FES) assisted walking on spatial and temporal characteristics in children with cerebral palsy. Phys Ther 1999; 78(5):S12.

Fishkind M, Haley SM. Independent sitting development and the emergence of associated motor compoments. Phys Ther 1986; 66:1509–1514.

Fisher AG. Assessment of Motor and Process Skills Manual. Fort Collins, CO: Colorado State University, 1994.

Fisk JD, Goodale MA. The organization of eye and limb movements during unrestricted reaching to targets in contralateral and ipsilateral visual space. Exp Brain Res 1985; 60:159–178.

Fisk JD. Sensory and motor integration in the control of reaching. In: Bard C, Fleury M, Hay L, eds. Developmental of Eye-Hand Coordination Across the Lifespan. Columbia, SC: University of South Carolina Press, 1990:75–98.

Fisk JD, Goodale MA. The effects of unilateral brain damage on visually guided reaching: hemispheric differences in the nature of the deficit. Exp Brain Res 1988; 72:425–435.

Fitts PM. The information capacity of the human motor system in controlling the amplitude of movement. J Exp Psychol 1954; 47:381–391.

Fitts PM, Posner MI. Human performance. Belmont, CA: Brooks/Cole, 1967.

Florence SL, Kaas JH. Large-scale reorganization at multiple levels of the somatosensory pathway follows therapeutic amputation of the hand in monkeys. J Neurosci 1995; 15:8083–8095.

Foerster O. The motor cortex in man in the light of Hughlings Jackson's Doctrines. In: Payton OD, Hirt S, Newman, R, eds. Scientific bases for neurophysiologic approaches to therapeutic exercise. Philadelphia: FA Davis, 1977:13–18.

Folio RM, Fewell RR. Peabody Developmental Motor Scales. DLM Teaching Resources, Allen TX, 1983.

Folstein MF, Folstein SE, McHugh PR. Mini-mental state: A practical method for grading the cognitive states for the clinician. J Psychiatric Res 1975; 12:188–198.

Ford-Smith CD, VanSant AF. Age differences in movement patterns used to rise from a bed in subjects in the third through fifth decades of age. Phys Ther 1993; 73:300–309.

Forlander DA, Bohannon RW. Rivermead Mobility Index: a brief review of research to date. Clinical Rehabilitation 1999; 13:97–100.

Forssberg H. Motor learning: A neurophysiological review. In: Berg K, Eriksson B, eds. Children and exercise, vol 9. Baltimore: University Park, 1980:13–22.

Forssberg H. Ontogeny of human locomotor control. I. Infant stepping, supported locomotion, and transition to independent locomotion. Exp Brain Res 1985; 57:480–493.

Forssberg H, Eliasson AC, Kinoshita H, Johansson RS, Westling G. Development of human precision grip I. basic coordination of forces. Exp Brain Res 1991; 85:451–457.

Forssberg H, Eliasson AC, Kinoshita H, Johansson RS, Westling G. Development of human precision grip IV. Tactile adaptation of isometric finger forces to the frictional condition. Exp Brain Res 1995; 104:323–330.

Forssberg H, Grillner S, Rossignol S. Phase dependent reflex reversal during walking in chronic spinal cats. Brain Res 1975; 85:103–107.

Forssberg H, Grillner S, Rossignol S. Phasic gain control of reflexes from the dorsum of the paw during spinal locomotion. Brain Res 1977;132:121–139.

Forssberg H, Hirschfeld H. Postural adjustments in sitting humans following external perturbations: muscle activity and kinematics. Exp Brain Res 1994; 97:515–527.

Forssberg H, Kinoshita H, Eliasson AC, Johansson RS, Westling G, Gordon AM. Development of human precision grip II. Anticipatory control of isometric forces targeted for object's weight. Exp Brain Res 1992; 90:393–398.

Forssberg H, Nashner L. Ontogenetic development of

postural control in man: adaptation to altered support and visual conditions during stance. J Neurosci 1982; 2:545–552.

Forsstrom A, von Hofsten C. Visually directed reaching in children with motor impairments. Dev Med Child Neuro 1982; 24(5):653–61.

Foster E, Sveistrup H, Woollacott MH. Transitions in visual proprioception: a cross-sectional developmental study of the effect of visual flow on postural control. Journal of Motor Behavior 1996; 28:101–112.

Foudriat BA, Di Fabio RP, Anderson JH. Sensory organization of balance responses in children 3–6 years of age: a normative study with diagnostic implications. Int J Pediatr Otorhinolaryngol 1993; 27:255–271.

Frank JS, Patla AE, Brown JE. Characteristics of postural control accompanying voluntary arm movement in the elderly. Society for Neuroscience Abstracts 1987; 13:335.

Frascarelli M, Mastrogregori L, Conforti L. Initial motor unit recruitment in patients with spastic hemiplegia. Electromyogr Clin Neurophysiol 1998; 38:267–271.

Fraser C, Wing A. A case study of reaching by a user of a manually-operated artificial hand. Prosthet Orthot Int 1981; 5:151–156.

Fredericks CM, Saladin LK. Clinical presentations in disorders of motor function. In: Fredericks CM, Saladin LK, eds. Pathophysiology of the Motor Systems. Principles and Clinical Presentations. Philadelphia: FA Davis, 1996.

Fries W, Danek A, Scheidtmann K, Hamburger C. Motor recovery following capsular stroke. Role of descending pathways from multiple motor areas. Brain 1993; 116: 369–382.

Frontera W, Meredith C, O'Reilly KP, et al. Strength conditioning in older men: Skeletal muscle hypertrophy and improved function. J Applied Physiol 1988; 64:1038–1044.

Fugl-Myer AR, Jaasko L, Leyman I, et al. The post-stroke hemiplegic patient: a method for evaluation of physical performance. Scand J Rehabil Med 1975; 7:13–31.

Fujii N, Mushiake H, Tanji J. An oculomotor representation area within the ventral premotor cortex. Proc Natl Acad Sci 1998; 95:12034–12037.

Fukuda T. Studies on human dynamic postures from the viewpoint of postural reflexes. Acta Otolaryngol (Suppl) 1961; 161:1–52.

Fuster JM. The prefrontal cortex: anatomy, physiology and neuropsychology of the frontal lobe, 2nd ed. New York: Raven, 1989.

Gabell A, Nayak USL. The effect of age on variability in gait. J Gerontol 1984; 39:662–666.

Gabell A, Simons MA, Nayak USL. Falls in the healthy elderly: predisposing causes. Ergonomics 1985; 28:965–975.

Gage JR. Gait analysis in cerebral palsy. New York: Mac Keith, 1991.

Gahery Y, Massion J. Coordination between posture and movement. Trends Neurosci 1981; 4:199–202.

Gallahue DL. Understanding motor development: infants, children, adolescents. Indianapolis: Benchmark, 1989.

Gallistel, CR. The organization of action: a new synthesis. Hillsdale, NJ: Lawrence Erlbaum, 1980.

Gard SA, Childress DS. The effect of pelvic list on the vertical displacement of the trunk during normal walking. Gait and Posture 1997; 5:233–238.

Gard SA, Childress DS. The influence of stance-phase knee flexion on the vertical displacement of the trunk during normal walking. Arch Phys Med Rehabil 1999; 80:26–32.

Gardner MF. Test of Visual-Perceptual Skills (n-m) Revised. Psychological and Educational Publications, Inc., 1996.

Garraghty PE, Hanes DP, Florence SL, Kaas JH. Pattern of peripheral deafferentation predicts reorganizational limits in adult primate somatosensory cortex. Somatosens Mot Res 1994; 11: 109–117.

Gauthier GM, Nommay D, Vercher JL. The role of ocular muscle proprioception in visual localization of targets. Science 1990; 249:58–61.

Gauthier GM, Vercher JL, Ivaldi FM, Marchetti E. Oculo-manual tracking of visual targets: control learning, coordination control and coordination model. Exp Brain Res 1988; 73:127–137.

Gehlsen GM, Whaley MH. Falls in the elderly: Part I, gait. Arch Phys Med Rehabil 1990:71:735–738.

Gentile A. Skill acquisition: action movement, and neuromotor processes. In: Carr J, Shepherd R, Gordon J, et al., eds. Movement science: foundations for physical therapy in rehabilitation. Rockville, MD: Aspen Systems, 1987.

Gentile A. The nature of skill acquisition: therapeutic implications for children with movement disorders. In: Forssberg H, Hirschfeld H, eds. Movement disorders in children. Med Sport Sci. Basel: Karger, 1992:31–40.

Georgiou, N, Iansek R, Bradshaw JL, et al. An evaluation of the role of internal cues in the pathogenesis of Parkinsonian hypokinesia. Brain 116: 1575–1587, 1993.

Georgopoulos AP, Kalaska JF, Caminiti R, Massey JT. On the relations between the direction of two-dimensional arm movements and cell discharge in primate motor cortex. J Neurosci 1982; 2:1527–1537.

Gesell A, Halverson HM, Thompson H, Ilg FL, Castner BM, Ames LB, Amatruda CS. The First Five Years of Life. New York: Harper & Row, 1940.

Gesell A. The ontogenesis of infant behavior. In: Carmichael L, ed. Manual of child psychology. New York: Wiley, 1946:335–373.

Gesell A. Behavior patterns of fetal-infant and child. In: Hooker D, Kare C, eds. Genetics and inheritance of neuropsychiatric patterns. Res Publ Assoc Res Nerv Ment Dis 1954; 33:114–126.

Gesell A, Amatruda CS. Developmental diagnosis. 2nd ed. New York: Paul B. Hoeber, 1947.

Ghez C. Contributions of central programs to rapid limb movement in the cat. In: Asanuma H, Wilson VJ, eds. Integration in the nervous system. Tokyo: Igaku-Shoin, 1979: 305–320.

Ghez C. The cerebellum. In: Kandel E, Schwartz JH, Jessell TM, eds. Principles of Neuroscience. 3rd ed. New York: Elsevier, 1991A:627–646.

Ghez C. Posture. In: Kandel ER, Schwartz JH, Jessell TM, eds. Principles of neural science. 3rd ed. New York: Elsevier, 1991B:596–607.

Ghez C. Voluntary movement. In: Kandel E, Schwartz JH, Jessell TM, eds. Principles of Neuroscience. 3rd ed. New York: Elsevier, 1991C:609–625.

Gibson E, Walker AS. Development of knowledge of visual-tactual affordance of substance. Child Dev 1984; 55:453–460.

Gibson JJ. The senses considered as perceptual systems. Boston, MA: Houghton Mifflin, 1966.

Giladi N, Kao R, Fahn S. Freezing phenomenon in patients with Parkinsonian syndromes. Mov Disord 1997; 12:302–305.

Gilbert PFC, Thach WT. Purkinje cell activity during motor learning. Brain Res 1977; 128:309–328.

Gill-Body KM, Popat RA, Parker SW, Krebs DE. Rehabilitation of balance in two patients with cerebellar dysfunction. Phys Ther 1997; 77:534–551.

Gilliam J, Barstow IK. Joint range of motion. In: Van Deusen J, Brunt D, eds. Assessment in Occupational and Physical Therapy. Philadelphia: WB Saunders. 1997:49–77.

Giulliani C, Genova PA, Purser KE, Light KE. Limb trajectory in non-disabled subjects under two conditions of external constraint compared with the nonparetic limb of subjects with hemiparesis. Neuroscience Abstracts 1993; 19:990.

Godges JJ, MacRae PG, Engelke KA. Effects of exercise on hip range of motion, trunk muscle performance and gait economy. Phys Ther 1993; 73:468–477.

Goldstein LB. Pharmacology of recovery after stroke. Stroke 1990; 21(suppl III): 139–142.

Goldstein LB. Basic and clinical studies of pharmacologic effects on recovery from brain injury. J Neural Transplantation Plasticity 1993; 4:175–192.

Goldstein LB. Common drugs may influence motor recovery after stroke. Neurology 1995; 45:865–871.

Goldstein LB, Davis JN. Physician prescribing patterns after ischemic stroke. Neurology 1988; 38: 1806–1809.

Gonshor A, Melvill-Jones G. Short-term adaptive changes in the human vestibulo-ocular reflex arc. J Physiol (Lond) 1976; 256:361–379.

Goodale MA, Milner AD. Separate visual pathways for perception and action. Trends in Neuroscience 1992; 15:20–25.

Goodale MA, Milner AD, Jakobson LS, Carey DP. A neurological dissociation between perceiving objects and grasping them. Nature 1991; 349:154–156.

Goode SL. The contextual interference effect in learning an open motor skill. Unpublished doctoral dissertation, Louisiana State University, Baton Rouge, LA, 1986.

Goodglass H, Kaplan E. The Assessment of Aphasia and Related Disorders. Philadelphia: Lea & Febiger, 1972.

Goodwin GM, McCloskey DI, Matthews PBC. The contribution of muscle afferents to kinaesthesia shown by vibration induced illusions of movement and by the effects of paralysing joint afferents. Brain 1972; 95:705–748.

Gordon AM. Task-dependent deficits during object release in Parkinson's disease. Exp Neuro 1998; 153:287–298.

Gordon AM, Charles J, Duff SV. Fingertip forces during object manipulation in children with hemiplegic cerebral palsy. II: Bilateral coordination. Dev Med Child Neurol 1999; 41:176–185.

Gordon AM, Duff SV. Fingertip forces during object manipulation in children with hemiplegic cerebral palsy I: Anticipatory scaling. Dev Med Child Neurol 1999a;41:166–175.

Gordon AM, Duff SV. (1999). Relationships between clinical measures and fine manipulative control in children with hemiplegic cerebral palsy. Dev Med Child Neurol 1999b;41:586–591.

Gordon AM, Forssberg H, Johansson RS, Westling G. Visual size cues in the programming of manipulative forces during precision grip. Exp Brain Res 1991; 83:477–482.

Gordon AM, Ingvarsson PE, Forssberg H. Anticipatory control of manipulative forces in Parkinson's disease. Exp Neurol 1997; 145:477–488.

Gordon J. Assumptions underlying physical therapy intervention: theoretical and historical perspectives. In: Carr JH, Shepherd, RB, Gordon J, et al., eds. Movement sciences: foundations for physical therapy in rehabilitation. Rockville, MD: Aspen, 1987:1–30.

Gordon J. Motor Control Workshop for Physical Therapists. Umea, Sweden: June 1997.

Gordon J, Ghez C. Muscle receptors and spinal reflexes: the stretch reflex. In: Kandel E, Schwartz JH, Jessell TM, eds. Principles of neuroscience. 3rd ed. New York: Elsevier, 1991:564–580.

Gormley ME, O'Brien CF, Yablon SA. A clinical overview of treatment decisions in the management of spasticity. Muscle Nerve 1997;Suppl6:S14-S20.

Gosh S, Porter R. Morphology of pyramidal neurones in monkey motor cortex and the synaptic actions of their intracortical axon collaterals. J Physiol 1988; 400:593–615.

Gowland C. Staging motor impairment after stroke. Stroke 1990; 21(suppl II):II-19–II-21.

Gracies JM, Elovic E, McGuire J, Simpson D. Traditional pharmacological treatments for spasticity: 1. Local treatments. Muscle Nerve 1997a;Supp 6:S61–83.

Gracies JM, Elovic E, McGuire J, Simpson D. Traditional pharmacological treatments for spasticity: 2. General and regional treatments. Muscle Nerve 1997b;Supp 6:S92–S97.

Granger CV, Albrecht GL, Hamilton BB. Outcome of comprehensive medical rehabilitation: Measurement of PULSES profile and the Barthel index. Arch Phys Med Rehabil 1979; 60:145–154.

Granger CV, Cotter AC, Hamilton BB, Fiedler RC, & Hens MM. Functional assessment skills: A study of persons with multiple sclerosis. Arch Phys Med Rehab 1990; 71:870–875.

Granger CV, Hamilton BB, Sherwin FS. Guide for use of the Uniform Data Set for medical rehabilitation. Buffalo, NY: Buffalo General Hospital, 1986.

Green LN, Williams K. Differences in developmental movement patterns used by active vs sedentary middle-aged adults coming from a supine position to erect stance. Phys Ther 1992; 72:560–568.

Gregson JM, Leathley M, Moor AP, et al. Reliability of the Tone Assessment Scale and the Modified Ashworth Scale as clinical tools for assessing poststroke spasticity. Arch Phys Med Rehabil 1999; 80:1013–1016.

Gresty MA. Coordination of head and eye movements to fixate continuous and intermittent targets. Vision Res 1974; 14:395–403.

Grieve DW. Gait patterns and the speed of walking. Biomed Eng 1968; 3:119–122.

Grillner S. Locomotion in the spinal cat. In: Stein RB, Pearson KG, Smith RS, Redford JB, eds. Control of posture and locomotion. New York: Plenum, 1973:515–535.

Grillner S. Control of locomotion in bipeds, tetrapods, and fish. In: Brooks VB, ed. Handbook of physiology: the nervous system. vol 2. Motor control. Baltimore: Williams & Wilkins, 1981:1179–1236.

Grillner S, Halbertsma J, Nilsson J, Thorstensson A. The adaptation to speed in human locomotion. Brain Res 1979; 165:177–182.

Grillner S, Rossignol S. On the initiation of the swing phase of locomotion in chronic spinal cats. Brain Res 1978; 146:269–277.

Grillner S, Wallen P. Central pattern generators for locomotion, with special reference to vertebrates. Annu Rev Neurosci 1985; 8:233–261.

Grillner S, Zangger P. On the central generation of locomotion in the low spinal cat. Exp Brain Res 1979; 34:241–261.

Gronley JK, Perry J. Gait analysis techniques: Rancho Los Amigos Hospital gait laboratory. Phys Ther 1984; 64:1831–1837.

Grossman GE, Leigh RJ. Instability of gaze during locomotion in patients with deficient vestibular function. Ann Neurol 1990; 27:528–532.

Guccione AA. Physical therapy diagnosis and the relationship between impairments and function. Phys Ther 1991; 71:499–504.

Guide for the Functional Independence Measure for Children (WeeFIM) of the Uniform Data System for Medical Rehabilitation. Version 4.0, Buffalo, NY: State University of New York at Buffalo, 1993.

Guiliani C. The relationship of spasticity to movement and considerations for therapeutic interventions. Neurol Report 1997; 21:78–84.

Guralnik JM, Ferrucci L, Simonsick EM, et al. Lower extremity function in persons over the age of 70 years as a predictor of subsequent disability. N Engl J Med 1995; 332:556–561.

Guralnik JM, LaCroix AZ, Abbott RD, et al. Maintaining mobility in late life: demographic characteristics and chronic conditions. Am J Epidemiol 1993; 127:845–857.

Guralnik JM, LaCroix AZ, Everett DF, Kovar MG. Aging in the eighties: the prevalence of comorbidity and its association with disability. Advance Data (Vital and Health Statistics of the National Center for Health Statistics) 1989; 170:1–8.

Guralnik JM, Simonsick EM, Ferrucci L, et al. A short physical performance battery assessing lower extremity function: association with self-reported disability and prediction of mortality and nursing home admission. J Gerontol Med Sci 1994; 49:M85–M94.

Gurfinkel VS, Levik YS. Sensory complexes and sensorimotor integration. Fiziolog Cheloveka 1978; 5:399–414.

Gurfinkel VS, Levick YS. Perceptual and automatic aspects of the postural body scheme. In: Paillard J, ed. Brain and space. New York: Oxford Science, 1991.

Gurfinkel VS, Lipshits MI, Popov KE. Is the stretch reflex the main mechanism in the system of regulation of the vertical posture of man? Biophysics 1974; 19:761–766.

Hadders-Algra, M, Brogren E, Forssberg H. Ontogeny of postural adjustments during sitting in infancy: variation, selection and modulation. J Physiol 1996a;493:273–288.

Hadders-Algra, M, Brogren E, Forssberg H. Training affects the development of postural adjustments in sitting infants. J Physiology 1996b;493:289–298.

Haffenden AM, Goodale MA. The effect of pictorial illusion on prehension and perception. J Cogn Neurosci 1998; 10:122–136.

Haley S. Sequential analyses of postural reactions in nonhandicapped infants. Phys Ther 1986; 66: 531–536.

Haley SM, Coster WJ, Binda-Sundberg K. Measuring physical disablement: the contextual challenge. Phys Ther 1994; 74:443–451.

Haley SM, Coster WJ, Ludlow LH, Haltiwanger JT, Andrellos PJ. Pediatric Evaluation of Disability Inventory (PEDI). Boston: New England Medical Center Hospitals, 1992.

Hallett M. Classification and treatment of tremor. JAMA 1991; 266:1115–1117.

Hallett M. Overview of human tremor physiology. Mov Disord 1998; 13:43–48.

Hallett M, Shahani BT, Young RR. EMG analysis of stereotyped voluntary movements in man. J Neurol Neurosurg Psychiatry 1975; 38:1154–1162.

Hamman R, Longridge NS, Mekjavic I, Dickinson J. Effect of age and training schedules on balance improvement exercises using visual feedback. J Otolaryngol 1995; 24: 221–229.

Hanlon RE. Motor learning following unilateral stroke. Arch Phys Med Rehabil 1996; 77:811–815.

Hansen PD, Woollacott MH, Debu B. Postural responses to changing task conditions. Exp Brain Res 1988; 73:627–636.

Harbourne RT, Giuliani C, MacNeela, J. A kinematic and electromyographic analysis of the development of sitting posture in infants. Dev Psychobiol 1993; 26:51–64.

Harburn K, Hill K, Kramer J, et al. An overhead harness and trolley system for balance and ambulation assessment and training. Arch Phys Med Rehabil 1993; 74:220–223.

Hass G, Diener HC. Development of stance control in children. In: Amblard B, Berthoz A, Clarac F, eds. Development, adaptation and modulation of posture and gait. Amsterdam: Elsevier, 1988:49–58.

Hass G, Diener HC, Bacher M, Dichgans J. Development of postural control in children: short-, medium-, and long-latency EMG responses of leg muscles after perturbation of stance. Exp Brain Res 1986; 64:127–132.

Hay L. Accuracy of children on an open-loop pointing task. Percept Mot Skills 1978; 47:1079–1082.

Hay L. Spatial-temporal analysis of movements in children: motor programs versus feedback in the development of reaching. J Motor Behav 1979; 11: 189–200.

Hay L. Developmental changes in eye-hand coordination behaviors: Preprogramming versus feedback control. In: Bard C, Fleury M, Hay L, eds. Development of eye-hand coordination across the lifespan. Columbia: University of South Carolina, 1990: 217–244.

Hay L, Bard C, Fleury M. Visuo-manual coordination from 6 to 10: specification, control and evaluation of direction and amplitude parameters of movement. In: Wade MG, Whiting HTA, eds. Motor development in children: aspects of coordination and control. Dordrecht: Martinus Nijhoff, 1986.

Hayes KC. Biomechanics of postural control. Exerc Sports Sci Rev 1982; 10:363–391.

Hayes KC, Riach CL. Preparatory postural adjustments and postural sway in young children. In: Woollacott MH, Shumway-Cook A, eds. Development of posture and gait across the life span. Columbia: University of South Carolina, 1989:97–127.

Hein A, Held R. Dissociation of the visual placing response into elicited and guided components. Science 1967; 158:390–392.

Heitmann DK, Gossman MR, Shaddeau SA, Jackson JR.

Balance performance and step width in non-institutionalized elderly female fallers and nonfallers. Phys Ther 1989; 69:923–931.

Held JM. Recovery of function after brain damage: theoretical implications for therapeutic intervention. In: Carr JH, Shepherd, RB, Gordon J, et al., eds. Movement sciences: foundations for physical therapy in rehabilitation. Rockville, MD: Aspen, 1987:155–177.

Held JM. Environmental enrichment enhances sparing and recovery of function following brain damage. Neurol Report 1998; 22:74–78.

Held JM, Gordon F, Gentile AM. Environmental influences on locomotor recovery following cortical lesions in rats. Behav Neurosci 1985; 99:678–690.

Held R, Hein A. Movement-produced stimulation in the development of visually guided behavior. J Compar Physiol Psychol 1963; 56:872–876.

Hellebrandt FA, Schode M, Carns ML. Methods of evoking the tonic neck reflexes in normal human subjects. Am J Phys Med 1962; 41:90–139.

Heniemann AW, Linacre JM, Wright BD, Hamilton BB, Granger CV. Relationships between impairment and physical disability as measured by the functional independence measure. Arch Phys Med Rehab 1993; 74:566–573.

Herdman S. Vestibular Rehabilitation. Philadelphia: FA Davis, 1999.

Herman R. Augmented sensory feedback in control of limb movement. In: Fields WS, ed. Neural organization and its relevance to prosthetics. New York: Intercontinental Medical Book, 1973.

Herman R, Cook T, Cozzens B, Freedman W. In: Stein RB, Pearson KG, Smith RS, Redford JB, eds. Control of posture and locomotion. New York: Plenum, 1973:363–388.

Herman R, Wirta R, Bampton S, Finley FR. Human solutions for locomotion: 1. Single limb analysis. In: Herman R, Grillner S, Stein P, Stuart D, eds. Neural control of locomotion. New York: Plenum, 1976:13–49.

Hesse S, Bertelt C, Jahnke MT, et al. Treadmill training with partial body weight support compared with physiotherapy in non ambulatory hemiparetic patients. Stroke 1995; 26:976–981.

Hesse S, Bertelt C, Schaffrin A, et al. Restoration of gait in non ambulatory hemiparetic patients by treadmill training with partial weight support. Arch Phys Med Rehabil 1994; 75:1087–1093.

Hesse S, Konrad M, Uhlenbroch D. Treadmill walking with partial body weight support versus floor walking in hemiparetic subjects. Arch Phys Med Rehabil 1999; 80:421–427.

Hesse S, Reiter F, Jahnke M, et al. Asymmetry of gait initiation in hemiparetic stroke subjects. Arch Phys Med Rehabil 1997; 78:719–724.

Higgins JR, Spaeth RA. Relationship between consistency of movement and environmental conditions. Quest 1979; 17:61–69.

Hirschfeld H. On the integration of posture, locomotion and voluntary movement in humans: normal and impaired development. Dissertation. Stockholm: Karolinska Institute, 1992.

Hirschfeld H, Forssberg, H. Epigenetic development of postural responses for sitting during infancy. Exp Brain Res 1994; 97:528–540.

Hirt S. The tonic neck reflex mechanism in the normal human adult. Am J Phys Med 1967; 46:56–65.

Hoehn MM, Yahr MD. Parkinsonism: onset, progression and mortality. Neurology 1967; 17:433–450.

Hoffer MM, Feiwell E, Perry R, et al. Functional ambulation in patients with myelomeningocele. J Bone Joint Surg 1973; 55A:137–148.

von Hofsten C. Eye-hand coordination in the newborn. Dev Psychol 1982; 18:450–461.

von Hofsten C. Developmental changes in the organization of pre-reaching movements. Dev Psychol 1984; 3;378–388.

von Hofsten C. Studying the development of goal-directed behavior. In: Kalverboer AF, Hopkins B, Geuze R, eds. Motor development in early and later childhood: longitudinal approaches. Cambridge, UK: Cambridge University, 1993:109–124.

von Hofsten C, Fazel-Zandy S. Development of visually guided hand orientation in reaching. J Exp Child Psychol 1984; 38:208–219.

von Hofsten C, Lindhagen K. Observations on the development of reaching for moving objects. J Exp Child Psychol 1979; 28:158–173.

von Hofsten C, Ronnqvist L. Preparation for grasping an object: a developmental study. J Exp Psychol 1988; 14:610–621.

von Hofsten C, Rosander K. The development of gaze control and predictive tracking in young infants. Vision Res 1996; 36:81–96.

von Hofsten C, Rosander K. Development of smooth pursuit tracking in young infants. Vision Res 1997; 37:1799–1810.

von Hofsten C, Woollacott M. Anticipatory postural adjustments during infant reaching. Neurosci Abstr 1989; 15:1199.

Hogan N, Bizzi E, Mussa-Ivaldi FA, Flash T. Controlling multijoint motor behavior. In: KB Pandolf, ed. Exerc Sport Sci Rev 1987; 15:153–190.

Holden MK, Gill KM, Magliozzi MR, et al. Clinical gait assessment in the neurologically impaired: reliability and meaningfulness. Phys Ther 1984; 64:35–40.

Hollerbach JM. Planning of arm movements. In: Osherson DN, Kosslyn SM, Hollerbach JM, eds. Visual cognition and action: an invitation to cognitive science, vol 2. Cambridge, MA: MIT, 1990:183–211.

Horak F. Clinical measurement of postural control in adults. Phys Ther 1987; 67:1881–1885.

Horak F. Assumptions underlying motor control for neurologic rehabilitation. In: Contemporary management of motor control problems. Proceedings of the II Step Conference. Alexandria, VA: APTA, 1991:11–27.

Horak FB. Comparison of cerebellar and vestibular loss on scaling of postural responses. In: Brandt T, Paulus IO, Bles W, et al., eds. Disorders of posture and gait. Stuttgart: George Thieme Verlag, 1990:370–373.

Horak FB. Effects of neurological disorders on postural movement strategies in the elderly. In: Vellas B, Toupet M, Rubenstein L, et al., eds. Falls, balance and gait disorders in the elderly. Paris: Elsevier, 1992:137–152.

Horak FB, Anderson M, Esselman P, Lynch K. The effects of movement velocity, mass displaced and task certainty on associated postural adjustments made by normal and hemiplegic individuals. J Neurol Neurosurg Psychiatry 1984; 47:1020–1028.

Horak F, Diener HC. Cerebellar control of postural scaling and central set in stance. J Neurophysiol 1994; 72:479–493.

Horak F, Diener H, Nashner L. Postural strategies associated with somatosensory and vestibular loss. Exp Brain Res 1990; 82:167–177.

Horak F, Diener HC, Nashner LM. Influence of central set on human postural responses. J Neurophysiol 1989a;62:841–853.

Horak F, Jones-Rycewicz C, Black FO, Shumway-Cook A. Effects of vestibular rehabilitation on dizziness and imbalance. Otolaryngol Head Neck Surg 1992; 106:175–180.

Horak FB, Macpherson JM. Postural orientation and equilibrium. In: Shepard J & Rowell L, eds. Handbook of physiology, section 12. Exercise: regulation and integration of multiple systems. New York, Oxford University, 1996:255–292.

Horak FB, Mirka A, Shupert CL. The role of peripheral vestibular disorders in postural dyscontrol in the elderly. In: Woollacott MH, Shumway-Cook A, eds. The development of posture and gait across the lifespan. Columbia: University of South Carolina, 1989b:253–279.

Horak F, Moore S. Lateral postural responses: the effect of stance width and perturbation amplitude. Phys Ther 1989; 69:363.

Horak F, Nashner L. Central programming of postural movements: adaptation to altered support surface configurations. J Neurophysiol 1986; 55:1369–1381.

Horak FB, Nashner LM, Nutt JG. Postural instability in Parkinson's disease: motor coordination and sensory organization. Neurol Report 1988a;12:54–55.

Horak FB, Nashner LM, Diener HC. Postural strategies associated with somatosensory and vestibular loss. Exp Brain Res 1990; 82:167–177.

Horak F, Shumway-Cook A. Clinical implications of postural control research. In: Duncan P, ed. Balance: proceedings of the APTA Forum. Alexandria, VA: APTA, 1990:105–111.

Horak FB, Shumway-Cook A, Crowe T, Black FO. Vestibular function and motor proficiency in children with hearing impairments and in learning disabled children with motor impairments. Dev Med Child Neurol 1988b;30:64–79.

Horak F, Shupert C. The role of the vestibular system in postural control. In: Herdman S, ed. Vestibular rehabilitation. New York: FA Davis, 1994:22–46.

Horak F, Shupert C, Mirka A. Components of postural dyscontrol in the elderly: a review. Neurobiol Aging 1989c;10:727–745.

Horowitz L, Sharby N. Development of prone extension postures in healthy infants. Phys Ther 1988; 68:32–39.

Hovda DA, Feeney DM. Haloperidol blocks amphetamine induced recovery of binocular depth perception after bilateral visual cortex ablation in the cat. Proc West Pharmacol Soc 1985; 28:209–211.

Hoy MG, Zernicke RF. Modulation of limb dynamics in the swing phase of locomotion. J Biomech 1985; 18:49–60.

Hoy MG, Zernicke RF. The role of intersegmental dynamics during rapid limb oscillations. J Biomech 1986; 19:867–877.

Hoy MG, Zernicke RF, Smith JL. Contrasting roles of inertial and muscle moments at knee and ankle during paw-shake response. J Neurophysiol 1985; 54: 1282–1294.

Hoyle G. Muscles and their neural control. New York: Wiley, 1983.

Hoyt DF, Taylor CR. Gait and energetics of locomotion in horses. Nature 1981; 292:239–240.

Hreljac A. Preferred and energetically optimal gait transition speeds in human locomotion. Med Sci Sports Exerc 1993a;25:1158–1162.

Hreljac A. Determinants of the gait transition speed during human locomotion: kinetic factors. Gait Posture 1993b;1:217–223.

Hreljac A. Determinants of the gait transition speed during human locomotion: kinematic factors. J Biomechanics 1995a;28:669–677.

Hreljac A. Effects of physical characteristics on the gait transition speed during human locomotion. Hum Mov Sci 1995b; 14:205–216.

Hu M, Woollacott M. Multisensory training of standing balance in older adults: 1. Postural stability and one-leg stance balance. J Gerontol 1994a;49:M52-M61.

Hu M, Woollacott M. Multisensory training of standing balance in older adults: 2. Kinetic and electromyographic postural responses. J Gerontol 1994b;49: M62-M71.

Hubel DH. Eye, brain and vision. New York: Scientific American, 1988.

Hubel DH, Wiesel TN. Receptive fields of single neurones in the cat's striate cortex. J. Physiol Lond 1959; 148:574–591.

Hubel DH, Wiesel TN. Receptive fields, binocular interaction and functional architecture in the cat's visual cortex. J Physiol Lond 1962; 160:106–154.

Hugon M, Massion J, Wiesendanger M. Anticipatory postural changes induced by active unloading and comparison with passive unloading in man. Pflugers Arch 1982; 393:292–296.

Hulliger M, Nordh E, Thelin AE, Vallbo AB. The responses of afferent fibers from the glabrous skin of the hand during voluntary finger movements in man. J Physiol 1979; 291:233–249.

Humphrey NK, Weiskrantz L. Vision in monkeys after removal of the striate cortex. Nature 1969; 215:595–597.

Imms FJ, Edholm OG. Studies of gait and mobility in the elderly. Age Ageing 1981; 10:147–156.

Inglin B, Woollacott MH. Age-related changes in anticipatory postural adjustments associated with arm movements. J Gerontol 1988; 43:M105–M113.

Inglis JT, Horak FB, Shupert CL, Rycewicz C. The importance of somatosensory information in triggering and scaling automatic postural responses in humans. Exp Brain Res 1994; 101:159–164.

Ingvarsson PE, Gordon AM, Forssberg H. Coordination of manipulative forces in Parkinson's disease. Exp Neuro; 1997; 145:489–501.

Inman VT, Ralston H, Todd F. Human walking. Baltimore: Williams & Wilkins, 1981.

International Classification of Impairments, Disabilities and Handicaps. Geneva: World Health Organization; 1980.

Ito M. The cerebellum and neural control. New York: Raven, 1984.

Ivry R. Representational issues in motor learning: phenomena and theory. In: Keele S, Heuer H, eds. Handbook of perception and action: motor skills. New York: Academic, 1997.

Ivry RB, Keele, SW. Timing functions of the cerebellum. J Cogn Neurosci 1989; 1:136–152.

Jackson RT, Epstein CM, De L'Amme WR. Abnormalities in posturography and estimations of visual vertical and horizontal in multiple sclerosis. Am J Otol 1995; 16:88–93.

Jacobs R, Macpherson J. Two functional muscle groupings during postural equilibrium tasks in standing cats. J Neurophysiol 1996; 76:2402–2411.

Jaffee R, Farne-Mokris S. Volumeter. In: Casannova J, ed. Clinical Assessment Recommendations. Chicago: American Society of Hand Therapists, 1992:13–19.

Jeannerod M. The timing of natural prehension movements. J Motor Behav 1984; 16(3):235–254.

Jeannerod M. Reaching and grasping: parallel specification of visuomotor channels. In: Handbook of perception and action, vol 2. London: Academic Press 1996:405–460.

Jeannerod M. The timing of natural prehension movements. J Motor Behav 1984; 16:235–254.

Jeannerod M. The formation of finger grip during prehension. A cortically mediated visuomotor pattern. Behav Brain Res 1986; 19:99–116.

Jeannerod M. The neural and behavioral organization of goal-directed movements. Oxford: Clarendon, 1990.

Jeannerod M. Arbib MA, Rizzolatti G, Sakata H. Grasping objects: the cortical mechanisms of visuomotor transformation. Trends Neurosci 1995;18:314–320.

Jeannerod M. The Neural and Behavioral Organization of Goal-Directed Movements. Clarendon Press: Oxford, 1990.

Jebsen RH, Taylor N, Trieschmann RB, Trotter MJ, Howard L. An objective and standard test of hand function. Arch Phys Med 1969; 50:311–319.

Jedlinsky BP, McCarthy CF, Michel TH. Validating pediatric pain measurement: Sensory and affective components. Ped Phys Ther 1999; 11:83–88.

Jeka JJ. Light touch contact as a balance aid. Phys Ther 1997; 77:477–487.

Jeka JJ, Lackner JR. Fingertip contact influences human postural control. Exp Brain Res 1994; 100:495–502.

Jeka JJ, Lackner JR. The role of haptic cues from rough and slippery surfaces in human postural control. Exp Brain Res 1995; 103:267–276.

Jenkins WM, Merzenich MM. Reorganization of neocortical representations after brain injury: a neurophysiological model of the bases of recovery from stroke. In: Weil FJ, Herbert E, Carlson BM, eds. Progr Brain Res 1987; 71:249–266.

Jenkins, WM, Merzenich MM, Och MT, et al. Functional reorganization of primary somatosensory cortex in adult owl monkeys after behaviorally controlled tactile stimulation. J Neurophysiol 1990; 63:82–104.

Jensen JL, Bothner KE, Woollacott MH. Balance control: the scaling of the kinetic response to accommodate increasing perturbation magnitudes. J Sport Exerc Psychol 1996; 18:S45.

Jette AM. Diagnosis and classification by physical therapists: a special communication. Phys Ther 1989; 69:967–969.

Jette AM. Physical disablement concepts for physical therapy research and practice. Phys Ther 1994; 74:380–386.

Jims C. Foot placement pattern, an aid in gait training: suggestions from the field. Phys Ther 1977; 57:286.

Johansson RS. Sensory control of dexterous manipulation in humans. In: Wing AM, Haggard P, Flanagan J, eds. Hand and Brain: The Neurophysiology and Psychology of Hand Movements. New York: Academic Press, 1996:381–414.

Johansson RS, Edin BB. Neural control of manipulation and grasp. In: Forssberg H, Hirschfeld H, eds. Movement disorders in children. Basel: Karger, 1992:107–112.

Johnson RH. Disorders of stretch reflex modulation during volitional movements. Brain 1991; 114:443–460.

Jordan T, Rabbitt P. Response times to stimuli of increasing complexity as a function of ageing. Br J Psychol 1977; 68:189–201.

Jouen F. Visual-vestibular interactions in infancy. Infant Behav Dev 1984; 7:135–145.

Jouen F. Early visual-vestibular interactions and postural development. In: Bloch H, Bertenthal BI, eds. Sensory-motor organizations and development in infancy and early childhood. Dordrecht: Kluwer, 1990:199–215.

Jouen F. Titres et travaux en vue de l'habilitation a diriger des recherches. State doctoral thesis. Paris: Universite Paris IV1993:104.

Judge JO, Underwood M, Gennosa T. Exercise to improve gait velocity. Arch Phys Med Rehabil 1993; 74:400–406.

Judge J, Whipple R, Wolfson L. Effects of resistive and balance exercises on isokinetic strength in older persons. J Am Geriatr Soc 1994; 42:937–946.

Kaas JH. Development of cortical sensory maps. In: Rakic P, Singer W, eds. Neurobiology of neocortex. New York: Wiley 1988; 115–136.

Kaas JH, Florence SL, Jain N. Reorganization of sensory systems of primates after injury. Neuroscientist 1997:3:123–130.

Kaminski T, Bock C, Gentile AM. The coordination between trunk and arm motion during pointing movements. Exp Brain Res 1995; 106(3):457–466.

Kamm K, Thelen E, Jensen J. A dynamical systems approach to motor development: In: Rothstein JM, ed. Movement science. Alexandria, VA: APTA, 1991: 11–23.

Kandel ER. Cellular basis of behavior: an introduction to behavioral neurobiology. San Francisco: Freeman, 1976.

Kandel E. Brain and Behavior. In: Kandel E, Schwartz JH, Jessell TM, eds. Principles of neuroscience. 3rd ed. New York: Elsevier, 1991a:5–17.

Kandel ER. Cellular mechanisms of learning and the biological basis of individuality. In: Kandel ER, Schwartz JH, Jessell TM, eds. Principles of neuroscience. 3rd ed. New York: Elsevier, 1991b: 1009–1031.

Kandel ER. Genes, nerve cells, and the remembrance of things past. J Neuropsychiatry 1989; 1:103–125.

Kandel ER. Perception of motion, depth and form. In: Kandel E, Schwartz JH, Jessell TM, eds. Principles of Neuroscience. 3rd ed. New York: Elsevier, 1991c:440–466.

Kandel E, Jessell TM. Touch. In: Kandel E, Schwartz JH, Jessell TM, eds. Principles of Neuroscience. 3rd ed. New York: Elsevier, 1991:367–384.

Kandel ER, Schwarz JH. Molecular biology of learning: modulation of transmitter release. Science 1982; 218:433–443.

Kane RA, Kane RL. Assessing the elderly: A practical guide to measurement. Lexington, MA: Lexington, 1981.

Kapteyn TS. Afterthought about the physics and mechanics of postural sway. Agressologie 1973; 14: 27–35.

Katoka S, Croll GA, Bles W. Somatosensory ataxia. In: Bles W, Brandt T, eds. Disorders of posture and gait. Amsterdam: Elsevier 1986:177–183.

Katz S, Downs TD, Cash JR, Grotz RC. Progress in development of the index of ADL. Gerontologist 1970:20–30.

Katz R, Rymer Z. Spastic hypertonia: mechanisms and measurement. Arch Phys Med Rehabil 1989; 70:144–155.

Kay D. An analysis of the home environment encountered by stroke patients (unpublished thesis). School of Physiotherapy, La Trobe University, Melbourne, Australia.

Keele S. Movement control in skilled motor performance. Psychol Bull 1968; 70:387–403.

Keele SW. Behavioral analysis of movement. In: Brooks VB, ed. Handbook of physiology. I: The nervous system, vol 2. Motor control, part 2. Baltimore: Williams & Wilkins, 1981:1391–1414.

Keele SW. Motor control. In: Kaufman L, Thomas J, Boff K, eds. Handbook of perception and performance. New York: Wiley, 1986:30.1–30.60.

Keele S, Ivry R. Does the cerebellum provide a common computation for diverse tasks? A timing hypothesis. In: Diamond A, ed. Developmental and neural bases of higher cognitive function. New York: New York Academy of Sciences, 1990:179–207.

Keele SW, Posner MI. Processing visual feedback in rapid movement. J Exp Psychol 1968; 77:155–158.

Keith RA, Granger CV, Hamilton BB, Sherwin FS. The functional independence measure: a new tool for rehabilitation. In: Eisentberg MG, Grzesiak RC, eds. Advances in clinical rehabilitation, vol 1. New York: Springer Verlag, 1987:6–18.

Kelly JP. The sense of balance. In: Kandel E, Schwartz JH, Jessell TM, eds. Principles of neuroscience. 3rd ed. New York: Elsevier, 1991:500–511.

Kelso JAS, Holt KJ. Exploring a vibratory systems analysis of human movement production. J Neurophysiol 1980; 43:1183–1196.

Kelso JAS, Southard DL, Goodman D. On the coordination of two-handed movements. J Exp Psychol Hum Percept 1979; 5:229–238.

Kelso JAS, Tuller B. A dynamical basis for action systems. In: Gazzaniga MS, ed. Handbook of cognitive neuroscience. New York: Plenum, 1984:321–356.

Kendall FP, McCreary EK. Muscles: testing and function. 3rd ed. Baltimore: Williams & Wilkins, 1983.

Kennard MA. Relation of age to motor impairment in man and in sub-human primates. Arch Neurol Psychiatry 1940; 44:377–398.

Kennard MA. Cortical reorganization of motor function: studies on a series of monkeys of various ages from infancy to maturity. Arch Neurol Psychiatr 1942; 48:27–240.

Kenshalo DR. Aging effects on cutaneous and kinesthetic sensibilities. In: Han SS and Coons DH, eds. Special senses in aging. Ann Arbor: University of Michigan, 1979.

Kerns K, Mateer CA, Walking and chewing gum: the impact of attentional capacity on everyday activities. In: Sbordone RJ, Long CJ, eds. Ecological validity of neuropsychological testing. Delray Beach, FL: GR, 1996.

Kerr R. Movement control and maturation in elementary-grade children. Percept Mot Skills 1975; 41:151–154.

Kerr R, Booth B. Skill acquisition in elementary school children and schema theory. In: Landers DM, Christina RW, eds. Psychology of motor behavior and sport, vol. 2. Champaign, IL: Human Kinetics, 1977.

Kerrigan DC, Schaufele M, Wen MN. Gait analysis. In: DeLisa JA, Gans BM. Rehabilitation medicine: principles and practice. ed 3. Philadelphia: Lippincott-Raven, 1998.

Keshner E, Allum J. Plasticity in pitch sway stabilization: normal habituation and compensation for peripheral vestibular deficits. In: Bles W, Brandt T, eds. Disorders of posture and gait. New York: Elsevier, 1986:289–314.

Kessler RM, Hertling D. Management of common musculoskeletal disorders. Philadelphia: Harper & Row, 1983.

Ketelaar M, Vermeet A, Helders P. Functional motor abilities of children with CP: a systematic literature review of assessment measures. Clin Rehabil 1998; 12:369–380.

Kipper S, Tuchman MM. Treatment of chronic post traumatic organic brain syndrome with dextroamphetamine: first reported case. J Nerv Ment Dis 1976; 162:366–371.

Klatzky RL, McCloskey B, Doherty S, et al. Knowledge about hand shaping and knowledge about objects. J Motor Behav 1987; 19:187–213.

Kluzik J, Fetters L, Coryell J. Quantification of control: a preliminary study of effects of neurodevelopmental treatment on reaching in children with spastic cerebral palsy. Phys Ther 1990; 2:65–78.

Knapp HD, Taub E, Berman J. Movements of monkeys with deafferented forelimbs. Exp Neurol 1963; 7:305–315.

Knutsson E. An analysis of parkinsonian gait. Brain 1972; 95:475–486.

Knutsson E. Gait control in hemiparesis. Scand J Rehabil Med 1981; 13:101–108.

Knutsson E. Can gait analysis improve gait training in stroke patients? Scand J Rehabil Med Suppl 1994; 30:73–80.

Knutsson E, Richards C. Different types of disturbed motor control in gait of hemiparetic patients. Brain 1979; 102:405–430.

Koester J. Passive membrane properties of the neuron. In: Kandel E, Schwartz JH, Jessell TM, eds. Principles of neuroscience. 3rd ed. New York: Elsevier, 1991:95–103.

Konczak J, Borutta M, Dichgans J. The development of goal-directed reaching in infants: 2. Learning to produce task-adequate patterns of joint torque. Exp Brain Res 1997; 113:465–474.

Konczak J, Borutta M, Topka H, Dichgans J. The development of goal-directed reaching in infants: hand trajectory formation and joint torque control. Exp Brain Res 1995; 106:156–168.

Konczak J, Dichgans J. The development toward stereotypic arm kinematics during reaching in the first 3 years of life. Exp Brain Res 1997; 117:346–354.

Kosnik W, Winslow L, Kline D, et al. Visual changes in daily life throughout adulthood. J Gerontol Psych Sci 1988; 43:63–70.

Kots YM, Syrovegin AV. Fixed set of variants of interactions of the muscles to two joints in the execution of simple voluntary movements. Biophysics 1966; 11:1212–1219.

Kraft GH, Fitts S, Hammond MC. Techniques to improve function of the arm and hand in chronic hemiplegia. Arch Phys Med Rehabil 1992; 73:220–227.

Kram R, Domingo, A, Ferris D. Effect of reduced gravity on the preferred walk-run transition speed. J Exper Biology 1997; 200:821–826.

Krebs DE, Edelstein JE, Fishman S. Reliability of observational kinematic gait analysis. Phys Ther 1985; 65:1027–1033.

Krebs DE, Jette AM, Assmann SF. Moderate exercise improves gait stability in disabled elders. Arch Phys Med Rehabil 1998; 79:1489–1495.

Kugler PN, Kelso JAS, Turvey MT. On the concept of coordinative structures as dissipative structures: 1. Theoretical line. In: Stelmach GE, Requin J, eds. Tutorials in motor behavior. Amsterdam: North-Holland, 1980:3–37.

Kugler PN, Kelso JAS, Turvey MT. On the control and coordination of naturally developing systems. In: Kelso JAS, Clark JE, eds. The development of movement control and coordination. New York: Wiley, 1982:5–78.

Kugler PN, Turvey MT. Information, natural law and self assembly of rhythmic movement. Hillsdale, NJ: Erlbaum, 1987.

Kunesch E, Schnitzler A, Tyercha C, Knecht S, Stelmach G. Altered force release control in Parkinson's disease. Behav Brain Res 1995; 67:43–49.

Kunkel A, DiplPsych, Kopp B, Müller G, Diplypsych, Villringer K, Villringer A, Taub E, Flor H. Constraint-induced movement therapy for motor recovery in chronic stroke patients. Arch Phys Med Rehabil 1999; 80:624–628.

Kupfermann I. Localization of higher cognitive and affective functions: the association cortices. In: Kandel E, Schwartz JH, Jessell TM, eds. Principles of neuroscience. 3rd ed. New York: Elsevier, 1991a:823–838.

Kupfermann I. Learning and memory. In: Kandel ER, Schwartz JH, Jessell TM, eds. Principles of neuroscience. 3rd ed. New York: Elsevier, 1991b: 997–1008.

Kuypers HGJM. Corticospinal connections: postnatal development in rhesus monkey. Science 1962; 138:678–680.

Kuypers HGJM. The descending pathways to the spinal cord, their anatomy and function. In: Eccles JC, ed. Organization of the spinal cord. Amsterdam: Elsevier, 1964.

Lackner JR, DiZio P. Visual stimulation affects the perception of voluntary leg movements during walking. Perception 1988; 17:71–80.

Lackner JR, DiZio P. Sensory-motor calibration processes constraining the perception of force and motion during locomotion. In: Woollacott MH, Horak FB, eds. Posture and gait: control mechanisms. Eugene, OR: University of Oregon, 1992:92–96.

Lafortune MA, Hennig EM, Lake MJ. Dominant role of interface over knee angle for cushioning impact loading and regulating initial leg stiffness. J Biomech 1996; 29:1523–1529.

LaJoie Y, Teasdale N, Bard C, Fleury M. Attentional demands for static and dynamic equilibrium. Exp Brain Res 1993; 97:139–144.

Lance JW. Symposium synopsis. In: Feldman RG, Young RR, Koella WP, eds. Spasticity: Disordered Motor Control. Chicago: Year Book, 1980.

Lang W, Obrig H, Lindinger G, et al. Supplementary motor area activation while tapping bimanually different rhythms in musicians. Exp Brain Res 1990; 79:504–514.

Larson MA, Lee SL, Vasque DE. Comparison of ATNR presence and developmental activities in 2–4 month old infants. Alexandria, VA: APTA conference proceedings, June, 1990.

Larsson LE. Neural control of gait in man. In: Eccles J, Dimitrijevic MR, eds. Recent achievements in restorative neurology. Basel: Karger, 1985:185–198.

Lasarus JC. Associated movement in hemiplegia: The effects of force exerted, limb usage and inhibitory training. Arch Phys Med Rehabil 1992; 73:1044 –52.

Lashley KS. In search of the engram. Symp Soc Exp Biol 1950; 4:454–482.

Lashley KS. Brain mechanism and intelligence. Chicago: University of Chicago, 1929.

Lavery JJ. Retention of simple motor skills as a function of type of knowledge of results. Can J Psych 1962; 16:300–311.

Law M. Self-care. In: Van Deusen J, Brunt D, eds. Assessment in Occupational Therapy and Physical Therapy. Philadelphia: WB Saunders, 1997:421–433.

Law M, Cadman D, Rosenbaum P, Walter S, Russell D, DeMatteo C. NDT therapy and upper extremity inhibitive casting for children with CP. Dev Med Child Neurol 1991; 33:379–387.

Lawrence DG, Hopkins DA. Developmental aspects of pyramidal motor control in the rhesus monkey. Brain Res 1972; 40:117–118.

Lawrence DG, Hopkins DA. The development of motor control in the rhesus monkey: evidence concerning the role of corticomotoneuronal connections. Brain 1976; 99:235–254.

Lawton MP. The functional assessment of elderly people. J Am Geriatr Soc 1971; 19:465–481.

Ledebt A, Bril B, Breniere Y. The build-up of anticipatory behavior: an analysis of the development of gait initiation in children. Exp Brain Res 1998; 120:9–17.

Ledebt A, Bril B, Wiener-Vacher S. Trunk and head stabilization during the first months of independent walking. Neuroreport 1995; 6:1737–1740.

Lee DN. The functions of vision. In: Pick H, Saltzman E, eds. Modes of perceiving and processing information. Hillsdale, NJ: Erlbaum, 1978.

Lee DN, Aronson E. Visual proprioceptive control of standing in human infants. Percept Psychophysics 1974; 15:529–532.

Lee TD. Transfer-appropriate processing: a framework for conceptualizing practice effects in motor learning. In: Meijer OG, Roth K, eds. Complex movement behavior: the motor-action controversy. Amsterdam: North Holland, 1988.

Lee DN, Lishman R. Visual proprioceptive control of stance. J Hum Mov Studies 1975; 1:87–95.

Lee I, Manson J, Hennekens C, Paffenbarger R. Body weight and mortality: a 27 year follow up of middle aged men. JAMA 1993; 270:2623–2628.

Lee RG, van Donkelaar P. Mechanisms underlying functional recovery following stroke. Can J Neurol Sci 1995; 22:257–263.

Lee DN, Young DS. Gearing action to the environment. Exp Brain Res Series 15. Berlin: Springer-Verlag, 1986:217–230.

Lee W, Buchanan T, Rogers M. Effects of arm acceleration and behavioral conditions on the organization of postural adjustments during arm flexion. Exp Brain Res 1987; 66: 257–270.

Lekhel H, Assaiante C, Cremieux J, Amblard B. Postural strategies in the frontal plane as revealed by a statistical analysis of accelerometric measurements. J Biomech 1993; 762.

Lemon RN, Mantel GWH, Muir RB. Corticospinal facilitation of hand muscles during voluntary movements in the conscious monkey. J Physiol 1986; 381:497–527.

Lemsky C, Miller CJ, Nevitt M, Winograd C. Reliability and validity of a physical performance and mobility examination for hospitalized elderly. Soc Gerontol 1991; 31:221.

Leonard CT, Hirshfeld H, Forssberg H. The development of independent walking in children with cerebral palsy. Dev Med Child Neurol 1991; 33:567–577.

Lerner-Frankiel MB, Vargas S, Brown MB, et al. Functional community ambulation: what are your criteria? Clin Manag 1990; 6:12–15.

Levin MF. Interjoint coordination during pointing movements is disrupted in spastic hemiparesis. Brain 1996; 119:281–293.

Levin MF, Horowitz M, Jurrius C, et al. Trajectory formation and interjoint coordination of drawing movements in normal and hemiparetic subjects. Neurosci Abstr 1993; 19:990.

Lewis C, Bottomley J. Musculoskeletal changes with age. In: Lewis C, ed. Aging: health care's challenge. 2nd ed. Philadelphia: FA Davis, 1990:145–146.

Lewis C, Phillippi L. Postural changes with age and soft tissue treatment. Phys Ther Forum 1993; 9:4–6.

Lezak MD. Neuropsycholoigcal Assessment. New York: Oxford University Press, 1976.

Liepert J, Miltner WH, Bauder H, et al. Motor cortex plasticity during constraint-induced movement therapy in stroke patients. Neurosci Lett 1998; 250:5–8.

Lin SI. Adapting to dynamically changing balance threats: differentiating young, healthy older adults and unstable older adults. Doctoral dissertation, University of Oregon, 1998.

Lindholm L. Weight-bearing splint: a method for managing upper extremity spasticity. Physical Therapy Forum 1985; 5:3.

Lipsitz LA, Jonsson PV, Kelley MM, Koestner JS. Causes and correlates of recurrent falls in ambulatory frail elderly. J Gerontol 1991; 46:M114–M122.

Livingstone M, Hubel D. Segregation of form, color, movement and depth: anatomy, physiology, perception. Science 1988; 240:740–749.

Llewellyn M, Prochazka A, Vincent S. Transmission of human tendon jerk reflexes during stance and gait. J Physiol Lond 1986; 382:82.

Lloyd DG. Environmental requirements for elderly people to have stability underfoot while walking. Proc. National Forum on Prevention of Falls and Injuries amongst Older People. Sydney, 1990.

Lord SE, Halligan PW, Wade DT. Visual gait analysis: the development of a clinical assessment and scale. Clin Rehabil 1998; 12:107–119.

Lord SR, Lloyd DG, Li SK. Sensorimotor function, gait patterns and falls in community-dwelling women. Age Ageing 1996a;25:292–299.

Lord SR, Lloyd DG, Nirui M, et al. The effect of exercise on gait patterns in older women: a randomized controlled trial. J Gerontol 1996B:51:M64–M70.

Lord S, Ward J, Williams P, Anstey K. An epidemiological study of falls in older community dwelling women: the Randwick falls and fracture study. Aust J Public Health 1993; 17:240–245.

Lovely RG, Gregor RJ, Edgerton VR. Effects of training on the recovery of full-weight-bearing stepping in the adult spinal cat. Exp Neurol 1986; 92:421–435.

Lucy SD, Hayes KC. Postural sway profiles: normal subjects and subjects with cerebellar ataxia. Physiother Can 1985; 37:140–148.

Lundin-Olsson L, Nyberg L, Gustafson Y. Stops walking when talking as a predictor of falls in elderly people. Lancet 1997; 349:617.

Lundin-Olsson L, Nyberg L, Gustafson Y. Attention, frailty and falls: the effect of a manual task on basic mobility. J Am Geriatr Soc 1998; 46:758–761.

Lundgren-Lindquist B, Aniansson A, Rundgren A. Functional studies in 79 year olds: 3. Walking performance and climbing ability. Scand J Rehabil Med 1983; 12:107–112.

Luria AR. Higher cortical functions in man. New York: Basic, 1966.

Lynch KB, Bridle MJ. Validity of the Jebsen-Taylor hand function test in predicting activities of daily living. Occup Ther J Res 1989; 5:316–318.

MacKay-Lyons M. Variability in spatiotemporal gait characteristics over the course of L-dopa cycle in people with advanced Parkinson disease. Phys Ther 1998; 78:1083–1094.

MacKinnon SE, Dellon AL. Two point discrimination test. Journal of Hand Surgery 1985; 10:906–907.

Macpherson J. The neural organization of postural control: do muscle synergies exist? In: Amblard B, Berthoz A, Clarac F, eds. Posture and gait: development, adaptation and modulation. Amsterdam: Elsevier, 1988: 381–390.

Macpherson J, Craig LS. Postural responses in cats to movements of the support surface in the horizontal plane: comparison of lateral and longitudinal displacements. Soc Neurosci Abstr 1986; 12:1300.

Macpherson JM, Fung J. Weight support and balance during postural stance in the chronic spinal cat. J Neurophysiol 1999;82:3060–3081.

Macpherson JM, Fung J, Jacobs R. Postural orientation, equilibrium and the spinal cord. In: Seil FJ, ed. Advances in neurology, vol 72: Neuronal regeneration, reorganization, and repair. Philadelphia: Lippincott-Raven, 1997:227–232.

Magee DJ. Orthopedic Physical Assessment. Philadelphia: Saunders, 1987.

Magill RA, Hall KG. A review of the contextual interference effect in motor skill acquisition. Hum Mov Sci 1990; 9:241–289.

Magnus R. Animal posture (Croonian lecture). Proc R Soc Lond 1925; 98:339.

Magnus R. Some results of studies in the physiology of posture. Lancet 1926; 2:531–585.

Mahoney RI, Barthel DW. Functional evaluation: the Barthel Index. Md Med J 1965; 14:61–65.

Maki B, Holliday PJ, Topper AK. Fear of falling and postural performance in the elderly. J Gerontol 1991; 46:M123-M131.

Maki BE, Holliday PJ, Topper AK. A prospective study of postural balance and risk of falling in an ambulatory and independent elderly population. J Gerontol 1994a;49:M72–84.

Maki B, McIlroy W, Perry S. Compensatory responses to multi-directional perturbations. In: Taguchi K, Igarashi M, Mori S, eds. Vestibular and neural front. Amsterdam: Elsevier, 1994b:437–440.

Malick M. Manual on Static Hand Splinting. Pittsburgh: Harmarville Rehab Center, 1980.

Manchester D, Woollacott M, Zederbauer-Hylton N, Marin O. Visual, vestibular and somatosensory contributions to balance control in the older adult. J Gerontol 1989; 44:M118–M127.

Manheim CJ, Lavett DK. The Myofascial Release Manual. Thorofare, NJ: Slack Inc., 1989.

Man'kovskii NB, Mints AY, Lysenyuk VP. Regulation of the preparatory period for complex voluntary movement in old and extreme old age. Hum Physiol Moscow 1980; 6:46–50.

Mann RA, Hagy JL, White V, Liddell D. The initiation of gait. J Bone Joint Surg 1979; 61A:232–239.

Mannheimer JS, Lampe GN. Clinical Transcutaneous Electrical Nerve Stimulation. Philadelphia: FA Davis Co., 1984.

Margaria R. Biomechanics and energetics of muscular exercise. Oxford: Clarendon, 1976:67–74.

Marque P, Felez A, Puel M, et al. Impairment and recovery of left motor function in patients with right hemiplegia. J Neurol Neurosurg Psychiatry 1997; 62:77–81.

Marsden CD. Slowness of movement in Parkinson's disease. Mov Disord 1989; 4:26–37.

Marsden CD. The dystonias. Br Med J 1990; 300:139–144.

Marsden CD, Fahn S. Problems in Parkinson's disease and other akinetic-rigid syndromes. In: Marsden CD, Fahn S, eds. Movement disorders, vol 3. Oxford: Butterworth-Heinemann, 1994:117–123.

Marsden CD, Merton PA, Morton HB. Anticipatory postural responses in the human subject. J Physiol 1977; 275: 47P–48P.

Marteniuk RG, Leavitt JL, Mackenzie CL, Athenes S. Functional relationships between grasp and transport components in a prehension task. Hum Mov Sci 1990; 9:149–176.

Marteniuk RG, Mackenzie CL, Jeannerod M, et al. Constraints on human arm movements trajectories. Can J Psychol 1987; 41:365–368.

Martin J. Coding and processing of sensory information. In: Kandel E, Schwartz JH, Jessell TM, eds. Principles of neuroscience. 3rd ed. New York: Elsevier, 1991:329–340.

Martin JP. The basal ganglia and posture. London: Pitman, 1967.

Martin JH, Jessell TM. Anatomy of the somatic sensory system. In: Kandel E, Schwartz JH, Jessell TM, eds. Principles of neuroscience. 3rd ed. New York: Elsevier, 1991:353–366.

Martin TA, Keating JG, Goodkin HP, et al. Storage of multiple gaze-hand calibrations. Neurosci Abstr 1993; 19:980.

Mason C, Kandel ER. Central visual pathways. In: Kandel E, Schwartz JH, Jessell TM, eds. Principles of neuroscience. 3rd ed. New York: Elsevier, 1991:420–439.

Massion J. Role of motor cortex in postural adjustments associated with movement. In: Asanuma H, Wilson VJ, eds. Integration in the nervous system. Tokyo: Igaku-Shoin, 1979:239–260.

Massion J. Movement, posture and equilibrium: Interaction and coordination. Prog Neurobiol 1992; 38(1):35–36.

Massion J, Woollacott M. Normal balance and postural control. In: Bronstein AM, Brandt T, Woollacott M. Clinical aspects of balance and gait disorders. London: Edward Arnold, 1996.

Mathias S, Nayak U, Issacs B. Balance in elderly patients: the "Get-up and Go" test. Arch Phys Med Rehabil 1986; 67:387–389.

Mathiowetz V, Kashmann N, Volland G, Weber K, Dowe M, Rogers S. Grip and pinch strength: Normative data for adults. Arch Phys Med Rehabil 1985; 66(2):69–74.

Mathiowetz V, Rogers SL, Dowe-Keval M, Donahue L, Rennells C. The Purdue Pegboard: Norms for 14 to 19 year olds. Am J Occup Ther 1986; 40(3):174–9.

Mathiowetz V, Wiemer DM, Federman SM. Grip and pinch strength: Norms for 6- to 19-year olds. Am J Occup Ther 1986; 40(10):705–11.

Mayer NH. Clinicophysiologic concepts of spasticity and motor dysfunction in adults with upper motoneuron lesion. Muscle Nerve 1997; 6 (Suppl):S1–S13.

Mayer NH, Esquenazi A, Childers MK. Common patterns of clinical motor dysfunction. Muscle Nerve 1997; 6:S21-S35.

Maynard CJ. Sensory reeducation following peripheral nerve injury. In: Hunter JM, Schneider LH, Mackin EJ, Bell JA, eds. Rehabilitation of the Hand. St. Louis: CV Mosby, 1978:318–323.

Mayston M. The Bobath concept: evolution and application. In: Forssberg H, Hirschfeld H, eds. Movement disorders in children. Med Sport Sci. Basel: Karger, 1992:1–6.

McCarter RJ, Kelly NG. Cellular basis of aging in skeletal muscle. In: Coe RM, Perry HM, eds. Aging, musculoskeletal disorders and care of the frail elderly. New York: Springer, 1993:45–60.

McCollum G, Leen T. The form and exploration of mechanical stability limits in erect stance. J Motor Behav 1989; 21:225–238.

McCoy AO, VanSant AF. Movement patterns of adolescents rising from a bed. Phys Ther 1993; 73:182–193.

McCullagh P, Weiss MR, Ross D. Modeling considerations in motor skill acquisition and performance: An integrated approach. In: Pandolf KB, ed. Exercise and Sport Sciences Reviews 1989; 17:475–513.

McDonnell PM. Patterns of eye-hand coordination in the first year of life. Can J Psychol 1979; 33:253–267.

McFadyen BJ, Winter DA. An integrated biomechanical analysis of normal stair ascent and descent. J Biomech 1988; 21:733–744.

McGavin CR, Gupta SP, McHardy GJR. Twelve minute walking test for assessing disability in chronic bronchitis. Br Med J 1976; 1:822–823.

McGraw M. Neuromuscular maturation of the human infant. New York: Hafner, 1945.

McGraw MB. From reflex to muscular control in the assumption of an erect posture and ambulation in the human infant. Child Dev 1932; 3:291.

McHorney CA, Haley SM, Ware JE. Evaluation of the MOS SF-36 Physical Functioning Scale (PF-10): II. Comparison of relative precision using Likert and Rasch scoring methods. J Clin Epidemiol 1997; 50(4):451–61.

McIlroy W, Maki B. Do anticipatory adjustments precede compensatory stepping reactions evoked by perturbation? Neurosci Lett 1993; 164:199–202.

McKinnon CD, Winter DA. Control of body balance in the frontal plane during human walking. J Biomech 1993; 26:633–644.

McLellan DL. Co-contraction and stretch reflex in spasticity during treatment with baclofen. Neurol Neurosurg Psychiatry 1973; 40:30–38.

McMahon TA. Muscles, reflexes and locomotion. Princeton, NJ: Princeton University, 1984.

McPherson J. Schild R, Spaulding SJ, Barsamian, Transon C, White SC. Analysis of upper extremity movement in four sitting positions: a comparison of persons with and without cerebral palsy. Am J Occup Ther 1991; 2:123–129.

Medina JJ. The clock of ages. New York, Cambridge University, 1996.

Meier A. Rehabilitation following falls of undetermined etiology: results of an intervention study. Schweiz Rundsch Med Prax 1992; 81:1405–1410.

Melville-Jones G, Mandl G. Neurobionomics of adaptive plasticity: integrating sensorimotor function with environmental demands. In: Desmedt JE, ed. Motor control mechanisms in health and disease. Adv Neurol 1983; 39:1047–1071.

Merbitz C, Morris J, Grip C. Ordinal scales and foundations of misinference. Arch Phys Med Rehab 1989; 70:308–312.

Melzack R. The McGill Pain Questionnaire: Major properties and scoring methods. Pain 1975; 1:277–299.

Merskey H, Lindblom U, Mumford JM, et al. Classification of chronic pain: Descriptions of chronic pain syndromes and definitions of pain terms. Pain 1986; Suppl 3:S215–S221.

Merzenich MM. Sources of intraspecies and interspecies cortical map variability in mammals: conclusions and hypotheses. In: Cohen MJ, Strumwasser F, eds. Comparative neurology: modes of communication in the nervous system. New York: Wiley, 1985:105–116.

Merzenich MM, Jenkins WM. Reorganization of cortical representation of the hand following alterations of skin inputs induced by nerve injury, skin island transfers & experience. J Hand Ther 1993; 6(2):89–104.

Merzenich MM, Kaas JH, Wall J, Nelson RJ, Sur M, Felleman D. Topographic reorganization of somatosensory cortical areas 3b and 1 in adult monkeys following restricted deafferentation. Neuroscience 1983; 8(1):33–55.

Merzenich MM, Kaas JH, Wall J, et al. Topographic reorganization of somatosensory cortical areas 3B and 1 in adult monkeys following restricted deafferentation. Neurosci 1983a;8:33–55.

Merzenich MM, Kaas JH, Wall JT, et al. Progression of change following median nerve section in the cortical representation of the hand in areas 3b and 1 in adult owl and squirrel monkeys. Neurosci 1983b;10:639–665.

Meyer DE, Abrams RA, Kornblum S, et al. Optimality in human motor performance: ideal control of rapid aimed movements. Psychol Rev 1988; 95:340–370.

Michlovitz S, Ziskin MC. Therapeutic ultrasound. In: Michlovitz S, ed. Thermal Agents in Rehabilitation. Philadelphia: FA Davis, 1986:141–176.

Middleton FA, Strick PL. Anatomical evidence for cerebellar and basal ganglia involvement in higher cognitive function. Science 1994; 266:458–461.

Milani-Comparetti A, Gidoni EA. Pattern analysis of motor development and its disorders. Dev Med Child Neurol 1967; 9:625–630.

Milezarek JJ, Kirby LM, Harrison ER, MacLeod DA. Standard and four-footed canes: their effect on the standing balance of patients with hemiparesis. Arch Phys Med Rehabil 1993; 74:281–284.

Miller OH. Theories of developmental psychology. San Francisco: WH Freeman, 1983:2.

Millington PJ, Myklebust BM, Shambes GM. Biomechanical analysis of the sit-to-stand motion in elderly persons. Arch Phys Med Rehabil 1992; 73:609–617.

Milner AD, Goodale MA. Visual pathways to perception and action. Progr Brain Res 1993; 95:317–337.

Milner AD, Ockleford EM, Dewar W. Visuo-spatial performance following posterior parietal and lateral frontal lesions in stumptail macaques. Cortex 1977; 13:350–360.

Milner B. Amnesia following operation on the temporal lobes. In: Whitty CWM, Zangwill OL, eds. Amnesia. London: Butterworths, 1966:109–133.

Miltner W, Bauder H, Sommer M, et al. Effects of constraint-induced movement therapy on patients with chronic motor deficits after stroke. Stroke 1999; 30:586–592.

Miltner WH, Bauder H, Sommer M, Dettmers C, Taub E. Effects of constraint-induced movement therapy on patients with chronic motor deficits after stroke: a replication. Stroke 1999; 30(3):586–92.

Mishkin MH, Malamut B, Bachevalier J. Memories and habits: two neural systems. In: McGaugh JL, Lynch G, Weinberger NM, eds. The neurobiology of learning and memory. New York: Guilford, 1984:65–77.

Moberg E. The unsolved problem—How to test the functional value of hand sensibility. J Hand Therapy 1991; 4:105–110.

Mochon S, McMahon TA. Ballistic walking. J Biomech 1980; 13:49–57.

Molen HH. Problems on the evaluation of gait. Dissertation. Amsterdam: Free University, Institute of Biomechanics and Experimental Rehabilitation, 1973.

Molnar GE. Analysis of motor disorder in retarded infants and young children. A J Ment Defic 1978; 83:213–222.

Montgomery J. Assessment and treatment of locomotor deficits in stroke. In: Duncan PW, Badke MB. Stroke rehabilitation: the recovery of motor control. Chicago: Year Book, 1987:223–259.

Moore S, Brunt D, Nesbitt ML, Juarez T. Investigation of evidence for anticipatory postural adjustments in seated subjects who performed a reaching task. Phys Ther 1992a;72:335–343.

Moore SP, Rushmer DS, Windus SL, Nashner LM. Human automatic postural responses: responses to horizontal perturbations of stance in multiple directions. Exp Brain Res 1988; 73:648–658.

Moore S, Sveistrup H, Massion M, et al. Postural control strategies for simultaneous control tasks. In: Woollacott M, Horak F, eds. Posture and gait: control mechanisms. Eugene, OR: University of Oregon, 1992b:218–221.

Morasso P. Spatial control of arm movements. Exp Brain Res 1981; 42:223–227.

Morgan MH. Ataxia and weights. Physiotherapy 1975; 61:332–334.

Morgan M, Phillips JG, Bradshaw JL, et al. Age-related motor slowness: simply strategic? J Gerontol 1994; 49:M133–M139.

Morris ME, Iansek R, Matyas TA, Summers JJ. Stride length regulation in Parkinson's disease: normalization strategies and underlying mechanisms. Brain 1996a;119:551–569.

Morris ME, Iansek R, Matyas TA, Summers JJ. Abnormalities in the stride length-cadence relation in Parkinsonian gait. Mov Disord 1998; 13:61–69.

Morris ME, Matyas TA, Iansek R, Summers JJ. Temporal stability of gait in Parkinson's disease. Phys Ther 1996b;76:763–789.

Morris RGM, Anderson E, Lynch GS, Baudry M. Selective impairment of learning and blockage of long-term potentiation by an N-methyl-D-aspartate receptor antagonist, AP5. Nature 1986; 319:774–776.

Mott FW, Sherrington CS. Experiments upon the influence of sensory nerves upon movement and nutrition of the limbs. Preliminary communication. Proc R Soc Lond Biol 1895; 57:481–488.

Mouchnino L, Aurenty R, Massion J, Pedotti A. Coordination between equilibrium and head-trunk orientation during leg movement: a new strategy built up by training. J Neurophysiol 1992; 67:1587–1599.

Msall ME, DiGaudio KM, Duff LL. Use of functional assessment in children with developmental disabilities. Phys Med Rehab Clinics of North Am 1993; 4:517–527.

Mudie MH, Matyas TA. Can simultaneous bilateral movement involve the undamaged hemisphere in reconstruction of neural networks damaged by stroke? Disabil Rehabil. 2000 Jan 10–20; 22(1-2):23–37.

Muir RB, Lemon RN. Corticospinal neurons with a special role in precision grip. Brain Res 1983; 261:312–316.

Mulcahey MJ, Betz RR, Smith BT, Weiss AA, Davis, SE. Implanted functional electrical stimulation hand system in adolescents with spinal injuries: An evaluation. Arch Phys Med Rehabil 1997; 78:597–607.

Mulder T, Berndt H, Pauwels J, Nienhuis B. Sensorimotor adaptability in the elderly and disabled. In: Stelmach G, Homberg V, eds. Sensori-motor impairment in the elderly. Dordrecht: Kluwer, 1993.

Murray MP. Gait as a total pattern of movement. Am J Phys Med 1967; 46:290–333.

Murray M, Kory R, Sepic S. Walking patterns of normal women. Arch Phys Med Rehabil 1970; 51:637–650.

Murray MP, Kory RC, Clarkson BH. Walking patterns in healthy old men. J Gerontol 1969; 24:169–178.

Murray MP, Kory RC, Clarkson BH, Sepic SB. Comparison of free and fast speed walking patterns of normal men. Am J Phys Med 1966; 45:8–24.

Murray MP, Mollinger LA, Gardner GM, Sepic SB. Kinematic and EMG patterns during slow, free, and fast walking. J Orthop Res 1984; 2:272–280.

Murray MP, Seireg A, Scholz RC. Normal postural stability and steadiness: quantitative assessment. J Bone Joint Surg 1975; 57A:510–516.

Mushiake H, Inase M, Tanji J. Neuronal activity in the primate premotor, supplementary and precentral motor cortex during visually guided and internally determined sequential movements. J Neurophysiol 1991;66:705–718.

Mushiake H, Strick P. Preferential activity of dentate neurons during limb movements guided by vision. J Neurophysiol 1993; 70:2660–2664.

Nadeau S, Gravel D, Arsenault AB, Bourbonnais D, Goyette M. Dynamometric assessment of the plantarflexors in hemiparetic subjects: relations between muscular, gait and clinical parameters. Scand J Rehabil Med 1997; 29:137–146.

Nagi SZ. Some conceptual issues in disability and rehabilitation. In: Sussman MD, ed. Sociology and rehabilitation. Washington: American Sociological Association, 1965:100–113.

Napier JR. The prehensile movement of the human hand. J Bone Joint Surg 1956; 38b:902–913.

Nashner L. Adapting reflexes controlling the human posture. Exp Brain Res 1976; 26:59–72.

Nashner LM. Fixed patterns of rapid postural responses among leg muscles during stance. Exp Brain Res 1977; 30:13–24.

Nashner LM. Balance adjustment of humans perturbed while walking. J Neurophysiol 1980; 44:650–664.

Nashner LM. Adaptation of human movement to altered environments. Trends Neurosci 1982; 358–361.

Nashner LM. Sensory, neuromuscular, and biomechanical contributions to human balance. In: Duncan P, ed. Balance: Proceedings of the APTA Forum. Alexandria, VA: APTA, 1989:5–12.

Nashner LM, Shumway-Cook A, Marin O. Stance posture control in select groups of children with cerebral palsy: deficits in sensory organization and muscular coordination. Experimental Brain Res 1983; 49:393–409.

Nashner L, Woollacott M. The organization of rapid postural adjustments of standing humans: an experimental-conceptual model. In: Talbott RE, Humphrey DR, eds. Posture and movement. New York: Raven, 1979:243–257.

Nashner L, Woollacott M, Tuma G. Organization of rapid responses to postural and locomotor-like perturbations of standing man. Experimental Brain Res 1979; 36:463–476.

National Advisory Board on Medical Rehabilitation Research, Draft V: Report and Plan for Medical Rehabilitation Research. Bethesda, MD: National Institutes of Health, 1992.

Nelson SR, DiFabio RP, Anderson JH. Vestibular and sensory interaction deficits assessed by dynamic platform posturography in patients with multiple sclerosis. Ann Otol Rhinol 1995; 104:62–68.

Neuhaus BE, Ascher B, Coullon M, et al. A survey of rationales for and against hand splinting in hemiplegia. Am J Occup Ther 1981; 35:83–95.

Nevitt MC, Cummings SR, Kidd S, Black D. Risk factors for recurrent nonsyncopal falls. JAMA 1989; 261:2663–2668.

Newell KM. Motor skill acquisition. Annu Rev Psychol 1991; 42:213–237.

Newell KM, Kennedy JA. Knowledge of results and children's motor learning. Dev Psych 1978; 14:531–536.

Newell K, van Emmerik REA. The acquisition of coordination: Preliminary analysis of learning to write. Hum Mov Sci 1989; 8:17–32.

Norman DA, Shallice T. Attention to action: willed and automatic control of behavior. In: Davidson RJ, Schwartz GE, Shapiro D, eds. Consciousness and self-regulation, vol 4. New York: Plenum, 1986.

Noronha J, Bundy A, Groll J. The effect of positioning on the hand function of boys with cerebral palsy. Am J Occup Ther 1989; 43:507–512.

Noth J. Trends in the pathophysiology and pharmacotherapy of spasticity. J Neurol 1991; 238:131–139.

Nudo RJ, Milliken GW, Jenkins WM, Merzenich MM. Use-dependent alterations of movement representations in primary motor cortex of adult squirrel monkeys. J Neuroscience 1996; 16:785–807.

Nutt JG, Horak FB. Gait and balance disorders. In: Watts R, Koller W, eds. Movement disorders: neurologic principles and practice. New York, McGraw-Hill, 1997.

Nutt JG, Marsden CD, Thompson PD. Human walking and higher-level gait disorders, particularly in the elderly. Neurology 1993; 43:268–279.

Nutt JG, Woodward WR, Hammerstad JP, et al. The "on-off" phenomenon in Parkinson's disease: relation to levodopa absorption and transport. N Engl J Med 1984; 310:483–488.

Nwaobi OM, Brubaker CE. Cusick B, Sussman M. Electromyographic investigation of extensor activity in cerebral palsied children in different seating positions. Dev Med Child Neurol 1983; 25:175–183.

Oatis CA, Perspectives on the evaluation and treatment of gait disorders. In: Montgomery PC, Connolly, BH, eds. Motor control and physical therapy: theoretical framework and practical applications. Hixson, TN: Chattanooga Corp., 1990:141–155.

Ochs AL, Newberry J, Lenhardt ML, Harkins SW. Neural and vestibular aging associated with falls. In: Birren JE, Schaie KW, eds. Handbook of psychology of aging. New York: Van Nostrand & Reinholdt, 1985:378–399.

Ogden R, Franz SI. On cerebral motor control: the recovery from experimentally produced hemiplegia. Psychobiology 1917; 1:33–49.

Okamoto T, Kumamoto M. Electromyographic study of the learning process of walking in infants. Electromyography 1972; 12:149–158.

Olney SJ, Griffin MP, McBride ID. Temporal, kinematic and kinetic variables related to gait speed in subjects with hemiplegia: a regression approach. Phys Ther 1994; 74:872–885.

Olney SJ, Griffin MP, Monga TN, et al. Work and power in gait of stroke patients. Arch Phys Med Rehabil 1991; 72:309–314.

Olney SJ, Richards C. Hemiparetic gait following stroke, part I characteristics. Gait Posture 1996; 4:136–148.

Olsen JZ. Handwriting Without Tears. 7th ed. Potomac MD, 1998.

Ornitz E. Normal and pathological maturation of vestibular function in the human child. In: Romand R, ed. Development of auditory and vestibular systems. New York: Academic, 1983:479–536.

O'Sullivan S. Clinical decision making: planning effective treatments. In: O'Sullivan S, Schmitz T, eds. Physical rehabilitation: assessment and treatment. 2nd ed. Philadelphia: FA Davis, 1988:1–7.

O'Sullivan S. Parkinson's disease: physical rehabilitation. In: O'Sullivan S, Schmitz T. Physical rehabilitation: assessment and treatment. 2nd ed. Philadelphia: FA Davis, 1994:481–493.

Oszkowski WJ, Barreca S. The Functional Independence Measure: Its use to identify rehabilitation needs in stroke survivors. Arch Phys Med Rehab 1993; 74:1291–1294.

Overstall PW, Exton-Smith AN, Imms FJ, Johnson AL. Falls in the elderly related to postural imbalance. Br Med J 1977; 1:261–264.

Pai YC, Patton J. Centre of mass velocity-position predictions for balance control. J Biomech 1997; 30:347–354.

Pai YC, Naughton BJ, Chang RW, Rogers MW. Control of body center of mass momentum during sit-to-stand among young and elderly adults. Gait Posture 1994; 2:109–116.

Paillard J. The contribution of peripheral and central vision to visually guided reaching. In: Ingle DJ, Goodale MA, Mansfield RJW, eds. Analysis of visual behavior. Cambridge, MA: MIT, 1982:367–385.

Paillard J. Cognitive versus sensorimotor encoding of spatial information. In: Ellen P, Thinus-Blanc C, eds. Cognitive processes and spatial orientation in animal and man: neurophysiology and developmental aspects. Hague: Martinus Nijhoff, NARO ASI Series 37, 1987, 43–77.

Paine RS. The evolution of infantile postural reflexes in the presence of chronic brain syndromes. Dev Med Child Neurol 1964; 6:345–361.

Palisano RJ. Neuromotor and developmental assessment. In: Wilhelm IJ, ed. Physical therapy assessment in early infancy. New York: Churchill Livingstone, 1993:173–224.

Palliyath S, Hallett M, Thomas SL, Lebiedowska MK. Gait in patients with cerebellar ataxia. Mov Disord 1998; 13:958–964.

Panzer VP, Hallett M. Biomechanical assessment of Parkinson's disease: A single-subject study. Clin Biomech 1990; 5:73–80.

Partridge CJ, Edwards SM, Mee R, van Langenberghe HVK. Hemiplegic shoulder pain: a study of two methods of physiotherapy treatment. Clin Rehabil 1990; 4:43–49.

Pascual-Leone A, Grafman J, Hallett M. Modulation of cortical motor output maps during development of implicit and explicit knowledge. Science 1994; 263:1287–1289.

Passingham RE. Premotor cortex: sensory cues and movement. Behav Brain Res 175–185, 1985.

Passinham RE, Chen YC, Thaler D. Supplementary motor cortex and self-initiated movement. In: Ito M, ed. Neural programming. Tokyo: Japan Scientific Society, 1989:13–24.

Pastalan LA, Mantz RK, Merrill J. The simulation of age-related sensory losses: a new approach to the study of environmental barriers. In: Preiser WFE, ed. Environment design research, vol 1. Stroudsberg, PA: Dowden, Hutchinson & Ross, 1973:383–390.

Patla AE. Understanding the control of human locomotion: a prologue. In: Patla AE, ed. Adaptability of human gait. Amsterdam: North-Holland, 1991:3–17.

Patla AE. Age-related changes in visually guided locomotion over different terrains: major issues. In: Stelmach G, Homberg V, eds. Sensorimotor impairment in the elderly. Dordrecht: Kluwer, 1993:231–252.

Patla A. A framework for understanding mobility problems in the elderly. In: Craik RL, Oatis CA, eds. Gait analysis: theory and application. St. Louis: Mosby, 1995.

Patla AE. Neurobiomechanical bases for the control of human locomotion. In: Bronstein AM, Brandt T, Woollacott MH, eds. Clinical aspects of balance and gait disorders. Kent, England: Edward Arnold Publishers, 1996; 19–40.

Patla AE. Understanding the roles of vision in the control of human locomotion. Gait Posture 1997; 5:54–69.

Patla AE, Prentice SD, Martin C, Rietdyk S. The bases of selection of alternate foot placement during locomotion in humans. In: Posture and gait: control mechanisms. Woollacott MH, Horak F, eds. Eugene: University of Oregon, 1992:226–229.

Patla AE, Shumway-Cook A. Dimensions of mobility: defining the complexity and difficulty associated with community mobility. J Aging Phys Activity 1999; 7:7–19.

Patla AE, Winter DA, Frank JS, et al. Identification of age-related changes in the balance-control system. In: Duncan P, ed. Balance: Proceedings of the APTA Forum, Alexandria, VA: APTA, 1990:43–55.

Patton HD, Fuchs A, Hille B, et al. Textbook of physiology, vol 1. 21st ed. Philadelphia: WB Saunders, 1989.

Paulignan Y, McKenzie C, Marteniuk R, Jeannerod M. The coupling of arm and finger movements during prehension. Exper Brain Res 1990; 79:431–436.

Paulus W, Straube A, Brandt T. Visual stabilisation of posture. Brain 1984; 107:1143–1163.

Pause M, Kunesch E, Binkofski F, Freund HG. Sensorimotor disturbances in patients with lesions of the parietal cortex. Brain 1989; 112:1599–1625.

Payton O, Melson C, Ozer M. Patient participation in program planning: a manual for therapists. FA Davis, Philadelphia, 1990.

Pearson KG. Proprioceptive regulation of locomotion. Curr Opin Neurobiol 1995; 5:786–791.

Pearson KG, Ramirez JM, Jiang W. Entrainment of the locomotor rhythm by group Ib afferents from ankle extensor muscles in spinal cats. Exp Brain Res 1992; 90:557–566.

Pedersen SW, Eriksson T, Oberg B. Effects of withdrawal of anti-Parkinson medication on gait and clinical score in the Parkinson patient. Acta Neurol Scand 1991; 84:7–13.

Pehoski C. Object manipulation in infants and children. In: Henderson A, Pehoski C., eds. Hand Function in the Child: Foundations for Remediation. Boston: Mosby, 1995:136–153.

Peiper A. Cerebral functions in infancy and childhood. New York: Consultants Bureau, 1963.

Penfield W. Functional localization in temporal and deep Sylvian areas. Res Publ Assoc Res Nerv Ment Dis 1958; 36:210–226.

Penfield W, Rasmussen T. The cerebral cortex of man: a clinical study of localization of function. New York: Macmillan, 1950.

Peoppel E. Letter to the editor. Nature 1973; 243:231.

Perenin MT, Jeannerod M. Residual vision in cortically blind hemifields. Neuropsychologia 1975; 13:1–7.

Perenin MT, Jeannerod M. Visual function within the hemianoptic field following early cerebral hemidecortication in man: 1. Spatial localization. Neuropsychologia 1978; 16:1–13.

Perry J. Gait analysis: normal and pathological function. Thorofare, NJ: Slack, 1992.

Perry RJ, Hodges JR. Attention and executive deficits in Alzheimer's Disease: A critical review. Brain 1999; 122:383–406.

Perry J, Garrett M, Gronley JK, Mulroy, SJ. Classification of walking handicap in the stroke population. Stroke 1995; 26:982–989.

Perry J, Newsam C. Function of the hamstrings in cerebral palsy. In: Sussman M, ed. The diplegic child. Rosemont, IL: American Academy of Orthopedic Surgeons, 1992:299–307.

Perry SB. Clinical implications of a dynamical systems theory. Neurol Report 1998; 22:4–10.

Peterka RJ, Black FO. Age-related changes in human posture control: sensory organization tests. J Vestib Res 1990; 1:73–85.

Pfeiffer E. Short portable mental status questionnaire. J Am Geriatric Soc 1975; 23:433–441.

Piaget J. The origins of intelligence in children. New York: WW Norton, 1954.

Pitts DG. The effects of aging on selected visual functions: dark adaptation, visual acuity, stereopsis, and brightness contrast. In: Sekular R, Kline D, Dismukes K, eds. Modern aging research: aging and human visual function. New York: Alan R. Liss, 1982:131–160.

Platt JR. Strong inference. Science 1964; 146:347–352.

Podsiadlo D, Richardson S. The timed "Up and Go" test: a test of basic functional mobility for frail elderly persons. J Am Geriatr Soc 1991; 39:142–148.

Poewe WH. Clinical aspects of motor fluctuations in Parkinson's disease. Neurology 1994; 44(suppl 6):S6–S9.

Pohl PS, Winstein CJ. Practice effects on the less-affected upper extremity after stroke. Arch Phys Med Rehabil 1999; 80:668–675.

Pohl PS, Winstein CJ, Fisher BE. The locus of age-related movement slowing: sensory processing in continuous goal-directed aiming. J Gerontol 1996; 51:P94–102.

Poizner H, Mack L, Verfaellie M, Rothi LJG, Heilman KM. Three-dimensional computergraphic analysis of apraxia. Brain 1990; 113:85–101.

Polit A, Bizzi E. Processes controlling arm movements in monkeys. Science 1978; 201:1235–1237.

Polit A, Bizzi E. Characteristics of motor programs underlying arm movements in monkeys. J Neurophysiol 1979; 42:183–194.

Pons TP, Garraghty PE, Mishkin M. Lesion induced plasticity in the second somatosensory cortex of adult macaques. Proc Natl Acad Sci U S A 1988; 85:5279–5281.

Poole JL, Gallagher J, Janosky J, Qualls C. The mechanisms for adult-onset apraxia and developmental dyspraxia: an examination and comparison of error patterns.

Poole JL, Whitney SL. Motor assessment scale for stroke patients: Concurrent validity and interrater reliability. Arch Phys Med Rehab 1988; 69:195–197.

Powell J, Pandyan AD, Granat M, et al. Electrical stimulation of wrist extensors in poststroke hemiplegia. Stroke 1999; 30:1384–1389.

Powers RK, Campbell DL, Rymer WZ. Stretch reflex dynamics in spastic elbow flexor muscles. Ann Neurol 1989; 25:32–42.

Pozzo T, Berthoz A, Lefort L. Head stabilization during various locomotor tasks in humans: 1. Normal subjects. Exp Brain Res 1990; 82:97–106.

Pozzo T, Berthoz A, Lefort L, Vitte E. Head stabilization during various locomotor tasks in humans: 2. Patients with bilateral peripheral vestibular deficits. Exp Brain Res 1991; 85:208–217.

Pozzo T, Levik Y, Berthoz A. Head stabilization in the frontal plane during complex equilibrium tasks in humans. In: Woollacott M, Horak F, eds. Posture and gait: control mechanisms. Eugene: University of Oregon, 1992:97–100.

Prechtl HFR. Continuity and change in early neural development. In: Prechtl HFR, ed. Continuity of neural functions from prenatal to postnatal life. Clinics in Developmental Medicine 94. Oxford: Blackwell Scientific, 1984:1–15.

Prechtl HFR, Prenatal motor development. In: Wade MC, Whiting HTA, eds. Motor development in children: aspects of coordination and control. Dordrecht: Martinus Nighoff, 1986:53–64.

Price DD, McGrath PA, Rafii A, Buckingham B. The validation of visual analogue scales as ratio scale measure for chronic and experimental pain. Pain 1983; 17:45–56.

Prigatano GP, Fordyce DJ. Cognitive dysfunction and psychological adjustment after brain injury, In: GP Prignatano, ed. Neuropsychological Rehabilitation after Brain Injury. Baltimore: Johns Hopkins University Press, 1986.

Prokop T, Berger W. Influence of optic flow on locomotion in normal subjects and patients with Parkinson's disease. Electroencephalogr Clin Neurophysiol 1996; 99:402.

Province M, Hadley E, Hornbrook M et al. The effects of exercise on falls in elderly patients: a preplanned meta-analysis of the FICSIT Trials. JAMA 1995; 273:1341–1347.

Quintana LA. Evaluation of perception and cognition. In: Tromby CA, ed. Occupational therapy for physical dysfunction. Baltimore: Williams & Wilkins, 1995.

Rabbit P, Birren JE. Age and responses to sequences of

repetitive and interruptive signals. J Gerontol 1967; 22:143–150.

Rabbit P, Rogers M. Age and choice between responses in a self-paced repetitive task. Ergonomics 1965; 8:435–444.

Rademaker GGJ. De Beteekenis der Roode Kernen en van de overige Mesencephalon voor Spiertonus, Lichaamshouding en Labyrinthaire Reflexen. Leiden: Eduarol Ijdo, 1924.

Raibert M. Symmetry in running. Science 1986; 231:1292–1294.

Ralston HJ. Energetics of human walking. In: Herman RM, Grillner S, Stein PSG, Stuart DG, eds. Neural control of locomotion. New York: Plenum, 1976:77–98.

Ramon y Cajal S. Degeneration and regeneration of the nervous system. May RM, translator. London: Oxford University, 1928.

Rankin JK, Woollacott MH, Shumway-Cook A, Brown LA. Cognitive influence on postural stability: a neuromuscular analysis in young and older adults. J Gerontol 2000; 55A: M112–119.

Rantanen T, Guralnik JM, Ferrucci L, et al. Coimpairments: strength and balance as predictors of severe walking disability. J Gerontol Med Sci 1999; 54A:M172–M176.

Rapcsak SZ, Ochipa C, Anderson KC, Poizner H. Progressive ideomotor apraxia: Evidence for a selective impairment of the action production system. Brain Cogn 1995; 27(2):213–36.

Rauschecker JP, Kniepert U. Auditory localization behavior in visually deprived cats. Eur J Neurosci 1994; 6:149–160.

Rawlings EI, Rawlings IL, Chen CS, Yilk MD. The facilitating effects of mental rehearsal in the acquisition of rotary pursuit tracking. Psychonom Sci 1972; 26:71–73.

Reed ES. An outline of a theory of action systems. J Motor Behav 1982; 14:98–134.

Rey A. Le freinage volontaire du mouvement graphique chez l'enfant. In: Epreuves d'intelligence pratique et de psychomotricite. Neuchatel: Delachaux & Niestle, 1968.

Richards CL, Malouin F, Wood-Dauphinee S, et al. Task-specific physical therapy for optimization of gait recovery in acute stroke patients. Arch Phys Med Rehabil 1993; 74:612–620.

Richards CL, Malouin F, Dumas F, et al. Gait velocity as an outcome measure of locomotor recovery after stroke. In: Craik RL and Oatis C, eds. Gait analysis: theory and applications. St. Louis: Mosby, 1995:355–364.

Richards CL, Malouin F, Dumas F, et al. Early and intensive treadmill locomotor training for young children with cerebral palsy: a feasibility study. Pediatr Phys Ther 1997; 9:158–165.

Richter A, Loscher W. Pathophysiology of idiopathic dystonia: findings from genetic animal models. Progr Neurobiol 1998; 54:633–677.

Richter RR, VanSant AF, Newton RA. Description of adult rolling movements and hypothesis of developmental sequences. Phys Ther 1989; 69:63–71.

Ring C, Nayak USL, Isaacs B. Balance function in elderly people who have and who have not fallen. Arch Phys Med Rehabil 1988; 69:261–264.

Rivet L. Functional capacity evaluation. In: Cassanova J, ed. Clinical Assessment Recommendations, 2nd ed. Chicago: American Society of Hand Therapists, 1992.

Rizzolatti G, Camarda R, Fogassi L, et al. Functional organization of inferior area 6 in the macaque monkey. Exp Brain Res 1988; 71:491–597.

Roberts TDM. Neurophysiology of postural mechanisms. London: Butterworths, 1979.

Robertson SL, Jones LA. Tactile sensory impairments and prehensile function in subjects with left-hemisphere cerebral lesions. Arch Phys Med Rehabil 1994; 75:1108–1117.

Robinson JL, Smidt GL. Quantitative gait evaluation in the clinic. Phys Ther 1981; 61:351–353.

Rogers MW. Control of posture and balance during voluntary movements in Parkinson's disease. In: Duncan P, ed. Balance: proceedings of the APTA Forum. Alexandria, VA: APTA, 1990:79–86.

Rogers MW. Motor control problems in Parkinson's disease. In: Contemporary management of motor control problems. Proceedings of the II Step Conference. Alexandria, VA: APTA, 1991:195–208.

Roland PE, Larsen B, Lassen NA, Skinhof E. Supplementary motor area and other cortical areas in organization of voluntary movements in man. J Neurophysiol 1980; 43:118–136.

Roll JP, Bard C, Paillard, J. Head orienting contributes to directional accuracy of aiming at distant targets. Hum Mov Sci 1986; 5:359–371.

Roll, JP, Roll R. From eye to foot: a proprioceptive chain involved in postural control. In: Amblard B, Berthoz A, Clarac F, eds. Posture and gait: development, adaptation and modulation. Amsterdam: Elsevier, 1988:155–164.

Romberg MH. Manual of nervous diseases of man. London: Sydenham Society, 1853:395–401.

Roncesvalles MNC, Jensen J. The expression of weight-bearing ability in infants between four and seven months of age. Sport Exerc Psychol 1993; 15:568.

Roncesvalles MNC, Woollacott MH, Jensen JL. Development of kinetic strategies in children. J Motor Behav (in press).

Roncesvalles MNC, Woollacott MH, Jensen JL. The development of compensatory stepping skills in children. J Motor Behav 2000; 32:100–111.

Rose DJ. A multilevel approach to the study of motor control and learning. Boston: Allyn & Bacon, 1997.

Rose SJ. Physical therapy diagnosis: role and function. Phys Ther 1989; 69:535–537.

Rose J, Haskell WL, Gamble JG, et al. Muscle pathology and clinical measures of disability in children with cerebral palsy. J Ortho Res 1994; 12:758–768.

Rosenbaum D. Human Motor control. New York: Academic, 1991.

Rosenhall U, Rubin W. Degenerative changes in the human vestibular sensory epithelia. Acta Otolaryngol 1975; 79:67–81.

Rosenrot P, Wall JC, Charteris J. The relationship between velocity, stride time, support time and swing time during normal walking. J Hum Mov Studies 1980; 6:323–335.

Rosenthal RB, Deutsch SD, Miller W, et al. A fixed-ankle, below-the-knee orthosis for the management of genu recurvatum in spastic cerebral palsy. J Bone Joint Surg 1975; 57A:545–547.

Rosin R, Topka H, Dichgans J. Gait initiation in Parkinson's disease. Mov Disord 1997; 12:682–690.

Rothstein J. Disability and our identity. Phys Ther 1994:74:375–377 (editor's note).

Rothstein JM, Echternach JL. Hypothesis-oriented algorithm for clinicians: a method for evaluation and treatment planning. Phys Ther 1986; 66:1388–1394.

Rothwell JC. Cerebral cortex. In: Rothwell JC, ed. Control of Human Voluntary Movement. 2nd ed. 1994:293–286.

Rothwell JC, Obeso JA, Day VL, Marsden CD. Pathophysiology of dystonias. In: Desmedt JE, ed. Motor control mechanisms in health and disease. New York: Raven, 1983:851–864.

Rothwell JC, Traub MM, Day BL, et al. Manual motor performance in a deafferented man. Brain 1982; 105:515–542.

Rowe JW, Kahn RL. Successful aging. New York: Pantheon, 1998.

Roy CW. Shoulder pain in hemiplegia: a literature review. Clin Rehabil 1988; 2:35–44.

Rozendal RH. Biomechanics of standing and walking. Amsterdam: Elsevier, 1986.

Rubenstein LZ, Robbins AS, Schulman BL, et al. Falls and instability in the elderly. J Am Geriatr Soc 1988; 36:266–278.

Ruff HA. Infants' manipulative exploration of objects: effects of age and object characteristics. Dev Psychol 1984; 20:9–20.

Runge CF, Shupert CL, Horak FB, Zajac FE. Postural strategies defined by joint torques. Gait Posture 1999; 10:161–170.

Russell DJ, Rosenbaum PL, Gowland C, et al. Manual for the gross motor function measure. Hamilton, Ontario, Canada: McMaster University, 1993.

Sadato N, Pascual-Leone A, Grafman J, et al. Activation of the primary visual cortex by Braille reading in blind subjects. Nature 1996; 380:526–528.

Sahrmann SA. Diagnosis by the physical therapist: a prerequisite for treatment. Special communication. Phys Ther 1988; 68:1703–1706.

Sahrmann SA, Norton BJ. The relationship of voluntary movement to spasticity in the upper motor neuron syndrome. Arch Neurol 1977; 2:460–465.

Sakata H, Shibutani H, Kawano K, Harrington TL. Neural mechanisms of space vision in the parietal association cortex of the monkey. Vision Res 1985; 25:453–463.

Salmoni AW, Schmidt RA, Walter CB. Knowledge of results and motor learning: a review and critical reappraisal. Psychol Bull 1984; 95:355–386.

Sanes JN, LeWitt PA, Mauritz KH. Visual and mechanical control of postural and kinetic tremor in cerebellar system disorders. J Neurol Neurosurg Psychiatry 1988; 51:934–943.

Sanes JN, Mauritz KH, Dalakas MC, Evarts EV. Motor control in humans with large-fiber sensory neuropathy. Hum Neurobiol 1985; 4:101–114.

Saunders D. Evaluation, Treatment and Prevention of Musculoskeletal Disorders. Minneapolis: Viking Press, 1991.

Saunders JBdeCM, Inman VT, Eberhart HD. The major determinants in normal and pathological gait. J Bone Joint Surg 1953; 35A:543–558.

Sauvage LR, Myklebust BM, Crow Pan J, et al. A clinical trial of strengthening and aerobic exercise to improve gait and balance in elderly male nursing home residents. Am J Phys Med Rehabil 1992; 71:333–342.

Schaltenbrand G. The development of human motility and motor disturbances. Arch Neurol Psychiatr 1928; 20:720.

Scheker LR, Chesher SP, Ramirez S. Neuromuscular electrical stimulation and dynamic bracing as a treatment for upper extremity spasticity in children with cerebral palsy. Brit J Hand Surg 1999; 2:226–232.

Schenkman M. Interrelationships of neurological and mechanical factors in balance control. In: Duncan P, ed. Balance: proceedings of the APTA Forum. Alexandria, VA: APTA, 1990:29–41.

Schenkman M, Butler RB. A model for multisystem evaluation, interpretation, and treatment of individuals with neurologic dysfunction. Phys Ther 1989; 69:538–547.

Schenkman MA, Berger RA, Riley PO, et al. Whole-body movements during rising to standing from sitting. Phys Ther 1990; 10:638–651.

Schenkman M, Butler RB. "Automatic Postural Tone" in posture, movement, and function. Forum on physical therapy issues related to cerebrovascular accident. Alexandria, VA: APTA, 1992:16–21.

Schneck CM, Henderson A. Descriptive analysis of the developmental progression of grip position for pencil and crayon control in nondysfunctional children. Am J Occup Ther 1990; 44(10):893–900.

Schloon H, O'Brien MJ, Scholten CA, Prechtl HE. Muscle activity and postural behavior in newborn infants: a polymyographic study. Neuropaediatrie 1976; 7:384–415.

Schmidt R. Motor and action perspectives on motor behaviour. In: Meijer OG, Roth K, eds. Complex movement behavior: the motor-action controversy. Amsterdam: Elsevier, 1988A:3–44.

Schmidt RA. A schema theory of discrete motor skill learning. Psychol Rev 1975; 82:225–260.

Schmidt RA. Motor control and learning. 2nd ed. Champaign, IL: Human Kinetics, 1988b.

Schmidt RA. Motor learning principles for physical therapy. Contemporary management of motor control problems. Proceedings of the II Step Conference. Alexandria, VA: APTA, 1991.

Schmidt RA. Motor learning principles for physical therapy. In: Contemporary management of motor control problems. Proceedings of the II Step Conference. Alexandria, VA: APTA, 1992:49–62.

Schmidt RA, Young DE. Augmented kinematic information feedback for skill learning: a new research paradigm. J Motor Behav 1987.

Schmidt RA, Zelaznik HN, Hawkins B, et al. Motor output variability: a theory for the accuracy of rapid motor acts. Psychol Rev 1979; 86:415–452.

Schmitz, TJ. Gait training with assistive devices. In: O'Sullivan S, Schmitz TM, eds. Physical rehabilitation: assessment and treatment. 2nd ed. Philadelphia: FA Davis 1998.

Schultz AB. Muscle function and mobility biomechanics in the elderly: an overview of some recent research. J Gerontol 1995; 50A(special issue):60–63.

Schultz A, Alexander NB, Gu MJ, Boismier T. Postural control in young and elderly adults when stance is challenged: clinical versus laboratory measurements. Ann Otol Rhinol Laryngol 1993; 102:508–517.

Schultz-Johnson K. Assessment of upper extremity injured persons' return to work potential. J Hand Surg 1987; 12A(5),950–957.

Schwab RS. Progression and prognosis in Parkinson's disease. J Nerv Ment Dis 1960; 130:556–572.

Schwartz MF, Reed ES, Montgomery M, et al. The quantitative description of action disorganization after brain damage: a case study. Cogn Neuropsychol 1991; 8:381–414.

Sea MJC, Henderson A, Cermak SA. Patterns of visual spatial inattention and their functional significance in stroke patients. Arch Phys Med Rehabil 1993; 74:355–360.

Seeger BR, Caudrey DJ, O'Mara NA. Hand function in cerebral palsy: The effect of hip flexion angle. Dev Med Child Neurol 1984; 26:601–606.

Seeley RR, Stephens TD, Tate P. Anatomy and physiology. St. Louis: Mosby, 1989.

Semmes J, Weinstein S. Somatosensory Changes After Penetrating Brain Wounds in Man. Cambridge: Harvard University Press, 1960.

Shaltenbrand G. The development of human motility and motor disturbances. Arch Neurol Pyschiatr 1928; 20:720–730.

Shambes GM, Gibson JM, Welker W. Fractured somatotopy in granule cell tactile areas of rat cerebellar hemispheres revealed by micromapping. Brain Behav Evol 1978; 15:94–140.

Shapiro DC, Schmidt RA. The schema theory: recent evidence and developmental implications. In: Kelso FAS, Clark JE, eds. The development of movement control and coordination. New York: Wiley, 1982:113–173.

Shea SL, Aslin RN. Oculomotor responses to step-ramp targets by young infants. Vision Res 1990; 30:1077–1092.

Shea CH, Shebilske W, Worchel S. Motor learning and control. Englewood Cliffs, NJ: Prentice Hall, 1993.

Sheldon JH. On the natural history of falls in older age. Br Med J 1960; 1685–1690.

Sheldon JH. The effect of age on the control of sway. Gerontol Clin 1963; 5:129–138.

Shellenkens JM, Scholten CA, Kalverboer AF. Visually guided hand movements in children with minor neurological dysfunction: Response time and movement organization. J Child Psych Psychiatry 1983; 24:89–102.

Shepard K. Theory: criteria, importance and impact. In: Contemporary management of motor control problems: proceedings of the II Step Conference. Alexandria, VA: APTA, 1991:5–10.

Shephard RJ. Benefits of exercise in the elderly. In: Coe RM, Perry HM, eds. Aging, musculoskeletal disorders and care of the frail elderly. New York: Springer, 1993:228–242.

Shepherd RB, Crosbie J, Squires T. The contribution of the ipsilateral leg to postural adjustments during fast voluntary reaching in sitting. Abstract of International Society for Biomechanics. 14th Congress. Paris: 1993.

Sherrington, C. The integrative action of the nervous system. 2nd ed. New Haven: Yale University, 1947.

Sherrington CS. Decerebrate rigidity, and reflex coordination of movements. J Physiol Lond 1898; 22:319–332.

Shik ML, Severin FV, Orlovsky GN. Control of walking and running by means of electrical stimulation of the mid-brain. Biophysics 1966; 11:756–765.

Shiverick D. Loss of gastrocnemius length in hemiplegic patients. Neurol Report 1990; 3:4–6.

Shumway-Cook A. Equilibrium deficits in children. In: Woollacott M, Shumway-Cook A, eds. Development of posture and gait across the life span. Columbia: University of South Carolina, 1989:229–252.

Shumway-Cook A. Retraining stability and mobility. Annual conference, Cincinnati. APTA, 1993.

Shumway-Cook A. Vestibular rehabilitation in traumatic brain injury. In: Herdman S, ed. Vestibular rehabilitation. Philadelphia: FA Davis, 1994:347–359.

Shumway-Cook A, Anson D, Haller S. Postural sway biofeedback for pretraining postural control following hemiplegia. Arch Phys Med Rehabil 1988a;69: 395–400.

Shumway-Cook A, Baldwin M, Pollisar N, Gruber W. Predicting the probability of falls in community dwelling older adults. Phys Ther 1997a;77:812–819.

Shumway-Cook A, Brauer S, Woollacott M. The effect of a secondary task on performance of the TUG in young vs. older adults. Phys Ther. In press.

Shumway-Cook A, Gruber W, Baldwin M, Liao S. The effect of multidimensional exercises on balance, mobility and fall risk in community dwelling older adults. Phys Ther 1997b;77:46–57.

Shumway-Cook A, Horak F. Assessing the influence of sensory interaction on balance. Phys Ther 1986; 66:1548–1550.

Shumway-Cook A, Horak FB. Vestibular rehabilitation: an exercise approach to managing symptoms of vestibular dysfunction. Semin Hearing 1989; 10:196–205.

Shumway-Cook A, Horak FB. Rehabilitation strategies for patients with vestibular deficits. Neurol Clin 1990; 8:441–457.

Shumway-Cook A, Horak F. Balance rehabilitation in the neurologic patient: course syllabus. Seattle: NERA, 1992.

Shumway-Cook A, Horak FB, Black FO. Critical examination of vestibular function in motor-impaired learning disabled children. Int J Pediatr Otorhinolaryngol 1988b;14:21–30.

Shumway-Cook A, McCollum G. Assessment and treatment of balance disorders in the neurologic patient. In: Montgomery T, Connolly B, eds. Motor control and physical therapy: theoretical framework and practical applications. Chattanooga, TN: Chattanooga Corp., 1990:123–138.

Shumway-Cook A, Olmscheid R. A systems analysis of postural dyscontrol in traumatically brain-injured patients. J Head Trauma Rehabil 1990; 5:51–62.

Shumway-Cook A, Woollacott M. The growth of stability: postural control from a developmental perspective. J Motor Behav 1985a;17:131–147.

Shumway-Cook A, Woollacott M. Postural control in the Down's syndrome child. Phys Ther 1985b;9: 211–235.

Shumway-Cook A, Woollacott M. Theoretical issues in assessing postural control. In: Wilhelm I, ed. Physical therapy assessment in early infancy. New York: Churchill Livingstone, 1993:161–171.

Shumway-Cook A, Woollacott M. Attentional demands and postural control: new insights for assessing and treating instability in older adults. Talk given at the APTA annual meeting, June, 1997.

Shumway-Cook A, Woollacott M, Baldwin M, Kerns K. The effects of cognitive demands on postural control in elderly fallers and non-fallers. J Gerontol 1997c;52:M232–240.

Simondson J, Goldie P, Brock K, Nosworthy J. The Mobility Scale for acute stroke patients: intrarater and interrater reliability. Clin Rehabil 1996; 10:295–300.

Simoneau GG, Cavanagh PR, Ulbrecht JS, et al. The influence of visual factors on fall-related kinematic variables during stair descent by older women. J Gerontol 1991; 46:188–195.

Singer RN. Motor learning and human performance. 3rd ed. New York: Macmillan, 1980.

Sinkjaer T, Andersen JB, Nielsen JF. Impaired stretch

reflex and joint torque modulation during spastic gait in multiple sclerosis patients. J Neurol 1996; 243:566–574.

Slavin MD, Laurence S, Stein DG. Another look at vicariation. In: Le Vere TE, Almli RB, Stein DG, eds. Brain injury and recovery: theoretical and controversial issues. New York: Plenum, 1988:165–179.

Sloane P, Baloh RW, Honrubia V. The vestibular system in the elderly. Am J Otolaryngol 1989; 1:422–429.

Smania N, Martini MC, Gambina G, et al. The spatial distribution of visual attention in hemineglect and extinction patients. Brain 1998; 121:1759–1770.

Smith JL. Programming of stereotyped limb movements by spinal generators. In: Stelmach GE, Requin J, eds. Tutorials in motor behavior. Amsterdam: North-Holland, 1980:95–115.

Smith JL, Smith LA, Dahms KL. Motor capacities of the chronic spinal cat: recruitment of slow and fast extensors of the ankle. Neurosci Abstr 1979; 5:387.

Smith JL, Zernicke RF. Predictions for neural control based on limb dynamics. Trends Neurosci 1987; 10:123–128.

Smith LH, Harris SR. Upper extremity inhibitive casting for a child with cerebral palsy. Phys Occup Ther Ped 1985; 5:71–79.

Smutok MA, Grafman J, Salazar AM, et al. Effects of unilateral brain damage on contralateral and ipsilateral upper extremity function in hemiplegia. Phys Ther 1989; 69:195–203.

Snow BJ, Tsui JK, Bhart MH, et al. Treatment of spasticity with botulinum toxin: a double blind study. Ann Neurol 1990; 28:512–515.

Sohlberg MM, Mateer CA. Introduction to Cognitive Rehabilitation. New York: Giford Press, 1989.

Sollerman C. Assessment of grip function: Evaluation of a new method. Sweden: MITAB, 1984

Southard D, Higgins T. Changing movement patterns: effects of demonstration and practice. Res Q Exerc Sport 1987; 58:77–80.

Speechley M, Tinetti M. Assessment of risk and prevention of falls among elderly persons: role of the physiotherapist. Physiother Can 1990; 2:75–79.

Speechley M, Tinetti M. Falls and injuries in frail and vigorous community elderly persons. J Am Geriatr Soc 1991; 39:46–52.

Sperle PA, Ottenbacher KJ, Braun SL, Lane SJ, Nochajski S. Equivalence reliability of the functional independence measure for children (WeeFIM) administration methods. Am J Occup Ther 1997; 51(1): 35–41.

Spielberg PI. Walking patterns of old people: cyclographic analysis. In: Bernstein NA, ed. Investigations on the biodynamics of walking, running, and jumping. Moscow: Central Scientific Institute of Physical Culture, 1940.

Spirduso W. Physical dimensions of aging. Champaign, IL: Human Kinetics, 1995.

Squire LR. Mechanisms of memory. Science 1986; 232:1612–1619.

Steenbergen B, Hulstijn W, Lemmens IHL, Meulenbroek RGJ. The timing of prehensile movements in subjects with cerebral palsy. Dev Med Child Neurol 1998; 40:108–114.

Stehouwer DJ, Farel PB. Development of hindlimb locomotor behavior in the frog. Dev Psychobiol 1984; 17:217–232.

Stein DG, Brailowsky S, Will B. Brain repair. New York: Oxford, 1995.

Stein RB. Reflex modulation during locomotion: functional significance. In: Patla A, ed. Adaptability of human gait. Amsterdam: North Holland, 1991: 21–36.

Steindler A. Kinesiology of the human body under normal and pathological conditions. Springfield, IL: CC Thomas, 1955.

Steinfeld EH, Danford GS. Environment as a mediating factor in functional assessment. In: Dittmar SS, Gresham GE, eds. Functional assessment and outcome measures for the rehabilitation health professional. Gaithersburg, MD: Aspen, 1997:37–56.

Stephens JM, Goldie PA. Walking speed on parquetry and carpet after stroke: effect of surface and retest reliability. Clin Rehabil 1999; 13(2):171–181.

Stern EB. Stability of the Jebsen-Taylor hand function test across three test sessions. Am J Occup Ther 1992; 7:647–649.

Stern EB. Volumetric comparison of seated and standing test postures. Am J Occup Ther 1991; 801–805.

Stern GM, Franklyn SE, Imms FJ, Prestidge SP. Quantitative assessments of gait and mobility in Parkinson's disease. J Neural Transm Park Dis Dement Sect 1983; 19:201–214.

Stern GM, Lander DM, Lee AJ. Akinetic freezing and trick movements in Parkinson's disease. J Neural Tranm 1980; 16(suppl):137–141.

Steward O. Reorganization of neuronal connections following CNS trauma: principles and experimental paradigms. J Neurotrauma 1989; 6:99–151.

Stockmyer S. An interpretation of the approach of Rood to the treatment of neuromuscular dysfunction. Am J Phys Med 1967; 46:950–955.

Stoffregen TA, Adolph K, Thelen T, et al. Toddlers' postural adaptations to different support surfaces. Motor Control 1997; 1:119–137.

Strick PL. Anatomical organization of multiple areas of frontal lobe: implications for recovery of function. Adv Neurol 1988;47:293–312.

Stone JH. Sensibility. In: Casanova J , ed. Clinical Assessment Recommendations, 1992:71–84.

Strub RL, Black FW. The Mental Status Examination in Neurology. Philadelphia: FA Davis, 1977.

Studenski S, Duncan PW, Chandler J. Postural responses and effector factors in persons with unexplained falls: results and methodologic issues. J Am Geriatr Soc 1991; 39:229–234.

Sudarsky L, Ronthal M. Gait disorders among elderly patients: a survey study of 50 patients. Arch Neurol 1983; 40:740–743.

Sudarsky L, Ronthal M. Gait disorders in the elderly: assessing the risk for falls. In: Vellas B, Toupet M, Rubenstein L, et al., eds. Falls, balance and gait disorders in the elderly. Amsterdam: Elsevier, 1992:117–127.

Sugden DA. Movement speed in children. J Motor Behav 1980; 12:125–132.

Sunderland A. Recovery of ipsilateral dexterity after stroke. Stroke 2000; 31(2):430–433.

Sundermier L, Woollacott M, Jensen J, Moore S. Postural sensitivity to visual flow in aging adults with and without balance problems. J Gerontol 1996; 51:M45–52.

Sundermier L, Woollacott M, Roncesvalles J, Jensen J. The development of balance control in children: Comparisons of EMG and kinetic variables, and chronological and developmental groupings. Exp Brain Res (in press).

Sur M, Pallas SL, Roe AW. Cross-modal plasticity in cortical development: differentiation and specification of sensory neocortex. Trends Neurosci 1990; 13:227–233.

Surberg PR. Aging and effect of physical-mental practice upon acquisition and retention of a motor skill. J Gerontol 1976; 31:64–67.

Sutherland DH, Olshen R, Cooper L, Woo S. The development of mature gait. J Bone Joint Surg 1980; 62A:336–353.

Suzuki E, Chen W, Kondo T. Measuring unilateral spatial during stepping. Arch Phys Med Rehabil 1997; 78:173–178.

Suzuki K, Yamada Y, Handa T, et al. Relationship between stride length and walking rate in gait training for hemiparetic stroke patients. Am J Phys Med Rehabil 1999; 78:147–152.

Svantesson U, Osterverg U, Grimby G, Sunnerhagen KS. The standing heel-rise test in patients with upper motor neuron lesion due to stroke. Scand J Rehabil Med 1998; 30:73–80.

Sveistrup H, Massion J, Moore S, et al. Are there differences in postural support strategies for simple balance tasks vs. tasks requiring precise hand stabilization? Neurosci Abstr 1991; 17:1388.

Sveistrup H, Woollacott MH. Longitudinal development of the automatic postural response in infants. J Motor Behav 1996; 28:58–70.

Sveistrup H, Woollacott M. Can practice modify the developing automatic postural response? Exp Brain Res 1997; 114:33–43.

Swanson AB, Goran-Hagert C, Swanson, GD. Evaluation of impairment of hand function. In: Hunter JM, Schneider LH, Mackin EJ, Bell JA, eds. Rehabilitation of the Hand. St. Louis: CV Mosby, 1978:31–69.

Sweatt JD, Kandel ER. Persistent and transcriptionally-dependent increase in protein phosphorylation in long-term facilitation of Aplysia sensory neurons. Nature 1989; 339:51–54.

Taguchi K, Tada C. Change of body sway with growth of children. In: Amblard B, Berthoz A, Clarac F, eds. Posture and gait: development, adaptation and modulation. Amsterdam: Elsevier, 1988:59–65.

Taira M, Milne S, Georgopoulos AP, et al. Parietal cortex neurons of the monkey related to the visual guidance of hand movement. Exp Brain Res 1990; 83:29–36.

Takebe D, Kukulka C, Narayan G, et al. Peroneal nerve stimulator in rehabilitation of hemiplegic patients. Arch Phys Med Rehabil 1975; 56:237–239.

Takahashi M, Hoshikawa H, Tjujita N, Akiyama I. Effect of labyrinthine dysfunction upon head oscillation and gaze during stepping and running. Acta Otolaryngol Stockh 1988; 106:348–353.

Tang PF, Woollacott MH. Inefficient postural responses to unexpected slips during walking in older adults. J Gerontol 1998; 53:M471–M480.

Tang PF, Woollacott MH. Phase-dependent modulation of proximal and distal postural responses to slips in young and older adults. J Gerontol 1999; 54: M89–M102.

Tang PF, Woollacott MH, Chong RKY. Control of reactive balance adjustments in perturbed human walking: roles of proximal and distal postural muscle activity. Exp Brain Res 1998; 119:141–152.

Tardieu C, Lespargot A, Tabary C, Bret MD. For how long must the soleus muscle be stretched each day to prevent contrature? Dev Med Child Neurol 1988; 30(1):3–10.

Tatton WG, Bedingham V, Verrier MC, et al. Defective utilization of sensory inputs as the basis for bradykinesia, rigidity, and decreased movement repertoire in Parkinson's disease: a hypothesis. Can J Neurol Sci 1984; 11:136–143.

Taub E, Wolf S. Constraint-induced movement techniques to facilitate upper extremity use in stroke patients. Topics Stroke Rehab 1997; 3(4):38–61.

Taub E. Motor behavior following deafferentation in the developing and motorically mature monkey. In: Herman S, Grillner R, Ralston HJ, et al., eds. Neural control of locomotion. New York: Plenum, 1976; 675–705.

Taub E. Some anatomical observations following chronic dorsal rhizotomy in monkeys. Neuroscience 1980; 5:389–401.

Taub E. Technique to improve chronic motor deficit after stroke. Arch Phys Med Rehabil 1993; 74:347–354.

Taub E, Berman AJ. Movement and learning in the absence of sensory feedback. In: Freedman SJ, ed. The neurophysiology of spatially oriented behavior. Homewood, NJ: Dorsey, 1968:173–192.

Taub E, Goldberg IA, Taub P. Deafferentation in monkeys: Pointing at a target without visual feedback. Exp Neurol 1975; 46:176–186.

Taub E, Miller NE, Novack TA, et al. Technique to improve chronic motor deficit after stroke. Arch Phys Med Rehabil 1993; 74:347–354.

Taub E, Miller NE, Novack TA. Technique to improve chronic motor deficit after stroke. Arch Phys Med Rehabil 1993; 74:347–354.

Taylor N, Sand PL, Jebsen RH. Evaluation of hand function in children. Arch Phys Med Rehabil 1973; 54(3):129–135.

Teasdale N, Bard C, LaRue J, Fleury M. On the cognitive penetrability of postural control. Exper Aging Res 1993; 19:1–13.

Teasdale N, Stelmach GE, Breunig A. Postural sway characteristics of the elderly under normal and altered visual and support surface conditions. J Gerontol 1991; 46:B238–B244.

Teixeira-Salmela LF, Olney SJ, Nadeau S, Brouwer B. Muscle strengthening and physical conditioning to reduce impairment and disability in chronic stroke survivors. Arch Phys Med Rehabil 1999; 80: 1211–1218.

Tessier-Lavigne M. Phototransduction and information processing in the retina. In: Kandel E, Schwartz JH, Jessell TM, eds. Principles of neuroscience. 3rd ed. New York: Elsevier, 1991:400–417.

Teulings H, Contreras-Vidal JL, Stelmach GE, Adler CH. Parkinsonism reduces coordination of fingers, wrist, and arm in fine motor control. Exp Neurol 1997; 146:159–170.

Thach WT. Correlation of neural discharge with pattern and force of muscular activity, joint position and direction of intended next movement in motor cortex and cerebellum. J Neurophysiol 1978; 41:654–676.

Thelen DG, Schultz AB, Alexander NB, Ashton-Miller JA. Effects of age on rapid ankle torque development. J Gerontol Med Sci 1996; 51:M226–232.

Thelen E, Corbetta D, Kamm K, et al. The transition to reaching: mapping intention and intrinsic dynamics. Child Dev 1993; 64:1058–1098.

Thelen E, Fisher DM. Newborn stepping: an explanation for a disappearing reflex. Dev Psychol 1982; 18:760–775.

Thelen E, Fisher DM, Ridley-Johnson R. The relationship between physical growth and a newborn reflex. Infant Behav Dev 1984; 7:479–493.

Thelen E, Kelso JAS, Fogel A. Self-organizing systems and infant motor development. Dev Rev 1987; 7:39–65.

Thelen E, Spencer JP. Postural control during reaching in young infants: a dynamic systems approach. Neurosci Biobehav Rev 1998; 22:507–514.

Thelen E, Ulrich BD. Hidden skills: a dynamic systems analysis of treadmill stepping during the first year. Monographs of the Society for Research in Child Development. Serial 223, vol 56, 1991.

Thelen E, Ulrich, BD, Jensen JL. The developmental origins of locomotion. In: Woollacott MH, Shumway-Cook A, eds. Development of posture and gait across the life span. Columbia: University of South Carolina, 1989:25–47.

Thilmann AF, Fellows SJ, Garms E. The mechanism of spastic muscle hypertonus. Brain 1991; 114: 233–244.

Thomas RL, Williams AK, Lundy-Ekman L. Supine to stand in elderly persons: relationship to age, activity level, strength and range of motion. Issues Aging 1998; 21:9–18.

Thorstensson A, Roberthson H. Adaptations to changing speed in human locomotion: speed of transition between walking and running. Acta Physiol Scand 1987; 131:211–214.

Tiffin J. Purdue Pegboard Examiner Manual. Chicago: Science Research Associates, 1968.

Timiras P. Aging of the skeleton, joints and muscles. In: Timiras PS, ed. Physiological basis of aging and geriatrics. 2nd ed. Ann Arbor, MI: CRS, 1994.

Tinetti ME. Performance oriented assessment of mobility problems in elderly patients. J Am Geriatr Soc 1986; 34:119–126.

Tinetti ME, Ginter SF. Identifying mobility dysfunctions in elderly patients: standard neuromuscular examination or direct assessment? JAMA 1988; 259: 1190–1193.

Tinetti ME, Richman D, Powell L. Falls efficacy as a measure of fear of falling. J Gerontol 1990; 45:P239-P243.

Tinetti ME, Speechley M, Ginter SF. Risk factors for falls among elderly persons living in the community. N Engl J Med 1988; 319:1701–1707.

Tinetti ME, Williams TF, Mayewski R. Fall risk index for elderly patients based on numbers of chronic disabilities. Am J Med 1986; 80:429–434.

Titus MND, Gall NG, Yerxa EJ, Robertson TA, Mack W. Correlation of perceptual performance and activities of daily living in stroke patients. Am J Occup Ther 1991; 45:410–418.

Tizard JPM, Paine RS, Crothers B. Disturbances of sensation in children with hemiplegia. JAMA 1954; 155:628–632.

Tobis JS, Lowenthal M. Evaluation and management of the brain damaged patient. Springfield IL: Charles C. Thomas, 1960.

Tokizane T, Murao M, Ogata T, Kordo T. Electromyographic studies on tonic neck, lumbar and labyrinthine reflexes in normal persons. Jpn J Physiol 1951; 2:130–146.

Toupet M, Gagey PM, Heuschen S. Vestibular patients and aging subjects lose use of visual input and expend more energy in static postural control. In: Vellas B, Toupet M, Rubenstein L, et al., eds. Falls, balance and gait disorders in the elderly. Paris: Elsevier, 1992:183–198.

Touwen B. Neurological development in infancy. Clinics in Developmental Medicine 58. Philadelphia: JB Lippincott, 1976.

Travis AM, Woolsey CN. Motor performance of monkeys after bilateral partial and total cerebral decortication. Am J Phys Med 1956; 35:273–310.

Treisman A. Features and objects: the fourteenth Bartlett Memorial Lecture. J. Exp Psychol 1988; 40A:201–237.

Trombly C. Anticipating the future: Assessment of occupational function. Am J Occup Ther 1993; 47(3):253–257.

Trombly C , Scott AD. Evaluation and treatment of somatosensory sensation. In: CA Trombly, ed. Occupational Therapy for Physical Disabilities. Baltimore: Williams & Wilkins, 1989:41–54.

Trombly CA. Theoretical foundations for practice. In: Tromby CA, ed. Occupational therapy for physical dysfunction. 4th ed. Baltimore: Williams & Wilkins, 1995:15–28.

Turton A, Wroe S, Trepte N, Fraser C, Lemon RN. Contralateral and ipsilateral EMG responses to transcranial magnetic stimulation during recovery of arm and hand function after stroke. Electroencephalogr Clin Neurophysiol. 1996 Aug;101(4):316–28.

Twitchell T. Reflex mechanisms and the development of prehension. In: Connolly K, ed. Mechanisms of motor skill development. New York: Academic, 1970.

Tyson SF. The support taken through walking aids during hemiplegic gait. Clin Rehabil 1998; 12:395–401.

Ungerleider LG, Brody BA. Extrapersonal spatial orientation: the role of posterior parietal, anterior frontal, and inferotemporal cortex. Exp Neurol 1977; 56:265–280.

Van Donkelaar P, Lee RG. Interactions between the eye and hand motor systems: disruptions due to cerebellar dysfunction. J Neurophysiol 1994; 72: 1674–1684.

Van Heest A, House J, Putnam M. Sensibility deficiencies in the hands of children with spastic hemiplegia, J Hand Surg Am 1993; 18:278.

VanSant AF. Concepts of neural organization and movement. In: Connolly BH, Montgomery PC, eds. Therapeutic exercise in developmental disabilities. Chattanooga, TN: Chattanooga Corp., 1987:1–8.

VanSant AF. Age differences in movement patterns used by children to rise from a supine position to erect stance. Phys Ther 1988a;68:1130–1138.

VanSant AF. Rising from a supine position to erect stance: description of adult movement and a developmental hypothesis. Phys Ther 1988b;68:185–192.

VanSant AF. Life-span development in functional tasks. Phys Ther 1990; 70:788–798.

van Woerkom TC, Minderhoud JM, Gottschal T, Micolai G. Neurotransmitters in the treatment of patients with severe head injuries. Eur Neurol 1982; 21:227–234.

Vaughan CL, Sussman MD. Human gait: From clinical interpretation to computer simulation. In: Grabiner MD, ed. Current issues in biomechanics. Champaign. IL: Human Kinetics, 1993:53–68.

Verbrugge L, Jette A. The disablement process. Soc Sci Med 1994; 38:1–14.

Vercher JL, Gauthier GM, Guedon O, et al. Self-moved target eye tracking in control and deafferented subjects: roles of arm motor command and proprioception in arm-eye coordination. J Neurophysiol 1996; 76:1133–1144.

Vereijken B, van Emmerik REA, Whiting HTA, Newell KM. Freezing degrees of freedom in skill acquisition. J Motor Behav 1992; 24:133–142.

Vinter A. Manual imitations and reaching behaviors: an illustration of action control in infancy. In: Bard C, Fleury M, Hay L, eds. Development of eye-hand coordination across the lifespan. Columbia: University of South Carolina 1990:157–187.

Vinogrand A, Taylor E, Grossmand S. Sensory retraining of the hemiplegic hand. Am J Occup Ther 1962; 5:246–256.

Voss D, Ionata M, Myers B. Proprioceptive Neuromuscular Facilitation: Patterns and Techniques. 3rd ed. Philadelphia: Harper & Row, 1985.

Vrtunski PB, Patterson MB. Psychomotor decline can be described by discontinuities in response trajectories. Int J Neurosci 1985; 27:265–275.

Vygotsky LS. Mind in Society: The Development of Higher Psychological Processes. Cambridge, MA: Harvard University Press, 1978.

Waagfjord J, Levangle PK, Certo CME. Effects of treadmill training on gait in a hemiparetic patient. Phys Ther 1990; 70:549–558.

Wade MG, Lindquist R, Taylor JR, Treat-Jacobson D. Optical flow, spatial orientation, and the control of posture in the elderly. J Gerontol 1995; 50B:P51-P58.

Wadsworth PT, Krishman R. Intrarater reliability of manual muscle testing and hand held dynamometric muscle testing. Physiological Review 1987; 67:1342–1347.

Wagenaar RC, Beek WJ. Hemiplegic gait: a kinematic analysis using walking speed as a basis. J Biomech 1992; 25:1007–1015.

Waksvik K, Levy R. An approach to seating for the cerebral palsied. Can J Occup Ther 1979; 46:147–152.

Walker-Batson D, Smith P, Unwin H, et al. Use of amphetamine in the treatment of aphasia. Restor Neurol Neurosci 1992; 4:47–50.

Wallace SA, Weeks DL, Kelso JAS. Temporal constraints in reaching and grasping behavior. Hum Mov Sci 1990; 9:69–93.

Wallen P. Cellular bases of locomotor behaviour in lamprey: coordination and modulatory control of spinal circuitry. In: WR Ferrell, U Proske, eds. Neural control of movement. New York: Plenum, 1995: 125–133.

Wanning T. Healing and the mind/body arts: massage, acupuncture, yoga, t'ai chi, and Feldenkrais. AAOHN J 1993; 41(7):349–511.

Warburg CL. Assessment and treatment planning strategies for perceptual deficits. In: O'Sullivan S, Schmitz T. Physical rehabilitation: assessment and treatment. 2nd ed. Philadelphia: FA Davis, 1994.

Warren WH Jr. Self-motion: visual perception and visual content. In: Epstein W, Rogers S, eds. Handbook of perception and cognition, vol 5: Perception of space and motion. New York: Academic, 1995:263–325.

Warren WH, Blackwell AW, Morris MW. Age differences in perceiving the direction of self-motion from optical flow. J Gerontol 1989; 44:P147-P153.

Wartenberg R. Pendulousness of the legs as a diagnostic test. Neurology 1951; 1:8–24.

Waters RL. Energy expenditure. In: Perry J. Gait analysis: normal and pathological function. Thorofare, NJ: Slack, 1992.

Waters RL, Lunsford BR, Perry J, Byrd R. Energy-speed relationship of walking: standard tables. J Orthop Res 1988; 6:215–222.

Waters R, McNeal DR. Tasto J. Peroneal nerve conduction velocity after chronic electrical stimulation. Arch Phys Med Rehabil 1975; 56:240–243.

Waters RL, Wilson DJ, Savinelli R. Rehabilitation of the upper extremity following stroke. In: Hunter J, Schneider LH, Mackin EJ, Bell JA, eds. Rehabilitation of the hand. St. Louis: Mosby, 1978; 505–520.

Weil MJ, Cunningham Amundson SJ. Relationship between visuomotor and handwriting skills of children in kindergarten. Am J Occup Ther 1995; 48(11):982–988.

Weiller C, Chollet F, Friston KJ, et al. Functional reorganization of the brain in recovery from striato-capsular infarction in man. Ann Neurol 1992; 31: 463–472.

Weiller C, Ramsay SC, Wise RJS, et al. Individual patterns of functional reorganization in the human cerebral cortex after capsular infarction. Ann Neurol 1993; 33:181–189.

Weinstein Enhanced Sensory Test (WEST). Connecticut: Bioinstruments, Inc.

Weinstein S. Fifty years of somatosensory research: from the Semmes-Weinstein monofilaments to the Weinstein Enhanced Sensory Test. J Hand Ther 1993; 6:11–22.

Weiskrantz L, Warrington ER, Sanders MD, Marshall J. Visual capacity in the hemianopic field following a restricted occipital ablation. Brain 1974; 97: 709–728.

Weisz S. Studies in equilibrium reaction. J Nerv Ment Dis 1938; 88:150–162.

Welford AT. Motor performance. In: Birren G, Schaie K, eds. Handbook of the psychology of aging. New York: Van Nostrand Reinhold, 1977:3–20.

Welford AT. Motor skills and aging. In: Mortimer J, Pirozzolo FJ, Maletta G, eds. The aging motor system. New York: Praeger, 1982:152–187.

Werner W, Dannenberg S, Hoffman KP. Arm-movement-related neurons in the primate superior colliculus and underlying reticular formation: comparison of neuronal activity with EMGs of muscles of the shoulder, arm and trunk during reaching. Exp Brain Res 1997; 115:191–205.

Westling G, Johansson RS. Factors influencing the force control during precision grip. Exp Brain Res 1984; 53:277–284.

Whanger A, Wang HS. Clinical correlates of the vibratory sense in elderly psychiatric patients. J Gerontol 1974; 29:39–45.

Whipple RH, Wolfson LI, Amerman PM. The relationship of knee and ankle weakness to falls in nursing home residents: an isokinetic study. J Am Geriatr Soc 1987; 35:13–20.

White BL, Castle P, Held R. Observations on the development of visually-directed reaching. Child Dev 1964; 35:349–364.

Wiener-Vacher SR, Toupet F, Narcy P. Canal and otolith vestibulo-ocular reflexes to vertical and off vertical axis rotations in children learning to walk. Acta Otolaryngol Stockh 1996; 116:657–665.

Wiley ME, Damiano DL. Lower-extremity strength profiles in spastic cerebral palsy. Dev Med Child Neurol 1998; 40:100–107.

Williams H. Aging and eye-hand coordination. In: Bard C, Fleury M, Hay L, eds. Development of eye-hand coordination across the lifespan. Columbia: University of South Carolina, 1990:327–357.

Williamson GL, Leiper CI, Mayer NH. Beaver College

Assessment of speed and accuracy of movement in older adults using Fitts' tapping test. Neurosci Abstr 1993; 19:556.

Wilson DM. The central nervous control of flight in a locust. J Exp Biol 1961; 38:471–490.

Wing AM, Allison S, Jenner JR. Retaining and retraining balance after stroke. Ballieres Clin Neurol 1993; 2:87–120.

Wing AM, Frazer C. The contribution of the thumb to reaching movements. Q J Exp Psychol 1983; 35A:297–309.

Winograd CH, Lemsky CM, Nevitt MC, et al. Development of a physical performance and mobility examination. J Am Geriatr Soc 1994; 42:743–749.

Winstein CJ. Designing practice for motor learning: clinical implications. Contemporary management of motor control problems. Proceedings of the II Step Conference. Alexandria, VA: APTA, 1991.

Winstein C, Gardner ER, McNeal DR, et al. Standing balance training: effect on balance and locomotion in hemiparetic adults. Arch Phys Med Rehabil 1989; 70:755–762.

Winstein CJ, Pohl PS. Effects of unilateral brain damage on the control of goal directed hand movements. Exp Brain Res 1995; 105:163–174.

Winstein CJ, Schmidt RA. Reduced frequency of knowledge of results enhances motor skill learning. J Exp Psychol Learn Memory Cogn 1990; 16:677–691.

Winter DA. Overall principle of lower limb support during stance phase of gait. J Biomech 1980; 13: 923–927.

Winter DA. Biomechanical motor patterns in normal walking. J Motor Behav 1983; 15:302–330.

Winter DA. Kinematic and kinetic patterns of human gait: variability and compensating effects. Hum Mov Sci 1984; 3:51–76.

Winter DA. Biomechanics and motor control of human movement. New York: Wiley, 1990:80–84.

Winter DA. Knowledge base for diagnostic gait assessment. Med Prog Tech 1993; 19:61–81.

Winter DA, McFadyen BJ, Dickey JP. Adaptability of the CNS in human walking. In: Patla AE, ed. Adaptability of human gait. Amsterdam: Elsevier, 1991: 127–144.

Winter DA, Patla AE, Frank JS, Walt SE. Biomechanical walking pattern changes in the fit and healthy elderly. Phys Ther 1990; 70:340–347.

Winter DA, Prince F, Steriou P, Powell C. Medial-lateral and anterior-posterior motor responses associated with centre of pressure changes in quiet standing. Neurosci Res Commun 1993; 12:141–148.

Wise SD, Evarts EV. The role of the cerebral cortex on movement. Trends Neurosci 1981; 4:297–300.

Wisleder D, Zernicke RF, Smith JL. Speed-related changes in hindlimb intersegmental dynamics during the swing phase of cat locomotion. Exp Brain Res 1990; 79: 651–660.

Wolf SL, Barnhart HX, Kutner NG, et al. Reducing frailty and falls in older persons: An investigation of Tai Chi and computerized balance training. J Am Geriatr Soc 1996; 44:489–497.

Wolf S, Kutner N, Green R, et al. The Atlanta FICSIT Study: Two exercise interventions to reduce frailty in elders. J Am Geriatr Soc 1993:41:329–332.

Wolf SL, LeCraw DE, Barton LA. Comparison of motor copy and targeted biofeedback training techniques for restitution of upper extremity function among patients with neurologic disorders. Phys Ther 1989a;69:719–735.

Wolf SL, Lecraw DE, Barton LA, Jann BB. Forced use of hemiplegic upper extremities to reverse the effect of learned nonuse among chronic stroke and head injured patients. Exp Neurol 1989b;104(2):125–132.

Wolfson L, Whipple R, Amerman P, et al. Gait and balance in the elderly. Clin Geriatr Med 1985; 1:649–659.

Wolfson L, Whipple R, Amerman P, Tobin JN. Gait assessment in the elderly: a gait abnormality rating scale and its relation to falls. J Gerontol 1990; 45:M12–M19.

Wolfson L et al. A dynamic posturography study of balance in healthy elderly. Neurology 1992; 42: 2069–2075.

Wolfson L, Judge J, Whipple R, King M. Strength is a major factor in balance, gait and the occurrence of falls. J Geronotol 1995; 50A:64–67.

Wolfson L, Whipple R, Derby C, et al. Balance strength training in older adults: Intervention gains and Tai Chi maintenance. J Am Geriatr Soc 1996; 44: 498–506.

Wong DL, Baker CM. Pain in hildren: Comparison of assessment scales. Pediatr Nurs 1988; 14:9–17.

Woo SLV, Matthews JV, Akerson WH, et al. Connective tissue response to immobility. Arthritis Rheum 1975; 18:257–264.

Woods BT. The restricted effects of right hemispheric lesions after age one: Wechsler test data. Neuropsychologia 1980; 18:65–70.

Woollacott M. Gait and postural control in the aging adult. In: Bles W, Brandt T, eds. Disorders of posture and gait. Amsterdam: Elsevier, 1986:325–336.

Woollacott M. Aging, posture control and movement preparation. In: Woollacott MH, Shumway-Cook A, eds. Development of posture and gait across the life span. Columbia: University of South Carolina, 1989:155–175.

Woollacott M, Burtner P, Jensen J, Jasiewicz J, et al. Development of postural responses during standing in healthy children and in children with spastic diplegia. Neurosci Biobehav Rev 1998; 22:583–589.

Woollacott M, Debu B, Mowatt M. Neuromuscular control of posture in the infant and child: is vision dominant? J Motor Behav 1987; 19:167–186.

Woollacott MH, Jensen J. Posture and locomotion. In: H Heuer, S Keele, eds. Handbook of perception and action, vol 2. New York: Academic, 1996:333–403.

Woollacott M, Moore S, Hu MH. Improvements in balance in the elderly through training sensory organization abilities. In: GE Stelmach, V Homberg, eds. Sensorimotor impairment in the elderly. Dordrecht: Kluwer, 1993:377–392.

Woollacott M, Roseblad B, Hofsten von C. Relation between muscle response onset and body segmental movements during postural perturbations in humans. Exp Brain Res 1988; 72:593–604.

Woollacott M, Shumway-Cook A. The development of the postural and voluntary motor control system in Down's syndrome children. In: Wade M, ed. Motor skill acquisition of the mentally handicapped: issues in research and training. Amsterdam: Elsevier, 1986:45–71.

Woollacott M, Shumway-Cook A. Changes in posture control across the life span: a systems approach. Phys Ther 1990; 70:799–807.

Woollacott M, Shumway-Cook A. Clinical research methodology for the study of posture and balance. In: JC Masdeu, L Sudarsky, L Wolfson, eds. Gait disorders of aging: falls and therapeutic strategies. Philadelphia: Lippincott-Raven, 1997:107–121.

Woollacott MH, Shumway-Cook A, Nashner L. Aging and posture control: changes in sensory organization and muscular coordination. Int J Aging Hum Dev 1986; 23:97–114.

Woollacott M, Shumway-Cook A, Williams H. The development of posture and balance control. In: Woollacott MH, Shumway-Cook A, eds. Development of posture and gait across the life span. Columbia: University of South Carolina, 1989:77–96.

Woollacott MH, Sundermier L. Postural sensitivity to visual flow in older adults: Electromyographic responses. J Gerontol (Submitted).

Woollacott MH, Sveistrup H. Changes in the sequencing and timing of muscle response coordination associated with developmental transitions in balance abilities. Hum Mov Sci 1992; 11:23–36.

Woollacott M, Tang PF, Lin SI. Dynamic balance control in older adults: does limited response capacity lead to falls? In: GN Gantchev, S Mori, J Massion, eds. Motor control, today and tomorrow. Sophia, Bulgaria: Academic Publishing House Prof. Marin Drinov, 1999:293–305.

Wright DL, Kemp TL. The dual-task methodology and assessing the attentional demands of ambulation with walking devices. Phys Ther 1992; 72:306–315.

Wu C, Trombly CA, Lin K, Tickle-Degnen L. Effects of object affordances on reaching in persons with and without cerebrovascular accident. Am J Occup Ther 1998; 52(6):447–456.

von Wright JM. A note on the role of "guidance" in learning. Br J Psychol 1957; 48:133–137.

Yan K, Fang J, Shahani BT. Motor unit discharge behaviors in stroke patients. Muscle Nerve 1998a;21: 1502–1506.

Yan K, Fang J, Shahani BT. An assessment of motor unit discharge patterns in stroke patients using surface electromyographic technique. Muscle Nerve 1998a;21:946–947.

Yasukawa A. Upper extremity casting: adjunct for a child with cerebral palsy hemiplegia. J Occup Ther 1990; 4:840–846.

Yasukawa A. Upper-extremity casting: adjunct treatment for the child with cerebral palsy. In: Case-Smith J, Pehoski C, eds. Development of Hand Skills in Children. Rockville, MD: American Occupational Therapy Association, 1992:111–123.

Young A. Exercise physiology in geriatric practice. Acta Scand 1986; 711(Suppl):227–232.

Yu BP, Masossro EJ, McMahan CA. Nutritional influences on aging of Fischer 344 rats: 1. Physical, metabolic and longevity characteristics. J Gerontol 1985; 40:657–670.

Zancolli EA, Goldner LJ, Swanson AB. Surgery of the spastic hand in cerebral palsy: Report of the committee on spastic hand evaluation. J Hand Surg 1983; 8:776–772.

Zarro VJ. Mechanisms of inflammation and repair. In: Michlovitz SL, ed. Thermal Agents in Rehabilitation. Philadelphia: FA Davis, 1986.

Zarrugh MY, Todd FN, Ralston HJ. Optimization of energy expenditure during level walking. Eur J Appl Physiol 1974; 33:293–306.

Zee DS. Vertigo. Curr Ther Neurol Dis 1985; 1–13.

Zeller W. Konstitution und Entwicklung. Gottingen: Verlag fur Psychologic, 1964.

Zihl J, Werth R. Contributions to the study of "blindsight": 2. The role of specific practice for saccadic localization in patients with postgeniculate visual field defects. Neuropsychologia 1984; 22:13–22.

Zizlis J. Splinting of the hand in a spastic hemiplegic patients. Arch Phys Med Rehabil 1964; 1:41–43.

Action potential—the dramatic jump in voltage across the cell membrane that is observed when a neuron is excited.

Adaptation requirement—one of the three major requirements for successful locomotion, reflecting the ability to adapt gait to meet the goals of the animal and the demands of the environment.

Adaptive postural control—modifying sensory and motor systems in response to changing task and environmental demands.

Agnosia—the inability to recognize. Lesions in the parietal lobe often cause agnosia or neglect of the contralateral side of the body, objects, and drawings.

Alpha-motor neurons—motor neurons within the spinal cord that innervate skeletal muscle fibers.

Anticipatory postural control—pretuning sensory and motor systems in expectation of postural demands based on previous experience and learning.

Assessment—the systematic acquisition of information that is relevant and meaningful in providing the clinician with a comprehensive picture of the patient's abilities and problems.

Associative stage—in the Fitts-Posner description of motor learning, this is the second stage. By this time, the person has selected the best strategy for the task and begins to refine the skill.

Asymmetrical tonic neck reflex—A reflex that produces a change in the position of the arms in response to change in head position. Turning the head produces extension in the face arm and flexion in the skull arm.

Autonomous stage—in the Fitts-Posner description of motor learning, this is the third stage. In this stage, there is automaticity in the skill, and a low degree of attention is required for its performance.

Body-on-body righting reaction—a mechanism that keeps the body oriented with respect to the ground regardless of the position of the head.

Body-on-head righting reaction—a mechanism that orients the head in response to proprioceptive and tactile signals from the body in contact with a supporting surface.

Cadence—the number of steps per unit of time, usually reported as steps per minute.

Classical conditioning—a form of association learning. An initially weak stimulus (the conditioned stimulus) becomes highly effective in producing a response when it becomes associated with another stronger stimulus (the unconditioned stimulus). After repeated pairing of the conditioned and the unconditioned stimulus, one begins to see a conditioned response to the conditioned stimulus.

Clinical decision-making process—a procedure for gathering information essential to developing a plan of care consistent with the problems and needs of the patient.

Closed-loop process—motor control processing in which sensory feedback is used for the ongoing production of skilled movement.

Cognitive processes—in this book, a broad category including high-level neural processes, such as planning, attention, motivation, and emotional aspects of motor control that underlie the establishment of intent or goals. It is difficult to make a distinction between higher-level perceptual/motor processing and cognitive processing, since there is a gradual transition and overlap between the processing levels.

Cognitive stage—in the Fitts-Posner description of motor learning, this is the first stage in the process. In it, the learner is concerned with understanding the nature of the task, developing strategies that can be used to carry out the task, and determining how the task should be evaluated.

Compensation—behavioral substitution, that is, alternative behavioral strategies adopted to complete a task.

Conceptual framework—a logical structure that helps the clinician organize clinical practices related to assessment and treatment into a cohesive and comprehensive plan.

Coordinative structure—neural commands that are temporally grouped so that signals are sent to muscles in a coherent fashion. This reduces the degrees of freedom to be controlled by the nervous system by constraining groups of muscles to act within functionally coherent units (the term synergy is often used as a synonym).

Decerebrate locomotor preparation—animal experimental preparation that leaves the spinal cord, brainstem, and cerebellum intact. An area in the brainstem called the mesencephalic locomotor region appears to be important in the descending control of locomotion. Decerebrate cats do not normally walk on a treadmill but begin to walk normally when tonic electrical stimulation is applied to the mesencephalic locomotor region.

Declarative learning—The process of learning knowledge that can be consciously recalled and thus requires processes such as awareness, attention, and reflection.

Decorticate locomotor preparation—animal experimental preparation with only the cerebral cortex removed. In this preparation, an external stimulus is not required to produce locomotor behavior, and the behavior is reasonably normal goal-directed behavior.

Degrees of freedom problem—a motor control problem involving how to control the many joints and muscles of the body.

Denervation supersensitivity—response that occurs when neurons show a loss of input from another brain region. The postsynaptic membrane of a neuron becomes hyperactive to a released transmitter substance.

Distributed practice—a training session in which the amount of rest between trials equals or is greater than the amount of time for a trial.

Excitatory postsynaptic potential (EPSP)—the change in membrane potential in the postsynaptic cell (typically depolarizing) made by the excitatory transmitter substance released from the presynaptic neuron.

Excitatory summation—outcome that occurs when a series of excitatory postsynaptic potentials continue to build up depolarization to the threshold voltage for the action potential in the next neuron.

Extrinsic feedback—information that supplements intrinsic feedback, such as when you tell a patient that he or she needs to pick up his or her foot higher to clear an object while walking.

Flexor withdrawal reflex—a cutaneous reflex caused by a sharp focal stimulus producing withdrawal, or flexion, and causing protection from injury. The typical pattern of response is ipsilateral flexion and contralateral extension, which allow the support of body weight on the opposite limb. The reflex is mediated by group III and IV afferents.

Forced-use paradigm—a therapeutic approach in which hemiplegic patients are forced to use their hemiplegic arm (the intact side is restrained) to facilitate the return of function in that arm.

Frozen gait pattern—a gait pattern of patients with Parkinson's disease characterized by an inability to generate sufficient momentum, so that forward progression is arrested.

Gamma-motor neurons—motor neurons from the spinal cord that innervate the muscle spindle muscle fibers.

General static reactions (called attitudinal reflexes)—changes in position of the whole body in response to changes in head position.

Glabrous skin—hairless skin.

Habituation—a decrease in responsiveness that occurs as a result of repeated exposure to a nonpainful stimulus (see synaptic defacilitation).

Intrafusal muscle fibers—Specialized muscle fibers found in muscle spindles (extrafusal fibers are normal skeletal muscle fibers).

HAT—head, arm, neck, and trunk segments that constitute the unit that must be balanced above the legs during locomotion.

Hierarchical processing—a system of neural processing in which higher levels of the brain are concerned with issues of abstraction of information. For example, higher brain centers integrate inputs from many senses and interpret incoming sensory information.

Hypothesis—a hypothetical explanation of the cause or causes of a problem.

Hypothesis-oriented clinical practice—a process used to systematically test assumptions about the nature and cause of a patient's problems.

Inertia—the tendency to remain at rest or in motion; the inability to move spontaneously.

Intrinsic feedback—feedback that comes to the individual through the various sensory systems as a result of the normal production of the movement, such as visual information concerning whether a movement was accurate or somatosensory information concerning the position of the limbs as one was moving.

Joint-based planning—one possible way the central nervous system may control movements toward a target: by using joint angle coordinates to program movements.

Knowledge of performance (KP)—feedback relating to the movement pattern that the performer has made.

Knowledge of results (KR)—a form of extrinsic feedback. It has been defined as verbal (or its equivalent) terminal feedback about the outcome of the movement in terms of the movement's goal.

Labyrinthine righting reaction—orientation of the head to an upright vertical position in response to vestibular signals.

Landau reaction—combination of the effect of the labyrinthine, optical, and body-on-head righting reactions.

Learning—the process of acquiring knowledge about the world.

Local static reactions—stiffness of the animal's limb for support of body weight against gravity.

Long-term memory—continuum of processes involving information storage. Initial stages reflect functional changes in the efficiency of synapses. Later stages reflect structural changes in synaptic connections. These memories are relatively resistant to disruption.

Long-term potentiation (LTP)—similar to sensitization. In the hippocampus, LTP occurs when a weak and an excitatory input arrive at the same region of a neuron's dendrite. The weak input is enhanced if it is activated in association with the strong one. LTP appears to require the simultaneous firing of both presynaptic and postsynaptic cells. After this occurs, LTP is maintained through an increase in presynaptic transmitter release.

Massed practice—a session in which the amount of practice time in a trial is greater than the amount of rest between trials.

Memory trace—in Adam's closed-loop theory of motor control, the mechanism used to select and initiate a movement.

Model of brain function—a simplified representation of the structure and function of the brain as it relates to the coordination of movement; related to motor control.

Model of disablement—an approach to ordering the effects of disease, enabling the clinician to develop a hierarchical list of problems toward which treatment can be directed.

Monosynaptic reflex—the simplest reflex pathway, consisting of a sensory neuron, the Ia afferent neuron from the muscle spindle, an interneuron, the Ia inhibitory interneuron, and a motor neuron, the alpha-motor neuron to the same muscle. The muscle contracts in response to stretch of the muscle spindle and activation of the Ia afferent neuron.

Motor learning—the acquisition and/or modification of movement; a set of processes associated with practice or experience leading to relatively permanent changes in the capability for producing skilled action. It emerges from a complex of perception, cognition, and action processes and involves the search for a task solution, which emerges from an interaction of the individual with the task and the environment.

Motor program—a central pattern generator, that is, a specific neural circuit like that for generating walking in the cat. In this case, the term represents neural connections that are stereotyped and hard-wired. Also used to describe higher-level hierarchically organized neural processes that store the rules for generating movements so that tasks can be performed with a variety of effector systems.

Muscle tone—the force with which a muscle resists being lengthened.

Neck-on-body righting reaction—orientation of the body in response to cervical afferents, which report changes in the position of the head and neck.

Neuronal shock (diaschisis)—the short-term loss of function in neuronal pathways at a distance from the lesion itself.

Operant conditioning—the process of learning to associate a certain response, from among many that have been made, with a consequence. Behaviors that are rewarded tend to be repeated, while behaviors followed by aversive stimuli are reduced in number.

Optical righting reaction—a contributor to the reflex orientation of the head using visual inputs.

Parachute or protective responses—actions that protect the body from injury during a fall.

Parallel distributed processing—neural processing in which the same signal is processed simultaneously among many different brain structures, though for different purposes.

Perceptual trace—in Adam's closed-loop theory of motor control, the perceptual trace is considered an internal reference of correctness built up over a period of practice.

Performance-based functional measures—assessment tools that focus on measuring performance on functional tasks.

Plasticity—the ability to show modification or change. Short-term functional plasticity refers to changes in the efficiency, or strength, of synaptic connections. Structural plasticity refers to changes in the organization and numbers of synaptic connections.

Postural control—regulation of the body's position in space for the dual purposes of stability and orientation.

Postural fixation reaction—action used to recover from perturbations other than to the supporting surface.

Postural motor strategy—the organization of movements appropriate for controlling the body's position in space.

Postural orientation—the ability to maintain an appropriate relationship between the body segments and between the body and the environment for a task.

Postural stability—the ability to maintain the position of the body and specifically the center of body mass within specific boundaries of space, referred to as stability limits.

Postural tone—increased level of activity in antigravity muscles that helps maintain the body vertically against the force of gravity.

Procedural learning—the process of learning tasks that can be performed automatically, without attention or conscious thought, like a habit.

Progression requirement—one of the three major requirements for successful locomotion, reflecting the need for a basic locomotor pattern that can move the body in the desired direction.

Propulsive gait pattern—gait pattern of patients with Parkinson's disease, characterized by inability to restrain momentum, leading to uncontrolled progression.

Reactive synaptogenesis (collateral sprouting)—process in which neighboring normal axons sprout to innervate synaptic sites that were previously activated by the injured axon.

Recall schema—in Schmidt's schema theory, when initiating a movement, it is used for the selection of a specific response. Inputs to this schema include the initial conditions, desired goal of the movement, and the abstract memory of previous response specifications in similar tasks.

Receptive field—the specific area of skin, retina, and so on, to which a cell is sensitive when the skin or retina is stimulated. The receptive field can be either excitatory or inhibitory.

Recognition schema—in Schmidt's schema theory, process for the evaluation of a response. The sensory consequences and outcomes of previous movements are combined with the current initial conditions to create a representation of the expected sensory consequences.

Recovery—stringently defined, achievement of the functional goal in the same way it was performed before injury, that is, using the same processes as prior to the injury. Less stringent definitions include the ability to achieve task goals using effective and efficient means but not necessarily those used before the injury.

Recovery of function—the reacquisition of movement skills lost through injury.

Recurvatum—hyperextension, which occurs when the knee has sufficient mobility to move posteriorly past neutral.

Reflex—a stereotyped muscle response to a sensory stimulus. The simplest reflex pathway is the monosynaptic stretch reflex pathway, consisting of a sensory neuron, the Ia afferent neuron from the muscle spindle, an interneuron, the Ia inhibitory interneuron, and a motor neuron, the alpha-motor neuron to the same muscle. The muscle contracts in response to stretch of the muscle spindle and activation of the Ia afferent neuron.

Regenerative synaptogenesis—sprouting of injured axons.

Response-produced feedback—all of the sensory information that is available as the result of a movement.

Resting potential—the negative electrical charge or potential on the inside of the cell with respect to the outside that is always present when the neuron is at rest.

Righting reactions—actions that allow the animal to assume or resume a species-specific orientation of the body with respect to its environment.

Schema—an abstract representation stored in memory following multiple presentations of a class of objects.

Segmental static reactions—reactions that involve more than one body segment; includes the flexor withdrawal reflex and the crossed extensor reflex.

Self-organizing system—a system that can spontaneously form movement patterns that arise simply from the interaction of the different parts of the system.

Sensitization—an increased responsiveness, often following a threatening or noxious stimulus.

Sensorimotor strategies—movement strategies that reflect the rules for coordinating sensory and motor aspects of postural control.

Sensory strategies—movement strategies that organize sensory information from visual, somatosensory, and vestibular systems for postural control.

Short-term memory—working memory, which has a limited capacity for information storage and lasts for a few moments only. This reflects momentary attentional processes.

Spared function—a function that is not lost following injury.

Spasticity—a motor disorder characterized by a velocity-dependent increase in tonic stretch reflexes (muscle tone) with exaggerated tendon jerks, resulting from hyperexcitability of the stretch reflex (it is one component of the upper motor neuron syndrome).

Spatial summation—summation that produces depolarization because of the simultaneous action potentials of multiple cells synapsing on the same postsynaptic neuron.

Spinal locomotor preparation—animal experimental preparation in which lesions are made at the low spinal level to allow the observation of the hind limbs only or at the high spinal level to allow the observation of all four limbs as part of the preparation. For this preparation, one needs an external stimulus, for example an electrical or pharmacological stimulus, to produce locomotor behavior.

Stability limits—boundaries of an area of space in which the body can maintain its position without changing the base of support.

Stability requirement—one of the three major requirements for successful locomotion, reflecting the ability to maintain stability, including the support of the body against gravity.

Step length—the distance from the foot strike of one foot to the foot strike of the other foot. For example, the right step length is the distance from the left heel to the right heel when both feet are in contact with the ground.

Strategy—a plan for action; an approach to organizing individual elements within a system into a collective structure.

Stride length—the distance covered by the same foot from one heel strike to the next heel strike; two steps.

Support moment—the algebraic sum of the joint moments at the hip, knee, and ankle during the stance phase of the step cycle. The support moment is an extensor torque. This net extensor torque keeps the limb from collapsing while bearing weight, allowing stabilization of

the body and thus accomplishing one of the requirements of locomotion.

Symmetrical tonic neck reflex—reflex that changes the position of the limbs in response to a change in head position. When the head is extended, extensor activity predominates in the upper extremities, while flexor activity predominates in the lower extremities. Flexion of the head reverses this; thus, there is an increase in flexion in the upper extremities and extensor activity in the lower extremities.

Synaptic defacilitation or habituation—reduced release of transmitter by a neuron that has been activated over time, often because of transmitter depletion, reducing effectiveness in influencing the postsynaptic neuron.

Synaptic facilitation—increased release of transmitter by a neuron that is activated over a short time with each action potential and therefore more easily depolarizes the next cell.

Synaptic transmission—process whereby each action potential in a neuron releases a small amount of transmitter substance. It diffuses across the cleft and attaches to receptors on the next cell, which open up channels in the membrane and depolarize the new cell. If the depolarization is sufficient, an action potential will be activated.

Synergy—functional coupling of groups of muscles so that they are constrained to act together as a unit (synonym: coordinative structure).

Task-oriented approach—a therapeutic approach to retraining the patient with movement disorders based on a systems theory of motor control.

Temporal summation—summation that results in depolarization because of synaptic potentials from a presynaptic neuron that occur close together in time.

Theory of motor control—a group of abstract ideas about the nature and cause of movement. Theories are often but not always based on models of brain function.

Tilting reactions—movements used for controlling the center of gravity in response to a tilting surface.

Tonic labyrinthine reflex—reflex that produces a change in body posture in response to vestibular inputs, signaling head position with respect to gravity. When the body is supine, extensor muscles are facilitated; conversely, the prone position results in facilitation of flexor muscles.

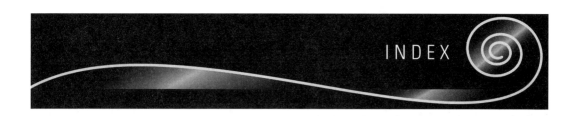

Page numbers in *italics* denote figures; those followed by a t denote tables; those followed by a b denote boxes.